TEXTBOOK of

Diagnostic
Ultrasonography

volume **ONE**

TEXTBOOK of
Diagnostic Ultrasonography

sixth edition

Sandra L. **Hagen-Ansert, MS, RDMS, RDCS**

Cardiology Department
Scripps Clinic — Torrey Pines
Former Office Manager and Clinical Cardiac Sonographer
University Cardiology Associates, Medical University of South Carolina

with 3217 illustrations

volume **ONE**

MOSBY
ELSEVIER

11830 Westline Industrial Drive
St. Louis, Missouri 63146

TEXTBOOK OF DIAGNOSTIC ULTRASONOGRAPHY

ISBN 13: 978-0-323-02803-5
ISBN 10: 0-323-02803-9

Copyright © 2006, 2001, 1995, 1989, 1983, 1978 by Mosby, Inc., an affiliate of Elsevier Inc.

Notice

Knowledge and best practice in this field are constantly changing. As new research and experience broaden our knowledge, changes in practice, treatment and drug therapy may become necessary or appropriate. Readers are advised to check the most current information provided (i) on procedures featured or (ii) by the manufacturer of each product to be administered, to verify the recommended dose or formula, the method and duration of administration, and contraindications. It is the responsibility of the practitioner, relying on their own experience and knowledge of the patient, to make diagnoses, to determine dosages and the best treatment for each individual patient, and to take all appropriate safety precautions. To the fullest extent of the law, neither the Publisher nor the Author assumes any liability for any injury and/or damage to persons or property arising out of or related to any use of the material contained in this book.

The Publisher

ISBN 13: 978-0-323-02803-5
ISBN 10: 0-323-02803-9

Publisher: Andrew Allen
Executive Editor: Jeanne Wilke
Developmental Editor: Linda Woodard
Publishing Services Manager: Pat Joiner
Project Manager: Gena Magouirk
Design Direction: Kathi Gosche

Printed in Canada

Last digit is the print number: 9 8 7 6 5 4 3 2 1

Contributors

DARLEEN CIOFFI-RAGAN, BS, RDMS
Instructor
Obstetrics and Gynecology
University of Colorado Health Sciences Center
Denver, Colorado

M. ROBERT De JONG, RDMS, RDCS, RVT
Radiology Technical Manager, Ultrasound
The Russell H. Morgan Department of Radiology and Radiological
  Science
The Johns Hopkins Hospital
Baltimore, Maryland

TERRY J. DuBOSE, MS, RDMS, FSDMS, FAIUM
Associate Professor and Director
Diagnostic Medical Sonography Program
University of Arkansas for Medical Sciences
Little Rock, Arkansas

M. ELIZABETH GLENN, MD
Women's Health Center at Baptist East
Memphis, Tennessee

**CHARLOTTE G. HENNINGSEN, MS, RT,
RDMS, RVT**
Chair and Professor
Diagnostic Medical Sonography Department
Florida Hospital College of Health Sciences
Orlando, Florida

MIRA L. KATZ, PhD, MPH
Assistant Professor
Division of Health Behavior and Health Promotion
School of Public Health
The Ohio State University
Columbus, Ohio

VALJEAN MacMILLAN, RDMS, RDSC
Sonographer
Shared Imaging Services
Madison, Wisconsin

DANIEL A. MERTON, BS, RDMS
Technical Coordinator of Research
Department of Radiology
The Jefferson Ultrasound Research and Education Institute
Thomas Jefferson University
Philadelphia, Pennsylvania

CAROL MITCHELL, PhD, RDMS, RDCS, RVT, RT(R)
Program Director
School of Diagnostic Medical Sonography
University of Wisconsin Hospitals & Clinics
Madison, Wisconsin

CINDY A. OWEN, RT, RDMS, RVT
Ultrasound Consultant
Diagnostic Ultrasound Services
Memphis, Tennessee

**SUSAN RAATZ STEPHENSON, MEd, BSRT-U,
RDMS, RT(R)(C)**
Clinical Product Specialist
Philips Ultrasound
Bothell, Washington

TAMARA L. SALSGIVER, RT(R), RDMS, RVT
Program Director
Diagnostic Medical Sonography
Kaiser Permanente School of Allied Health Sciences
Richmond, California

JEAN LEA SPITZ, MPH, RDMS, FSDMS, FAIUM
Professor
College of Allied Health
University of Oklahoma Health Sciences Center
Oklahoma City, Oklahoma

DENISE SPRADLEY, BSRT, RDMS, RDCS, RVT
Lead Sonographer
Perinatal Center of Oklahoma
Oklahoma City, Oklahoma

DIANA M. STRICKLAND, BSBA, RDMS, RDCS
Clinical Assistant Professor and Co-Director
Ultrasound Program
Department of Obstetrics and Gynecology
Brody School of Medicine
East Carolina University
Greenville, North Carolina

BARBARA TRAMPE, RN, RDMS
Chief Sonographer
Meriter/University of Wisconsin Perinatal Ultrasound
Madison, Wisconsin

BARBARA J. VANDER WERFF, RDMS, RDCS, RVT
Chief Sonographer
University of Wisconsin-Madison Hospitals and Clinics
Madison, Wisconsin

KERRY WEINBERG, RDMS, RDCS
Director
Diagnostic Medical Sonography Program
New York University
New York, New York

Reviewers

BETH ANDERHUB, MEd, RDMS, RSDMS
Program Director
Diagnostic Medical Sonography
St. Louis Community College
St. Louis, Missouri

GINA M. AUGUSTINE, MLS, RT(R)
Director
School of Radiography and Specialty Programs
Jameson Health System
New Castle, Pennsylvania

KEVIN BARRY, MEd, RDMS, RDCS, RT(R)
Department Head
Diagnostic Medical Imaging
New Hampshire Technical Institute
Concord, New Hampshire

KATHI BOROK, BS, RDMS, RDCS
Clinical Coordinator
Diagnostic Medical Sonography Department
Florida Hospital College of Health Sciences
Orlando, Florida

PAMELA BROWER, RVT, RVS, CRT
Department Chair
Diagnostic Medical Sonography
Tyler Junior College
Tyler, Texas

JAN BRYANT, MS, RDMS, RT(R)
Program Director
Ultrasound
El Centro College
Dallas, Texas

ERIC CADIENTE, AS, RDCS, RVT
Diagnostic Medical Sonography Department
Florida Hospital College of Health Sciences
Orlando, Florida

LYNN CARLTON, MS, RDMS, RT(R)(M)
Staff Sonographer
Metropolitan Hospital
Grand Rapids, Michigan

JOAN M. CLASBY, BvE, RDMS, RT, RDCS
Professor and Director
Diagnostic Medical Sonography Program
Orange Coast College
Costa Mesa, California

**JANICE DIANE DOLK, MA, RT(R), RDMS
(abdomen, ob/gyn, breast)**
Director of Allied Health Education
University of Maryland—Baltimore County
UMBC Training Enterprises
Baltimore, Maryland

KEVIN EVANS, PhD, RT(R)(M)(BD), RDMS, RVT
Assistant Professor and Director
Ohio State University
Columbus, Ohio

JANET M. FELDMEIER, BSRT, RDMS
Staff Ultrasonographer
Cardinal Glennon Children's Hospital
St. Louis, Missouri

THOMAS J. GERVAISE, BS, RT, RDMS
Ultrasound Division Director
Modern Division Director
Anaheim, California

TIM S. GIBBS, RT(R,F), RDMS, RVT, CTNM
Senior Sonographer
West Anaheim Medical Center
Anaheim, California

CHARLOTTE G. HENNINGSEN, MS, RT, RDMS, RVT
Chair and Professor
Diagnostic Medical Sonography Department
Florida Hospital College of Health Sciences
Orlando, Florida

FELICIA JONES, MSEd, RDMS, RCDS, RVT
Director
Diagnostic Medical Sonography
Tidewater Community College
Virginia Beach, Virginia

RUBEN MARTINEZ, BS, RDCS, RVT
Cardiovascular Ultrasound Instructor
Florida Hospital College of Health Sciences
Orlando, Florida

CAROL MITCHELL, PhD, RDMS, RDCS, RVT, RT(R)
Program Director
School of Diagnostic Medical Sonography
University of Wisconsin Hospitals & Clinics
Madison, Wisconsin

JOSEPH B. MORTON III, MBA, RT(R), RDMS
Sonographer/Clinical Instructor
Columbia—St. Mary's Hospitals
Milwaukee, Wisconsin

KATHLEEN MURPHY, MBA, RDMS, RT
Program Director
Diagnostic Ultrasound
Gateway Community College
Phoenix, Arizona

SUSANNA OVEL, RDMS, RVT
Senior Sonographer/Trainer
Radiological Associates of Sacramento (RAS)
Sacramento, California

CRAIG PENOFF, BSAS, RDMS, RVT
Assistant Professor and Program Director
Diagnostic Medical Sonography
Lorain County Community College
Elyria, Ohio

CYNTHIA REBER-BONHALL, BS, RDMS, RVT
Clinical Faculty
Orange Coast College
Costa Mesa, California

DANA SALMONS, BS, RT, RDMS
Sonographer
Florida Hospital
Orlando, Florida

LISA STROHL, BS, RT(R), RDMS, RVT
Marketing Manager
Jefferson Center City Imaging
Thomas Jefferson University
Philadelphia, Pennsylvania

REGINA SWEARENGIN, BS, RDMS (AB, OB, NE)
Sonography Department Chair
Austin Community College
Austin, Texas

ELLEN T. TUCHINSKY, BA, RDMS, RDCS
Clinical Education Coordinator
Diagnostic Medical Sonography Program
School of Continuing Professional Studies
New York University
New York, New York

CHERYL L. ZELINSKY, MM, ARRT(R), RDMS
Associate Professor and Director
Diagnostic Medical Sonography
Oregon Institute of Technology
Klamath Falls, Oregon

To our own little sonic boomers:
Rebecca, Alyssa, and **Katrina,**
who are growing up to make their own waves

Preface

A LOOK BACK

Medicine has always fascinated me. I had my first introduction to this field of study in 1963 when Dr. Charles Henkelmann provided me the opportunity to learn radiography while I was still in high school. Although radiographic technology was interesting, it did not provide the opportunity to evaluate patient history or to follow through on more complex cases, which seemed to be the most intriguing aspect of medicine and my primary concern.

Shortly after I finished my radiographic training in 1968 at UCSD Medical Center, I was assigned to the radiation therapy department. I was introduced to a very quiet, young, dedicated radiologist, whom I would later grow to admire and respect as one of the foremost authorities in diagnostic ultrasound. Convincing Dr. George Leopold that he needed another hand to assist him was difficult in the beginning, and it was through the efforts of his resident, Dr. Dan MacDonald, that I was able to learn what eventually developed into an exciting new medical modality.

Using high-frequency sound waves, diagnostic ultrasound provides a unique method for the visualization of soft tissue anatomic structures. Identifying such structures and correlating the results with clinical symptoms and patient data presents an ongoing challenge to the sonographer. The art of sonography demands expertise in scanning techniques and maneuvers to demonstrate the anatomic structures, for without high-quality images, limited diagnostic sonographic information is available to the physician.

At UCSD, our initial experience in ultrasound took us through the era of A-mode techniques, identifying aortic aneurysms through pulsatile reflections, trying to separate splenic reflections from upper-pole left renal masses, and, in general, attempting to echo every patient with a probable abdominal or pelvic mass. Of course, the one-dimensional A-mode techniques were difficult for me to conceptualize, let alone trust. However, with repeated success and the experience gained from mistakes, I began to believe in this method. The conviction that Dr. Leopold had about this technique was a strong indicator of its success in our laboratory.

In 1969, when our first 2-D ultrasound unit arrived in the laboratory, the "skeptics" started to believe a little more in this modality. I must admit that those early images looked like weather maps to me for several months. The repeated times I asked, "What is that?" were enough to try anyone's patience.

I can recall when Siemens installed our first real-time unit and we saw our first obstetrical case. It was such a thrill for us to see the fetus move, wave his hands, and show us fetal heart pulsations!

We scouted the clinics and various departments in the hospital for interesting cases to scan. With our success rate surpassing our failures, the caseload increased, and soon we were involved in all aspects of ultrasound. There was not enough material for us to read to learn about new developments. It was for this reason that excitement in clinical research soared, attracting young physicians throughout the country to develop techniques in diagnostic ultrasound.

Because Dr. Leopold was so intensely interested in ultrasound, it became the diagnostic method of choice for our patients. It was not long before conferences were incomplete without the mention of the technique. Later, local medical meetings and eventually national meetings grew to include discussion of this new modality. A number of visitors were attracted to our laboratory to learn the technique, and thus we became swamped with a continual flow of new physicians, some eager to work with ultrasound and others skeptical at first, but believers in the end.

In 1970, the beginning of ultrasound education progressed slowly, with many laboratories offering a one-on-one teaching experience. Commercial companies thought the only way to push the field was to develop their own national training programs, and thus several of the leading manufacturers were the first to put forth a dedicated effort in the development of ultrasound education.

The combined efforts of our laboratory and the commercial interests precipitated my involvement in furthering ultrasound education. Seminars, weekly sessions, local and national meetings, and consultations became a vital part of the growth of ultrasound.

As ultrasound grew in popularity, more intense training was desperately needed to maintain the quality that the pioneers strove for. Working with one of the commercial ultrasound companies conducting national short-term training programs, I became acquainted with Dr. Barry Goldberg and his enthusiasm for quality education in ultrasound. His organizational efforts and pioneer spirit led me to the East Coast to further develop more intensive educational programs in ultrasound. The challenge grew in establishing new programs and continuing education in diagnostic medical sonography as we ventured across the United States and Canada in the years to follow.

There are very few moments in life when one is in the right place at the right time, but this was one of those moments for me. I had the opportunity to begin when the field was in its infancy and to work with some of the stellar ultrasound scholars along the way. This textbook is a culmination of knowledge gained throughout the years as I have taught students in sonography.

INTRODUCING THE NEW SIXTH EDITION

The sixth edition of the *Textbook of Diagnostic Ultrasonography* continues the tradition of excellence begun when the first edition was published in the 1978. Each new edition brings impressive updates and vital reorganization. The field of diagnostic ultrasound has changed dramatically over the past 50 years, reflecting the changing approaches to many procedures. Phenomenal strides in transducer design, instrumentation, color flow Doppler, tissue harmonics, contrast applications, and 3-D imaging continue to provide increased resolution in the ultrasound image.

The primary goal of this textbook is to serve as an in-depth resource for students studying sonography, as well as for practitioners in hospitals, clinics, and private radiology, cardiology, and obstetric settings. This sixth edition strives to keep abreast of the rapid advancements, providing students and practitioners with the most complete and up-to-date information in the field of medical sonography.

ORGANIZATION

The *Textbook of Diagnostic Ultrasonography* remains divided into two volumes to compensate for its expanded coverage and to make the book more convenient to use. The content has been critically reviewed, reorganized, and improved to provide a better flow for the reader. Volume One covers general ultrasound applications, techniques, and scan protocols and introduces abdominal anatomy and physiology and the general health history analysis. Sonography of the abdomen, superficial structures, and pediatrics are also found in Volume One. Volume Two focuses on cardiovascular applications and obstetrics and gynecologic sonography. A comprehensive glossary is found at the end of each volume, and a reference of common medical and ultrasound abbreviations is located on the inside covers of each volume.

Each chapter begins with *learning objectives*, a *chapter outline*, and *key terms* and *definitions* to aid the reader. Sonographic concepts are presented in a logical and consistent manner in each chapter. To help the student and the sonographer understand the patient's total clinical picture before the sonographic examination, discussions on anatomy, physiology, laboratory data, clinical signs and symptoms, pathology, and sonographic findings are found within each chapter. The sonographic evaluation of the organ (to include normal measurements) is included in the chapters. Each chapter also offers discussion of the pathology of the organ, including clinical symptoms, gross pathology, ultrasound findings, and differential considerations. Tables throughout the text summarize the pathology discussed in each chapter and break the information

down into Clinical Findings, Sonographic Findings, and Differential Considerations. Key points are also pulled out into numerous boxes in the chapters, making it easy to find important information quickly. References and a Selected Bibliography are found at the ends of the chapters, as relevant. The review questions have been moved into the Instructor's Manual that accompanies the textbook

ILLUSTRATIONS AND VISUALS

Hundreds of beautifully drawn full-color illustrations highlight anatomical information important when performing the different ultrasound examinations presented. Color Doppler illustrations are also included in relevant chapters. Tables and boxes continue to highlight important areas of knowledge throughout both volumes.

One-third of the more than 3000 illustrations in this edition are new. Almost 800 new images have been incorporated, including color Doppler, 3-D, and contrast images. The anatomic illustrations—almost 200 of which are new—clearly add to the understanding of each of the organ structures discussed throughout the textbook. Gross pathology images have also been added to help the reader visually image the particular type of pathology presented.

Sonographic findings for particular pathologic conditions are preceded by the following special heading:

Sonographic Findings. This icon makes it very easy for students and practicing sonographers to find this information.

NEW TO THE SIXTH EDITION

This edition has been completely revised and expanded to offer student and practicing sonographers a comprehensive textbook of general ultrasound.

Chapter 1, *Foundations of Sonography,* was revised to provide more background information for students just entering the field of ultrasound. New to this chapter is the section "Medical Terms for the Sonographer," which introduces students to common medical terms they will encounter in their field. This chapter also introduces key physical principles of sonography.

Chapter 2, *Introduction to Physical Findings, Physiology, and Laboratory Data of the Abdomen,* exposes the student to the clinical assessment that the patient experiences prior to arriving in the ultrasound department. Although in many busy labs the student does not have an opportunity to perform such a thorough evaluation of the patient, an understanding of which questions may be appropriate for specific complaints can be invaluable during the ultrasound examination. Also included in this chapter is an introduction to laboratory tests relevant to various disease processes.

Chapter 14, *Abdominal Applications of Ultrasound Contrast Agents,* by Daniel Merton, provides an excellent introduction to the clinical applications of contrast in ultrasound. This chapter lists and discusses the various types of contrast that are available and includes illustrated examples of how contrast has aided in the diagnostic accuracy of the ultrasound examination.

Chapter 15, *Ultrasound-Guided Interventional Techniques,* by Robert DeJong, offers an excellent step-by-step analysis of how to perform invasive procedures with ultrasound guidance. DeJong has exquisitely illustrated the different types of needles, transducer devices, and protocols for performing the procedure. Guidelines for finding the needle tip for the biopsy procedures are clearly outlined.

Chapter 16, *Emergent Abdominal Ultrasound Procedures,* is a new chapter that focuses on the FAST scan technique used in Emergency Departments throughout the country. A few of the more common "STAT" ultrasound procedures are also included in this chapter for easy reference in an on-call situation.

Chapter 17, *The Breast,* was completely rewritten and updated to provide the student and sonographer with a solid foundation of the applications of ultrasound of the breast.

Chapter 19, *The Scrotum,* by Cindy Owen, is a new chapter that includes many images of normal scrotal anatomy as well as scrotal pathology. This chapter also offers practical tips on scanning techniques as well as discussion of Doppler principles as they relate to scrotal imaging.

Chapter 20, *The Musculoskeletal System,* by Susan Raatz Stephenson, is a new chapter with exquisite images and anatomical drawings. The author shares her practical experience in ultrasound imaging of the musculoskeletal system with excellent descriptions and protocols for performing multiple examinations. Because this is a new area for most sonographers, readers may encounter some new terminology. I recommend reviewing the drawings and images before reading through the text material.

Part IV, Pediatric Applications, was updated with the addition of three new introductory chapters that focus on the basic anatomy and common pathology that sonographers may encounter: Chapter 22, *The Pediatric Abdomen: Jaundice and Common Surgical Conditions;* Chapter 25, *The Neonatal Hip;* and Chapter 26, *The Neonatal Spine.*

Part V, Cardiology, contains four chapters that provide readers with a basic foundation of hemodynamics with an introduction to echocardiography. The subject of fetal echocardiography is now divided into two chapters: Chapter 29, *Introduction to Fetal Echocardiography,* and Chapter 30, *Fetal Echocardiography: Congenital Heart Disease.*

Part VI, Vascular, offers four chapters that help students understand vascular applications within a general ultrasound department.

Part VII, Gynecology, was completely rewritten and reorganized. Tami Salsgiver opens this part of the textbook with the excellent, illustrated Chapter 35, *Normal Anatomy and Physiology of the Female Pelvis.* Barb Vander Werff rewrote and updated four chapters in Part VII. Finally, Carol Mitchell and Valjean MacMillan added an excellent new chapter called *The Role of Ultrasound in Evaluating Female Infertility.*

Several additions have been made to Part VIII, Foundations of Obstetric Sonography. Jean Lea Spitz rewrote Chapter 41, *The Role of Ultrasound in Obstetrics;* Chapter 42, *Clinical Ethics for Obstetric Sonography;* and Chapter 45, *Sonography of the Second and Third Trimesters.* Terry DuBose reevaluated Chapter 46, *Obstetric Measurements and Gestational Age.* Chapter 48, *Ultrasound and High-Risk Pregnancy,* was rewritten by Carol Mitchell and Barbara Trampe. A brief introduction to the clinical applications of 3D ultrasound was contributed by Darleen Cioffi-Ragan (Chapter 50). Chapter 54, *The Fetal Face and Neck,* is beautifully illustrated and rewritten by Diana Strickland.

Each of these chapters was reviewed by numerous sonographers currently working in various areas of ultrasound. Their comments, critiques, and suggestions for change have been incorporated into this edition in an effort to make this textbook practical in a clinical setting and useful for both the student and the practicing sonographer. It continues to be my hope that this textbook will not only introduce the reader to the field of ultrasound but also allow readers to go a step beyond to what I have found to be the very stimulating and challenging experience of diagnostic patient care.

Also Available. *Workbook for Textbook of Diagnostic Ultrasonography* is available for separate purchase and has been created to provide the learner with ample opportunities to practice and apply the information presented in the text. Each workbook chapter covers all the material presented in the textbook. Each chapter includes exercises and activities on image identification, anatomy identification, key term definition, and sonographic technique. Case reviews and self tests are also included at the end of the workbook.

For the Instructor. An *Instructor's Electronic Resource (IER)* has also been created to assist instructors in preparing classroom lectures and activities. This resource consists of:

- Instructor's Manual, which includes detailed chapter outlines, chapter objectives, in-depth lecture notes, and critical thinking questions and exercises.
- Test Bank, which includes 1500 multiple-choice questions in Examview and Word format.
- Electronic Image Collection, which includes all of the images from the text in PowerPoint and jpeg formats.

The IER is also posted on Evolve, which also includes a Course Management system for instructors and WebLinks for students.

Evolve Online Course Management. Evolve is an interactive learning environment designed to work in coordination with *Textbook of Diagnostic Ultrasonography.* Instructors may use Evolve to provide an Internet-based course component that reinforces and expands on the concepts delivered in class. Evolve may be used to publish the class syllabus, outlines, and lecture notes; set up "virtual office hours" and email communication; share important dates and information through the online class Calendar; and encourage student participation through Chat Rooms and Discussion Boards. Evolve allows instructors to post exams and manage their grade books online. An online version of the Instructor's Resource Manual is also available on Evolve. For more information, visit http://www.evolve.elsevier.com/HagenAnsert/diagnostic/ or contact an Elsevier sales representative.

Sandra L. Hagen-Ansert, MS, RDMS, RDCS

Acknowledgments

I would like to express my gratitude and appreciation to a number of individuals who have served as mentors and guides throughout my years in ultrasound. Of course it all began with Dr. George Leopold at UCSD Medical Center. His quest for knowledge and his perseverance for excellence have been the mainstay of my career in ultrasound. I would also like to recognize Drs. Dolores Pretorius, Nancy Budorick, Wanda Miller-Hance, and David Sahn for their encouragement throughout the years at the UCSD Medical Center in both Radiology and Pediatric Cardiology.

I would also like to acknowledge Dr. Barry Goldberg for the opportunity he gave me to develop countless numbers of educational programs in ultrasound in an independent fashion and for his encouragement to pursue advancement. I would also like to thank Dr. Daniel Yellon for his early-hour anatomy dissection and instruction; Dr. Carson Schneck, for his excellent instruction in gross anatomy and sections of "Geraldine;" and Dr. Jacob Zutuchni, for his enthusiasm for the field of cardiology.

I am grateful to Dr. Harry Rakowski for his continued support in teaching fellows and students while I was at the Toronto Hospital.

Dr. William Zwiebel encouraged me to continue writing and teaching while I was at the University of Wisconsin Medical Center, and I appreciate his knowledge, which found its way into the liver physiology section of this textbook.

I would like to acknowledge the feedback from several individuals as I contemplated changes for this edition: Kerry Weinberg, Jean Lea Spitz, and Tami Salsgiver. I would also like to extend gratitude to Misty Johnson and Charlene Fessler from MUSC Medical Center.

My good fortune in learning about and understanding the *total patient* must be attributed to a very dedicated cardiologist, James Glenn, with whom I had the pleasure of working while I was at MUSC in Charleston, South Carolina. It was through his compassion and knowledge that I grew to appreciate the total patient beyond the transducer, and for this I am grateful.

For their continual support, feedback, and challenges, I would like to thank and recognize all the students I have taught in the various Diagnostic Medical Sonography programs: Episcopal Hospital, Thomas Jefferson University Medical Center, University of Wisconsin-Madison Medical Center, UCSD Medical Center, Baptist College of Health Science, and Trident Technical College. These students continually work toward the development of quality ultrasound techniques and protocols and have given back to the ultrasound community tenfold.

I would like to thank the very supportive and capable staff at Elsevier who have guided me though yet another edition of this textbook. Jeanne Wilke and her excellent staff are to be commended on their perseverance to make this an outstanding textbook. Linda Woodard was a constant reminder to me to stay on task and was there to offer assistance when needed. Gena Magouirk, Project Manager, has done an excellent job with the manuscript. She is to be commended on her eye for detail. Also, Jennifer Moorhead has been a tremendous aid in working with this project. Finally, Luke Held, Editorial Assistant, worked on the test bank questions for the Instructor's Manual.

I would like to thank my family, Art, Becca, Aly, and Kati, for their patience and understanding, as I thought this edition would never come to an end.

I think that you will find the 6th Edition of the *Textbook of Diagnostic Ultrasonography* reflects the contribution of so many individuals with attention to detail and a dedication to excellence. I hope you will find this educational experience in ultrasound as rewarding as I have.

Contents

TEXTBOOK of

Diagnostic Ultrasonography

volume **ONE**

PART I

Foundations of Sonography

•••

CHAPTER 1

Foundations of Sonography

Sandra L. Hagen-Ansert

KEY TERMS

acoustic impedance – measure of a material's resistance to the propagation of sound; expressed as the product of acoustic velocity of the medium and the density of the medium

amplitude – strength of the ultrasound wave measured in decibels

angle of incidence – angle at which the sound beam strikes the interface

angle of reflection – angle at which the beam of the sound is reflected from an interface; the angle of reflection equals the angle of incidence

attenuation – reduction in the amplitude and intensity of a sound wave as it propagates through a medium; attenuation of ultrasound waves in tissue is caused by absorption and by scattering and reflection

axial resolution – refers to the minimum distance between two structures positioned along the axis of the beam where both structures can be visualized as separate objects

bulk modulus – amount of pressure required to compress a small volume of material a small amount

compression – region of increased particle density

crystal – special material in the transducer that has the ability to convert electrical impulses into sound waves

cycle – a sequence of events occurring at regular intervals; a wavelength cycle is that of a particle density that varies from maximum in the compression zone to a minimum in the reflection zone and back to maximum in the successive compression zone to complete one cycle

decibel (dB) – unit used to quantitatively express the ratio of two amplitudes or intensities; decibels are not absolute units, but express one sound level or intensity in terms of another or in terms of a reference (e.g., the amplitude 10 cm from the transducer is 10 dB lower than the amplitude 5 cm from the transducer)

dynamic range – ratio of the largest to smallest signals that an instrument or component of an instrument can respond to without distortion

focal zone – the region over which the effective width of the sound beam is within some measure of its width at the focal distance

frame rate – rate at which images are updated on the display; dependent on frequency of the transducer and depth selection

Fraunhofer zone – the field farthest from the transducer during the formation of the sound beam

frequency – number of cycles per second that a periodic event or function undergoes; number of cycles completed per unit of time; the frequency of a sound wave is determined by the number of oscillations per second of the vibrating source

Fresnel zone – the field closest to the transducer during the formation of the sound beam

gain – measure of the strength of the ultrasound signal; can be expressed as a simple ratio or in decibels; overall gain amplifies all signals by a constant factor regardless of the depth

gray scale – B-mode scanning technique that permits the brightness of the B-mode dots to be displayed in various shades of gray to represent different echo amplitudes

hertz (Hz) – unit for frequency, equal to 1 cycle per second

intensity – power per unit area

interface – surface forming the boundary between media having different properties

kilohertz (kHz) – 1000 Hz

lateral resolution – the minimum distance between two objects where they still can be displayed as separate objects

megahertz (MHz) – 1,000,000 Hz

period – duration of a single cycle of a periodic wave or event

piezoelectric effect – generation of electric signals as a result of an incident sound beam on a material that has piezoelectric properties; in the converse (or reverse) piezoelectric effect, the material expands or contracts when an electric signal is applied

power – rate of energy flow over the entire beam of sound; in general terms it is the rate at which energy is transmitted and is often measured in watts (W) or milliwatts (mW)

pulse duration – the time interval required for generating the transmitted pulse; the pulse duration is calculated by multiplying the number of cycles in the pulse times the period

pulse repetition frequency (PRF) – in pulse-echo instruments, it is the number of pulses launched per second by the transducer

real-time – ultrasound instrumentation that allows the image to be displayed many times per second to achieve a "real-time" image of anatomic structures and their motion patterns

refraction – change in the direction of propagation of a sound wave transmitted across an interface where the speed of sound varies

resolution – ability of the transducer to distinguish between two structures adjacent to one another

slice thickness – thickness of the section in the patient that contributes to echo signals on any one image

spatial pulse length – the product of a number of cycles in the pulse and wavelength of the pulse

temporal resolution – ability of the system to accurately depict motion

time gain compensation (TGC) – also referred to as *depth gain compensation (DGC)*; ability to compensate for attenuation of the transmitted beam as the sound wave travels through tissues in the body; usually, individual POT (potentiometer) controls allow the operator to manually change the amount of compensation necessary for each patient to produce a quality image

transducer – any device that converts energy from one form to another

velocity – in ultrasound, the tissue density determines the speed (velocity) of the ultrasound wave

wave – propagation of energy that moves back and forth or vibrates at a steady rate

wavelength – distance over which a wave repeats itself during one period of oscillation

DOPPLER KEY TERMS

Following are important terms related to Doppler imaging:

aliasing – technical artifact occurring when the frequency change is so large that it exceeds the sampling view and pulse repetition frequency

color flow – velocity in each direction is quantified by allocating a pixel to each area; each velocity frequency is allocated a color; flow toward the transducer may be red; flow away from the transducer may be blue

continuous wave (CW) Doppler – one transducer continuously transmits sound, and one continuously receives sound; used in higher-velocity flow patterns

Doppler angle – the angle that the reflector path makes with the ultrasound beam; the most accurate velocity is recorded when the beam is parallel to flow

Doppler shift – change in frequency of a reflected wave; caused by motion between the reflector and the transducer's beam

frequency shift – amount of change in the returning frequency compared with the transmitting frequency when the sound wave hits a moving target, such as blood in an artery

gate – the sample site from which the signal is obtained with pulsed Doppler

laminar – normal pattern of vessel flow; flow in the center of the vessel is faster than it is at the edges

Nyquist sampling limit – in pulsed Doppler, the Doppler signal must be sampled at least twice for each cycle in the wave if the Doppler frequencies are to be detected accurately

pulsed wave (PW) Doppler – sound is transmitted and received intermittently with one transducer

rarefaction – region of decreased particle density

resistance – passive force in opposition to another active force; occurs when tissue exerts pressure against the flow

spectral analysis – analysis of the entire frequency spectrum

spectral broadening – echo fill-in of the spectral window that is proportional to the severity of the stenosis (may also be due to poor technique or *gain* that is too high)

HISTORICAL OVERVIEW OF ACOUSTICS

Acoustics is the branch of physics that deals with sound and sound waves. It is the study of generating, propagating, and receiving sound waves. Within the field of acoustics, *ultrasound* is defined as sound frequencies beyond (*ultra* means *beyond*) the upper limits of human hearing, that is, greater than 20 kilohertz.

The Greeks were the first to describe the relationship between sound pitch and frequency when Pythagoras invented the sonometer, an instrument used to study musical sounds, in 500 BC. Several hundred years later, in 1500 AD, Leonardo da Vinci discovered sound traveled in waves and discovered the angle of reflection is equal to the angle of incidence. In 1638 Galileo demonstrated that the frequency of sound waves determined the pitch. Shortly thereafter, Sir Isaac Newton announced the derivation of the theory of velocity, and Robert Boyle announced the theory of elasticity of air.

Additional highlights of the history of the study of sound are included in this time line:

1793   Lazzaro Spallanzani, an Italian priest and scientist, studies the activities of bats and theorizes that bats were listening to something he could not hear.

1794   Augustin Fresnel forms a theory of wave diffraction. Sir Francis Galton invents the ultrasonic whistle.

1845   Christian Johann Doppler discovers the effect of motion on the pitch of sounds: When a source of wave motion itself moves, the apparent frequency of the emitted wave changes.

1880   Jacques and Pierre Curie observe the phenomenon of piezoelectricity. They find that certain crystals expand and contract slightly when placed in an alternating field. The reverse piezoelectricity permits the same crystals to create an electrical potential, or voltage, making the crystals useful both as receivers and sources of sound waves, from audible to ultrasonic frequencies.

1890   Lord Rayleigh writes his "Theory of Sound."

1900s   Paul Langevin studies controlled sound frequency and intensity and discovers a way to use the property of echoing sound waves to detect underwater objects. This is known as SONAR.

1938   G.W. Pierce invents the sonic detector, which picks up high-frequency vibrations of bats to convert into audible sound. Floyd Firestone develops the ultrasonic machine called the "Reflectoscope," which is a metallic flaw detector and cleansing machine.

DIAGNOSTIC MEDICAL SONOGRAPHY

The terms *diagnostic medical ultrasonography, sonography, ultrasound,* and *ultrasonography* have been used to describe an imaging technique used to visualize soft tissue structures of the body by recording the returning reflection of ultrasonic waves directed into the body. The term *echocardiography* applies to the ultrasound examination of the cardiac structures.

The development of materials, testing techniques, and sonar provided a major impetus in the development of diagnostic ultrasound. World War II brought sonar equipment to the forefront for defense purposes, and ultrasound was influenced by the success of sonar instrumentation. The research of several key individuals greatly advanced the knowledge of ultrasound and its medical applications. One of the pioneers in the clinical investigation and development of ultrasound was Dr. Joseph Holmes from the University of Colorado. His vivid accounts of those early days of ultrasound are summarized in the following paragraphs.

In the 1940s, Karl Dussik made one of the earliest applications of ultrasound to medical diagnosis when he used two transducers positioned on opposite sides of the head to measure ultrasound transmission profiles. He also discovered that tumors and other intracranial lesions could be detected by this technique.

Dussik went on to join Drs. R.H. Bolt and H.T. Ballantyne at the Massachusetts Institute of Technology acoustic laboratory in the early 1950s. The group continued to use through-transmission techniques and computer analysis to diagnose brain lesions through the intact skull. They discontinued their studies after concluding that the technique was too complicated for routine clinical use.

Around the same time, Dr. W. Fry, an electrical engineer who worked for the Office of Naval Research during World War II, became head of the Department of Electrical Engineering at the University of Illinois and selected ultrasound as his field of study. His primary research used ultrasound to pinpoint lesions within the central nervous system of animals by arranging several transducers to focus on a single point. Thus a destructive lesion could be produced at a selected distance without destroying normal tissue along the path of the beam. In addition, Dr. Fry observed that local heating by a second ultrasound beam would enhance echo reflection from adjacent structures.

Along with Dr. R. Meyers, chief of neurosurgery at the University of Iowa, Dr. Fry applied his "pinpoint" lesion technique to treat Parkinson's syndrome and other brain lesions. Questions arose as to whether this destruction technique was the most suitable for patients with Parkinson's syndrome, and because highly skilled investigators were required to perform the procedure, the project was terminated in 1959.

Between 1948 and 1950 three investigators, Drs. D. Howry (radiology), J. Wild, a clinician interested in tissue characterization, and G. Ludwig, who was interested in reflections from gallstones, all demonstrated independently that when ultrasound waves generated by a piezoelectric crystal transducer were transmitted into the body, ultrasound waves of different acoustic impedances would be returned to the transducer. Equipment development subsequently occurred in efforts to transform the naval sonar equipment into a clinically useful tool.

In 1948 Dr. Howry developed the first ultrasound scanner; it consisted of a cattle watering tank with a wooden rail anchored along the side. The transducer carriage moved along the rail in a horizontal plane, whereas the object to be scanned and the transducer were positioned inside the water tank. Dr. Howry developed the compound (back and forth) double scanning motion in an attempt to produce a more realistic anatomic image. The transducer carriage was moved in a 360-degree path around the object to produce reflections from all angular and curved surfaces (Figure 1-1). Many of the subjects were surgical candidates so that actual comparison of the tissue could be made with the ultrasound images.

The water bath ultrasound device was modified for patient use by building a half-pan scanner with a plastic window along its flat side. The membrane was then oiled, and the patient pressed his or her abdomen flush against it. The transducer rotated through a 180-degree arc with a 4-inch compound sector.

Along with medical applications of ultrasound, the technique was also used to determine the lean to fat ratio of cattle and other animals ready for slaughter. The cattle were greased with 30-weight motor oil instead of mineral oil to provide a coupling for the transducer and the skin.

In 1950 three faculty members from the University of Washington, R. Rushmer, D. Franklin, and D. Baker, developed sophisticated flow meters known as continuous wave Doppler. E. Strandness later developed peripheral vascular Doppler systems.

In 1954 echocardiographic ultrasound applications were developed by Drs. C. H. Hertz and I. Edler in Sweden. These investigators soon found they were able to distinguish normal heart valvular motion from the thickened, calcified valve motion that was observed in patients with rheumatic heart disease.

The early obstetric contact compound scanner was built by Tom Brown and Dr. Ian Donald in Scotland in 1957. Dr. Donald went on to discover many fascinating image patterns in the obstetric patient, and his work is still referred to today. Meanwhile, in Philadelphia, Dr. Stuart Lehman designed a real-time obstetric ultrasound system (Figure 1-2).

The development of the contact static scanner in North America came in 1962 from the University of Colorado. The instrument was constructed so the transducer moved in a mechanical sector scan 30 degrees to each side of the perpendicular while the carriage moved over the surface to be scanned. The initial ultrasound examination of a pregnant woman revealed the localization of the placenta, fetal age, and gross abnormalities of the fetus.

Shortly thereafter the grants terminated for the various ultrasound projects, and the engineers left the University of Colorado to build the first commercial Physionics ultrasound

Figure 1-1   One of the early ultrasound scanning systems used a B-52 gun turret tank with the transducer carriage moved in a 360-degree path around the patient.

Figure 1-2   Dr. Lehman used a water path system to scan his obstetric patients.

system, which was later acquired by the Picker Corp. for distribution to major medical centers throughout the country.

In 1959 G. Kossoff, H. P. Robinson, and W. Garrett at the Commonwealth Acoustic Laboratories in Australia developed diagnostic B-scanners with the use of a water bath to improve resolution of the image (Figures 1-3 and 1-4). This group was also responsible for the introduction of the new revolutionary gray scale imaging in 1972. Kossoff and colleagues were the pioneers in the development of large-aperture, multitransducer technology in which the transducers are automatically programmed to operate independently or as a whole to provide a panoramic image in seconds. This technique provided high-quality images without operator intervention as found with the contact static scanners.

At the same time, real-time scanners were being developed for the market. These provided a quick assessment of the area in question without "physically creating an image" (e.g., with the contact static scanner). The flexible real-time transducers

Figure 1-3 The Octoson used eight transducers mounted in a 180-degree semicircle and completely covered with water. The patient would lie on top of the covered waterbed, and the transducers would automatically scan the patient.

Figure 1-4 Real-time image of the neonatal head. *TV,* Third ventricle.

are now universally accepted in performing high-quality ultrasound examinations. The mobile real-time systems quickly overtook the automated multitransducer systems, which were bulky and permanently fixed in their location.

Today, nearly every hospital and medical clinic has some form of ultrasound instrumentation to provide the clinician with an inside look at the soft tissue structures within the body. Manufacturers are still defining better image acquisition, improved transducer design, and updated computer assessment of the acquired information. The two-dimensional information can now be recreated in a three- or four-dimensional format to provide a surface rendering of the area in question. Color flow Doppler, harmonics, tissue characterization, and spectral analysis have added to the understanding of ultrasound imaging.

To obtain even more information from the ultrasound image, various medical centers and manufacturers have been developing contrast agents that may be ingested or administered intravenously into the bloodstream to facilitate the detection and diagnosis of specific pathologies. Early attempts at producing a contrast effect with ultrasound imaging involved administration of aerated saline or carbon dioxide. The research today focuses on the development of gas microspheres, which are injected into the patient to provide a visual contrast during the ultrasound study. Specific applications of ultrasound contrast are found in Chapter 14.

THE ROLE OF THE SONOGRAPHER

What is the role of the sonographer as a member of the allied health profession? A *role* is a specific behavior that an individual demonstrates to others. A *function* involves the tasks or duties one is obligated to perform in carrying out a role. Therefore a *sonographer* is one who performs ultrasound studies and gathers diagnostic data under the direct or indirect supervision of a physician. Sonographers are known as the "image makers" with the ability to create images of soft tissue structures and organs inside the body, such as the liver, pancreas, biliary system, kidneys, heart, vascular system, uterus, and fetus. In addition, sonographers are able to record hemodynamic information with velocity measurements through the use of Doppler spectral analysis to determine if a vessel or cardiac valve is patent or restricted.

Sonographers work directly with patients as part of a team member of a medical facility. They also interact with physicians and other members as part of the health care team. The sonographer must be able to review the patient's records to assess clinical history and clinical symptoms; to interpret lab values; and to understand other diagnostic examinations. The sonographer is required to operate complex ultrasound instrumentation.

To produce the highest quality sonographic image for interpretation, the sonographer must possess an in-depth understanding of anatomy and pathophysiology and be able to evaluate the patient's problem. Sonographers use their skills to provide the physician with information such as the evaluation of a trauma victim's injury, or the detection of fetal anomalies, or to measure fetal growth and progress, or even to evaluate the patient for cardiac abnormalities or injury.

QUALITIES OF A SONOGRAPHER

The sonographer must possess the following qualities and talents:

- *Intellectual curiosity* to keep abreast of developments in the field
- *Perseverance* to obtain high-quality images and the ability to recognize an artifact from structural anatomy
- *Ability to conceptualize two-dimensional images into a three-dimensional format*
- *Quick and analytical mind* to continually analyze image quality while keeping the clinical situation in mind
- *Technical aptitude*
- *Good physical health* because continuous scanning may cause strain on back, shoulder, or arm
- *Independence and initiative* to analyze the patient, the history, the clinical findings and tailor the examination to answer the clinical question
- *Emotional stability* to deal with patients in times of crisis; this means the ability to understand the patient's concerns without losing objectivity
- *Communication skills* for interactions with peers, clinicians, and patients; this includes the ability to clearly communicate ultrasound findings to physicians and the ability *not* to disclose or speculate on findings to the patient during the examination
- *Dedication.* A willingness to go beyond the "call of duty" is typically required of the sonographer

ADVANTAGES AND DISADVANTAGES OF A SONOGRAPHY CAREER

Sonographers with specialized education in ultrasound have demonstrated their ability to produce high-quality consistent ultrasound images, thereby earning the respect of other allied health professionals and clinicians. Every day, sonographers are faced with varied human interactions and opportunities to solve problems. These experiences give sonographers an outlet for their creativity by requiring them to come up with innovative ways to meet the challenge of performing quality ultrasound examinations on difficult patients. New applications in ultrasound and improvements in instrumentation also create a continual challenge for the sonographer. Flexible schedules and varieties in examinations and equipment make each day interesting and unique. Certified sonographers find that employment opportunities are abundant, schedule flexibility is high, and salaries are attractive.

On the other hand, some sonographers find their position to be stressful and demanding, with the constant changes facing medical care and decreased staffing causing increased workloads. Hours of continual scanning may lead to tendinitis, arm and shoulder pain, and back strain. Sonographers may become frustrated dealing with terminally ill patients, which can lead to fatigue and depression.

Employment. Sonographers may find employment in traditional settings of a hospital or medical clinic. Staffing positions within the hospital or medical setting may include the following: chief sonographer or office manager, clinical staff sonographer, research sonograhper, or clinical instructor. Clinical research opportunities are found in the major medical centers throughout the country. Sonographers with advanced degrees (i.e., BS, MS, or PhD) may serve as faculty in diagnostic medical sonography as a program director, department head, or dean of allied health. Many sonographers have entered the commercial world as application specialists and directors of education, continuing education, marketing, product design/engineering, sales, service, or quality control. Other sonographers have become independent business partners in medicine by offering mobile ultrasound services to smaller community hospitals.

Resource organizations. Specific organizations devoted to developing standards and guidelines for ultrasound are listed below:

- AIUM: American Institute of Ultrasound in Medicine *www.aium.org*
- ASE: American Society of Echocardiography *www.asecho.org*
- SDMS: Society of Diagnostic Medical Sonography *www.sdms.org*. This is the principal organization for sonographic affairs. The website contains information regarding the SDMS position statement on the code of ethics for the profession of diagnostic medical ultrasound; the non-diagnostic use of ultrasound; the scope of practice for the diagnostic ultrasound professional; and the diagnostic ultrasound clinical practice standards.
- SVU: Society for Vascular Ultrasound *www.svunet.org*

The National Examination for Ultrasound is:

- ARDMS: American Registry for Diagnostic Medical Sonography *www.ardms.org*.

The national review boards for educational programs in sonography are:

- JRC-DMS: Joint Review Committee on Education in Diagnostic Medical Sonography (includes general ultrasound, echocardiology, and vascular technology) www.jrcdms.org
- JRC-CVT: Joint Review Committee on Education in Cardiovascular Technology (includes noninvasive cardiology, invasive cardiology, and vascular technology)

There are several journals devoted to ultrasound; however, the three journals that are connected to the national organizations are:

- JDMS: *Journal of Diagnostic Medical Sonography*
- JUM: *Journal of Ultrasound in Medicine*
- JASE: *Journal American Society of Echocardiography*
- JVU: *Journal for Vascular Ultrasound*

MEDICAL TERMS FOR THE SONOGRAPHER

The sonographer is responsible for assessing the patient's request for the ultrasound examination, reading the patient's chart, and discussing any specific requests with the referring physician. Therefore, a familiarity with basic medical terminology and abbreviations is necessary. Common medical and ultrasound abbreviations are listed on the inside covers of this book for quick reference.

One of the sonographer's primary responsibilities is the identification and description of normal and abnormal anatomy. The following list of key terms will help the sonographer describe the results obtained from various ultrasound examinations.

anechoic or sonolucent—(opposite of echogenic) without internal echoes; the structure is fluid-filled and transmits sound easily (Figure 1-5, *A*); examples: vascular structures, distended urinary bladder, gallbladder, and amniotic cavity

echogenic or hyperechoic—(opposite of anechoic) echo-producing structure; reflects sound with a brighter intensity (Figure 1-5, *B*); examples: gallstone, renal calyx, bone, fat, fissures, and ligaments

enhancement, increased through-transmission—sound that travels through an anechoic (fluid-filled) substance and is not attenuated; there is increased brightness directly beyond the posterior border of the anechoic structure as compared with the surrounding area (see Figure 1-5, *A*).

fluid-fluid level—interface between two fluids with different acoustic characteristics; this level will change with patient position; example: dermoid with fluid level

heterogeneous—not uniform in texture or composition (Figure 1-5, *C*); example: many tumors have characteristics of both decreased and increased echogenicity

homogeneous—(opposite of heterogeneous) completely uniform in texture or composition (Figure 1-5, *D*); examples: the texture of the liver, thyroid, testes, and myometrium are generally considered homogeneous

hypoechoic—low-level echoes within a structure (Figure 1-5, *E*); example: lymph nodes and the gastrointestinal tract

infiltrating—usually refers to a diffuse disease process or metastatic disease (Figure 1-5, *F*)

irregular borders—borders are not well defined, are ill defined, or are not present (Figure 1-5, *G*); examples: abscess, thrombus, and metastases

isoechoic—very close to the normal parenchyma echogenicity pattern (Figure 1-5, *H*); example: metastatic disease

loculated mass—well-defined borders with internal echoes; the septa may be thin (likely benign) or thick (likely malignant) (Figure 1-5, *I*)

shadowing—the sound beam is attenuated by a solid or calcified object; this reflection or absorption may be partial or complete; air bubbles in the duodenum may cause a "dirty shadow" to occur secondary to reflection; a stone would cause a sharp shadow posterior to its border (see Figure 1-5, *B*)

CRITERIA FOR IDENTIFYING ABNORMALITIES

After the sonographer has delineated the normal landmarks and anatomic structures, careful evaluation is made for the presence of pathologies. The abnormality is identified and evaluated according to a number of criteria (Figure 1-6), which include the following:

- The *border* of the structure may be smooth and well defined, or irregular.
- The *texture* (parenchyma) of the structure is either homogeneous or heterogeneous.
- The *characteristic* of an organ or of a mass is said to be anechoic, hypoechoic, isoechoic, hyperechoic, or echogenic to the rest of the parenchyma.
- The *transmission* of the sound is either increased, decreased, or unchanged. An anechoic mass will show increased transmission of sound, whereas a dermoid tumor will show decreased transmission.

Structures may be identified as cystic, complex, or solid. Transmission is altered depending on what the mass is.

Cystic: A cyst has smooth, well-defined borders, anechoic, increased through-transmission (Figure 1-7)
Complex: Has characteristics of both a cyst and a solid structure
Solid: Irregular borders, internal echoes, decreased through-transmission (Figure 1-8)

Table 1-1 summarizes these ultrasound criteria for identifying abnormalities.

INTRODUCTION TO BASIC ULTRASOUND PRINCIPLES

To produce high quality images that are free of artifacts, sonographers must have a firm understanding of the basic principles of ultrasound. This section introduces sonographers to some basic principles of ultrasound physics, including common terminology, measurement units, and the fundamentals of sound generation.

Sound is generated by a vibrating source, such as a tuning fork or a violin string. When this source vibrates, adjacent particles are displaced. These particles in turn push against other adjacent particles. This constant "pushing" is known as particle vibration (Figure 1-9). Ultrasound refers to sound waves beyond the human audible range. Diagnostic applications of ultrasound use frequencies of 1 to 10 million cycles/sec, or 1 to 10 MHz. Ultrasound is used to examine soft tissue anatomic structures within all areas of the body (Table 1-2). In medical ultrasound, the vibrating source is a ceramic element that vibrates in response to an electrical signal. The vibrating motion of the ceramic element in the transducer causes the particles in the surrounding tissue to vibrate (Figure 1-10). As the source vibrates, it periodically presses against and pulls away from the adjacent medium with resultant particle **compression** and expansion (**rarefaction**) in the medium. This

Figure 1-5 **A,** Anechoic (simple cyst). **B,** Echogenic (stone with shadowing). **C,** Heterogeneous (Baker cyst with mixture of fluid, debris, and bright echo reflectors). **D,** Homogeneous (renal parenchyma). **E,** Hypoechoic (hemorrhagic cyst). **F,** Infiltrating (HIV systemic disease process involving the kidney).

Figure 1-5, cont'd   **G,** Irregular borders (thrombus within the renal pelvis). **H,** Isoechoic (one half of renal parenchyma has lower level echoes). **I,** Loculated (complex renal mass with septations).

TABLE 1-1	ULTRASOUND CRITERIA FOR IDENTIFYING ABNORMAL STRUCTURES

Border	Texture	Characteristic	Transmission of Sound	Structures that Affect Transmission
Smooth, well defined	*Homogeneous*—uniform texture within	*Anechoic*—without internal echoes	Increased	Cyst • Smooth • Well-defined borders
Irregular	*Heterogeneous*—nonuniform texture within	*Hypoechoic*—low-level echoes	Decreased	• Anechoic • Increased through-transmission
		Isoechoic—close to normal parenchyma	Unchanged	Complex Structure • Has characteristics both of cystic and of solid structures
		Hyperechoic/echogenic—echo-producing (bright) structure		Solid Structure • Irregular borders • Internal echoes • Decreased through transmission

Figure 1-6   Ultrasound criteria for describing a mass. **A,** Simple cyst: smooth borders, anechoic, increased transmission. **B,** Hypoechoic mass: few to low-level internal echoes, smooth border, no increased transmission. **C,** Complicated cyst: mixed pattern of cystic and solid, fluid, debris, blood, transmission may or may not increase. **D,** Lobulated cyst: well defined with thin septa, increased transmission. **E,** Loculated cyst: well defined with thick septa. **F,** Abscess: may have irregular borders, debris within, transmission may or may not be increased. **G,** Homogeneous mass: uniform texture within. **H,** Heterogeneous mass: nonuniform texture within. **I,** Infiltrating mass: distorted architecture, irregular borders, decreased transmission.

Figure 1-7   Gross pathology of a simple ovarian cyst showing smooth borders, well-defined; straw-colored fluid was found inside.

TABLE 1-2	APPLICATIONS OF SOUND FREQUENCY RANGES	
Frequency Range	Manner of Production	Application
Infrasound		
0–25 Hz	Electromagnetic vibrators	Vibration analysis of structures
Audible		
20 Hz–20 kHz	Electromagnetic vibrators, musical instruments	Communications, signaling
Ultrasound		
20–100 kHz	Air whistles, electric devices	Biology, sonar
100 kHz–1 MHz	Electric devices	Flaw detection, biology
1–20 MHz	Electric devices	Diagnostic ultrasound

Hz, Hertz; *kHz,* kilohertz; *MHz,* megahertz.

movement of energy through the anatomical structures is called a wave.

Patients are examined with a transducer that converts electrical energy into mechanical energy. As the sound beam is directed into the body at various angles to the organs, reflection, absorption, and scatter cause the returning signal to be weaker than the initial impulse. Over a short period of time, multiple anatomic images are acquired in a real-time format.

SOUND WAVES

A **wave** is a propagation of energy that moves back and forth or vibrates at a steady rate. Sound waves are mechanical oscillations that are transmitted by particles in a gas, liquid, or solid medium. Generated by an external source, ultrasound is the transmission of high frequency mechanical vibrations greater than 20 kilohertz (kHz) through a medium.

Waves are generated over a period of time. The time required to produce each **cycle** depends on the frequency of the transducer. Frequency is equal to the number of cycles per second by the sound source and the particles of the medium. The speed of the wave depends upon the properties of the medium. There are many forms of energy that travel in the forms of waves such as sound. Generally speaking there are two types of waves: mechanical (sound waves) and electromagnetic (x-rays or light waves). The mechanical waves are characterized by physical motion of particles in the medium and cannot travel through a vacuum. This is the reason why sonographers use a gel coupling medium between the transducer and the skin. On the other hand, electromagnetic waves can travel through a vacuum.

Waves may be further classified into longitudinal and transverse waves. Sound waves are considered longitudinal waves as the particles in the medium vibrate parallel to the direction that the sound wave is traveling. Transverse waves mean the particles in a medium vibrate perpendicular to the direction the sound wave is traveling.

Longitudinal Waves. Ultrasound is a form of nonionizing radiation in which longitudinal pressure waves of high frequency are transmitted through a medium. These waves are formed by the oscillation of particles or molecules parallel to the axis of wave propagation. Part of the molecules are "squeezed" closer together, or *compressed*, and part undergo expansion, or *rarefaction*, by which the molecules are pulled farther apart. As sound travels through a material, alternate regions of compression and rarefaction occur.

Along with wave properties, such as frequency and intensity, the medium that carries the sound is a major contributor

Figure 1-8   Gross pathology of a solid ovarian mass shows the irregular borders with complex tissue throughout.

Tuning fork

Figure 1-9   Particle vibration. When a tuning fork vibrates, multiple particles move back and forth to produce a wave which we can hear as a high-pitched hum sound.

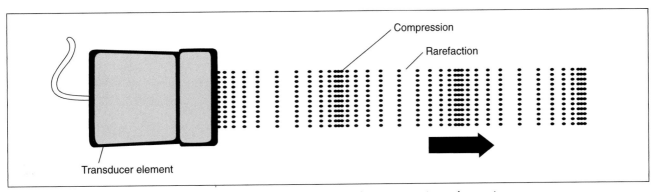

Compression

Rarefaction

Transducer element

Figure 1-10   As the transducer element vibrates, waves undergo compression and expansion, or rarefaction, by which the molecules are pulled apart.

in defining the ultrasound transmission properties. The medium can best be understood in forms of its bulk modulus and acoustic impedance characteristics. The **bulk modulus** is the amount of pressure required to compress a small amount of material. In part, the compressibility or density of a material determines the way sound is carried along with the material.

Wavelength. As noted earlier, the sound wave pulls and presses against the multiple structures in its line of travel causing compressions and rarefactions. In addition, there are pressure fluctuations that accompany the sound wave. The wavelength is the distance between two peaks over a period of time (Figure 1-11). The **wavelength** represents the distance occupied by each cycle, the operating frequency of the **transducer,** and the **velocity** of sound. The total distance occupied by a sound pulse is the wavelength multiplied by the number of cycles in the pulse and is called the *spatial pulse length.* The wavelength is inversely related to frequency, which means that the higher the frequency, the shorter the wavelength. Conversely the lower the frequency the longer the wavelength.

Pressure amplitude is the amount that the pressure increases or decreases in the medium as the sound wave travels through. As the energy in a sound wave increases, so does the pressure amplitude. Pressure amplitude is measured in units called pascals (Pa) or megapascals (MPa).

This time interval is the **period** of the wave. The *pulse duration* is the total time of each sound pulse multiplied by the number of cycles in each pulse. As frequencies become higher, the pulse duration decreases, yielding a decrease in the depth of field.

Measurement of Sound. The **decibel (dB)** unit is often used to measure the strength or intensity, amplitude, and power of an ultrasound wave. Decibels allow the sonographer to compare the intensity or amplitude of two signals.

Power refers to the rate at which energy is transmitted. Power is the rate of energy flow over the entire beam of sound

and is often measured in watts (W) or milliwatts (mW). **Intensity** is defined as power per unit area. It is the rate of energy flow across a defined area of the beam and can be measured in watts per square meter (W/m^2) or milliwatts per square centimeter. Power and intensity are related: If you double the power, the intensity also doubles.

Intensity is also related to pressure amplitude. Intensity is proportional to the square of the pressure amplitude: If you double the amplitude, the intensity increases four times.

Frequency. Sound is characterized according to its frequency. Frequency may be explained by the following analogy. If a stick were moved in and out of a pond at a steady rate, the entire surface of the water would be covered with waves radiating from the stick. If the number of vibrations made in each second were counted, the frequency of vibration could be determined. In ultrasound, **frequency** refers to the number of oscillations per second performed by the particles of the medium in which the wave is propagating:

1 oscillation/sec = 1 cycle/sec = 1 **hertz** (1 **Hz**)

1000 oscillations/sec = 1 kilocycle/sec = 1 **kilohertz** (1 **kHz**)

1,000,000 oscillations/sec = 1 megacycle/sec = 1 **megahertz** (1 **MHz**)

The sonographer should be familiar with the units of measurement commonly used in the profession (Table 1-3).

PROPAGATION OF SOUND THROUGH TISSUE

Velocity of Sound. The velocity of sound in a medium is determined by the *density* and elastic properties of the medium. The velocity of sound differs greatly between air, bone, and soft tissue. It travels slowly through gas (air), intermediate speed through liquids, and quickly through solids (metal). On the other hand, the velocity of sound varies by only a few percent from one soft tissue to another. Air-filled structures,

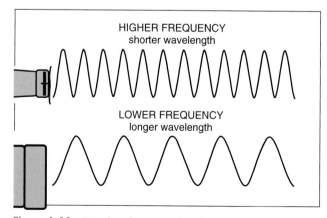

Figure 1-11 Wavelength is inversely related to frequency. The higher the frequency, the shorter the wavelength and the less depth of penetration. The longer wavelength has a lower frequency and greater depth of penetration.

TABLE 1-3	UNITS COMMONLY USED IN ULTRASOUND	
Quantity	Unit	Abbreviation
Amplifier gain	Decibels	dB
Area	Meters squared	m^2
Attenuation	Decibels	dB
Attenuation coefficient	Decibels per centimeter	dB/cm
Frequency	Hertz (cycles per second)	Hz
Intensity	Watts per square meter	W/m^2
Length	Meter	m
Period	Microseconds	μs
Power	Watts	W
Pressure amplitude	Pascals	Pa
Relative power	Decibels	dB
Speed	Meters per second	m/s
Time	Seconds	s
Volume	Meters cubed	m^3

such as the lungs and stomach, or gas-filled structures, such as the bowel, impede the sound transmission. Likewise, sound is attenuated through most bony structures. Small differences between fat, blood, and organ tissues, as seen on an ultrasound image, may be better delineated with higher frequency transducers that improve resolution. The stiffness and the density of a medium determine how fast sound waves will travel through the structure.

Piezoelectric Effect. The sound beam used in diagnostic ultrasound is produced from a transducer by the **piezoelectric effect** (Figure 1-12). The transducer is a means for converting one form of energy into another (e.g., electrical energy into mechanical sound waves). The Curie brothers first described the piezoelectric effect in 1880. They observed that when certain **crystals**, such as quartz, undergo mechanical deformation, a potential difference develops across the two surfaces of the crystals. Synthetic ceramic crystals have been developed for medical use that can be molded into various shapes and sizes and focused for ultrasound applications. Each ceramic crystal has a resonant frequency that depends on the thickness of the crystal.

Most diagnostic applications use short, pulsed ultrasound waves for optimum resolution. As a pulse of ultrasound is emitted, the pulse travels through tissue. When the pulse strikes an interface, part of the energy is reflected. The returning echo is a sound pressure wave that causes a slight mechanical deformation of the ceramic as it impinges on the transducer face, resulting in an electrical pulse.

Pulse-Echo. There are two basic modes of transducer operation that are used in medical diagnostic applications: continuous wave and pulsed wave. Doppler instrumentation uses both continuous and pulse-wave operations. Real-time instrumentation uses only the pulse-echo function, which means it sends out short bursts of sound energy and then listens for return echo information. The signal is converted to an electrical signal after it returns to the transducer. The ultrasound equipment measures the time it takes to receive the echoes after each transmitted pulse. The system keeps track of these pulses

and returning echo to determine the distance to various reflectors. Most systems are calibrated to 1540 m/sec, which is the average velocity of sound through human tissue.

Acoustic Impedance. The characteristic acoustic impedance is a property of substances that influences the strength or amplitude of reflected echoes. It is the opposition that particles in a medium present to acoustic vibration. The ultrasound wave is very similar to a light beam in that it may be focused, refracted, reflected, or scattered at interfaces between different media (Figure 1-13). At the junction of two media of different acoustic properties, an ultrasound beam may be reflected depending on the difference in **acoustic impedance** between the two media and the angle at which the beam hits the **interface** (**angle of incidence**) (Table 1-4).

In biologic tissues, with the exception of air-tissue and bone interfaces, the differences in acoustic impedance are so slight that only a small component of the ultrasound beam is reflected at each interface.

The lung and bowel have a detrimental effect on the ultrasound beam, causing poor transmission of sound. Therefore,

TABLE 1-4	CHARACTERISTIC ACOUSTIC IMPEDANCE AND VELOCITY OF ULTRASOUND	
Material	Acoustic Impedance (g/cm/sec × 10)	Velocity
Air	0.0001	331
Fat	1.38	1450
Water	1.50	1430
Blood	1.61	1570
Kidney	1.62	1560
Liver	1.65	1550
Muscle	1.70	1580
Skull	7.80	4080

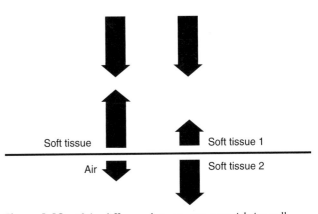

Figure 1-13   If the difference between two materials is small, most of the energy in a sound wave will be transmitted across an interface between them, while the reflected echo will be weak. If the difference is large, little energy will be transmitted; most will be reflected.

Piezoelectric Effect   Reverse Piezoelectric Effect

Electrical signal   Electrical signal

Sound waves   Sound waves
A   **B**

Figure 1-12   Piezoelectric effect. **A,** In certain crystals, when a sound wave is applied perpendicular to its surface, an electric charge is created. **B,** If the element is exposed to an electric shock, the elements will begin to vibrate and transmit a sound wave.

anatomy beyond these two areas cannot be imaged because of air interference. Bone conducts sound at a much faster speed than soft tissue. Normal transmission of sound through soft tissue travels at 1540 m/sec. Much of the sound beam is absorbed or scattered as it travels through the body, undergoing progressive attenuation. The sound is reflected according to the acoustic impedance. Acoustic impedance is related to tissue density; the greater the difference in density between two structures, the stronger are the returning interface echoes defining the boundaries between two structures on the ultrasound image.

Most of the sound is passed into tissues deeper in the body and reflected at other interfaces. The acoustic impedance is the product of the *velocity of sound* in a medium and the *density* of that medium. The acoustic impedance increases if the density or propagation speed increases.

Sound Reflections. Reflections most frequently received are those that occurred at a perpendicular incidence. The **angle of reflection** is equal to the angle of incidence (Figure 1-14). This occurs at most specular interfaces where the boundary is smooth and where the dimensions of the interface are larger than the wavelength (i.e., diaphragm and walls of vessels).

Sound not reflected is transmitted through the interface. Refraction (change in direction of sound) can occur if the incident angle is not zero and if the velocities of sound of the two materials forming the boundary are not equal.

Nonspecular reflectors are interfaces that are smaller than the wavelength or not smooth (rough). Examples include red blood cells and liver parenchyma (Figure 1-15).

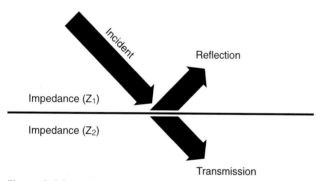

Figure 1-14 Reflection occurs when a sound wave strikes an interface between two objects with different acoustic impedances, causing some of the energy to be transmitted across the interface and some of it to be reflected.

Attenuation is the sum of acoustic energy losses resulting from absorption, scattering, and reflection. It refers to the reduction in intensity and amplitude of a sound wave as it travels through a medium (Figure 1-16). Some of the energy is absorbed, some is reflected or scattered. Thus, as the sound beam travels through the body, the beam becomes progressively weaker. In human soft tissue, sound is attenuated at the rate of 0.5 dB/cm per million hertz. If air or bone is coupled with soft tissue, more energy will be attenuated. Attenuation through a solid calcium interface, such as a gallstone, will produce a shadow with sharp borders on the ultrasound image.

Image Resolution. **Resolution** is the ability to separate the smallest reflectors from one another. Axial resolution is the minimum reflector separation along the sound path required to produce separate echoes. Lateral resolution is the ability to produce separate echoes perpendicular to the sound path and is affected by transducer diameter and focusing.

SOUND BEAM FORMATION

The sound beam that emerges from a transducer has analogous characteristics. The near field is called the **Fresnel zone** and is the area closest to the face of the transducer. The far field, or the **Fraunhofer zone**, is farther from the transducer face and is where the beam diverges (Figure 1-17). The frequency and diameter of a transducer determine the length of its near field. As the transducer diameter increases in size, the near field becomes longer. As the beam wavelength increases, the near field becomes shorter. As the beam frequency increases, the near field becomes longer. Most transducers will have some type of focus applied to the element to help shape the beam for a sharper beam formation. The focus may be a mechanical focus or a multiple element array electronic focus. Remember—the wider the diameter, the poorer the resolution of the beam.

BEAM WIDTH AND LATERAL RESOLUTION

Beam width determines lateral resolution (Figure 1-18). If two reflectors are closer together than the diameter or width of the beam, they will not be resolved. The best lateral resolution is in the **focal zone** (sharpest imagery point) of the transducer. This is the point at which the beam is the narrowest. Lateral resolution is affected by transducer frequency, diameter, and focusing.

The **spatial resolution** of an ultrasound system refers to the minimum distance between two objects where they can be

Figure 1-15 Nonspecular reflectors reflect, or scatter, the sound wave in many directions.

ATTENUATION

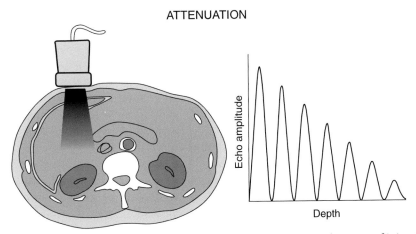

Figure 1-16   As the sound travels through the abdomen, it becomes attenuated as some of it is reflected, scattered, and absorbed.

FOCAL ZONE CHARACTERISTICS

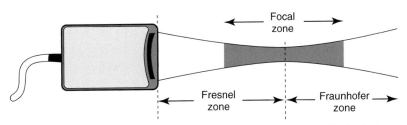

Figure 1-17   The near field, Fresnel zone, is the area closest to the transducer. The far field, Fraunhofer zone, is farthest from the transducer.

BEAM WIDTH AND
LATERAL RESOLUTION

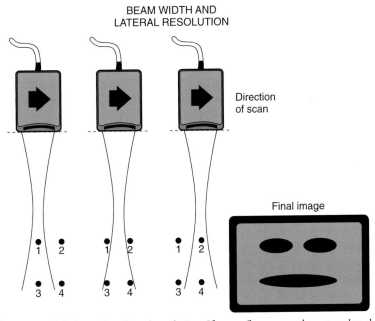

Figure 1-18   Beam width determines lateral resolution. If two reflectors are closer together than the diameter or width of the transducer, they will not be resolved.

displayed as separate structures. (Box 1-1 summarizes typical values for spatial resolution.) The better the spatial resolution, the sharper the detail. One aspect of spatial resolution is **lateral resolution** (Figure 1-19). This is defined as the minimum distance between two objects positioned along a line perpendicular to the beam, where both objects can be distinguished as separate structures by the ultrasound system.

Axial resolution refers to the minimum distance between two structures positioned along the axis of the beam, where both structures can be visualized as separate objects (Figure 1-20). Axial resolution is calculated from the spatial pulse length:

$$\text{Axial resolution} = \frac{1}{2} \text{ spatial pulse length}$$

Pulse duration is the time that a piezoelectric element vibrates after electrical stimulation (i.e., when the pulse duration is shorter than the interval between arrival times of two echoes at the transducer, the reflectors producing those echoes will be resolved as separate structures) (Figure 1-21). Therefore, the shorter the pulse duration, the better the axial resolution.

Slice thickness refers to the thickness of the section in the patient that contributes to echo signals on any one image (Figure 1-22).

INSTRUMENTATION

TRANSDUCER SELECTION

The majority of transducers used today are not a single element but a combination of elements that form an array. The transducer array scan head contains multiple small piezoelectric elements, each with its own electrical circuitry (Figure 1-23). Thus these elements are very small in diameter and therefore beam divergence is greatly reduced. This capability leads to beam steering and focusing. The focus of the array trans-

ducers occurs on reception and on transmission (Figure 1-24). The focusing is done dynamically during reception. Shortly after pulse transmission, the received focus is set close to the transducer. As time elapses and the echoes from the distant targets return, the focal distance is gradually lengthened. Some instruments will have multiple transmit focal zones to allow better control of the resolution of the beam at certain depths of field in the image.

To summarize, there are two important features of transducer arrays that determine the resolution of the image (Figure 1-25):

1. Electronic beam steering uses time delays between channels (phased arrays) or switching between groups of channels (liner, curvilinear) to control the beam direction. The annular array's electronic focus affects both the lateral resolution and the slice thickness.

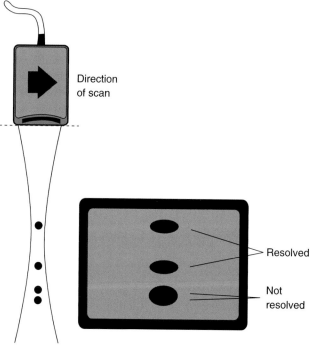

Figure 1-20   Axial resolution refers to the minimum distance between two structures positioned along the axis of the beam where both structures can be visualized as separate objects.

BOX 1-1	**TYPICAL VALUES FOR SPATIAL RESOLUTION**	
Axial resolution		0.1 mm–1 mm
Lateral resolution		1.0 mm–5 mm
Slice thickness		2.0 mm–12 mm

Figure 1-19   Lateral resolution is improved with a small diameter transducer.

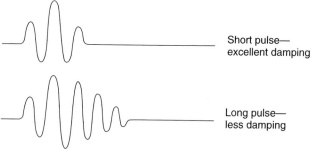

Figure 1-21   Pulse duration and damping. The more damping, the better the axial resolution.

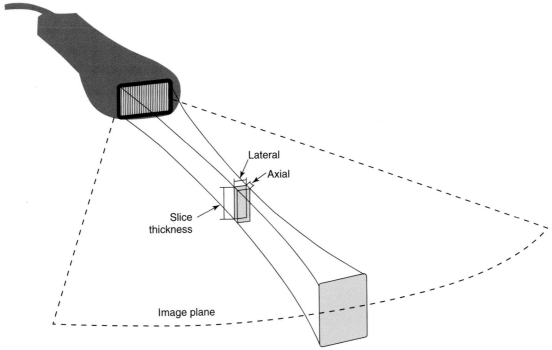

Figure 1-22 Slice thickness refers to the thickness of the section in the patient that contributes to the echo signals on any one image.

Figure 1-23 Single element transducer design.

METHODS OF FOCUSING

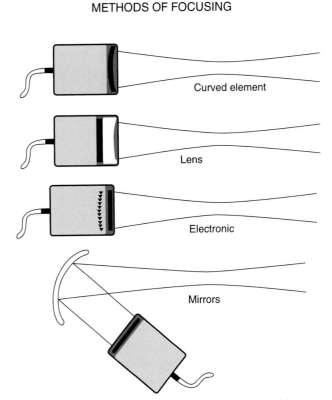

Figure 1-24 Focusing effectively narrows the ultrasound beam. There are multiple methods that can be used to achieve this effect.

2. Electronic focusing uses time delays between channels to focus each individual beam; this applies to all types of transducers. Electronic focusing is applied in the scanning plane, affecting the lateral resolution; the slice thickness is with a mechanical lens.

Types of transducers include the following:

Curved or curvilinear array—linear array transducer with a curved scan head and electronic focusing to produce a trapezoidal field of view (Figure 1-26)

Linear sequential array—multiple small transducer elements electronically coordinated to produce a rectangular image (see Figure 1-26)

Figure 1-25 Comparison of transducer models. **A,** Electronically scanned arrays may be curved or linear. **B,** Annular array has a larger diameter with multiple rings of focus. **C,** Sector array with multiple small elements within the transducer face.

Annular array—superior spatial resolution at some depths due to electronic focusing in the slice thickness; steering the beam requires mechanical manipulation of the array and difficult to interlace color and spectral Doppler

Sector phased array—small transducer head with multiple pinpoint elements that produces a pie-shaped image (Figure 1-27)

Single element—mechanical lens and mechanical beam steering

Endorectal transducer—special transducer that is introduced into the rectum to examine the prostate, bladder, and rectum

Endovaginal transducer—a high frequency probe that is inserted into the vagina to image the uterus, ovaries, and adnexal area (Figure 1-28)

Intraoperative transducer—specialized transducers designed specifically for intraoperative procedures

Transesophageal transducer—a special probe that is inserted into the esophagus to image the cardiac struc-

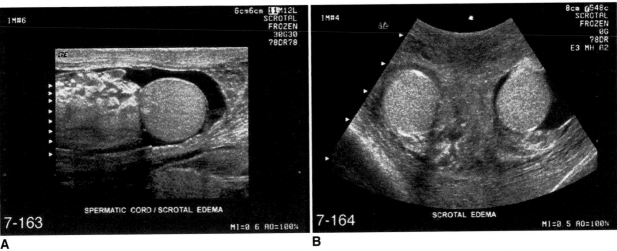

Figure 1-26 Comparison of linear array (**A**) to curved array (**B**) images of the scrotal sac. The linear array produces a "rectangular" image display, whereas the curved array shows a wide "pie" curve display.

Figure 1-27 Small sector array has small footprint to get in between ribs; however, there is limited visualization of the near field.

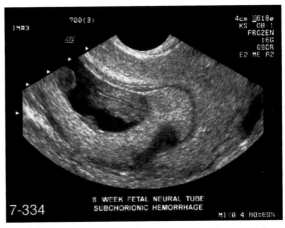

Figure 1-28 Endovaginal probe may provide 90- to 120-degree sector field of view to image this 8-week gestation with a subchorionic hemorrhage.

tures or to image the pancreas, pancreatic duct, and common bile duct

The type of transducer selected for a particular examination depends upon several factors: the type of examination, the size of the patient, and the amount of fatty or muscular tissue present. High frequency linear array probes are generally used for smaller structures (carotid artery, thyroid, scrotum, breast). The abdomen is usually scanned with a curved linear array and/or a sector array; the frequency will depend on the size of the patient. The echocardiographic examination is performed with a small head sector transducer to allow the probe to scan in between the ribs. The transesophageal studies are obtained with the transesophageal probe to image detailed anatomy of the cardiac structures or pancreatic areas. Obstetric and gynecologic scans are usually performed with a linear or curved

array transducer. The endovaginal probe is used to scan inter-cavity areas.

PULSE-ECHO INSTRUMENTATION

The critical component of the pulse-echo instrument is the B-mode (2-D) imager (Figure 1-29). The beam former includes the electronic transmit and receive focusing. The transmitter supplies the electrical signals to the transducer for producing the sound beam. The transducer may be connected to the transmitter and receiver through a beam-former system. Echoes picked up by the transducer are applied to the receiver. At this point, the echoes are amplified and processed into a suitable format for display. An image memory (scan converter) retains data for viewing or storage on digital media.

Pulsing Characteristics. In the pulse-echo instruments, a short burst of ultrasound is emitted repeatedly by the transducer at specific, well-defined intervals. As soon as the pulse is

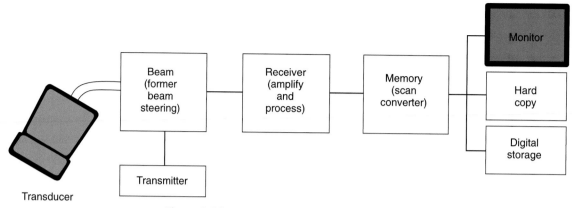

Figure 1-29   Components of an ultrasound system.

PULSING CHARACTERISTICS

Time ➤

Pulse Repetition Frequency (PRF) = Number of pulses per second

Figure 1-30   The PRF may be adjusted in Doppler applications to record the lower or higher velocity signals.

emitted, the transducer also acts as a receiver for the echoes reflected back and for the scattered echoes along the beam path. The **pulse repetition frequency (PRF)** is the number of pulses launched per second (Figure 1-30). The transducer emits sound for only a very small percentage of time; it spends about 99% of the time receiving echoes.

The power and intensity of the ultrasound equipment is varied by the output power control. As one increases the power on the ultrasound equipment, the acoustic pulse transmitted contains more energy and the amplitude of all the echoes increases. However, the acoustic exposure to the patient likewise increases.

The receiver **gain** allows the sonographer to amplify or boost the echo signals. It may be compared with the volume control on a radio—as one increases the volume, the sound becomes louder. The acoustic exposure to the patient is not changed when the receiver gain is increased. If the gain is set too high, artifactual echo noise will be displayed throughout the image.

Recall the discussion of how the signal is absorbed, reflected, and attenuated as the beam traverses the body. The **time gain compensation (TGC)** control, sometimes referred to as *DGC (depth gain compensation)*, allows the sonographer to amplify the receiver gain gradually at specific depths (Figure 1-31). Thus the echoes well seen in the near field may be

reduced in amplitude, while the echoes in the far field may be amplified with the TGC controls.

The reject control eliminates both electronic noise and low-level echoes from the display.

All of these instrumentation controls are best understood with the use of a phantom in the ultrasound scanning lab. A complete understanding of all these controls is critical to performing an adequate, high-quality diagnostic ultrasound examination.

Frame Rate. The **frame rate** is the rate at which images are updated on the display. The frame rate depends on the frequency of the transducer and depth selection. Each complete scan of the sound beam produces an image on the display that is called a frame. Each frame consists of scan lines (scan lines depend on the number of times the transducer is pulsed).

The pulse repetition frequency (PRF), the number of lines per frame, and the number of frames per second (frame rate) are all related to each other:

$$PRF \text{ (Hz)} = \text{lines per frame} \times \text{frame rate}$$

Furthermore, the relationship among the lines per frame, frame rate, and maximum imaging depth in soft tissue is as follows:

$$\text{Maximum depth (cm)} \times \text{lines per frame} \times \text{frame rate} = 77{,}000$$

TIME GAIN COMPENSATION (TGC)

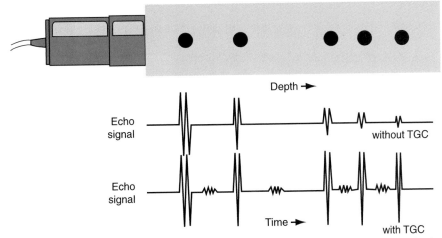

Figure 1-31 The TGC allows the sonographer to amplify the receiver gain gradually at specific depths to adjust for attenuation.

This means if the maximum imaging depth is 20 cm and the frame rate is 20 frames per second, there will be approximately 200 lines per frame. If a greater depth is required, either the frame rate or the lines per frame will have to be reduced.

Dynamic Range. The **dynamic range** of a device is the range of input signal levels that produce noticeable changes in the output of the device. The dynamic range capabilities will vary among the different ultrasound machines. The sonographer usually notes the low dynamic range as one of high contrast (echocardiography and peripheral vascular), whereas the high dynamic range shows more shades of gray and lower contrast (abdominal and obstetrics).

Tissue Harmonic Imaging. As discussed previously, sound waves contain many component frequencies. Harmonics are those components whose frequencies are integral multiples of the lowest frequency (the "fundamental" or "first harmonic"). Harmonic imaging involves transmitting at frequency f and receiving at frequency $2f$, the second harmonic. Because of the finite bandwidth constraints of transducers, the transducer insonates at half of its nominal frequency (e.g., 3 MHz for a 6 MHz transducer) in harmonic mode and then receives at its nominal frequency (6 MHz in this example). The harmonic beams generated during pulse propagation are narrower and have lower side-lobe artifacts than the fundamental beam. The strength of the harmonics generated depends on the amplitude of the incoming beam. Therefore, the image-degrading portions of the fundamental beam (i.e., scattered echoes, reverberations, and slice-thickness side lobes) are much weaker than the on-axis portions of the beam and therefore generate weaker harmonics.

Harmonic formation increases with depth so few harmonics are generated within the near field of the body wall. Therefore, filtering out the fundamental frequency and creating an image from the echoes of the second harmonic should result in an image that is relatively free of the noise formed during the passage of sound through the distorting layers of the body wall.

PULSE-ECHO DISPLAY MODES

A-Mode (Amplitude Modulation). A-mode, or amplitude modulation, produces a one-dimensional image displaying the amplitude strength of the returning echo signals along the vertical axis and the time (distance) along the horizontal axis. The **amplitude** display represents the time or distance it takes the beam to strike an interface and return the signal to the transducer. The greater the reflection at the interface, the taller the amplitude spike will appear (Figure 1-32).

B-Mode (Brightness Modulation). The B-mode, or brightness modulation, method displays the intensity (amplitude) of an echo by varying the brightness of a dot to correspond to echo strength. *Gray scale* refers to the condition of assigning each level of amplitude a particular shade of gray. The B-mode is the basis for all real-time imaging in ultrasound (Figure 1-33). In B-mode imaging, the ultrasound beam is sent in various directions into the region of interest to be scanned. Each beam interrogates the reflectors along a different line. The echo data picked up along the beam line is displayed in a B-mode format. The B-mode display "tracks" the ultrasound beam line as it scans the region, "sketching out the 2-D image" of the body. As many as 200 beam lines may be used to construct each image.

M-Mode (Motion Mode). The M-mode, or motion mode, displays time along the horizontal axis and depth along the vertical axis to depict movement, especially in cardiac structures (Figure 1-34).

A

Figure 1-32   **A,** Amplitude is shown along the vertical axis, and time is shown along the horizontal axis. **B,** Earlier instrumentation used the A-mode display to help determine proper settings for the two-dimensional image. The bottom images show the A-mode and time gain compensation scale below.

A   **B**

Final B-Mode 2-D Image

Figure 1-33   **A,** Acquisition of multiple image planes over a period of time is made to produce a B-mode image. **B,** B-mode image of the liver with a hemangioma in the center of the right lobe. The auto-optimize control is used in the right-hand display to show improved focus.

Real-time. **Real-time** imaging provides a dynamic presentation of multiple image frames per second over selected areas of the body. The frame rate is dependent on the frequency and depth of the transducer and depth selection. Typical frame rates are 30 frames per second or less. The principal barrier to higher scanning speeds is the speed of sound in tissue, dictating the time required to acquire echo data for each beam line. The **temporal resolution** refers to the ability of the system to accurately depict motion.

Three-Dimensional Ultrasound. Conventional ultrasound offers a two-dimensional visualization of anatomical structures with the flexibility of visualizing images from different orientations or "windows" in real-time. The sonographer acquires these two-dimensional images in at least two different scanning planes and thus forms a three-dimensional image in his or her head. Recent developments in technology have allowed ultrasound images to be acquired on their x, y, and z axes, manually realigned, and then reconstructed into

Figure 1-34 A, M-mode imaging. From the B-mode image, one line of site may be selected to record a motion image of a moving structure over time and distance. **B,** The M-mode is recorded through the stenotic mitral valve to show decreased opening and closing of the valve leaflet over time. On the M-mode, the vertical scale represents depth and the space between the markers represents time. The distance between these two markers is 1 second. *ALMV,* Anterior leaflet mitral valve; *LV,* left ventricle; *PLMV,* posterior leaflet mitral valve; *RV,* right ventricle.

a three-dimensional format. This technique has been useful in reconstructing the fetal face, ankle, and extremities in the second- and third-trimester fetus. Clinical investigations are currently underway to discover additional applications of three-dimensional imaging (Figure 1-35).

DOPPLER ULTRASOUND

DOPPLER EFFECT

The *Doppler effect* refers to a change in frequency of a sound wave when either the source or the listener is moving relative to one another (Figure 1-36). This is most generally applied when the motion of laminar or turbulent flow is detected within a vascular structure. When the source moves toward the listener, the perceived frequency is higher than the emitted fre-

quency, thus creating a higher pitched sound. If the sound moves away from the listener, the perceived frequency is lower than the transmitted frequency, and the sound will have a lower pitch.

In the medical application of the Doppler principle, the frequency of the reflected sound wave is the same as the frequency transmitted only if the reflector is stationary. If the red blood cell (RBC) moves along the line of the ultrasound beam (parallel to flow), the Doppler shift is directly proportional to the velocity of the RBC. If the RBC moves away from the transducer in the plane of the beam, the fall in frequency is directly proportional to the velocity and direction of the red blood cell movement (Figure 1-37). The frequency of the echo will be higher than the transmitted frequency if the reflector is moving toward the transducer, and lower if the reflector is moving away.

DOPPLER SHIFT

The difference between the receiving echo frequency and the frequency of the transmitted beam is called the **Doppler shift.** This change in the frequency of a reflected wave is caused by relative motion between the reflector and the transducer's beam. Generally the Doppler shift is only a small fraction of the transmitted ultrasound frequency.

The Doppler shift frequency is proportional to the velocity of the moving reflector or blood cell. The frequency at which a transducer transmits ultrasound influences the frequency of the Doppler shift. The higher the original, or transmitted, frequency, the greater is the shift in frequency for a given reflector velocity. The returning frequency increases if the red blood cell is moving toward the transducer and decreases if the blood cell is moving away from the transducer. The Doppler effect produces the shift that is the reflected frequency minus the transmitted frequency. When interrogating the same blood vessel with transducers of different frequencies, the higher frequency transducer will generate a larger Doppler shift frequency.

The angle that the reflector path makes with the ultrasound beam is called the **Doppler angle.** As the Doppler angle increases from 0 to 90 degrees, the detected Doppler frequency shift decreases. At 90 degrees the Doppler shift is zero, regardless of flow velocity. The frequency of the Doppler shift is proportional to the cosine of the Doppler angle. The beam should be parallel to flow to obtain the maximum velocity. The closer the Doppler angle is to zero, the more accurate the flow velocity (Figure 1-38). If the angle of the beam to the reflector exceeds 60 degrees, velocities will no longer be accurate.

SPECTRAL ANALYSIS

Blood flow through a vessel may be laminar or turbulent (Figure 1-39). **Laminar** flow refers to the pattern of blood flow through a vessel at different velocities. When the range of velocities increases significantly, the flow pattern becomes turbulent. The audio of the Doppler signal enables the sonographer to distinguish laminar flow from turbulent flow patterns. The process of **spectral analysis** allows the instrumentation to break down the complex multifrequency Doppler signal into individual frequency components by way of a fast Fourier transform (FFT) processor. The fast Fourier transform processor is a mechanical algorithm designed to break down a waveform into various frequency components. The spectral analysis of the Doppler signal identifies the Doppler shifts and their relative importance.

The spectral display shows the distribution of Doppler frequencies versus time (Figure 1-40). This is displayed as velocity on the vertical axis and time on the horizontal axis. Flow towards the transducer is displayed above the baseline, while flow away from the transducer is displayed below the baseline.

Figure 1-35 Three-dimensional reconstruction of the face from the two-dimensional fetal profile image in a third-trimester fetus.

Figure 1-36 The Doppler effect refers to a change in frequency of a sound wave when either the source or the listener is moving relative to the other.

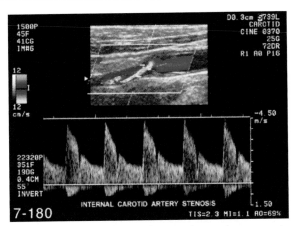

Figure 1-37   Color Doppler with spectral wave shows stenosis of the internal carotid artery and increased velocity through the area of stenosis.

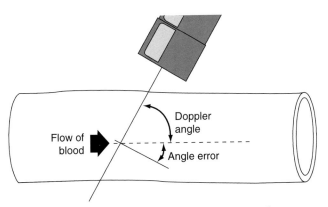

Figure 1-38   The closer the Doppler angle is to zero, the more accurate the flow velocity. Thus the more parallel the transducer is to flow, the more accurate the velocity.

Figure 1-39   Laminar flow is smooth and has uniform velocity, whereas turbulent flow has multiple flow velocity characteristics.

VELOCITIES ON SPECTRAL WAVEFORM

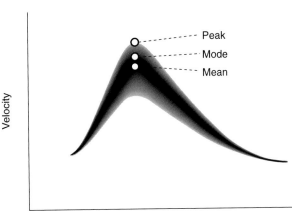

Figure 1-40   The spectral display shows the distribution of Doppler frequencies versus time.

When the area of the vessel that is examined contains red blood cells moving at similar velocities, they will be represented on the spectral display by a narrow band. This area under the band is called the "window." As flow becomes more turbulent or disturbed, the velocity increases, producing **spectral broadening** on the display. A very stenotic (high flow velocity) lesion would cause the window to become completely filled in.

CONTINUOUS WAVE DOPPLER

Continuous wave (CW) Doppler contains two piezoelectric elements: one for sending and one for receiving. The sound is transmitted continuously rather than in short pulses. Continuous wave is used to record the higher velocity flow patterns, usually above 2 m/sec and is especially useful in cardiology (Figure 1-41). Unlike pulsed wave Doppler, continuous wave cannot pinpoint exactly where along the beam axis flow is occurring, as it samples all of the flow along its path. In the example of a five-chamber view of the heart, a sample volume placed in the left ventricular outflow tract will sample all the flow along that "line" to include the flows in the outflow tract and in the ascending aorta.

PULSED WAVE DOPPLER

Pulsed wave (PW) Doppler is used for lower flows and has one crystal that pulses to transmit and signal and also listens or receives the returning signal. The pulsed wave Doppler uses brief bursts of sound like those used in echo imaging. These bursts are usually of a longer duration and produce well-defined frequencies. The sonographer may set the so-called **gate** or Doppler window to a specific area of interest in the vascular structure so interrogated. This means that a specific area of interest may be examined at the point the gate or sample volume is placed. For example, in a five-chamber view of the heart, the sample volume may be placed directly in the outflow tract and recordings only from that particular area "within the gate or window" will be measured.

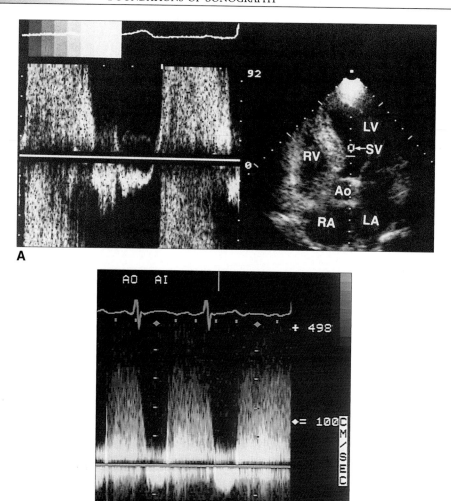

Figure 1-41   A, The sample volume *(SV)* is placed in the left ventricular outflow tract. There is aortic insufficiency that exceeds the Nyquist limit of the pulsed wave Doppler (flow is seen above and below the baseline). When the continuous wave transducer is used **(B),** the velocity measures 3.5 m per second. *Ao,* Aorta; *LA,* left atrium; *LV,* left ventricle; *RA,* right atrium; *RV,* right ventricle.

With pulsed Doppler, for accurate detection of Doppler frequencies to occur, the Doppler signal must be sampled at least twice for each cycle in the wave. This phenomenon is known as the **Nyquist sampling limit**. When the Nyquist limit is exceeded, an artifact called aliasing occurs. **Aliasing** presents on the spectral display as an apparent reversal of flow direction and a "wrapping around" of the Doppler spectral waveform. The highest velocity, therefore, may not be accurately demonstrated when aliasing occurs; this usually happens when the flows are greater than 2 m/sec. One can avoid aliasing by changing the Doppler signal from pulsed wave to continuous wave to record the higher velocities accurately.

COLOR FLOW DOPPLER

With **color flow** Doppler, velocity detection and display include multiple locations along a beam line. Velocities are quantitated by allocating a pixel to flow toward the transducer and flow away from the transducer. Each velocity frequency change is allocated a color. Color maps may be adjusted to

obtain different color assignments for the velocity levels; usually red is assigned to flow toward the transducer and blue to flow away from the transducer (Figure 1-42). Flow velocity is indicated by color brightness. The higher the velocity, the brighter the color. Aliasing also occurs in color flow imaging when Doppler frequencies exceed the Nyquist limit, just as in spectral Doppler. This appears as a wrap-around of the displayed color. The velocity scale (PRF) may be adjusted to avoid the aliasing. Color arising from sources other than moving blood is referred to as flash artifact or ghosting.

ARTIFACTS

Artifacts are structures and features of an image that do not correspond to the object being imaged. The sonographer must understand the appearance and characteristics of artifacts that may be encountered in the ultrasound examination. Artifacts in ultrasonic images can be classified into the following four categories: (1) equipment artifacts, (2) tech-

A   **B**

Figure 1-42 Color Doppler has been helpful to outline the direction and velocity of flow. The color box **(A)** shows which color assignment has been made for the image. The color toward the transducer is blue. **B,** This image shows that the color bar has been assigned red, as flow toward the transducer.

Figure 1-43 Absence of focusing shows overall blurring of the image.

Figure 1-44 Grating lobes show a linear echo *(arrows)* within the inferior vena cava.

nique-dependent artifacts, (3) movement artifacts, and (4) sound-tissue artifacts.

EQUIPMENT ARTIFACTS

Equipment artifacts are related to instrument problems, which occur when the equipment is not functioning properly.

1. Artifactual noise: 60-cycle interference may occur if ultrasound equipment is plugged into the same outlet as another high-powered piece of equipment (e.g., in surgery, the bovi [the surgical instrument used to cauterize vessels] unit should not be plugged into the same outlet as the ultrasound equipment).
2. Absence of focusing: if the proper focus is not used, the image may appear blurry or "fuzzy." The solution is to adjust the focal zone (Figure 1-43).
3. Grating lobes: caused by periodic spacing of the phased or linear array elements; the echoes travel at an angle to the main beam. The solution is to find a better acoustic window (Figure 1-44).

4. Side lobes: caused by secondary echoes outside the main beam; therefore, a "noisy" image is created. The solution is to adjust the focal zone.

TECHNIQUE ARTIFACTS

Technique artifacts are produced by unsatisfactory operator technique:

1. Noise: caused by excess gain (e.g., noise within the vascular structures or along the anterior wall of bladder). The solution is to decrease gain or adjust the TGC to clean up the image (Figure 1-45).
2. Banding: caused by finely focused transducer or inaccurate TGC settings. The solution is the change the transducer and/or the TGC (Figure 1-46).

MOVEMENT ARTIFACTS

Movement artifacts occur when patients fail to hold their breath properly.

1. Breathing: Image distorted and blurred. The solution is to *always* ask the patient either to take in a breath or stop

Figure 1-45 Noise is seen with "fill-in" of anechoic vascular structures. *Ao*, Aorta; *SMA*, superior mesenteric artery.

Figure 1-46 Banding is caused by incorrect time gain compensation settings; the near gain is too low, the midfield is too high, and the far field is attenuated.

breathing to obtain your images. If the patient takes in a breath and holds it, the patient ends up doing a slight Valsalva maneuver at the end of breath holding and causes the venous structures to dilate for improved imaging (Figure 1-47).

SOUND-TISSUE ARTIFACTS

This type of artifact is unavoidable because it results from the way tissues affect sound.

1. Shadowing is caused when sound strikes a strong interface, such as gas or bowel, with secondary reverberations or "ring down" of ill-defined echoes. The solution is to change to a higher frequency to delineate a sharp shadow (that may be pathologic versus gas) or compress the tissue gently to displace the shadow. The patient may be rolled into a different position or sat upright and rescanned to see if the shadow changes (Figure 1-48).

2. Reverberation is caused by sound passing out of a structure with acoustic impedance that is markedly different from its neighbor causing a large amount of sound returned to the transducer. This usually occurs when the transducer is placed over the ribs and causes a repeated duplication of the original echo at equal distance between the echoes.

Figure 1-47 Breathing is best seen in the area of the diaphragm. *Arrows*, diaphragm in inspiration and expiration.

A   B

Figure 1-48 **A,** Shadowing posterior to bowel may be seen as a "dirty" shadow. **B,** Shadowing beyond a stone or rib is sharply defined.

Figure 1-49   Reverberation artifact from a rib.

Figure 1-50   Mirror image artifact seen at the junction of the spleen-diaphragm interface shows "splenic parenchyma" to appear in the pleural cavity.

The solution is to try different acoustic windows, rotate the patient, or change transducer frequency (Figure 1-49).

3. Mirror image occurs if a structure has a curved surface; it causes the returning echo to focus and reflect sound like a mirror (e.g., diaphragm/liver interface). The solution is to scan the patient in another position (Figure 1-50).

4. Enhancement occurs when sound passes easily through an anechoic fluid-filled structure, without attenuation. The enhancement appears as bright echoes posterior to the fluid-filled structure. The solution is to diminish the overall gain or slightly adjust the TGC or change to a higher frequency transducer. This will not totally eliminate the enhancement, but will prove that it is anechoic (Figure 1-51).

5. Slice thickness is caused when an interface between a fluid-filled cyst and soft tissue is acutely angled and the beam strikes both the tissue and fluid simultaneously. Low-level echoes are displayed in the fluid (e.g., gallbladder and cyst

Figure 1-51   Enhancement appears as increased transmission through a cystic structure.

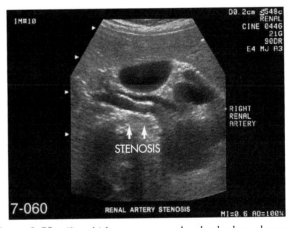

Figure 1-52   Slice thickness appears as low-level echoes along a cystic type of structure (vessels or bladder).

Figure 1-53   Comet effect appears as a strong acoustic interface from the air-filled bowel.

or abscess adjacent to one another). The solution is to scan from a different angle (Figure 1-52).

6. Comet effect is a strong acoustical interface from an air-bubble or metallic suture. The solution is to scan from a different angle or rotate the patient (Figure 1-53).

SELECTED BIBLIOGRAPHY

Craig M: Introduction to ultrasonography and patient care, Philadelphia, 1993, WB Saunders.

Curry R, Tempkin B, editors: Ultrasonography: an introduction to normal structure and functional anatomy, Philadelphia, 2004, WB Saunders.

Holmes JH: Perspectives in ultrasonography: early diagnostic ultrasonography, J Ultrasound Med 2:33, 1983.

Melany ML, Grant EG: Clinical experience with sonographic contrast agents, Semin Ultrasound CT MR 18(1):3, 1997.

Miner NS: Basic principles. In Sanders RC, editor: Clinical sonography, Boston, 2001, Little, Brown.

Nelson TR, Downey DD, Pretorius DH and others: Three-dimensional ultrasound, Philadelphia, 1999, Lippincott Williams & Wilkins.

Robinette WB: Ultrasound contrast agents: an overview, J Diagn Med Sonogr 13:29S, 1997.

Sanders RC, editor: Clinical sonography, Boston, 1997, Little, Brown.

Zagzebski J, Parks J: Ultrasound Physics and Instrumentation, Advanced Ultrasound Seminars, 1997.

CHAPTER 2

Introduction to Physical Findings, Physiology, and Laboratory Data of the Abdomen

Sandra L. Hagen-Ansert

OBJECTIVES

- Explain how to obtain a health history
- Learn about the interview process
- Learn how to perform the physical assessment
- Explain the clinical signs and symptoms of various diseases
- Describe the physiology of the abdominal structures
- List the various laboratory tests pertinent to the sonographic examination

---

KEY TERMS

acidic – a type of solution that contains more hydrogen ions than hydroxyl ions

alkaline – a type of solution that contains more hydroxyl ions than hydrogen ions

anemia – abnormal condition where blood lacks either a normal number of red blood cells or normal concentration of hemoglobin

auscultation – procedure of listening to the heart sounds with a stethoscope

bile – bile pigment, old blood cells, and the by-products of phagocytosis are known together as *bile*

buffer – chemical compound that can act as a weak acid or a base to combine with excess hydrogen or hydroxyl ions to neutralize the pH in blood

dysuria – painful or difficult urination

epigastric – above the umbilicus and between the costal margins

erythrocytes – red blood cells

erythropoiesis – production of red blood cells

hematochezia – passage of bloody stools

hematocrit – the percent of the total blood volume containing the red blood cells, white blood cells, and platelets

hemoglobin – protein in red blood cells that picks up oxygen and releases it in the capillaries of tissue

hypertension – high blood pressure >130/90

hypotension – low blood pressure

incontinence – see urinary incontinence

Kupffer cells – special hepatic cells that remove bile pigment, old blood cells, and the by-products of phagocytosis from the blood and deposit them into the bile ducts

leucopoiesis – white blood cell formation stimulated by presence of bacteria

leukocytes – white blood cells

polycythemia – overproduction of red blood cells

sphygmomanometer – device used to measure blood pressure

suprapubic – above the symphysis pubis

tachycardia – heart rate more than 100 beats per minute

thrombocytes – platelets in blood

tympany – predominant sound heard over hollow organs (stomach, intestines, bladder, aorta, gallbladder)

umbilical – around the navel

urinary incontinence – the uncontrollable passage of urine

The sonographer soon discovers that good patient history and pertinent clinical information are very important in planning the approach to each sonographic examination. Slight changes in the laboratory data (i.e., white blood cell differential, serum enzymes, or fluctuations in liver function tests) may enable the sonographer to tailor the examination to provide the best information possible to answer the clinical question. Specific questions related to the current health status of the patient will direct the sonographer to examine the critical area of interest with particular attention as part of the routine protocol. Knowledge of the patient's previous surgical procedures will also help tailor the examination. This way, the sonographer will not spend time looking for the gallbladder or ovaries that have been removed.

THE HEALTH ASSESSMENT

Obtaining a health history and performing a physical assessment are essential steps to analyzing the patient's medical problem. Although the health assessment is done by the health care practitioner before the patient's arrival at the ultrasound department, an understanding of the health assessment helps the sonographer better understand patient symptoms and lab values. Any health assessment involves collecting two types of data: objective and subjective. Objective data is obtained through observation and is verifiable. For example, a red swollen leg in a patient experiencing leg pain is data that can be seen and verified by someone other than the patient. Subjective data is derived from the patient alone and includes such statements as "I have back pain" or "My stomach hurts."

THE INTERVIEW PROCESS

The purpose of the health history is to gather subjective data about the patient and to explore previous and current problems. This information is gathered during a patient interview that typically occurs in a limited amount of time just before the ultrasound examination.

Be sure to introduce yourself to the patient and explain that the purpose of the assessment is to identify the problem and provide information for the ultrasound examination. Ask patients first about their general health, and then specifically about body systems and structures, with questions tailored to the ordered examination. Remember that your interviewing techniques will improve and become smoother with practice.

Successful patient interviews include the following considerations:

- Reassure the patient that everything will be kept confidential.
- Be sure the patient understands English and can hear well.
- Use language that the patient can understand and avoid many medical terms. If the patient does not understand, repeat the question in a different format using different words or examples. For example, instead of asking, "Did you have gastrointestinal difficulty after eating?" ask "What foods make you sick to your stomach?"
- Always address the patient respectfully by a formal name, such as Mr. Delado or Ms. Peligrino.
- Listen attentively and make notes of pertinent information on the ultrasound data sheet.
- Remember that the patient may be worried that a problem will be found. Explain the procedure that will occur after the examination is complete (i.e., the images will be shown to the clinician and the patient may contact his or her referring physician to find out the results).
- Briefly explain what you are planning to do, why you are doing it, how long it will take, and what equipment you will use.

Professional Demeanor. Remember to maintain professionalism throughout the interview process and examination. Remain neutral by avoiding sarcasm and keeping jokes in good taste. Do not let your personal opinions interfere with your assessment, and do not share your own medical problems with the patient. Do not offer advice. Know enough to answer questions the patient may have about ultrasound examination, but leave the diagnostic interpretation to the physician. Be careful if the patient asks how everything looks. If you respond, "It looks fine," meaning the technique was good, the patient will likely think you mean the examination is normal when it may not be.

Two Ways to Ask Questions. Questions may be characterized as either open-ended or closed. Open-ended questions require the patient to express feelings, opinions, and ideas. They may also help to gather further information. Such a question as "How would you describe the problems you have had with your abdomen?" is an example of an open-ended question.

Closed questions are short answer responses and may help you to zoom in on a specific point. These questions would include "Do you ever get short of breath?" or "Do you have nausea and vomiting after fatty meals?"

Important Interview Questions. The sonographer usually does not have a great deal of time to obtain extensive histories and thus it is important to ask the right questions:

- **Biographical data.** The patient's name, address, phone number, birth date, marital status, religion, and nationality likely have been obtained already. Be sure to always check the patient's name with the patient you are interviewing to make sure it is the correct patient. The primary care physician is important for contact information.

- **Chief Complaint.** Try to pinpoint why the patient is here for the ultrasound examination. Ask what his/her symptoms are and what prompted him/her to seek medical attention.
- **Medical History.** Ask the patient about past and current medical problems and hospitalizations that may be pertinent to the examination.

Questions Specific to Body Structures and Systems. The structures and systems that are most frequently encountered by the sonographer are presented below.

Neck. Do you have swelling, soreness, lack of movement, or abnormal protrusions in your neck? How long have you had the problem? Have you done anything specific to aggravate the condition?

Respiratory system. Do you have shortness of breath on exertion or while lying in bed? Do you have a productive cough? Do you have night sweats? Have you been treated for a respiratory condition before? Have you ever had a chest x-ray?

Cardiovascular system. Do you have chest pain, palpitations, irregular heartbeat, fast heartbeat, shortness of breath, or a persistent cough? Have you ever had an electrocardiogram or echocardiogram or nuclear exercise study before? Do you have high blood pressure, peripheral vascular disease, swelling of the ankles and hands, varicose veins, cold extremities, or intermittent pain in your legs?

Breasts. Do you perform monthly breast self-examinations? Have you noticed a lump, a change in breast contour, breast pain, or discharge from your nipples? Have you ever had breast cancer? If not, has anyone else in your family had it? Have you ever had a mammogram?

Gastrointestinal tract. Have you ever had nausea, vomiting, loss of appetite, heartburn, abdominal pain, frequent belching, or passing of gas? Have you lost or gained weight recently? How frequent are your bowel movements, and what color, odor, and consistency are your stools? Have you noticed a change in your regular pattern? Have you had hemorrhoids, rectal bleeding, hernias, gallbladder disease, or a liver disease, such as hepatitis?

Urinary system. Do you have urinary problems, such as burning during urination, incontinence, urgency, retention, reduced urinary flow, or dribbling? Do you get up during the night to urinate? What color is your urine? Have you ever noticed blood in it? Have you ever had kidney stones?

Female reproductive system. Do you have regular periods? Do you have clots or pain with them? What age did you stop menstruating? Have you ever been pregnant? How many live births? How many miscarriages? Have you ever had a vaginal infection or a sexually transmitted disease? When did you last have a gynecologic examination and Pap test?

Male reproductive system. Do you perform monthly testicular self-examinations? Have you ever noticed penile pain, discharge, or lesions, or testicular lumps? Have you had a vasectomy? Have you ever had a sexually transmitted disease?

Musculoskeletal system. Do you have difficulty walking, sitting, or standing? Are you steady on your feet, or do you lose your balance easily? Do you have arthritis, gout, a back injury, muscle weakness, or paralysis?

Endocrine system. Have you been unusually tired lately? Do you feel hungry or thirsty more than usual? Have you lost weight for unexplained reasons? How well can you tolerate heat and cold? Have you noticed changes in your hair texture or color? Have you been losing hair? Do you take hormonal medications?

PERFORMING THE PHYSICAL ASSESSMENT

The physical assessment is another important part of the health assessment. It is a good idea to do this in a well-lighted room to physically assess the patient's appearance, color of scleroderma, skin tone, etc. Performing a physical assessment usually includes the following:

Height and Weight. These measurements are important for evaluating nutritional status, calculating medication dosages, and assessing fluid loss or gain.

Body Temperature. Body temperature is measured in degrees Fahrenheit (F) or degrees Celsius (C). Normal body temperature ranges from 96.7° F to 100.5° F (35.9° C to 38° C) depending on the route used for measurement.

Pulse. The patient's pulse reflects the amount of blood ejected with each heartbeat. To assess the pulse, palpate one of the patient's arterial pulse points (usually at the wrist, on the radial side of the forearm) and note the rate, rhythm, and amplitude (strength) of the pulse. A normal pulse for an adult is between 60 to 100 beats/min. To palpate for a pulse, use the pads of your index and middle fingers. Press lightly over the area of the artery until you feel pulsations. If the rhythm is regular, count the beats for 10 seconds and multiply by 6 to obtain the number of beats per minute.

Although the radial pulse is the most easily accessible pulse site (on the wrist, same side as the thumb), the femoral or carotid pulse may be more appropriate in cardiovascular emergencies because these sites are larger and closer to the heart and more accurately reflect the heart's activity.

Respirations. Along with counting respirations, note the depth and rhythm of each breath. To determine the respiratory rate, count the number of respirations for 15 seconds and multiply by 4. A rate of 16 to 20 breaths/min is normal for an adult.

Blood Pressure. Systolic and diastolic blood pressure readings are helpful in evaluating cardiac output, fluid and circulatory status, and arterial resistance. The systolic reading reflects the maximum pressure exerted on the arterial wall at the peak of the left ventricular contraction. Normal systolic pressure ranges from 100 to 130 mm Hg.

The diastolic reading reflects the minimum pressure exerted on the arterial wall during left ventricular relaxation. This reading is usually more notable because it evaluates the arterial pressure when the heart is at rest. Normal diastolic pressure ranges from 60 to 80 mm Hg.

The *sphygmomanometer*, a device used to measure blood pressure, consists of an inflatable cuff, a pressure manometer, and a bulb with a valve. To record a blood pressure, the cuff is centered over an artery just above the elbow, inflated, and deflated slowly. As it deflates, listen with a stethoscope for Korotkoff sounds, which indicate the systolic and diastolic pressures. Blood pressures can be measured from most extremity pulse points, but the brachial artery is commonly used because of accessibility.

Auscultation. **Auscultation** is usually the last step in physical assessment. It involves listening for various breath, heart, and bowel sounds with a stethoscope. Hold the diaphragm (flat surface) firmly against the patient's skin, enough to leave a slight ring afterwards. Hold the bell lightly against the skin, enough to form a seal. Do not try to auscultate over the gown or bed linens because they can interfere with sounds. Be sure to warm the stethoscope in your hand.

FURTHER EXPLORATION OF SYMPTOMS

A clear understanding of the patient's symptoms is essential for guiding the specific examination. If the symptoms are acute and severe, you may need to pay particular attention to a specific area. If the symptoms seem mild to moderate, you may be able to take a more complete history.

The following five areas should be assessed:

1. Provocative or palliative. Your questions should be directed to finding out what causes the symptom and what makes it better or worse.
   - What were you doing when you first noticed it?
   - What seems to trigger it? Stress? Position? Activity?
   - What relieves the symptom? Diet? Position? Medication? Activity?
   - What makes the symptom worse?
2. Quality or quantity. Try to find out how the symptom feels, looks, or sounds.
   - How would you describe the symptom?
   - How often are you experiencing the symptom now?
3. Region or radiation. It is important to pinpoint the location of the patient's symptom. Ask the patient to use one finger to point to the area of discomfort.
   - Where does the symptom occur?
   - If pain is present, does it travel down (radiate from) your back or arms, up your neck, to your shoulder, etc.
4. Severity. The acuity of the symptom will impact the timeliness of further assessments. The patient may be asked to rate the symptom on a scale of 1 to 10, with 10 being the most severe.
   - How bad is the symptom at its worst? Does it force you to lie down, sit down, or slow down?
   - Does the symptom seem to be getting better, getting worse, or staying the same?
5. Timing. Determine when the symptom began and how it began, whether gradually or suddenly. If it is intermittent, find out how often it occurs.

GASTROINTESTINAL SYSTEM

The gastrointestinal (GI) system consists of two major divisions: the GI tract and the accessory organs. The GI tract is a hollow tube that begins at the mouth and ends at the anus. About 25 feet long, the GI tract includes the pharynx, esophagus, stomach, small intestine, and large intestine. Accessory GI organs include the liver, pancreas, gallbladder, and bile ducts. The abdominal aorta and the gastric and splenic veins also aid the GI system.

The major functions of the gastrointestinal (GI) system include ingestion and digestion of food and elimination of waste products. Gastrointestinal complaints can be especially difficult to assess and evaluate because the abdomen has so many organs and structures that may influence pain and tenderness.

NORMAL FINDINGS FOR THE GI SYSTEM

Visual Inspection
- Skin is free from vascular lesions, jaundice, surgical scars, and rashes.
- Faint venous patterns (except in thin patients) are apparent.
- Abdomen is symmetrical, with a flat, round, or scaphoid contour.
- Umbilicus is positioned midway between the xiphoid process and the symphysis pubis, with a flat or concave hemisphere.
- No variations in the color of the patient's skin are detectable.
- No bulges are apparent.
- The abdomen moves with respiration.

Auscultation
- High-pitched, gurgling bowel sounds are heard every 5 to 15 seconds through the diaphragm of the stethoscope in all four quadrants of the abdomen.
- A venous hum is heard over the inferior vena cava.
- No bruits, murmurs, friction rubs, or other venous hums are apparent.

Percussion
- **Tympany** is the predominant sound over hollow organs, including the stomach, intestines, bladder, abdominal aorta, and gallbladder.
- Dullness can be heard over solid masses, including the liver, spleen, pancreas, kidneys, uterus, and a full bladder.

Palpation
- No tenderness or masses are detectable.
- Abdominal musculature is free from tenderness and rigidity.
- No guarding, rebound tenderness, distention, or ascites are detectable.
- The liver is impalpable, except in children.
- The spleen is impalpable.
- The kidneys are impalpable, except in thin patients or those with a flaccid abdominal wall.

INSPECTING THE ABDOMEN

When visually inspecting the abdomen as part of the physical assessment, mentally divide the abdomen into four quadrants.

Keep in mind these three terms: *epigastric* (above the umbilicus and between the costal margins), *umbilical* (around the navel), and *suprapubic* (above the symphysis pubis).

- Observe the abdomen for symmetry, checking for bumps, bulges, or masses.
- Note the patient's abdominal shape and contour.
- Assess the umbilicus; it should be midline and inverted. Pregnancy, ascites, or an underlying mass can cause the umbilicus to protrude.
- The skin of the abdomen should be smooth and uniform in color.
- Note any dilated veins.
- Note any surgical scars.
- Note the abdominal movements and pulsations. Visible rippling waves may indicate bowel obstruction. In thin patients the aortic pulsations may be seen.

GUIDELINES FOR GI ASSESSMENT

- **Temperature:** Fever may be a sign of infection or inflammation.
- **Pulse: Tachycardia** may occur with shock, pain, fever, sepsis, fluid overload, or anxiety. A weak, rapid, and irregular pulse may point to hemodynamic instability, such as that caused by excessive blood loss.
- Diminished or absent distal pulses may signal vessel occlusion from embolization associated with prolonged bleeding.
- **Respirations:** Altered respiratory rate and depth can result from hypoxia, pain, electrolyte imbalance, or anxiety. Respiratory rate also increases with shock. Increased respiratory rate with shallow respirations may signal fever and sepsis. Absent or shallow abdominal movement on respiration may point to peritoneal irritation.
- **Blood Pressure:** Decreased blood pressure may signal compromised hemodynamic status, perhaps from shock caused by GI bleed. Sustained severe **hypotension** results in diminished renal blood flow, which may lead to acute renal failure. Moderately increased systolic or diastolic pressure may occur with anxiety or abdominal pain. *Hypertension* can result from vascular damage caused by renal disease or renal artery stenosis. A blood pressure drop of greater than 30 mm Hg when the patient sits up may indicate fluid volume depletion.

COMMON SIGNS AND SYMPTOMS OF GASTROINTESTINAL DISEASES AND DISORDERS

The most significant signs and symptoms related to gastrointestinal diseases and disorders are abdominal pain, diarrhea, bloody stools, nausea, and vomiting (Table 2-1).

Abdominal Pain. Abdominal pain usually results from a GI disorder, but it can be caused by a reproductive, genitourinary, musculoskeletal, or vascular disorder; use of certain drugs; or exposure to toxins.

- Constant, steady abdominal pain suggests organ perforation, ischemia, or inflammation or blood in the peritoneal cavity.
- Intermittent and cramping abdominal pain suggests the

patient may have obstruction of a hollow organ. Ask if the pain radiates to other areas. Ask if eating relieves the pain.

- Abdominal pain arises from the abdominopelvic viscera, the parietal peritoneum, or the capsule of the liver, kidney, or spleen, and may be acute or chronic, diffuse or localized.
- Visceral pain develops slowly into a deep, dull, aching pain that is poorly localized in the epigastric, periumbilical, or hypogastric region.
- Mechanisms that produce abdominal pain, including stretching or tension of the gut wall, traction on the peritoneum or mesentery, vigorous intestinal contraction, inflammation, ischemia, and sensory nerve irritation.

Diarrhea. Diarrhea is usually a chief sign of intestinal disorder. Diarrhea is an increase in the volume, frequency, and liquidity of stools compared with the patient's normal bowel habits. It varies in severity and may be acute or chronic.

- Acute diarrhea may result from acute infection, stress, fecal impaction, or use of certain drugs.
- Chronic diarrhea may result from chronic infection, obstructive and inflammatory bowel disease, malabsorption syndrome, an endocrine disorder, or GI surgery.
- The fluid and electrolyte imbalance may precipitate life-threatening arrhythmias or hypovolemic shock.

Hematochezia. Hematochezia is the passage of bloody stools and may be a sign of GI bleeding below the ligament of Treitz. It may also result from a coagulation disorder, exposure to toxins, or a diagnostic test. It may lead to hypovolemia.

Nausea and Vomiting. *Nausea* is a sensation of profound revulsion to food or of impending vomiting. *Vomiting* is the forceful expulsion of gastric contents through the mouth. This is usually preceded by nausea.

- Nausea and vomiting may occur with fluid and electrolyte imbalance, infection, metabolic, endocrine, labyrinthine, and cardiac disorders, use of certain drugs, surgery, and radiation.
- They may also arise from severe pain, anxiety, alcohol intoxication, overeating, or ingestion of distasteful food or liquids.

GENITOURINARY AND URINARY SYSTEMS

Although this chapter focuses on the urinary system, it is important to recognize that a disorder of the genitourinary system can affect other areas of the body systems. For example, ovarian dysfunction can alter endocrine balance, or kidney dysfunction can affect the production of certain hormones that regulate red blood cell production.

The primary functions of the urinary system are the formation of urine and the maintenance of homeostasis. These functions are performed by the kidneys. Kidney dysfunction can cause trouble with concentration, memory loss, or disorientation. Progressive chronic kidney failure can also cause

TABLE 2-1 SIGNS AND PROBABLE INDICATIONS OF GASTROINTESTINAL DISEASES AND DISORDERS

Sign or Symptom	Probable Indication	Sign or Symptom	Probable Indication
Abdominal Pain		**Hematochezia**	
• Localized abdominal pain, described as steady, gnawing, burning, aching, or hungerlike, high in the midepigastrium slightly off center, usually on the right • Pain begins 2 to 4 hours after a meal • Ingestion of food or antacids brings relief • Changes in bowel habits • Heartburn or retrosternal burning	Duodenal ulcer	• Moderate to severe rectal bleeding • Epistaxis (nosebleed) • Purpura (skin rash resulting from bleeding into the skin from small blood vessels)	Coagulation disorders
• Pain and tenderness in the right or left lower quadrant, may be sharp and severe on standing or stooping • Abdominal distention • Mild nausea and vomiting • Occasional menstrual irregularities • Slight fever	Ovarian cyst	• Bright-red rectal bleeding with or without pain • Diarrhea or ribbon-shaped stools • Stools may be grossly bloody • Weakness and fatigue • Abdominal aching and dull cramps	Colon cancer
		• Chronic bleeding with defecation • Painful defecation	Hemorrhoids
• Referred, severe upper abdominal pain, tenderness, and rigidity that diminish with inspiration • Fever, shaking, chills, aches, and pains • Blood-tinged or rusty sputum • Dry, hacking cough • Dyspnea	Pneumonia	**Nausea and Vomiting**	
		• May follow or accompany abdominal pain • Pain progresses rapidly to severe, stabbing pain in the right lower quadrant (McBurney sign) • Abdominal rigidity and tenderness • Constipation or diarrhea • Tachycardia	Appendicitis
Diarrhea		• Nausea and vomiting of undigested food • Diarrhea • Abdominal cramping • Hyperactive bowel sounds • Fever	Gastroenteritis
• Diarrhea occurs within several hours of ingesting milk or milk products • Abdominal pain, cramping, and bloating • Flatus	Lactose intolerance	• Headache with severe, constant, throbbing pain • Fatigue • Photophobia • Light flashes • Increased noise sensitivity	Migraine headache
• Recurrent bloody diarrhea with pus or mucus • Hyperactive bowel sounds • Cramping lower abdominal pain • Occasional nausea and vomiting	Ulcerative colitis		

lethargy, confusion, disorientation, stupor, convulsions, and coma. Observation of the patient's vital signs may give indication of **hypertension**, which may be related to renal dysfunction if the hypertension is uncontrolled.

ANATOMY AND PHYSIOLOGY OF THE URINARY SYSTEM

The urinary system consists of the kidneys, ureter, bladder, and urethra.

Kidneys. The kidneys are highly vascular organs that function to produce urine and maintain homeostasis in the body. The kidneys measure approximately 12 cm long by 5.5 cm wide. The two bean-shaped organs of the kidneys are located in the retroperitoneal cavity along either side of the vertebral column. The peritoneal fat layer protects the kidneys. The right kidney lies slightly lower than the left because it is displaced by the liver. Each kidney contains about 1 million nephrons. Urine gathers in the collecting tubules and ducts

and eventually drains into the ureters, then the bladder, and through the urethra (via urination).

Ureters. The ureters are 25 to 30 cm long. The narrowest part of the ureter is at the ureteropelvic junction. The other two constricted areas occur as the ureter leaves the renal pelvis and at the point it enters into the bladder wall. The ureters carry urine from the kidneys to the bladder by peristaltic contractions that occur one to five times per minute.

Bladder. The bladder is the vessel where urine collects. The bladder capacity ranges from 500 to 1000 ml in healthy adults. Children and older adults have less bladder capacity. When the bladder is empty, it lies behind the symphysis pubis; when it is full, it becomes displaced under the peritoneal cavity and serves as an excellent "window" for the sonographer to view the pelvic structures.

Urethra. The urethra is a small duct that carries urine from the bladder to the outside of the body. It is only 2.5 to 5 cm long and opens anterior to the vaginal opening. In the male, the urethra measures about 15 cm as it travels through the penis.

COMMON SIGNS AND SYMPTOMS RELATED TO URINARY DYSFUNCTION

The most common symptom of urinary dysfunction for both women and men is urinary incontinence. For women, a common symptom is dysuria, which often means a urinary tract infection. For men, common signs of urinary dysfunction include urethral discharge and urinary hesitancy. Tables 2-2 and 2-3 summarize the most common symptoms and probable causes of urinary dysfunction for women and men, respectively.

TABLE 2-2 SIGNS AND PROBABLE INDICATIONS OF URINARY DYSFUNCTION IN WOMEN	
Signs or Symptoms	Probable Indication
Dysuria	
• Urinary frequency • Nocturia • Straining to void • Hematuria • Perineal or low-back pain • Fatigue • Low-grade fever	Cystitis
• Dysuria throughout voiding • Bladder distention • Diminished urinary stream • Urinary frequency and urgency • Sensation of bloating or fullness in the lower abdomen or groin	Urinary system obstruction
• Urinary urgency • Hematuria • Cloudy urine • Bladder spasms • Feeling of warmth or burning during urination	Urinary tract infection
Urinary Incontinence	
• Urge or overflow incontinence • Hematuria • Dysuria • Nocturia • Urinary frequency • Suprapubic pain from bladder spasms • Palpable mass on bimanual examination	Bladder cancer
• Overflow incontinence • Painless bladder distention • Episodic diarrhea or constipation • Orthostatic hypotension • Syncope • Dysphagia	Diabetic neuropathy
• Urinary urgency and frequency • Visual problems • Sensory impairment • Constipation • Muscle weakness	Multiple sclerosis

Dysuria. Dysuria is painful or difficult urination and is commonly accompanied by urinary frequency, urgency, or hesitancy. This symptom usually reflects a common female disorder of a lower urinary tract infection (UTI).

Pertinent questions for the patient would include how long she has noticed the symptoms, whether anything precipitated them, if anything aggravates or alleviates them, and where exactly she feels the discomfort. You might also ask if she has undergone a recent invasive procedure such as a cystoscopy or urethral dilatation.

Urinary Incontinence. Urinary incontinence is the uncontrollable passage of urine. Incontinence results from either a bladder abnormality or a neurologic disorder. A common urologic sign may involve large volumes of urine or dribbling.

This condition would be important for the sonographer if a full bladder were required. It may be difficult for the patient to withhold large volumes of fluid to fill the bladder full enough for proper visualization.

Male Urethral Discharge. Male urethral discharge is discharge from the urinary meatus that may be purulent, mucoid, or thin; sanguineous or clear. It usually develops suddenly. The patient may have other signs of fever, chills, or perineal fullness. Previous history of prostate problems, sexually transmitted disease, or urinary tract infections may be associated with this condition.

Male Urinary Hesitancy. Male urinary hesitancy is a condition that usually arises gradually with a decrease in urinary stream. When the bladder becomes distended, the discomfort increases. Often prostate problems, previous urinary tract infection or obstruction, or neuromuscular disorders are associated with this condition.

PHYSIOLOGY AND LABORATORY DATA FOR THE ABDOMINAL CAVITY

THE CIRCULATORY SYSTEM

Fundamental to understanding human physiology is knowledge of the circulatory system. The circulation of the blood throughout the body serves as a vital connection to the cells, tissues, and organs to maintain a relatively constant environment for cell activity.

Functions of the Blood. The blood is responsible for a variety of functions to include transportation, defense against infection, and maintenance of body fluid (pH). Blood is thicker than water and therefore flows more slowly than water. The specific gravity of blood may be calculated by comparing the weight of blood to water; with water being 1.00, blood is in the range of 1.045 to 1.065.

Acidic versus alkaline. The hydrogen ion and the hydroxyl ion are found within water. When a solution contains more hydrogen than hydroxyl ions, it is called an **acidic** solution. Likewise, when it contains more hydroxyl ions than hydrogen

TABLE 2-3 SIGNS AND PROBABLE INDICATIONS OF URINARY DYSFUNCTION IN MEN

Signs or Symptoms	Probable Indication	Signs or Symptoms	Probable Indication
Scrotal Swelling		**Urinary Hesitancy**	
• Swollen scrotum that is soft or unusually firm • Bowel sounds may be heard in the scrotum	Hernia	• Reduced caliber and force of urinary stream • Perineal pain • Feeling of incomplete voiding • Inability to stop the urine stream • Urinary frequency • Urinary incontinence • Bladder distention	Benign prostatic hyperplasia
• Gradual scrotal swelling • Scrotum may be soft and cystic or firm and tense • Painless • Round, nontender scrotal mass on palpation • Glowing when transilluminated	Hydrocele		
		• Urinary frequency and dribbling • Nocturia • Dysuria • Bladder distention • Perineal pain • Constipation • Hard, nodular prostate palpated on digital rectal exam	Prostate cancer
• Scrotal swelling with sudden and severe pain • Unilateral elevation of the affected testicle • Nausea and vomiting	Testicular torsion		
Urethral Discharge			
• Purulent or milky urethral discharge • Sudden fever and chills • Lower back pain • Myalgia (muscle pain) • Perineal fullness • Arthralgia • Urinary frequency and urgency • Cloudy urine • Dysuria • Tense, boggy, very tender, and warm prostate palpated on digital rectal exam	Prostatitis	• Dysuria • Urinary frequency and urgency • Hematuria • Cloudy urine • Bladder spasms • Costovertebral angle tenderness • Suprapubic, low back, pelvic, or flank pain • Urethral discharge	Urinary tract infection
• Opaque, gray, yellowish, or blood-tinged discharge that is painless • Dysuria • Eventual anuria	Urethral neoplasm		
• Scant or profuse urethral discharge that is either thin and clear, mucoid, or thick and purulent • Urinary hesitancy, frequency, and urgency • Dysuria • Itching and burning around the meatus	Urethritis		

ions, it is referred to as an **alkaline** solution. This concentration of hydrogen ions in a solution is called the pH, with the scale ranging up to 14.0.

In water, an equal concentration of both ions exists and is thus a neutral solution, or 7.0 on the pH scale. Human blood has a pH of 7.34 to 7.44, being slightly alkaline. A blood pH below 6.8 would be called *acidosis*, and above 7.8 would be called *alkalosis*. Both conditions can lead to a serious illness and eventual death unless a proper balance is restored. To help in this process, blood plasma is supplied with chemical compounds called **buffers.** These buffers can act as weak acids or bases to combine with the excess hydrogen or hydroxyl ions to neutralize the pH. Plasma is the basic supporting fluid and transporting vehicle of the blood. It constitutes 55% of the total blood volume.

The volume of blood in the body depends on the body surface area; however, the total volume may be estimated as approximately 9% of total body weight. Therefore, the blood volume is approximately 5 qt in a normal-sized man.

The red blood cells (**erythrocytes**), the white blood cells (**leukocytes**), and the platelets (**thrombocytes**) make up the remainder of the blood. The percent of the total blood volume containing these three elements is called the **hematocrit.** Normally the hematocrit is described as 45, or 45% of the total blood volume (with plasma comprising the remaining 55%).

Red blood cells. The red blood cells are disk shaped, biconcave cells without a nucleus. They are formed in the bone marrow and are the most prevalent of the formed elements in the blood. Their primary role is to carry oxygen to the cells and tissues of the body. Oxygen is picked up by a protein in the red cell called **hemoglobin.** Hemoglobin releases the oxygen in the capillaries of the tissues.

The production of red blood cells is called *erythropoiesis.* Their life span is approximately 120 days. Vitamin B_{12} is necessary for complete maturity of the red blood cells. The inner mucosal lining of the stomach secretes a substance called the *intrinsic factor,* which promotes absorption of vitamin B_{12} from ingested food. **Anemia** is an abnormal condition where the blood lacks either a normal number of red blood cells or normal concentration of hemoglobin. If too many red blood cells are produced, **polycythemia** results.

As old red blood cells are destroyed in the liver, part of the hemoglobin is converted to bilirubin, which is excreted by the liver in the form of bile. When excessive amounts of hemoglobin are broken down or when biliary excretion is decreased by liver disease or biliary obstruction, the plasma bilirubin level rises. This rise in plasma bilirubin results in a yellow-skin condition known as jaundice.

White blood cells. These cells are the body's primary defense against infection. The WBCs lack hemoglobin, are colorless, contain a nucleus, and are larger than RBCs. The white cells are extremely active and move with an ameboid motion, often against the flow of blood. They can pass from the blood stream into intracellular spaces to phagocytize foreign matter found between the cells. A condition called *leucopoiesis* is WBC formation stimulated by the presence of bacteria.

Leukocytes. The neutrophils, eosinophils, and basophils are the group of leukocytes called **granulocytes** because of the presence of granules in their cytoplasm. Their function is to ingest and destroy the bacteria with the formation of pus.

The basophils contain heparin and control clotting. The eosinophils increase in patients with allergic diseases.

Lymphocytes and monocytes. The lymphocytes are WBCs formed in lymphatic tissue and enter the blood by way of the lymphatic system. They contain antibodies responsible for delayed hypersensitivity reactions. Monocytes are large white cells capable of phagocytosis and are quite mobile. Their numbers are few and are produced in the bone marrow.

The blood test that is responsible for stating specific values for all these subgroups of white blood cells is called a differential CBC.

The white cells have two main sources: (1) red bone marrow (granulocytes) and (2) lymphatic tissue (lymphocytes). When an increase in the white cells stems from a tumor of the bone marrow, it is called *myelogenous leukemia* and is noted as an increase in granulocytes. On the other hand, an increase in WBCs caused by overactive lymphoid tissue is called *lymphatic leukemia,* with an increase in lymphocytes. Splenomegaly and prominent lymph nodes may be imaged during an ultrasound examination.

In bacterial infections, the white cells increase in number (leukocytosis), with most of the increase in the neutrophils. A decrease in the total white cell count (leukopenia) is a result of a viral infection.

Thrombocytes. Thrombocytes or blood platelets are formed from giant cells in the bone marrow. They initiate a chain of events involved in blood clotting together with a plasma protein called *fibrinogen.* Thrombocytes are destroyed by the liver and have a life span of 8 days.

Blood composition. Plasma is 55% of the total blood volume and consists of about 92% water. The remaining 8% is numerous substances suspended or dissolved in this water. Hemoglobin of the red cells comprises two thirds of the blood proteins, with the remaining consisting of plasma proteins.

These include serum albumin, globulin, fibrinogen, and prothrombin.

Serum album constitutes 53% of the total plasma proteins and is produced in the liver. It is concerned with the regulation of blood volume. Globulin can be separated into alpha, beta, and gamma globulin. The latter is involved in immune reactions in the body's defense against infection. Fibrinogen is concerned with coagulation of blood. Prothrombin is produced in the liver and also participates in blood coagulation. Vitamin K is essential for prothrombin production.

THE LIVER AND THE BILIARY SYSTEM

The liver and the biliary system play a role in the digestive and circulatory systems. As food enters the small intestine, the nutrients are absorbed by the walls of the intestine. These nutrients enter the blood through the walls of the portal system. The portal venous system is a special transporting system that serves to carry nutrient-rich blood from the intestines to the liver for metabolic and storage purposes. The hepatic artery supplies nutrient-rich blood to the liver through the porta hepatis, whereas the biliary system drains the bile products from the liver and gallbladder through the porta hepatis.

The liver consists of rows of cubical cells that radiate from a central vein. On one side of these cells lie blood vessels that are slightly larger than capillaries and are called *sinusoids*. Blood from the portal vein and hepatic artery is brought into the liver to be filtered by these sinusoids, which in turn empty into the central vein. The bile ducts lie on The other side of the sinusoids. The bile pigment—old, worn-out blood cells and materials derived from phagocytosis—is removed from the blood by special hepatic cells called *Kupffer cells* and deposited into the bile ducts as **bile.**

The Kupffer cells are located in the sinusoids and are capable of ingesting bacteria and other foreign matter from the blood. These cells are part of the reticuloendothelial system of the liver and spleen.

The bilirubin arises from the hemoglobin of disintegrating red blood cells, which have been broken down by the Kupffer cells. After the bilirubin is formed, it combines with plasma albumin. The primary function of albumin is to maintain the osmotic pressure of the blood. When this serum albumin is lowered, conditions—such as liver disease, malnutrition, and chronic nephritis—should be considered.

The combination of bilirubin with plasma albumin is considered as either unconjugated or indirect bilirubin. The parenchyma cells of the liver excrete this bile pigment into the bile canaliculi. It is during this process that the bilirubin-plasma albumin chemical bond is broken and thus becomes conjugated or direct bilirubin is excreted into the biliary passages. This conjugation process occurs only in the hepatic parenchymal cells. Excreted bilirubin forced back into the bloodstream in cases of biliary obstruction results in elevated serum bilirubin of the direct type. If an abnormal amount of indirect bilirubin is found, it is probably caused by an increase in red blood cell breakdown and hemoglobin conversion.

Direct bilirubin enters the small bowel by way of the common bile duct and is acted upon by bacteria to form urobilinogen (urine) or stercobilinogen (feces). A portion of the pigment is reabsorbed and is carried to the liver by the portal circulation where it is reconverted into bilirubin. A small amount escapes into the general circulation and is excreted by the kidneys. The pooling of these bile pigments as a result of biliary obstruction or liver disease causes spillover into the tissues and general circulation, causing jaundice.

Jaundice. Jaundice is identified by its site of disruption of normal bilirubin metabolism: prehepatic, hepatic, or posthepatic. In prehepatic jaundice, there is no intrinsic disease in the liver or biliary tract. It is simply increased amounts of bilirubin being presented to the liver for excretion. There is no obstruction and therefore bilirubin is not forced back into the bloodstream; therefore, no significant increase in direct bilirubin is found. However, there are increased amounts of urobilinogen in the intestinal tract and subsequently in the feces and urine.

Hepatic jaundice is due to intrinsic hepatic parenchymal injury or disease. This may be the result of infections with hepatitis, drugs, tumor growth, or injury from toxic agents. The lack of bilirubin transfer by the hepatic cells results in a piling up of unconjugated bilirubin and increased amounts of conjugated bilirubin in the body's circulation. Clinically the patient has an enlarged and tender liver (with or without splenomegaly). Also noted are decreased appetite, nausea, and vomiting. The laboratory data would show elevation of the total serum bilirubin, positive urinary bilirubin, urinary urobilinogen as normal or elevated, and fecal urobilinogen as normal or decreased.

Posthepatic jaundice is a partial or complete blockage of the biliary tract by calculi, tumor, fibrosis, or extrinsic pressure that results in a conjugated bilirubin. Biliary calculi are classically manifested by colicky upper abdominal pain in the right upper quadrant that radiates to the shoulder. It may be accompanied by intermittent or increasing jaundice. On the other hand, tumor obstruction at the common bile duct tends to be painless, with increasing and unremitting jaundice. The total serum bilirubin is elevated, the urinary bilirubin is positive, the urinary urobilinogen is decreased or normal, and the fecal urobilinogen is decreased.

In addition to the transport and nourishment of nutrients to the body, the liver also provides energy for the body tissues. This process is done through the use of carbohydrates and their storage and release of sugars. After the nutrient sugars are absorbed by the small intestine, the sugars are transported to the liver by way of the portal system (superior mesenteric vein). The hepatic cells convert most of the sugars into glycogen (*glycogenesis*) for storage.

If the levels of available glucose in the blood are lower than normal, the liver can break down the available glycogen back into glucose (glycogenolysis) to maintain a normal blood glucose level. The most important use of glucose is the oxidation of glucose by the tissue cells. When glucose is oxidized by the tissues, carbon dioxide and water are formed and energy is released. Most tissues use glucose for their supply of energy.

The Pancreas. The pancreas plays an important role in the regulation of these carbohydrates. The secretion of insulin and glucagons from the islets of Langerhans provides for cellular control by promoting oxidation of glucose by the tissue cells. Inside the cell, released energy is stored as ATP (adenosine triphosphate) in the mitochondria. Only small molecules can enter the mitochondrial membrane; this can occur only by breaking down nutrient molecules to pyruvic acid and then to acetic acid. Once inside the mitochondria, the components combine to form citric acid. This series of reactions is called the *Krebs cycle*. The result is the release of carbon dioxide and energy. The Krebs cycle is also involved in the metabolism of fat and proteins. This is the principal energy cycle in the body.

Fat. Fat enters the system in the form of fatty acids, glycerol, phospholipids, and cholesterol. A small amount is produced in the liver, but most is synthesized in adipose tissue. The fat deposits in the body provide a concentrated source of energy and furnish about 40% of the energy used. The absorbed fats are acted upon by special cells in the liver (lipolysis) and the resultant products are channeled into the Krebs cycle for the release of energy. The production of fats (lipogenesis) results from an excess of fatty acids and glycerol, which combine to form triglyceride.

Besides being a source of energy, stored fats act as a cushion for the internal organs. The phospholipids are used in the formation of plasma membranes. Fats are completely broken down to carbon dioxide and water with a release of energy, and this process occurs predominantly in the liver. The end product of fatty acid oxidation is ketone or acetone bodies, which are secreted in the urine. In patients with uncontrolled diabetes, the sugar is not used properly and excessive fat metabolizes.

Cholesterol. Cholesterol is the last major plasma lipid to be discussed. It is found in fats and is derived from a diet of animal foods, such as egg yolks and meats. Cholesterol may serve as the substance from which various hormones are synthesized. High cholesterol levels have an adverse effect on the cardiovascular system. An increase in the cholesterol levels is seen in liver disease, whereas a decrease in serum cholesterol is found in acute infections, malnutrition, and anemias.

Amino Acids. Amino acids absorbed from the intestine are used in the production of proteins. They may be converted to fatty acids and glycogen, or they may be oxidized as an energy source. The transfer of the amino group to other substances is called transamination. Several enzymes associated with this process are useful in the diagnosis of hepatic disease. These enzymes are found in the blood: aspartate aminotransferase (AST) (formerly serum glutamic-oxaloacetic transaminase [SGOT]) and alanine aminotransferase (ALT) (formerly serum glutamic-pyruvic transaminase [SGPT]). There is an increase in these enzymes in the presence of hepatic cell necrosis caused by viral hepatitis and toxic hepatitis. However, there is not a significant increase in chronic liver disease or in obstructive jaundice.

Another important enzyme is alkaline phosphatase. This is normally found in the serum in either an acid or alkaline state. (Acid phosphatase is used primarily in assessing prostate cancer.) Alkaline phosphatase is helpful in determining disorders of the liver and biliary tract. An increase may be found in patients with biliary obstruction.

Lactic dehydrogenase (LDH) is another enzyme found in the liver. This level may be increased in conditions such as liver disease, acute leukemia, malignant lymphoma, and carcinoma. LDH is also found in cardiac tissue, and an increase may indicate myocardial infarction.

Blood Clotting. Another important function of the liver is the production of various factors involved in blood clotting. Prothrombin is converted to thrombin in the clotting process. The prothrombin content in the blood is lower in liver diseases, drug therapy, and vitamin K deficiency.

Detoxification. An essential function of the liver is detoxification. The liver breaks down a variety of toxins by way of chemical reactions.

The Gallbladder. Bile is constantly being secreted by the liver cells, beginning in the tiny channels in the liver called bile canaliculi. From these tiny channels, the canaliculi converge into right and left hepatic ducts. These ducts then drain into the right and left hepatic ducts and finally into the common bile duct. The common bile duct joins the pancreatic duct where it enters the duodenum at the ampulla of Vater. If no food is in the upper digestive tract, then most of the bile is diverted into the gallbladder. The gallbladder stores and concentrates the bile. After food is consumed, three functions occur: (1) the bile enters the small bowel because of the relaxation of the sphincter of Oddi, (2) the gallbladder contracts, and (3) increases in liver secretions occur. This process is initiated by the enzyme cholecystokinin, which is released when fats and proteins reach the duodenum. Therefore, bile plays an important role in the intestinal breakdown and absorption of fat and is the vehicle of excretion of the end product of hemoglobin breakdown.

The daily amount of bile excreted ranges from 250 to 1000 ml. Bile is made up of mostly water, bile salts, and other organic substances in small amounts, including cholesterol. Bile salts are derived from metabolism of hemoglobin. In addition to digesting and absorbing fats, bile also emulsifies fats into minute particles. This provides the pathway for the pancreatic lipase to act upon the fats to further aid in digestion. At the completion of their digestive function, the bile salts are returned via the portal system to the liver for reuse. Gallstones may form as the result of excessive cholesterol and bile salt deposits.

Obstruction of a bile duct prevents flow of bile, and the increases in liver secretions cause a backflow of bile in the liver, with a spillover into the blood and tissue that results in jaundice. As a result of obstruction, excessive excretion of fat is found in the feces because of a lack of digestion and absorption in the intestine secondary to the absence of bile salts.

Laboratory Tests for Hepatic and Biliary Function

No single laboratory test can fully evaluate liver function in a healthy or diseased state. The most commonly used tests to evaluate hepatic and biliary function are presented in Table 2-4. The normal lab values should be obtained from your respective laboratory.

The Pancreas

Endocrine Function. The pancreas functions as an exocrine and an endocrine gland. Endocrine function is carried out by small areas of specialized tissue called the *islets of Langerhans,* which are scattered throughout the gland. Two important hormones secreted are insulin and glucagon. Insulin is responsible for causing an increase in the rate of glucose metabolism.

Glucose does not readily pass through the cell pores without the help of some transport mechanism provided by insulin. In the absence of insulin, the rate of glucose transport is about one fourth the normal value. Conversely, an excess of insulin multiplies the normal rate. Insulin is also responsible for regulation of blood glucose levels.

In the presence of insulin, glucose is transported to the tissue cells so fast that the blood glucose level may drop. Diabetes mellitus is a disease caused by inadequate secretion of insulin by the pancreas. This results in the cells' inability to use glucose and an increase in the blood sugar level (hyperglycemia).

Glucagon mobilizes glucose from the liver, which causes an increase in blood glucose concentration. When the blood glucose concentration falls, the pancreas secretes large quantities of glucagons to compensate.

Exocrine Function. The pancreas is the most active and versatile of the digestive organs. In the absence of other digestive secretions, its enzymes alone are capable of almost completing total digestion. Pancreatic juice consists of three basic groups of enzymes: carbohydrate, fat, and trypsin.

The carbohydrate enzyme is pancreatic amylase, which acts upon starch and glycogen and produces the sugar maltose. The fat enzyme is pancreatic lipase and is capable of breaking down fats to monoglycerides and fatty acids. Trypsin ultimately digests proteins and peptides partially digested in the stomach. The end products of trypsin digestion are amino acids and polypeptides.

The digestion of food is incomplete without the action of the pancreatic enzymes. Lack of these enzymes may be due to obstruction in the pancreatic duct or to diseases that impair the ability of the pancreas to produce these enzymes in proper amounts. If inadequate digestion and absorption do not occur, amounts of carbohydrates increase, and protein is found in the feces.

Pancreatic juice also contains a high concentration of sodium bicarbonate, which is responsible for neutralization of gastric acid and a decrease in chloride concentration. The release of pancreatic juice is stimulated by secretin and pancreozymin (similar to cholecystokinin in the gallbladder). These hormones increase the volume of pancreatic secretion and increase the amount of bicarbonate in secretion. They also increase sodium levels, but decrease chloride and potassium. Incompletely digested proteins and peptides are found as increased amounts of total fecal nitrogen.

TABLE 2-4 LABORATORY TESTS FOR HEPATIC AND BILIARY FUNCTION

Laboratory Test	Description and Possible Indications
Bilirubin	Bilirubin is derived from the breakdown of hemoglobin in red blood cells and is excreted by the liver in the bile. When destruction of red cells increases greatly or when the liver is unable to excrete the normal amounts of bilirubin produced, the concentration in the serum rises. If it rises too high, jaundice may appear. The bilirubin test will spot the increase early before the onset of jaundice. Intrahepatic and extrahepatic obstruction may be determined by knowing the levels of direct and indirect bilirubin. This may be seen by an increase in conjugated or direct bilirubin. An increase in unconjugated or indirect bilirubin is indicative of an increase in red blood cell destruction or hemolysis.
Cholesterol	Cholesterol is found in the blood and in all cells. Hepatic disease may alter its metabolism. Total cholesterol is normal or decreased in hepatitis or cirrhosis, but increased in primary biliary cirrhosis and extrabiliary obstruction.
Glucose	This test may indicate the liver's ability to metabolize glucose. Chronic liver disease and severe diabetes will cause an increase in the blood glucose level. There may be a decrease in glucose with tumors of the islets of Langerhans.
Alkaline phosphatase	This is found in the serum and the value rises in disorders of the liver and biliary tract when excretion is impaired (i.e., obstruction). Alkaline phosphatase levels are elevated typically in obstructive jaundice, biliary cirrhosis, acute hepatitis, and granulomatous liver disease.
Aspartate aminotransferase (AST) (formerly SGOT)	This enzyme is increased in the presence of liver cell necrosis secondary to viral hepatitis, toxic hepatitis, and other acute forms. There is usually no significant increase in chronic liver disease, such as cirrhosis or obstructive jaundice.
Alanine aminotransferase (ALT) (formerly SGPT)	This enzyme rises higher than AST in cases of hepatitis. It falls slowly and reaches normal levels in 2 to 3 months.
Prothrombin time	Prothrombin is converted to thrombin in the clotting process. This is made possible by the action of vitamin K that is absorbed in the intestine and stored in the liver.
Urinary bile and bilirubin	There may be spillover into the blood in obstructive liver disease or where there is an excess of red blood cell destruction. Bile pigments are found in the urine when there is obstruction of the biliary tract. Bilirubin is found alone when there is excessive breakdown of red blood cells.
Urinary urobilinogen	This test may be used to differentiate between complete and incomplete obstruction of the biliary tract. Urobilinogen is a product of hemoglobin breakdown and may be found in hemolytic diseases, liver damage, and severe infections. In cases of complete obstructive jaundice, there is usually no excess of urobilinogen in the urine.
Fecal urobilinogen	Considerable amounts of urobilinogen are found in the feces, but an increase or decrease in normal amounts may indicate hepatic digestive abnormalities. In completed obstruction of the biliary tree, values are decreased, whereas an increase in fecal urobilinogen may suggest an increase in hemolysis.

TABLE 2-5 LABORATORY TESTS FOR PANCREATIC FUNCTION

Laboratory Test	Description and Possible Indications
Serum amylase	An increase in serum amylase levels may be a result of pancreatic disease, which causes the digestive enzymes to escape into the surrounding tissue and results in necrosis and severe pain with inflammation. Example: acute pancreatitis and obstruction, acute cholecystitis—high serum amylase
Serum lipase	In diseases such as acute pancreatitis and carcinoma of the pancreas, both amylase and lipase rise at the same rate, but lipase persists for a longer time.
Glucose tolerance test (GTT)	Large amounts of glucose are administered and blood sugar levels are monitored. The glucose should be metabolized in less than 3 hours, otherwise diabetes is suspected. If slow to return to normal, liver disease may also be involved.
Urinary amylase	Amylase in the serum is excreted in the urine and can be measured. Will remain higher in abnormal disease states than the serum amylase.
Ketone bodies	Ketone bodies are excreted in the urine as a result of faulty metabolism. Sugar is not used properly and excessive fat metabolizes. The fats produce ketone bodies and acetone, and when these levels rise there is a spillover into the urine. This is usually due to improperly controlled or uncontrolled diabetes.

LABORATORY TESTS FOR PANCREATIC FUNCTION

The most commonly used tests to evaluate pancreatic function are presented in Table 2-5.

THE KIDNEYS

The renal arteries carry approximately 25% of the cardiac output to the kidneys. This ensures the maintenance of an increased level of blood pressure as it reaches the cortical portion of the kidneys via the interlobar and arcuate arteries. These arteries branch into smaller afferent arterioles, which lead to a complex network of capillaries, called the glomeruli. From this point, the capillaries branch into the efferent arterioles to the peritubular capillaries and course through the venules to the returning blood supply of the renal veins and inferior vena cava.

The vascular anatomy is critical in supplying the vital nutrients for the important functional unit of the kidney, the *nephron.* There are at least 1 million nephrons in each normal adult kidney. Within the nephron complex, a diffusion process takes place to maintain continual homeostasis of blood plasma and other nutrient components for the body.

The two major parts of the nephron are the glomerulus and the renal tubules. These structures have a direct role in the production of urine by means of three processes: filtration, reabsorption, and secretion.

1. Glomerular filtration is the first step of urine formation. This filtration process takes place through the glomerular capsular membrane, which surrounds the glomerulus. The glomerular filtration is directly affected by the blood pressure of the glomerular arterial capillaries, which forces an essentially protein-free filtrate consisting mainly of blood plasma through the permeable glomerular capsular membrane, *Bowman's capsule.*

2. *Bowman's capsule* is the basis for determining the filtration permeability factor and the glomerular filtration rate.

3. Most of the filtered volume is reabsorbed back into the renal tubules along with many vital components of the filtrate, such as glucose, sodium, potassium, chlorides, and other essential nutrients in extracellular fluid.

4. As the remaining filtrate continues through the renal tubules, more solutes are added by secretions from the tubular epithelial cells.

5. Some of these cells are excreted with the remaining constituents of urine.

LABORATORY TESTS FOR THE KIDNEY

The detection of urinary tract disorders is usually performed through the analysis of urine (urinalysis). Urine samples may be collected randomly or over a prolonged period of time. Table 2-6 lists the most common laboratory tests for urinary disease.

TABLE 2-6 LABORATORY TESTS FOR URINARY DISEASE

Laboratory Test	Description and Possible Indications
Urine pH	• pH refers to the strength of the urine as a partly acidic or alkaline solution. • Abundance of hydrogen ions in a solution is called pH. When urine has more hydrogen ions than hydroxyl ions, it is acidic. It is alkaline when it has more hydroxyl ions. • Important in diagnosing and managing bacteriuria and renal calculi. Renal calculi are somewhat dependent on pH of urine. • Alkaline urine associated with renal tubular acidosis, chronic renal failure, and other urinary tract disorders.
Specific gravity	• Measurement of kidney's ability to concentrate urine. • The urine concentration factor is dependent upon the amount of dissolved waste products within it. • Excessive intake of fluids or decrease in perspiration may cause large output of urine and decrease in specific gravity. (Also low in renal failure, glomerular nephritis, and pyelonephritis.) • Low fluid intake, excessive perspiration, or diarrhea will cause the output of urine to be low and the specific gravity to increase. (May also be high in nephrosis.)
Blood (hematuria)	• Appearance of blood cell casts in the urine. • Can be associated with early renal disease.
Protein (albuminuria)	• Found when glomerular damage is apparent—albumin and other plasma proteins may be filtered in excess—allows overflow to enter the urine which lowers the blood serum albumin concentration. • Found with benign and malignant neoplasms, nephritis, calculi, chronic infection, and pyelonephritis.
Red cell casts	• Occurs when red blood cells in lumen of nephron tubule become trapped and elongated gelled proteins. • Indicates bleeding has occurred into the nephrons. • Abundance of casts may indicate renal trauma, calculi, or pyelonephritis.
White cells and white cell casts	• Leukocytes may be present whenever there is inflammation, infection, or tissue necrosis originating from anywhere within the genitourinary tract.
Creatinine clearance	• Specific measurements of creatinine concentrations in urine and blood serum are considered an accurate index for determining the glomerular filtration rate (GFR). • A decreased urinary creatinine clearance indicates renal dysfunction because it prevents the normal excretion of creatinine.
Hematocrit	• Refers to the relative ratio of plasma to packed cell volume in the blood. • Decrease in hematocrit will occur with acute hemorrhagic process secondary to disease or blunt trauma.
Hemoglobin	• Presence of hemoglobin in urine occurs whenever there is extensive damage or destruction of functioning erythrocytes. • Hemoglobinuria can cause acute renal failure.
Blood urea nitrogen (BUN)	• Concentration of urea nitrogen in blood—end product of cellular metabolism. • Urea is formed in the liver and carried to the kidneys through the blood to be excreted in the urine. • Impairment of renal function and increased protein catabolism will result in BUN elevation in relation to the degree of renal impairment and rate of urea nitrogen excreted by the kidneys.
Serum creatinine	• Renal dysfunction will result in elevation of serum creatinine. • More sensitive than BUN in determining renal impairment.

SELECTED BIBILIOGRAPHY

Diagnostic Tests: *A prescriber's guide to test selection and interpretation*, Philadelphia, 2004, Lippincott Williams & Wilkins.

McMinn RM, Gaddum-Rosse P, Hutchings RT and others: *McMinn's functional & clinical anatomy*, St Louis, 1995, Mosby.

Skill Masters: *3-minute assessment*, Philadelphia, 2002, Lippincott Williams & Wilkins.

PART II

Abdomen

CHAPTER 3

Anatomic and Physiologic Relationships within the Abdominal Cavity

Sandra L. Hagen-Ansert

OBJECTIVES

- Learn the key medical terminology
- Describe the organization of the body
- Name the body systems and their functions
- Know the anatomic directions in the body
- Describe the abdominal quadrants of the body
- List the organs located in each major body cavity
- Name the membranes associated with the thoracic and abdominopelvic cavities
- Name the types of abdominal muscles in the body
- Describe the potential spaces in the body
- Properly use the sonographic terms that describe relative positions, body sections, and body regions

FROM ATOM TO ORGANISM
METABOLISM
HOMEOSTASIS

BODY SYSTEMS

ANATOMIC DIRECTIONS

PLANES OR BODY SECTIONS

ABDOMINAL QUADRANTS AND REGIONS

BODY CAVITIES

THE ABDOMINAL CAVITY
ABDOMINAL VISCERA
OTHER ABDOMINAL STRUCTURES
ABDOMINAL MUSCLES

THE PELVIC CAVITY
FALSE PELVIS
TRUE PELVIS

ABDOMINOPELVIC MEMBRANES AND LIGAMENTS
PERITONEUM
MESENTERY
OMENTUM
GREATER AND LESSER SAC
EPIPLOIC FORAMEN
LIGAMENT

POTENTIAL SPACES IN THE BODY
SUBPHRENIC SPACES
PERITONEAL RECESSES
PARACOLIC GUTTERS
INGUINAL CANAL
ABDOMINAL HERNIAS

THE RETROPERITONEUM
RETROPERITONEAL SPACES

ANATOMIC TERMS

PREFIXES AND SUFFIXES

KEY TERMS

anterior pararenal space – located between the anterior surface of the renal fascia and the posterior area of the peritoneum

ascites – accumulation of fluid

diaphragm – broad muscle that separates the thoracic and abdominopelvic cavities and forms the floor of the thoracic cavity

epiploic foramen – opening to the lesser sac

falciform ligament – attaches the liver to the anterior abdominal wall and undersurface of the diaphragm

gastrosplenic ligament – ligament between the stomach and the spleen; helps support stomach and spleen

greater omentum – attaches to the greater curvature of the stomach

greater sac – primary compartment of the peritoneal cavity; extends across the anterior abdomen from the diaphragm to the pelvis

homeostasis – maintenance of normal body physiology

inguinal ligament – ligament between the anterior superior iliac spine and the pubic tubercle

intertubercular plane – lowest horizontal line joins the tubercles on the iliac crests

lateral arcuate ligament – thickened upper margin of the fascia covering the anterior surface of the quadratus lumborum muscle

left crus of the diaphragm – arises from the sides of the bodies of the first two lumbar vertebrae

lesser omentum – attaches to the lesser curvature of the stomach

lesser sac – peritoneal pouch located behind the lesser omentum and stomach

lienorenal ligament – ligament between the spleen and kidney

ligamentum teres – termination of the falciform ligament; seen in the left lobe of the liver

linea alba – fibrous band of tissue that stretches from the xiphoid to the symphysis pubis

linea semilunaris – extends from the ninth costal cartilage to the pubic tubercle

medial arcuate ligament – thickened upper margin of the fascia covering the anterior surface of the psoas muscle

median arcuate ligament – connects the medial borders of the two crura as they cross anterior to the aorta

mesothelium – single layer of cells that forms the peritoneum

metabolism – physical and chemical changes that occur within the body

Morison's pouch – right posterior subphrenic space lies between the right lobe of the liver, anterior to the kidney

parietal peritoneum – layer of the peritoneum that lines the abdominal wall

pelvic cavity – lower portion of the abdominopelvic cavity that contains part of the large intestine, the rectum, urinary bladder, and reproductive organs

perirenal space – located directly around the kidney; completely enclosed by renal fascia

peritoneal cavity – potential space between the parietal and visceral peritoneal layers

peritoneal recess – slitlike spaces near the liver; potential space for fluid to accumulate

posterior pararenal space – found between the posterior renal fascia and the muscles of the posterior abdominal wall

rectouterine space – posterior pouch between the uterus and rectum

rectus abdominis muscle – muscle of the anterior abdominal wall

right crus of the diaphragm – arises from the sides of the bodies of the first three lumbar vertebrae

scrotal cavity – in the male, a small outpocket of the pelvis cavity containing the testes

subcostal plane – upper horizontal line joins the lowest point of the costal margin on each side of the body

superficial inguinal ring – triangular opening in the external oblique aponeurosis

transpyloric plane – horizontal plane that passes through the pylorus, the duodenal junction, the neck of the pancreas, and the hilum of the kidneys

uterovesical space – anterior pouch between the uterus and bladder

viscera – the internal organs

visceral peritoneum – layer of peritoneum that covers the abdominal organs

vital signs – medical measurements to ascertain how the body is functioning

————————

To understand the complexity of the human body and how the parts work together to function as a whole is to gain an appreciation of anatomy and physiology. The science of body structure (anatomy) and the study of body function (physiology) are intricately related, for each structure of the human body system carries out a specific function. There are many forms of anatomy and physiology: *gross anatomy* studies the body by dissection of tissues; *histology* studies parts of the tissues under the microscope; *embryology* studies the development before birth; and *pathology* is the study of the disease process.

FROM ATOM TO ORGANISM

A review of the composition of the human body begins with an understanding that all materials consist of chemicals. The basic units of all matter are the tiny invisible particles called atoms. An atom is the smallest amount of a chemical element that retains the characteristic properties of that element. Atoms can combine chemically to form the larger particles called *molecules*. For example, two atoms of hydrogen combine with one atom of oxygen to produce a molecule of water.

The next level of complexity in the human body is a microscopic unit called a *cell*. Although they share common traits, cells can vary in size, shape, and specialized function. In the human body, atoms and molecules associate in specific ways to form cells, and there are trillions of different types of cells within the body. All cells have specialized tiny parts called *organelles*, which carry on specific activities. These organelles consist of aggregates of large molecules, including those of such substances as proteins, carbohydrates, lipids, and nucleic acids. One organelle, the *nucleus*, serves as the information and control center of the cell.

Cells that are organized into layers or masses that have common functions are known as *tissue*. The four primary types of tissue in the body are muscle, nervous, connective, and epithelial tissues.

Groups of different tissue combine together to form *organs*—complex structures with specialized functions, such as the liver, pancreas, or uterus. One organ may have more than one type of tissue (i.e., the heart is mainly muscle tissue, but it is also covered by epithelial tissue and contains connective and nervous tissue).

A coordinated group of organs are arranged into organ or *body systems*. For example, the digestive system consists of the mouth, esophagus, stomach, intestines, liver, gallbladder, and pancreas. Body systems make up the total part or *organism* that is the human body.

METABOLISM

All of the physical and chemical changes that occur within the body are referred to as **metabolism.** The metabolic process is essential to digestion, growth and repair of the body, and conversion of food energy into forms useful to the body. Other metabolic processes maintain the routine operations of the nerves, muscles, and other body parts.

HOMEOSTASIS

The anatomic structure and functions of all body parts are directed toward maintaining the life of the organism. To sustain life, the organisms must have the proper quantity and quality of water, food, oxygen, heat, and pressure. Maintenance of life depends on the stability of these factors. **Homeostasis** is the ability to maintain a steady and stable internal environment. Stressful stimuli, *stressors*, disrupt homeostasis.

Vital signs are medical measurements used to ascertain how the body is functioning. These vital signs include measuring body temperature and blood pressure and observing rates and types of pulse and breathing movements. There is a close relationship between these signs and the homeostasis of the body, as vital signs are the results of metabolic activities. Death is the absence of such signs.

BODY SYSTEMS

A body system consists of a group of tissues and organs that work together to perform specific functions. Each system contributes to the dynamic, organized, and carefully balanced state of the body. The sonographer should be familiar with the integumentary, skeletal, muscular, and nervous systems of the body. The remaining systems—endocrine, digestive, circulatory, lymphatic, urinary, and reproductive—should be thoroughly understood by the sonographer. Table 3-1 lists the components and functions of the human body systems.

ANATOMIC DIRECTIONS

The anatomic position assumes that the body is standing erect, the eyes are looking forward, arms are at the sides with the palms and toes directed forward. Refer to Figure 3-1 for the four anatomic directions of the body discussed below.

1. **Superior/inferior.** The top of the head is the most superior point of the body. The inferior point of the body is the

TABLE 3-1 SYSTEMS IN THE HUMAN BODY

System	Components	Functions
Integumentary	Skin, hair, nails, sweat glands	Covers and protects tissues, regulates body temperature, and supports sensory receptors.
Skeletal	Bones, cartilage, joints, ligaments	Supports the body, provides framework, protects soft tissues, provides attachments for muscles, produces blood cells, and stores inorganic salts; provides calcium storage.
Muscular	Skeletal, cardiac, smooth muscle	Moves parts of skeleton, provides locomotion; pumps blood; aids movement of internal materials; and produces body heat.
Nervous	Nerves and sense organs, brain, and spinal cord	Receives stimuli from external and internal environment, conducts impulses, integrates activities of other systems.
Endocrine	Pituitary, adrenal, thyroid, pancreas, parathyroid, ovaries, testes, pineal, and thymus gland	Regulates body chemistry and many body functions.
Lymphatic	Lymph nodes	Returns the tissue fluid to the blood, carries specific absorbed food molecules, and defends the body against infection.
Circulatory	Heart, blood vessels, blood; lymph and lymph structures	Moves the blood through the vessels and transports substances throughout the body.
Respiratory	Lungs, bronchi, and air passageways	Exchanges gases between blood and external environment.
Digestive	Mouth, tongue, teeth, salivary glands, pharynx, esophagus, stomach, liver, gallbladder, pancreas, and small and large intestines	The primary function of the digestive system is to receive, break down, and absorb food and eliminate unabsorbed material from the body.
Urinary	Kidney, bladder, ureters	Excretes waste from the blood, maintains water and electrolyte balance, and stores and transports urine.
Reproductive	Testes, scrotum, spermatic cord, vas deferens, ejaculatory duct, penis, epididymis, prostate, uterus, ovaries, fallopian tubes, vagina, breast	Reproduction; provides for continuation of the species.

Figure 3-1   A, Anterior view of the body in the anatomic position. Note the directions and body planes. **B,** Lateral view of the body.

bottom of the feet. All anatomic structures are designated relative to these two terms. The liver is considered to be superior to the bladder because the liver is closer to the head. The gallbladder is inferior to the diaphragm because it is closer to the feet. Other terms that are interchanged with superior are *cephalic* and *cranial* (towards the head). Caudal (towards the tail) is sometimes used instead of inferior.

2. **Anterior/posterior.** The front (belly) surface of the body is anterior, or *ventral.* The back surface of the body is posterior, or *dorsal.* This concept is very important to sonographers and their understanding of sectional anatomy. If the patient is lying supine (face up), the aorta would be anterior to the vertebral column. The right kidney would be posterior to the head of the pancreas.

3. **Medial/lateral.** The body axis is an imaginary line from the center of the top of the head to the groin. *Medial* is described as the superior-inferior body axis as it goes right through the midline of the body. Structures are said to be medial if they are closer to the midline of the body than to another structure (i.e., the hepatic artery is medial to the common duct). The structure is *lateral* if it is towards the side of the body. The adnexa are lateral to the uterus.

4. **Proximal/distal.** When a structure is closer to the body midline or point of attachment to the trunk, it is described as *proximal* (i.e., the hepatic duct is proximal to the common bile duct). *Distal* means farther from the midline or point of attachment to the trunk (i.e., the sphincter of Oddi is distal to the common bile duct).

Additionally, structures are identified as being superficial or deep. Structures located toward the surface of the body are *superficial.* The rectus abdominus muscles are superficial to the transverse abdominis muscles. Structures located farther inward (away from the body surface) are *deep.*

PLANES OR BODY SECTIONS

The sonographer observes the body in three different planes: transverse, sagittal, and coronal (see Figure 3-1).

1. **Transverse.** The transverse plane is horizontal to the body. This plane divides the body or any of its parts into upper and lower portions.
2. **Sagittal.** The sagittal plane is a lengthwise plane running from front to back. It divides the body or any of its parts

into right and left sides, or two equal halves. This is also known as the midsagittal plane.

3. **Coronal.** The coronal plane is a lengthwise plane running from side to side, dividing the body into anterior and posterior portions.

ABDOMINAL QUADRANTS AND REGIONS

To identify specific abdominal structures or refer to an area of pain, the abdomen may be divided into four quadrants or nine abdominal regions.

The abdominopelvic cavity is divided into four quadrants that include the right upper quadrant (RUQ), left upper quadrant (LUQ), right lower quadrant (RLQ), and left lower quadrant (LLQ). The quadrant is determined by a midsagittal and a transverse plane that pass through the umbilicus.

The abdomen is commonly divided into nine regions by two vertical and two horizontal lines. The surface landmarks of the anterior abdominal wall help to define the specific abdominal regions (Figure 3-2). Each vertical line passes through the midinguinal point (i.e., the point that lies on the inguinal ligament halfway between the pubic symphysis and anterior superior iliac spine. The upper horizontal line, referred to as the **subcostal plane**, joins the lowest point of the costal margin on each side of the body. The lowest horizontal line, the **intertubercular plane**, joins the tubercles on the iliac crests. The **transpyloric plane** is a horizontal plane that passes through the pylorus, the duodenal junction, the neck of the pancreas, and the hilum of the kidneys.

The nine abdominal regions include the following: (1) upper abdomen/right hypochondrium, (2) epigastrium, (3) left hypochondrium, (4) middle abdomen/right lumbar, (5) umbilical, (6) left lumbar, (7) lower abdomen/right iliac fossa, (8) hypogastrium, and (9) left iliac fossa (Figure 3-3).

Table 3-2 provides a list of additional terms that the sonographer is likely to encounter when identifying specific body regions or structures.

TABLE 3-2	**TERMS FOR COMMON BODY REGIONS AND STRUCTURES**
Term	Body Region or Structure
Abdominal	Portion of trunk below the diaphragm
Axillary	Area of armpit
Brachial	Arm
Celiac	Abdomen
Cervical	Neck region
Costal	Ribs
Femoral	Thigh: the part of the lower extremity between the hip and the knee
Groin/inguinal	Depressed region between the abdomen and the thigh
Leg	Lower extremity, especially from the knee to the foot
Lumbar	Loin; the region of the lower back and side, between the lowest rib and the pelvis
Mammary	Breasts
Pelvic	Pelvis; the bony ring that girdles the lower portion of the trunk
Perineal	Region between the anus and the pubic arch; includes the region of the external reproductive structures
Popliteal	Area behind the knee
Thoracic	Chest; the part of the trunk below the neck and above the diaphragm

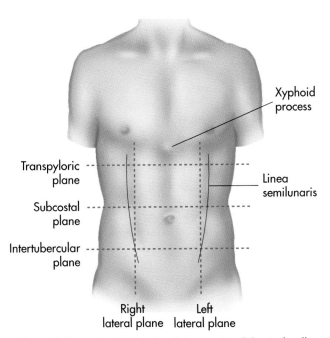

Figure 3-2   Surface landmarks of the anterior abdominal wall.

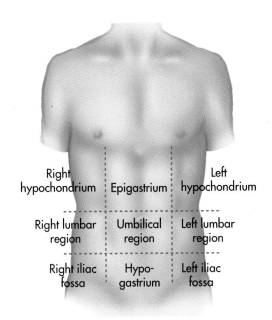

Figure 3-3   Regions of the abdominal wall.

BODY CAVITIES

There are many cavities within the human body. These body cavities contain the internal organs, or **viscera**. The two principal body cavities are the dorsal cavity and the ventral cavity (Figure 3-4). The bony dorsal cavity may be subdivided into the *cranial cavity*, which holds the brain, and the *vertebral or spinal canal*, which contains the spinal cord. The ventral cavity is located near the anterior body surface and is subdivided into the *thoracic cavity* and the *abdominal cavity*.

The thoracic and abdominopelvic cavities are separated by a broad muscle called the **diaphragm**. The diaphragm forms the floor of the thoracic cavity. Divisions of the thoracic cavity are the pleural sacs, each containing a lung, with the mediastinum between them. Within the mediastinum lie the heart, thymus gland, and part of the esophagus and trachea. The heart is surrounded by another cavity called the pericardial sac.

THE ABDOMINAL CAVITY

The abdominal cavity is the upper portion of the abdominopelvic cavity, excluding the retroperitoneum and the pelvis. It is bounded superiorly by the diaphragm; anteriorly by the abdominal wall muscles; posteriorly by the vertebral column, ribs, and iliac fossa; and inferiorly by the pelvis. The abdominal cavity contains the stomach, small intestine, much of the large intestine, liver, pancreas, gallbladder, spleen, kidneys, and ureters.

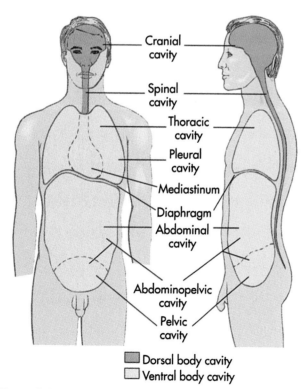

Dorsal body cavity
Ventral body cavity

Figure 3-4   Body cavities. Location and divisions of the dorsal and ventral body cavities as viewed from anterior and lateral. (From Thibodeau GA, Patton KT: *The human body in health and disease*, ed 5, St Louis, 2005, Mosby.)

ABDOMINAL VISCERA

The visceral organs within the abdominal cavity include the liver, gallbladder, spleen, pancreas, kidneys, stomach, small intestine, and part of the large intestine (Figure 3-5). Throughout the ultrasound examination, the sonographer will observe respiratory and positional variations in the abdominal viscera as they occur from patient to patient.

Liver.   The liver lies posterior to the lower ribs, with the majority of the right lobe in the right hypochondrium and epigastrium; the left lobe lies in the epigastrium/left hypochondrium.

Gallbladder.   The fundus of the gallbladder usually lies opposite the tip of the right ninth costal cartilage.

Spleen.   The spleen lies in the left hypochondrium under cover of the ninth, tenth, and eleventh ribs. Its long axis corresponds to the tenth rib, and in adults it usually does not project forward of the midaxillary line.

Pancreas.   The pancreas lies in the epigastrium. The head usually lies below and to the right, the neck lies on the transpyloric plane, and the body and tail lie above and to the left.

Kidneys.   The right kidney lies slightly lower than the left. Each kidney moves about 1 inch in a vertical direction during full respiratory movement of the diaphragm. The hilus of the kidney lies on the transpyloric plane, about three fingers width from the midline.

Aorta and Inferior Vena Cava.   The aorta lies anterior to the spine, slightly to the left of the midline in the abdomen. It bifurcates into the right and left common iliac arteries opposite the fourth lumbar vertebra on the intercristal plane. The inferior vena cava is formed by the confluence of the right and left common iliac veins. The inferior vena cava lies to the right of the spine.

Stomach.   The stomach lies in the transpyloric plane between the esophagus and the small intestine.

Small Intestine.   This tubular organ extends from the pyloric sphincter to the beginning of the large intestine.

Large Intestine.   The large intestine extends from the small intestine to the anal canal.

Bladder and Uterus.   The bladder and uterus lie in the lower pelvis in the hypogastric plane.

OTHER ABDOMINAL STRUCTURES

Diaphragm.   The diaphragm is a dome-shaped muscle that separates the thorax from the abdominal cavity (Figures 3-4 and 3-6). Its muscular component arises from the margins of the thoracic outlet. The **right crus of the diaphragm** arises from the sides of the bodies of the first three lumbar vertebrae;

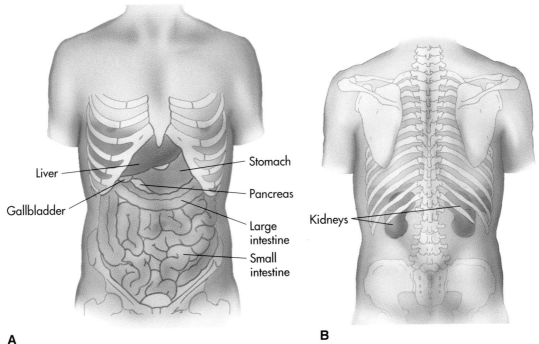

Liver — Stomach

Gallbladder — Pancreas

Large intestine

Small intestine

Kidneys

A

B

Figure 3-5   **A,** Basic abdominal landmarks and viscera viewed from anterior. **B,** Landmarks of the posterior torso.

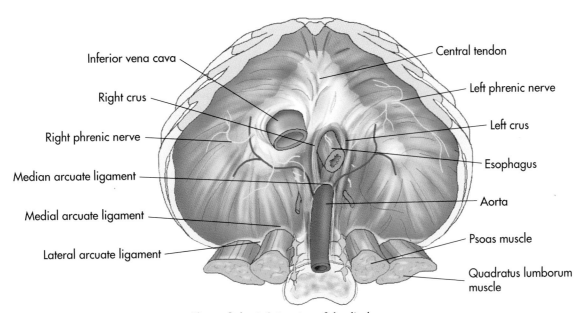

Inferior vena cava — Central tendon

Right crus — Left phrenic nerve

Right phrenic nerve — Left crus

Median arcuate ligament — Esophagus

Medial arcuate ligament — Aorta

Lateral arcuate ligament — Psoas muscle

Quadratus lumborum muscle

Figure 3-6   Inferior view of the diaphragm.

the **left crus of the diaphragm** arises from the sides of the bodies of the first two lumbar vertebrae.

Lateral to the crura, the diaphragm arises from the medial and lateral arcuate ligaments. The **medial arcuate ligament** is the thickened upper margin of the fascia covering the anterior surface of the psoas muscle. It extends from the side of the body of the second lumbar vertebra to the tip of the transverse process of the first lumbar vertebra. The medial arcuate ligament connects the medial borders of the two crura as they cross anterior to the aorta.

The **lateral arcuate ligament** is the thickened upper margin of the fascia covering the anterior surface of the quadratus lumborum muscle. It extends from the tip of the transverse process of the first lumbar vertebra to the lower border of the twelfth rib.

The diaphragm inserts into a central tendon. The superior surface of the tendon is partially fused with the inferior surface of the fibrous pericardium. Fibers of the right crus surround the esophagus to act as a sphincter to prevent regurgitation of the gastric contents into the thoracic part of the esophagus.

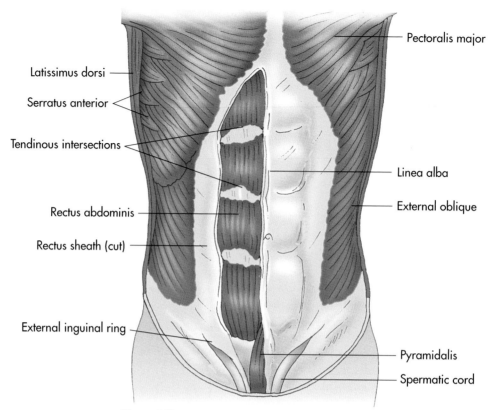

Figure 3-7 Anterior view of the abdominal muscles.

Abdominal Wall. Superiorly the abdominal wall is formed by the diaphragm. Inferiorly it is continuous with the pelvic cavity through the pelvic inlet. Anteriorly the wall is formed above by the lower part of the thoracic cage and below by several layers of muscles: the rectus abdominis, external oblique, internal oblique, and transversus abdominis (Figure 3-7). The **linea alba** is a fibrous band that stretches from the xiphoid to the symphysis pubis. It is wider at its superior end and forms a central anterior attachment for the muscle layers of the abdomen. It is formed by the interlacing of fibers of the aponeuroses of the right and left oblique and transversus abdominis muscles.

Posteriorly the abdominal wall is formed in the midline by five lumbar vertebrae and their disks (Figure 3-8). Posterolaterally, it is formed by the twelfth ribs, upper part of the bony pelvis, psoas muscles, quadratus lumborum muscles, and the aponeuroses of origin of the transversus abdominis muscles.

Laterally the wall is formed above by the lower part of the thoracic wall, including the lungs and pleura, and below by the external and internal oblique muscles and the transversus abdominis muscles.

ABDOMINAL MUSCLES

External Oblique Muscle. The external oblique muscle arises from the lower eight ribs and fans out to be inserted into the xiphoid process, the linea alba, the pubic crest, the pubic tubercle, and the anterior half of the iliac crest (Figure 3-9, A).

The **superficial inguinal ring** is a triangular opening in the external oblique aponeurosis and lies superior and medial to the pubic tubercle. The spermatic cord or the round ligament of the uterus passes through this opening.

The **inguinal ligament** is formed between the anterior superior iliac spine and the pubic tubercle, where the lower border of the aponeurosis is folded backward on itself. The lateral part of the posterior edge of the inguinal ligament gives origin to part of the internal oblique and transverse abdominal muscles.

Internal Oblique Muscle. The internal oblique muscle lies very deep to the external oblique muscle (Figure 3-9, B). The majority of its fibers are aligned at right angles to the external oblique muscle. It arises from the lumbar fascia, the anterior two thirds of the iliac crest, and the lateral two thirds of the inguinal ligament. The muscle inserts into the lower borders of the ribs and their costal cartilages, the xiphoid process, the linear alba, and the pubic symphysis. The internal oblique has a lower free border that arches over the spermatic cord or the round ligament of the uterus and then descends behind it to be attached to the pubic crest and the pectineal line. The lowest tendinous fibers are joined by similar fibers from the transversus abdominis to form the conjoint tendon.

Transversus Muscle. The transversus muscle lies deep to the internal oblique muscle, and its fibers run horizontally

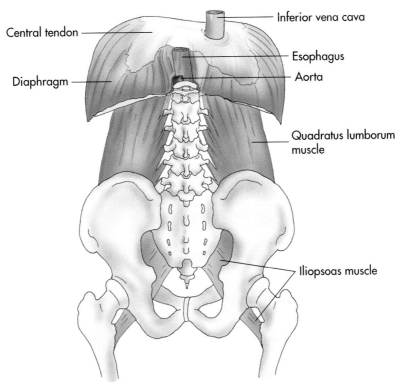

Figure 3-8　Posterior view of the diaphragm and abdominal muscles.

forward (Figure 3-9, *C*). The muscle arises from the deep surface of the lower six costal cartilages (interlacing with the diaphragm), the lumbar fascia, the anterior two thirds of the iliac crest, and the lateral third of the inguinal ligament. It inserts into the xiphoid process, the linear alba, and the pubic symphysis.

Rectus Sheath. The **rectus abdominis muscle** is a sheath formed by the aponeuroses of the muscles of the lateral group (Figure 3-10). The rectus muscle arises from the front of the symphysis pubis and from the pubic crest. It inserts into the fifth, sixth, and seventh costal cartilages and the xiphoid process. On contraction, the lateral margin forms a palpable curved surface, termed the **linea semilunaris,** which extends from the ninth costal cartilage to the pubic tubercle. The anterior surface of the rectus muscle is crossed by three tendinous intersections and is firmly attached to the anterior wall of the rectus sheath.

Linea Alba. The linea alba is a fibrous band stretching from the xiphoid to the symphysis pubis (see Figure 3-7). It is wider above than below and forms a central anterior attachment for the muscle layers of the abdomen. It is formed by the interlacing of the aponeuroses of the right and left oblique muscles and transversus abdominis muscles.

Back Muscles. The deep muscles of the back help to stabilize the vertebral column. They also influence the posture and curvature of the spine. The muscles have the ability to

extend, flex laterally, and rotate all or part of the vertebral column.

THE PELVIC CAVITY

The lower portion of the abdominopelvic cavity is the **pelvic cavity** (see Figure 3-4). The pelvis is divided into a pelvis major (*false pelvis*) and pelvis minor (*true pelvis*). The pelvis major is part of the abdominal cavity proper and lies between the iliac fossae, superior to the pelvic brim. The pelvis minor (which actually contains the pelvic cavity) is found inferior to the brim of the pelvis. The cavity of the pelvis minor is continuous at the pelvic brim with the cavity of the pelvis major.

The pelvic cavity contains several pelvic organs: part of the large intestine, the rectum, urinary bladder, and reproductive organs. In the female, the peritoneum descends from the anterior abdominal wall to the level of the pubic bone onto the superior surface of the bladder. It passes from the bladder to the uterus to form the vesicouterine pouch. The peritoneum covers the fundus and body of the uterus and extends over the posterior fornix and the wall of the vagina. Between the uterus and the rectum, the peritoneum forms the deep rectouterine pouch. In the male, the pelvic cavity has a small outpocket called the **scrotal cavity**, which contains the testes.

FALSE PELVIS

The false pelvis is bound posteriorly by the lumbar vertebrae, laterally by the iliac fossae and iliacus muscles, and anteriorly by the lower anterior abdominal wall. The sacral promontory

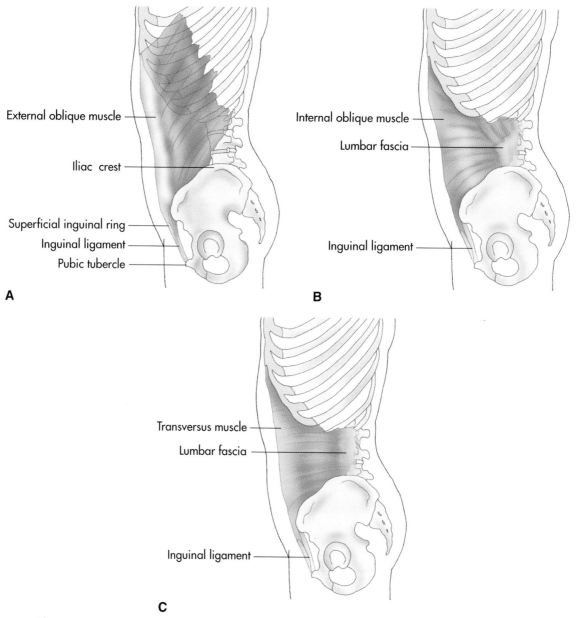

Figure 3-9 **A,** External oblique muscle of the anterior and lateral abdominal wall. **B,** Internal oblique muscle of the anterior and lateral abdominal wall. **C,** Transversus muscle of the anterior and lateral abdominal wall.

and the iliopectineal line form the boundary between the false pelvis and the true pelvis to delineate the boundary of the abdominal and pelvic cavities.

The uterus lies anterior to the rectum and posterior to the bladder and divides the pelvic peritoneal space into anterior and posterior pouches. The anterior pouch is termed the **uterovesical space,** and the posterior pouch is called the **rectouterine space,** or pouch of Douglas (Figure 3-11). The rectouterine pouch is a common location for accumulation of fluids, such as pus or blood.

The fallopian tubes extend laterally from the fundus of the uterus and are enveloped by a fold of peritoneum known as the broad ligament. This ligament arises from the floor of the

pelvis and contributes to the division of the peritoneal space into anterior and posterior pouches.

TRUE PELVIS

The true pelvis protects and contains the lower parts of the intestinal and urinary tracts and the reproductive organs. The true pelvis has an inlet, outlet, and cavity and is bounded posteriorly by the sacrum and coccyx (Figure 3-12). The anterior and lateral margins are formed by the pubis, the ischium, and a small portion of the ilium. A muscular "sling" consisting of the coccygeus and levator ani muscles forms the inferior boundary of the true pelvis and separates it from the perineum.

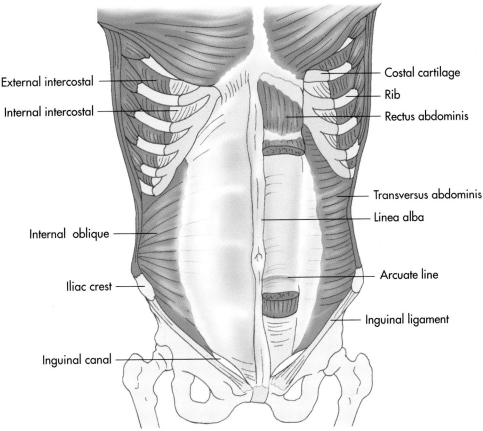

Figure 3-10   Anterior view of the rectus abdominis muscle and rectus sheath.

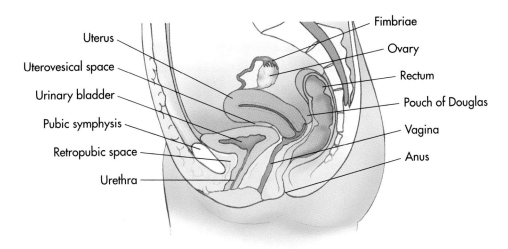

Figure 3-11   Lateral midsagittal view of the female pelvis.

The true pelvis is divided into anterior and posterior compartments. The anterior compartment contains the bladder and reproductive organs. The posterior compartment contains the posterior cul-de-sac, rectosigmoid muscle, perirectal fat, and presacral space.

The walls of the pelvis are formed by bones and ligaments, which are partly lined with muscles covered with fascia and parietal peritoneum. The pelvis has anterior, posterior, and lateral walls and an inferior floor. The obturator internus muscle lines the lateral pelvic wall; these muscles are symmetrically aligned along the lateral border of the pelvis with a concave medial border (see Figure 3-12).

The psoas and iliopsoas muscles lie along the posterior and lateral margins of the pelvis major (Figure 3-13). The fan-shaped iliacus muscles line the iliac fossae in the false pelvis. The psoas and iliacus muscles merge in their inferior portions to form the iliopsoas complex. The posterior border of the iliopsoas lies along the iliopectineal line and may be

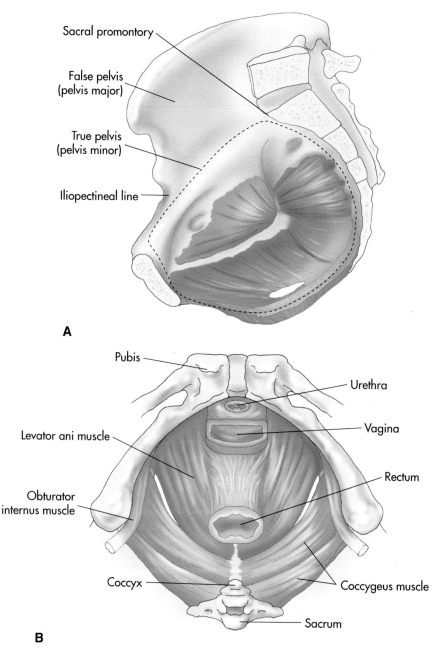

Figure 3-12   A, Lateral view of the pelvis, demonstrating the true pelvis and false pelvis. **B,** Inferior view of the pelvic diaphragm muscles.

used as a separation landmark of the true pelvis from the false pelvis.

The piriformis muscles form the posterior pelvic wall (Figure 3-14). The pelvic floor stretches across the pelvis and divides it into the main pelvic cavity, which contains the pelvic viscera and the perineum below. The levator ani muscles and pubococcygeus muscles form the pelvic diaphragm. The coccygeus muscles are rounded, concave muscles that lie more posterior than the obturator internus muscles.

Perineum.   The pelvic diaphragm is formed by the levatores ani and coccygeus muscles. The perineum has the following surface relationships: anterior is the pubic symphysis, posterior

is the tip of the coccyx, and lateral are the ischial tuberosities. The region is divided into two triangles formed by joining the ischial tuberosities with an imaginary line. The posterior triangle is the anal triangle, and the anterior triangle is the urogenital triangle.

ABDOMINOPELVIC MEMBRANES AND LIGAMENTS

PERITONEUM

The peritoneum is a serous membrane lining the walls of the abdominal cavity and clothing the abdominal viscera. The peritoneum is formed by a single layer of cells called the

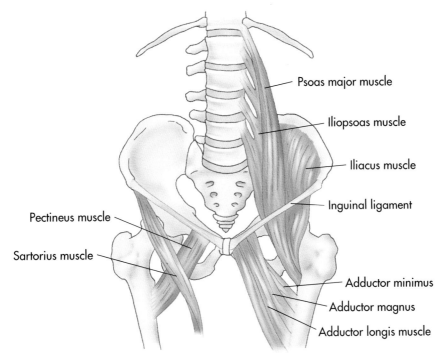

Figure 3-13   Anterior view of the psoas and iliopsoas muscles.

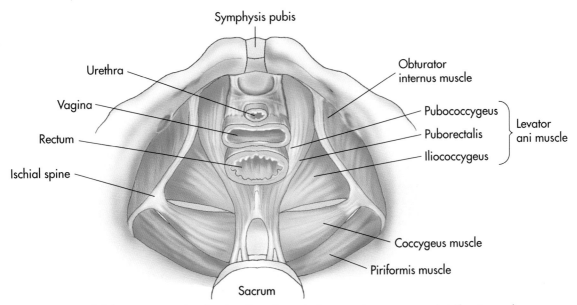

Figure 3-14   View of the female pelvic floor shows the levator ani, coccygeus, and piriformis muscles.

mesothelium, which rests on a thin layer of connective tissue (Figure 3-15). If the mesothelium is damaged or removed in any area (such as in surgery), there is danger that two layers of peritoneum may adhere to each other and form an adhesion. This adhesion may interfere with the normal movements of the abdominal viscera.

The peritoneum is divided into two layers. The **parietal peritoneum** is the portion that lines the abdominal wall, but does not cover a viscus; the **visceral peritoneum** is the portion that covers an organ (Figure 3-16). The **peritoneal cavity** is the potential space between the parietal and visceral peritoneum. This cavity contains a small amount of lubricating serous fluid to help the abdominal organs move on one another without friction. With certain pathologies, the potential space of the peritoneal cavity may be distended into an actual space containing several liters of fluid. This accumulation of fluid is known as **ascites.** Other fluid substances, such as blood from a ruptured organ, bile from a ruptured duct, or fecal matter from a ruptured intestine, also may accumulate in this cavity.

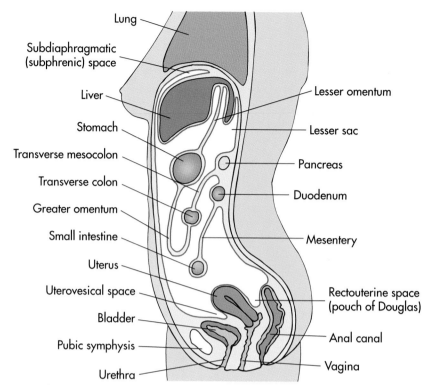

Figure 3-15   Lateral view of the peritoneum (*white area,* peritoneal cavity).

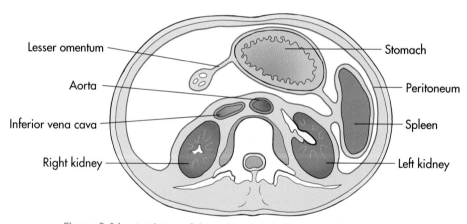

Figure 3-16   Axial view of the peritoneum (*white area,* peritoneal cavity).

The peritoneal cavity forms a completely closed sac in the male; in the female, there is a communication with the exterior through the fallopian tubes, uterus, and vagina.

Retroperitoneal organs and vascular structures remain posterior to the cavity and are covered anteriorly with peritoneum. These include the urinary system, aorta, inferior vena cava, colon, pancreas, uterus, and bladder. The other abdominal organs are located within the peritoneal cavity.

MESENTERY

A mesentery is a two-layered fold of peritoneum that attaches part of the intestines to the posterior abdominal wall and includes the mesentery of the small intestine, the transverse mesocolon, and the sigmoid mesocolon.

OMENTUM

The omentum is a two-layered fold of peritoneum that attaches the stomach to another viscus organ. The **greater omentum** is attached to the greater curvature of the stomach and hangs down like an apron in the space between the small intestine and anterior abdominal wall (Figure 3-17). The greater omentum is folded back on itself and is attached to the inferior border of the transverse colon. The **lesser omentum** slings the lesser curvature of the stomach to the undersurface of the liver. The gastrosplenic omentum ligament connects the stomach to the spleen (Figure 3-18).

GREATER AND LESSER SAC

The peritoneal cavity may be divided into two parts known as the greater and lesser sacs. The **greater sac** is the primary

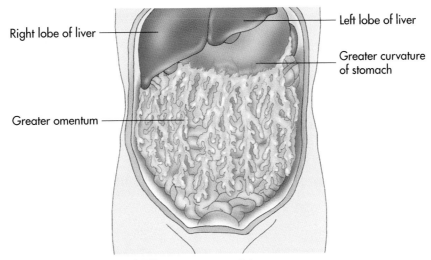

Figure 3-17   Anterior view of the greater omentum.

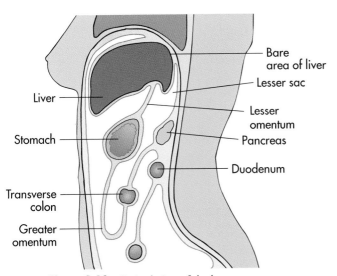

Figure 3-18   Sagittal view of the lesser omentum.

compartment of the peritoneal cavity and extends across the anterior abdomen and from the diaphragm to the pelvis.

The **lesser sac** is an extensive peritoneal pouch located behind the lesser omentum and stomach (Figure 3-19). It extends upward to the diaphragm and inferior between the layers of the greater omentum. The left margin is formed by the spleen and the gastrosplenic and lienorenal ligaments. The right margin of the lesser sac opens into the greater sac through the epiploic foramen.

EPIPLOIC FORAMEN
The **epiploic foramen** is the opening to the lesser sac in the abdomen and has the following boundaries: anteriorly, the free border of the lesser omentum containing the common bile duct, hepatic artery, and portal vein; posteriorly, the inferior vena cava; superiorly, the caudate process of the caudate lobe of the liver; and inferiorly, the first part of the duodenum (see Figure 3-19).

LIGAMENT
The peritoneal ligaments are two-layered folds of peritoneum that attach the lesser mobile solid viscera to the abdominal walls. For example, the liver is attached by the **falciform ligament** to the anterior abdominal wall and to the undersurface of the diaphragm (Figure 3-20). The **ligamentum teres** lies in the free borders of this ligament. The peritoneum leaves the kidney and passes to the hilus of the spleen as the posterior layer of the **lienorenal ligament**. The visceral peritoneum covers the spleen and is reflected onto the greater curvature of the stomach as the anterior layer of the **gastrosplenic ligament.**

POTENTIAL SPACES IN THE BODY
SUBPHRENIC SPACES
The subphrenic spaces are the result of the complicated arrangement of the peritoneum in the region of the liver (Figure 3-21). The right and left anterior subphrenic spaces lie between the diaphragm and the liver, one on each side of the falciform ligament. The sonographer should become very familiar with the right posterior subphrenic space that lies between the right lobe of the liver, the right kidney, and the right colic flexure. This is also called **Morison's pouch.** It is a frequent location for fluid collections, such as ascites, blood, and infection to accumulate.

PERITONEAL RECESSES
The omental bursa normally has some empty places. Parts of the peritoneal cavity near the liver are so slitlike that they are also isolated. These areas are known as **peritoneal recesses** and are clinically important because infections may collect in them. Two common sites are where the duodenum becomes the jejunum and where the ileum joins the cecum.

PARACOLIC GUTTERS
The arrangement of the ascending and descending colon, the attachments of the transverse mesocolon, and the mesentery of the small intestine to the posterior abdominal wall result in the

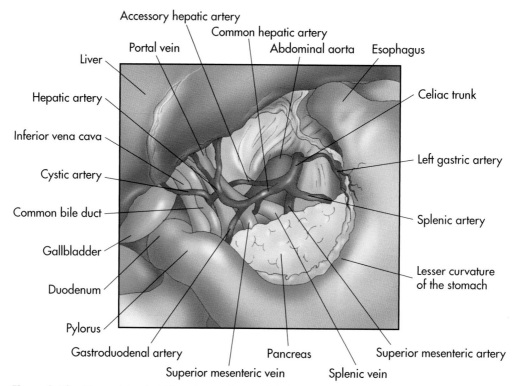

Figure 3-19 Upper abdominal dissection, with part of the left lobe of the liver and the lesser omentum removed to show the area of the epiploic foramen. Posterior to the foramen lie the celiac trunk, portal vein, bile duct, and related structures; one of the most important regions in the abdomen.

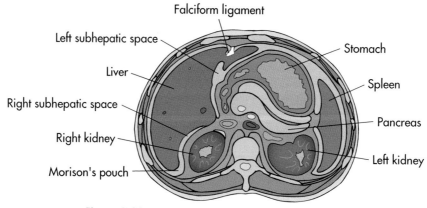

Figure 3-20 Transverse view of the falciform ligament.

formation of four paracolic gutters (Figure 3-22). The clinical significance of these gutters is their ability to conduct fluid materials from one part of the body to another. Materials—such as abscess, ascites, blood, pus, bile, or metastases—may be spread through this network.

The gutters are on the lateral and medial sides of the ascending and descending colon. The right medial paracolic gutter is closed off from the pelvic cavity inferiorly by the mesentery of the small intestine. The other gutters are in free communication with the pelvic cavity. The right lateral paracolic gutter communicates with the right posterior subphrenic space. The left lateral gutter is separated from the area around the spleen by the phrenicocolic ligament.

INGUINAL CANAL

The inguinal canal is an oblique passage through the lower part of the anterior abdominal wall. In the male, it allows structures to pass to and from the testes to the abdomen. In the female, it permits the passage of the round ligament of the uterus from the uterus to the labium majus (Figure 3-23).

ABDOMINAL HERNIAS

A hernia is the protrusion of part of the abdominal contents beyond the normal confines of the abdominal wall. It has the following three parts: the sac, the contents of the sac, and the coverings of the sac. The hernial sac is a diverticulum of the peritoneum and has a neck and a body. The hernial con-

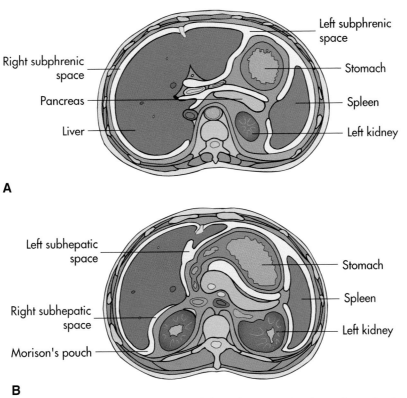

A

B

Figure 3-21   The supracolic compartment is located above the transverse colon and contains the right and left subphrenic spaces and the right and left subhepatic spaces. **A,** Transverse view of the subphrenic spaces. **B,** Transverse view of the subhepatic spaces.

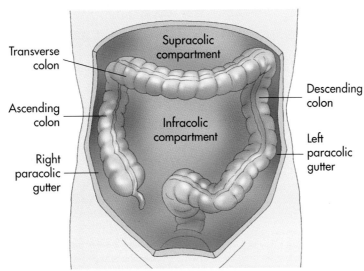

Figure 3-22   The infracolic compartment is found below the transverse colon. The right and left paracolic gutters are troughlike spaces located lateral to the ascending and descending colon.

tents may consist of any structure found within the abdominal cavity and may vary from a small piece of omentum to a large viscus organ. The hernial coverings are formed from the layers of the abdominal wall through which the hernial sac passes. Abdominal hernias are one of the following types: inguinal, femoral, umbilical, epigastric, or rectus abdominis.

THE RETROPERITONEUM

The retroperitoneal cavity contains the kidneys, ureters, adrenal glands, pancreas, aorta, inferior vena cava, bladder, uterus, and prostate gland. The ascending and descending colon and most of the duodenum are also located in the retroperitoneum.

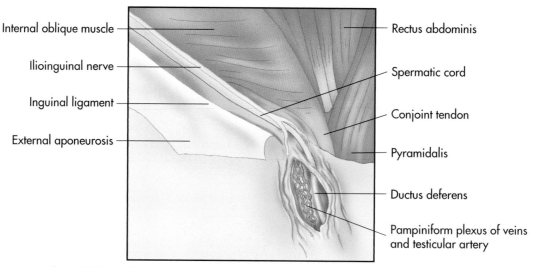

Figure 3-23   Right inguinal canal, spermatic cord, ductus deferens, and pampiniform plexus.

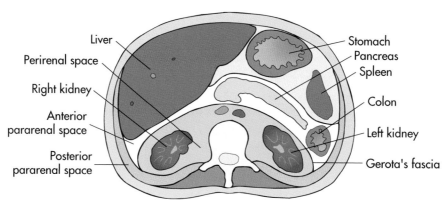

Figure 3-24   Transverse view of the retroperitoneum.

RETROPERITONEAL SPACES

The **anterior pararenal space** (Figure 3-24) is located between the anterior surface of the renal fascia (Gerota's fascia) and the posterior area of the peritoneum. Within this area are the ascending and descending colon, the pancreas, and the duodenum. The **posterior pararenal space** is found between the posterior renal fascia and the muscles of the posterior abdominal wall. Only fat and vessels are found within this space. The **perirenal space** is located directly around the kidney and is completely enclosed by renal fascia. Within this space lie the kidneys, adrenal glands, lymph nodes, blood vessels, and perirenal fat.

ANATOMIC TERMS

The ability of the sonographer to understand anatomy as it relates to the cross sectional, coronal, oblique, and sagittal projections is critical in performing a quality sonogram. Normal anatomy has many variations in size and position, and it is the responsibility of the sonographer to be able to demonstrate these findings on the sonogram. To complete this task, the sonographer must have a thorough understanding of anatomy

as it relates to the anteroposterior relationships and the variations in sectional anatomy. The following list contains anatomic terms grouped loosely by category:

anatomic position—individual is standing erect, arms are by the sides with the palms facing forward, face and eyes are directed forward, and heels are together, with the feet pointed forward

median plane—vertical plane that bisects the body into right and left halves

sagittal plane—any plane parallel to the median plane

coronal plane—any vertical plane at right angles to the median plane

transverse plane—any plane at right angles to both the median and coronal planes

supine—lying face up

prone—lying face down

anterior (ventral)—toward the front of the body or in front of another structure

posterior (dorsal)—toward the back of the body or in back of another structure

medial—nearer to or toward the midline

lateral—farther from the midline or to the side of the body

proximal—closer to the point of origin or closer to the body

distal—away from the point of origin or away from the body

internal—inside

external—outside

superior—above

inferior—below

cranial—toward the head

caudal—toward the feet

PREFIXES AND SUFFIXES

The sonographer should be familiar with the prefixes and suffixes that are commonly used in medical terminology.

a-, an- without; away from; not

ab-, abs- from; away from; absent

ad- toward

adipo- fat

angio- blood or lymph vessels

antero- anterior; front, before

-ase—enzyme

-asis, esis, iasis, -isis, -osis—condition; pathologic state

-cele—tumor, swelling

cephal- head

cran- helmet; *cranial:* pertaining to the portion of the skull that surrounds the brain

dextra- right

dors- back; *dorsal:* position toward the back of the body

-dynia—pain

dys- difficult, bad; painful

-emia—blood

end, endo- within, inside

eryth- red

ex-, exo- out, outside of

hem-, hema-, hemato- blood

hepato- liver

homeo-, homo- same; *homeostasis:* maintenance of a stable internal environment

hydra-, hydro- hydr- water

hyp-, hyph-, hypo- less than; under

hyper- excessive

hyster- uterus

infra- below, under, beneath; inferior to; after

inter- between

intra- within

ipsi- same

-itis—inflammation of

juxta- close proximity

lip-, lipo- fat

-lite, -lith, litho- stone, calculus

mega-, megalo- large, of great size

meio-, mio- less, smaller

mesio- toward the middle

meta- change; *metabolism:* chemical changes that occur within the body

necr-, necro- death; necrosis

neo- new

nephr-, nephra-, nephro- kidney

olig-, oligo- few; small

-ology—study of; *physiology:* study of body functions

-oma—tumor

omphal-, omphalo- navel

oophor- ovary

orchi- testicle

pariet- wall; *parietal membrane:* membrane that lines the wall of a cavity

pelv- basin; *pelvic cavity:* basin-shaped cavity enclosed by the pelvic bones

peri- around

pleur- rib; *pleural membrane:* membrane that encloses the lungs within the rib cage

-poiesis, -poietic—production; formation

pre- before, in front of

pseudo- false

py-, pyo- pus

pyelo- pelvis

retro- backward, back, behind

-rhage, rhagia—rupture; profuse fluid discharge

sebo- fatty substance

-stasis—standing still; *homeostasis:* maintenance of a relatively stable internal environment

sub- under; beneath

super, supra- above; beyond; superior; on top

thrombo- blood clot; thrombus

-tomy—cutting; *anatomy:* study of structure, which often involves cutting or removing body parts

trans- across, over; beyond; through

-trophin—stimulation of a target organ by a substance, especially a hormone

-uria, urin- urine

vaso- vessel (blood vessel)

veno- vein

ventro-, ventr-, ventri- abdomen; anterior surface of body

vesico—bladder; vesicle

xeno- strange, foreign

SELECTED BIBLIOGRAPHY

Netter F: The CIBA collection: digestive system, West Caldwell, NJ, 1989, CIBA.

Snell RS: *Clinical anatomy for medical students,* Boston, 2004, Little, Brown.

Swobodnik W and others: *Atlas of ultrasound anatomy,* New York, 1991, George Thieme.

CHAPTER 4

Introduction to Abdominal Scanning Techniques and Protocols

Sandra L. Hagen-Ansert

OBJECTIVES

- Name the scanning techniques used in ultrasound
- Describe how to properly label a sonogram
- Describe the correct orientation of an ultrasound image
- List the criteria for an adequate scan
- Describe the sectional anatomy in the transverse and longitudinal planes
- Describe the general abdominal protocol
- List the patient preparation, transducer selection, patient position, and images that should be obtained for all abdominal and soft tissue structures
- Describe the use of Doppler in the abdomen
- List the Doppler scanning techniques for abdominal vessels

BEFORE YOU BEGIN TO SCAN PATIENTS
ORIENTATION TO THE CLINICAL LABORATORY
SCANNING TECHNIQUES
PATIENT POSITIONS
TRANSDUCER SELECTION
TRANSDUCER POSITIONS
INITIAL SURVEY OF THE ABDOMEN

LABELING SCANS AND PATIENT POSITION

CRITERIA FOR AN ADEQUATE SCAN

SECTIONAL ANATOMY
TRANSVERSE PLANE
LONGITUDINAL PLANE

GENERAL ABDOMINAL ULTRASOUND PROTOCOLS
TRANSVERSE SCANS
LONGITUDINAL SCANS
LIVER AND PORTA HEPATIS PROTOCOL
BILIARY SYSTEM PROTOCOL
PANCREAS PROTOCOL
SPLEEN PROTOCOL
RENAL PROTOCOL
AORTA AND ILIAC ARTERY PROTOCOL
THYROID PROTOCOL
PARATHYROID PROTOCOL
BREAST PROTOCOL
SCROTAL PROTOCOL

ABDOMINAL DOPPLER
DOPPLER SCANNING TECHNIQUES
AORTA
INFERIOR VENA CAVA
PORTAL VENOUS SYSTEM
PORTAL HYPERTENSION

KEY TERMS

Arteries

aorta – largest arterial structure in the body; arises from the left ventricle to supply blood to the head, upper and lower extremities, and abdominopelvic cavity

celiac axis (CA) – first major anterior artery to arise from the abdominal aorta inferior to the diaphragm; it branches into the hepatic, splenic, and left gastric arteries

common femoral arteries – vessels originating from the iliac arteries and seen in the inguinal region into the upper thigh

gastroduodenal artery (GDA) – branch of the common hepatic artery to supply the stomach and duodenum

hepatic artery (HA) – common hepatic artery arises from the celiac trunk and courses to the right of the abdomen and branches into the GDA and proper HA

iliac arteries (IA) – originate from the bifurcation of the aorta at the level of the umbilicus

inferior mesenteric artery (IMA) – arises from the anterior aortic wall at the level of the third or fourth lumbar vertebra to supply the left transverse colon, descending colon, sigmoid colon, and rectum

left gastric artery (LGA) – small branch of the celiac axis that feeds the stomach

left renal artery (LRA) – arises from the posterolateral wall of the aorta directly into the hilus of the kidney

right renal artery (RRA) – leaves the posterolateral wall of the aorta; travels posterior to the inferior vena cava to enter the hilum of the kidney

splenic artery (SA) – arises from the celiac trunk to supply the spleen

superior mesenteric artery (SMA) – arises inferior to the celiac axis from the anterior wall of the abdominal aorta; travels parallel to the aorta to supply the small bowel, cecum, ascending colon, and transverse colon; lies posterior to the body of the pancreas

Veins

collateral vessels – ancillary vessels that develop when portal hypertension occurs

confluence of the splenic and portal veins – junction of the splenic and portal veins that occurs in the midabdomen and serves as a posterior border of the pancreas

femoral veins – upper part of the venous drainage system of the lower extremity found in the upper thigh and groin

hepatic veins (HV) – largest tributaries that drain the liver and empty into the inferior vena cava at the level of the diaphragm

iliac veins – receive tributaries from the lower extremities and drain into the inferior vena cava

inferior vena cava (IVC) – principle venous vessel that returns blood from the lower half of the body from the confluence of the right and left common iliac veins; flows posterior to the liver to enter the right atrium of the heart

left portal vein (LPV) – the main portal vein bifurcates into the right and left portal veins; the left portal vein supplies the left lobe of the liver

left renal vein (LRV) – leaves the renal hilum and travels anterior to the aorta, posterior to the superior mesenteric artery to empty into the lateral wall of the inferior vena cava

main portal vein (MPV) – formed by the union of the splenic vein and superior mesenteric vein; serves as the posterior border of the pancreas

portal venous system – comprises the splenic, inferior mesenteric, superior mesenteric, and portal veins

right portal vein (RPV) – the main portal vein bifurcates into right and left branches; the right portal vein supplies the right lobe of the liver

right renal vein (RRV) – leaves the renal hilum to flow directly into the inferior vena cava

splenic vein (SV) – drains blood from the spleen and part of the stomach; forms the posteromedial border of the pancreas as it travels horizontally across the abdomen; joins the superior mesenteric vein to form the main portal vein

superior mesenteric vein (SMV) – drains the small bowel and cecum, transverse and sigmoid colon; travels vertically to join the splenic and portal veins; serves as a posterior landmark to the body of the pancreas and anterior border to the uncinate process of the head

Ligaments and Other Structures

caudate lobe – smallest lobe of the liver; lies posterior to the left lobe and anterior to the inferior vena cava; superior border is the ligamentum venosum

crus of the diaphragm – muscular structure seen in the upper abdomen at the level of the celiac axis; aligns the vertebral column before crossing the midline posterior to the inferior vena cava and anterior to the aorta; may be mistaken for the right renal artery

dome of liver – most superior aspect of the liver at the level of the diaphragm

falciform ligament (FL) – attaches the liver to the anterior abdominal wall and undersurface of the diaphragm

ligamentum teres (LT) – termination of the falciform ligament, seen in the left lobe of the liver

ligamentum venosum (LV) – echogenic linear structure found anterior to the caudate lobe and posterior to the left lobe of the liver

Morison's pouch – small peritoneal recess located anterior to the right kidney and inferior to the liver

porta hepatis – where the triad of the portal vein, common bile duct, and hepatic artery enter the liver; this triad makes the area appear slightly more echogenic

portal confluence – see confluence of splenic and portal veins

psoas major muscle – group of muscles that originate at the hilum of the kidneys and lie lateral to the spine

splenic hilum – central area of the spleen that allows the vascular and lymph structure to emerge or enter

---

The art of scanning demands a lot from the sonographer: a high degree of manual dexterity and hand-eye coordination; the ability to conceptualize two-dimensional information into a three-dimensional format; and a thorough understanding of anatomy, physiology, pathology, instrumentation, artifact production, and transducer characteristics. Ultrasound equipment today is so sophisticated that producing quality images requires a greater understanding of the physical principles of sonography and computers than ever before. Moreover, sonographers should be aware of how Doppler techniques, color flow mapping, and three-dimensional imaging have enhanced modern medicine's understanding of anatomy and physiology as it relates to blood-flow dynamics and reconstruction.

Although one-on-one, hands-on training in a clinical setting is an essential part of the sonographer's experience of producing high-quality scans, this chapter will take you a long way toward mastering the foundations of abdominal scanning. Because correlation of ultrasound images with sectional anatomy is critical for producing consistent, quality images, the chapter focuses on normal sectional anatomy and normal abdominal ultrasound anatomy protocol. Specific organ protocol is discussed in the respective chapters. Just as the anatomic structures will vary, so too will the protocol for an abdominal scan differ among ultrasound departments. The protocols presented here are generic and may be adapted to the particular laboratory situation. Also included in this chapter are special scanning techniques and specific applications of abdominal scanning.

BEFORE YOU BEGIN TO SCAN PATIENTS

Remember that your ultimate goal as a sonographer is to produce diagnostic images that can be interpreted by the physician to answer a clinical question. To create images that are diagnostically useful, you must be familiar with ultrasound instrumentation and the clinical considerations of the patient exam. Clinical considerations include knowing which patient position should be used for specific examinations, transducer selection and scanning techniques, patient breathing techniques, and how to perform a sonographic survey of the abdomen.

As a sonographer, be sure you are very familiar with various types of ultrasound equipment. Know where the operator's manual is and how to find what you need in the manual. (Every manufacturer places the power supply in a different position, so make sure you know how to turn the machine on and off!) Become familiar with the transducers available for each machine, how to activate the transducers, and how to change transducers (some of the plug-in formats take some practice to master). Be sure you understand where the critical knobs are to operate the ultrasound instrumentation (e.g., TGC, power, gain, depth, angle, focus, Doppler, color flow, etc.). Know where the text keys are to label the image. If you are new to the instrument, it may be a good idea for one sonographer to work the controls, while the other scans until you become used to a particular ultrasound machine.

It is highly recommended that the student sonographer practice in a supervised laboratory setting (away from patients) before you begin working with patients. This way the student sonographer can become familiar with the ultrasound equipment by scanning phantoms or even building phantoms to be scanned. The next step should be to scan the students in the sonography lab. This allows the actual experience of feeling how "cold that gel really is" when applied to the abdomen and also to experience what the probe feels like with different individuals' scan techniques. You can see first hand how a light touch does not make as pretty an image as a moderate touch with the transducer adjacent to the skin. You may also experience the agony of the heavy hand as it scrapes across the rib cage. The student will also learn how much scanning gel is the "right amount." If it drips down your wrist and onto your clothes, it is too much gel! Controlled scanning should also emphasize how important it is to take in a breath to obtain the highest quality images. A recommended patient breathing technique tip is to have the patient inhale through the nose to reduce air going into the stomach. Breathing is probably the weakest learning link for the student. Respiration is critical to

making a beautiful scan versus an image that is not easy to interpret.

The student sonographer should also begin to understand the specific protocols required for each examination. Many protocols are outlined in this chapter that have been used in many labs across the country. The sonographer may also find universal protocols developed by the Society for Diagnostic Medical Sonography, the American Institute of Ultrasound in Medicine (AIUM), and the American College of Radiology (ACR) for ultrasound examinations. Likewise, the American College of Ob/Gyn has developed guidelines for the female patient and the American Society of Echocardiography has developed guidelines for echocardiography. The Society for Vascular Ultrasound has likewise established guidelines for vascular examinations. Each of these protocols may be found on the websites for the respective organization.

Of course, the student will not be able to completely remember all the protocols when they first begin their clinical scanning experience. Suggested building steps to help the student master the protocols are included in the workbook that accompanies this textbook.

ORIENTATION TO THE CLINICAL LABORATORY

When students arrive in the clinical ultrasound laboratory, they should take a few days to become familiar with the particular ultrasound department. The following points may make their entrance into the clinical world a little smoother:

- Learn the ultrasound equipment in the department. This means that every free minute should be spent with the equipment, finding the working knobs necessary to perform the examination.
- Know where the operator's manuals are for each piece of equipment so you may have a reference for troubleshooting.
- Find out what protocols are used for each examination.
- Understand how to read the patient request and know which items are relevant for patient identification.
- When you call for patients, be sure to check their I.D. bracelet or ask them to say their name.
- Introduce yourself and explain briefly the procedure you are going to do. Also explain the procedure the department will follow to notify the patient's physician of the results of the examination.
- Keep your conversation professional.
- Discuss the case only with your mentor or the physician responsible for interpreting the study.

SCANNING TECHNIQUES

Ultrasound can distinguish interfaces among soft tissue structures of different acoustic densities. The strength of the echoes reflected depends upon the acoustic interface and the angle at which the sound beam strikes the interface. The sonographer must determine which "window" on the patient is the best to record optimal ultrasound images and which transducer will best fit into that window. The curved array transducer provides a large field of view, but it may be difficult to scan between the patient's ribs in some examinations. The small footprint transducer allows the sonographer to scan between intercostal spaces with the patient in a supine, coronal, decubitus, or upright position but limits the near field of view.

PATIENT POSITIONS

The typical abdominal examination is primarily done in the supine position. However, the oblique, lateral decubitus, upright, and prone positions have also been used to demonstrate specific areas of interest (Figure 4-1). These positions will be discussed further in the specific protocols.

TRANSDUCER SELECTION

Know the types of transducers available for each piece of ultrasound equipment and be familiar with which transducer is used for specific examinations (Figure 4-2). The size of the patient will influence what megahertz transducer will be used. If the endovaginal transducer is used, be familiar with the decontamination process for the transducer.

TRANSDUCER POSITIONS

The sonographer will use multiple wrist actions throughout the study. Remember the beam is ideally reflected when the transducer is perpendicular to the surface. However, the body

Supine

Prone

Right lateral decubitus

Left lateral decubitus

Right posterior oblique

Left posterior oblique

Sitting semi-erect

Sitting erect

Figure 4-1   Various standard patient positions for the ultrasound examination.

Figure 4-2   Transducer designs in multiple shapes and sizes are used for specific ultrasound examinations.

has many angles, curves, and rib interferences causing the sonographer to use intercostal spaces, subcostal windows, multiple degrees of angulation, and many rotations of the transducer to obtain anatomic images (Figure 4-3).

INITIAL SURVEY OF THE ABDOMEN

Before you begin the protocol for the specific examination, take a minute to survey the area in question. This will give you an opportunity to see how the patient images with "routine" instrument settings, to see where the organs are in relationship to the patient's respiration pattern, and to see if the patient has a good "scanning window" in the supine position, or if the patient position needs to be altered into a decubitus or upright position. In a general abdominal survey, ask the patient to take in a deep breath, begin at the level of the xiphoid in the midline with the transducer angled steeply towards the patient's head so as to be perpendicular to the diaphragm (Figure 4-4). Slowly angle the transducer inferiorly to "sweep" through the liver, gallbladder, head of pancreas, and right kidney. The transducer may then be redirected in the same manner, only angled towards the left shoulder and a gradual angulation made inferiorly to see the stomach, spleen, pancreas, and left kidney. Likewise, a quick survey of the abdomen may be done with the transducer in the midline sagittal position (Figure 4-5). Remember to ask the patient to take in a breath and hold it in. Image the aorta first with the vertebral column posterior to the aorta. Then slowly angle the transducer to the right to image the dilated inferior vena cava and liver. Continue to angle towards the right to image more of the liver, gallbladder, and right kidney. If good penetration is seen with adequate TGC and overall gain adjustments, then you can proceed with the routine protocol for the abdominal study found later in this chapter.

LABELING SCANS AND PATIENT POSITION

Ultrasound images are labeled as *transverse* or *longitudinal* for a specific organ, such as the liver, gallbladder, pancreas, spleen, or uterus. The smaller organs that can be imaged on a single

plane, such as the kidney, are labeled as *long-midline, -lateral,* or *medial,* whereas the transverse scans are labeled as *transverse-low, -middle,* and *-high.*

All transverse supine scans are oriented with the liver on the left of the screen; this means the sonographer will be viewing the body from the feet up to the head ("optimistic view") (Figure 4-6). Longitudinal scans display the patient's head to the left and feet to the right of the screen and use the xiphoid, umbilicus, or symphysis to denote the midline of the scan plane (Figure 4-7).

All scans should be appropriately labeled for future reference. This includes the patient's name, date, and anatomic position. Body position markers are available on many ultrasound machines and may be used in the place of written labels.

The position of the patient should be described in relation to the scanning table (e.g., a right decubitus would mean the right side down; a left decubitus would indicate the left side down). If the scanning plane is oblique, the sonographer should merely state that it is an oblique view without specifying the exact degree of obliquity.

CRITERIA FOR AN ADEQUATE SCAN

With the use of real-time ultrasound, it is sometimes difficult to become oriented to all of the anatomic structures on a single image. It is therefore critical to obtain as much anatomy as possible in a single image.

Avoiding rib interference is important to eliminate artifact attenuation/reverberation that may destroy information. The small-footprint transducer allows the sonographer to scan in between the ribs but limits near-field visualization. Variations in the patient's respiration may also help eliminate rib interference and improve image quality. The sonographer can easily watch in real time how much interference is caused by patient breathing and ask the patient either to take in a breath and hold it or stop breathing at critical points to capture particular parts of the anatomy.

Patients should be instructed not to eat or drink anything for 6 to 8 hours before the abdominal ultrasound procedure. This will enable the gallbladder to be distended and to prevent unnecessary bowel gas that may interfere with the visualization of the smaller abdominal and vascular structures.

SECTIONAL ANATOMY

The sonographer must have a solid knowledge of both gross anatomy and sectional anatomy, as well as the normal anatomic variations that may occur in the body. The sonographer should carefully evaluate organ and vascular relationships to the neighboring structures rather than memorizing where in the abdomen a particular structure "should" be: It is better to recall the location of the gallbladder as anterior to the right kidney and medial to the liver than to remember it is found 6 cm above the umbilicus.

Perpendicular
The transducer is straight up and down.

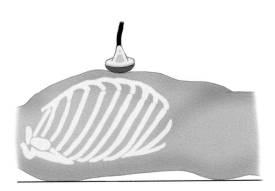

Subcostal
The transducer is angled superiorly just beneath the inferior costal margin.

Intercostal
The transducer is between the ribs. It can be perpendicular, subcostal, or angled.

Angled
The transducer is angled superiorly, inferiorly, or right and left laterally at varying degrees.

Rotated
The transducer is rotated varying degrees to oblique the scanning plane.

Figure 4-3   The sonographer must use a number of different transducer positions and angulations to complete the ultrasound examination.

TRANSVERSE PLANE

The transverse sectional illustrations (Figures 4-8 through 4-22) are presented in descending order from the dome of the diaphragm to the symphysis pubis. The sonographer should review the relationship of each organ to its neighboring struc-

tures, proceeding in a caudal direction. Specific detail is listed below each illustration with a thumbnail sketch of expected anatomy outlined below:

Dome of the liver (Figure 4-8). The **splenic artery (SA)** enters as the **splenic vein (SV)** leaves the splenic hilum. The

Figure 4-4   Most abdominal ultrasound examinations are performed initially in the supine position. The curved array probe is shown in the transverse position.

Figure 4-5   Longitudinal scan. The probe has now been rotated to the midline sagittal position.

A

B

Figure 4-6   **A,** The curved array probe is held in a transverse position just under the costal margin with a steep angulation to be perpendicular to the dome of the liver. Patient is supine. **B,** All transverse supine scans are oriented as looking up from the feet, with the liver on the left side of the screen (right side of the patient is on the left of the screen).

A

B

Figure 4-7   **A,** The curved array probe has been rotated 180 degrees to perform a sagittal scan of the abdomen. **B,** The longitudinal scans for the abdomen and pelvis are oriented with the patient's head toward the left of the screen and feet toward the right.

abdominal portion of the esophagus lies to the left of the midline and opens into the stomach through the cardiac orifice. The liver extends to the left mammillary line. The **falciform ligament (FL)** extends into the diaphragm.

Level of the caudate lobe (Figure 4-9). The right **hepatic vein** enters the lateral margin of the **inferior vena cava (IVC).** The fundus of the stomach is shown with the hepatogastric and gastrocolic ligaments. The lesser omental cavity is posterior to the stomach. The upper border of the splenic flexure of the colon is seen. The **caudate lobe** of the liver is anterior to the IVC and demarcated by the **ligamentum venosum (LV).** The body and tail of the pancreas are seen near the splenic hilum. The adrenal glands are lateral to the **crus of the diaphragm.**

Level of the caudate lobe and celiac axis (CA) (Figure 4-10). The **celiac axis (CA)** (branches into **left gastric artery [LGA]**, splenic artery, and **hepatic artery**) should be found near this section as it arises from the anterior wall of the **aorta (Ao).** The transverse and descending colon are shown inferior to the splenic flexure. The caudate lobe of the liver is shown. The body of the pancreas is anterior to the splenic vein. Both kidneys and the adrenal glands are shown lateral to the spine and crus of the diaphragm. The IVC is shown anterior to the crus, and the aorta is posterior to the crus of the diaphragm.

Level of the superior mesenteric artery and pancreas (Figure 4-11). The **psoas major muscles** are lateral to the spine. The

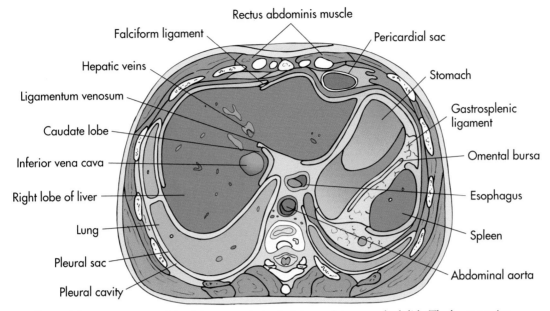

Figure 4-8 Cross section of the abdomen at the level of the tenth intervertebral disk. The lower portion of the pericardial sac is seen. The splenic artery enters the spleen, and the splenic vein emerges from the splenic hilum. The abdominal portion of the esophagus lies to the left of the midline and opens into the stomach through the cardiac orifice. The liver extends to the left mammillary line. The falciform ligament extends into the section above this. The spleen is shown to lie alongside the ninth rib.

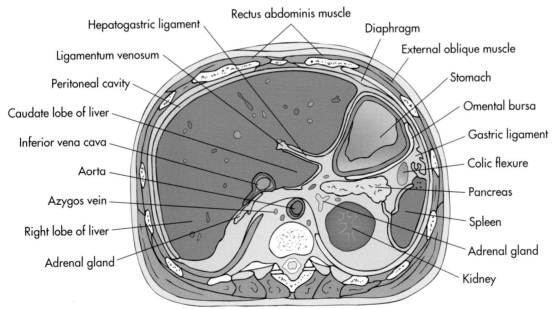

Figure 4-9 Cross section of the abdomen at the level of the eleventh thoracic disk. The hepatic vein is shown to enter the inferior vena cava. The renal artery and vein of the left kidney are shown. The left branch of the portal vein is seen to arch upward to enter the left lobe of the liver. The upper part of the stomach is shown with the hepatogastric and gastrocolic ligaments. The lesser omental cavity is posterior to the stomach. The upper border of the splenic flexure of the colon is seen. The caudate lobe of the liver is in this section. The tail and body of the pancreas are shown anterior to the left kidney. The spleen is shown to lie along the left lateral border. The adrenal glands are lateral to the crus of the diaphragm.

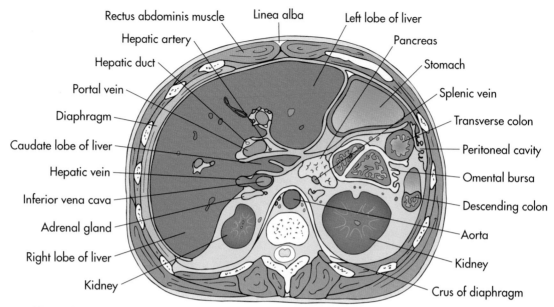

Figure 4-10 Cross section of the abdomen at the level of the twelfth thoracic vertebra. The celiac axis arises in the middle of this section from the anterior abdominal aorta. The right renal artery originates at this level. The hepatic vein is shown to enter the inferior vena cava. The greater curvature of the stomach and the pylorus are shown. The transverse and descending colon are shown inferior to the splenic flexure. The caudate lobe of the liver is well seen. The body of the pancreas, both kidneys, and the lower portions of the adrenal glands are shown.

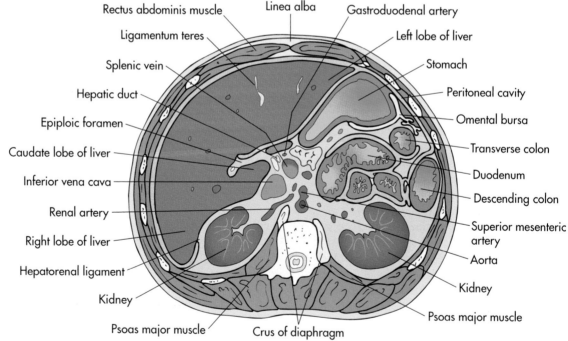

Figure 4-11 Cross section of the abdomen at the first lumbar vertebra. The psoas major muscle is seen. The crura of the diaphragm are shown on either side of the spine. The right renal artery is seen. The left renal artery arises from the lateral wall of the aorta. Both renal veins enter the inferior vena cava. The portal vein is seen to be formed by the union of the splenic vein and the superior mesenteric vein. The lower portions of the stomach and the pyloric orifice are seen, as is the superior portion of the duodenum. The duodenojejunal flexure and descending and transverse colon are shown. The greater omentum is very prominent. The small, nonperitoneal area of the liver is shown anterior to the right kidney. The round ligament of the liver and the umbilical fissure, which separates the right and left lobes of the liver, are seen. The neck of the gallbladder (not shown) is found just inferior to this section, between the quadrate and caudate lobes of the liver. The cystic duct is cut in two places. The hepatic duct lies just anterior to the cystic duct. The cystic and hepatic ducts unite in the lower part of the section to form the common bile duct. The pancreatic duct is found within the pancreas at this level. Both kidneys are seen just lateral to the psoas muscles.

right renal artery is shown posterior to the IVC. The **left renal artery** would arise from the posterolateral wall of the aorta; the **right** and **left renal veins** are inferior to the renal arteries. The **portal confluence** (also called **confluence of the splenic and portal veins**) is formed by the splenic vein and **superior mesenteric vein**. The superior portion of the duodenum is shown posterior to the stomach. Part of the transverse colon is shown. The hepatic duct is anterior to the portal vein.

Level of the gallbladder and right kidney (Figure 4-12). The kidneys are lateral to the psoas muscles. The **gastroduodenal artery (GDA)** lies along the anterolateral border of the head of the pancreas, and the duodenum surrounds the lateral border. The stomach and transverse colon fill the left upper quadrant, and the liver fills the right upper quadrant. The gallbladder is medial to the liver. The common bile duct is seen along the posterior lateral border of the pancreatic head.

Level of the liver, gallbladder, and right kidney (Figure 4-13). The **inferior mesenteric artery** originates from the abdominal aorta at this level. The greater omentum is shown on the left side of the abdomen. The descending and ascending portions of the duodenum lie between the aorta and the superior mesenteric artery and vein. The gallbladder is seen along the medial border of the right lobe of the liver. Both lower poles of the kidneys are seen lateral to the psoas muscles.

Level of the right lobe of the liver (Figure 4-14). The lower portion of the right lobe of the liver and the duodenum are shown.

Level of the bifurcation of the aorta (Figure 4-15). The psoas major muscles are lateral to the spine. The **iliac arteries** are anterior to the spine. The common **iliac veins** unite to form the inferior vena cava.

Level of the external iliac arteries (Figure 4-16). The external iliac arteries are well seen. The ileum is seen throughout this level, and the mesentery terminates at this level.

Level of the external iliac veins (Figure 4-17). The internal and external iliac veins have united to form the common iliac vein.

Level of the male pelvis (Figure 4-18). The external iliac arteries become the **common femoral arteries** in this section. The **femoral veins** become the external iliac veins. The cecum and rectum are seen.

Level of the male pelvis (Figure 4-19). The pelvic muscles are shown; the rectum is seen in the midline. The trigone of the bladder and urethral orifice are shown, and the seminal vesicles and the ampulla of the vasa deferentia can be identified. The ejaculatory ducts enter the urethra in the lower portion of this section.

Level of the male pelvis (Figure 4-20). The rectum, prostate gland, penis, and corpus cavernosum are seen.

Level of the female pelvis (Figure 4-21). The bladder is anterior to the uterus. The pouch of Douglas is posterior to the uterus, anterior to the rectum. The ovaries are seen along the fundal border of the uterus.

Level of the female pelvis (Figure 4-22). The pelvic diaphragm muscles are shown.

LONGITUDINAL PLANE

The longitudinal sectional illustrations (Figures 4-23 through 4-33) are presented from the right abdominal border, proceeding across the abdominal wall to the left border.

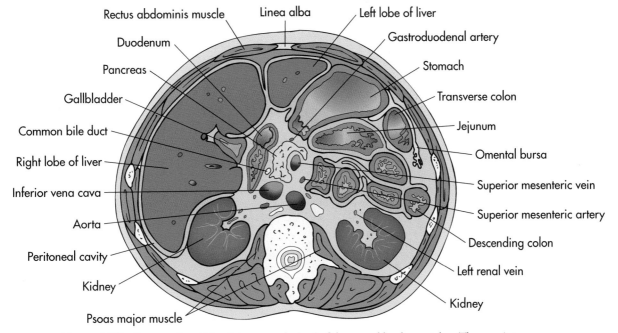

Figure 4-12   Cross section of the abdomen at the level of the second lumbar vertebra. The superior pancreaticoduodenal artery originates as shown in Figure 3-6 and shows some of its branches in this section. The lower portion of the stomach is found in this section, and the hepatic flexure of the colon is seen. The lobes of the liver are separated by the round ligament. The left lobe of the liver ends at this level. The head and neck of the pancreas drape around the superior mesenteric vein. Both kidneys and the psoas muscles are shown.

Text continues on p. 82

Figure 4-13 Cross section of the abdomen at the level of the third lumbar vertebra. The inferior mesenteric artery originates from the abdominal aorta at this level. The greater omentum is shown mostly on the left side of the abdomen. The descending and ascending portions of the duodenum lie between the aorta and the superior mesenteric artery and vein. The fundus of the gallbladder lies in the lower portion of this section. The lower poles of both kidneys lie lateral to the psoas muscles.

Figure 4-14 Cross section of the abdomen at the level of the third lumbar disk. The lower portion of the duodenum is shown. The lower margin of the right lobe of the liver is seen along the right lateral border.

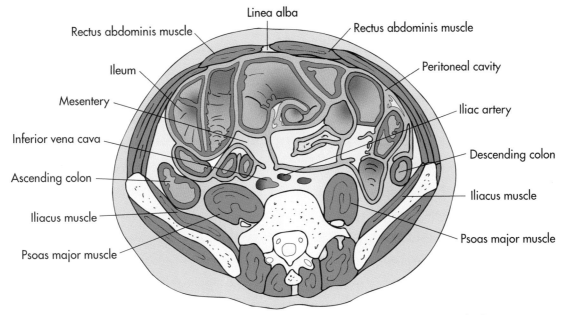

Figure 4-15 Cross section of the abdomen at the level of the fifth lumbar vertebra. It cuts the ileum through the upper part of the iliac fossa and passes just above the wings of the sacrum. The gluteus medius and iliacus muscles are shown. The right common iliac artery bifurcates into the external and internal iliac arteries. The common iliac veins are shown to unite to form the inferior vena cava. The lower part of the greater omentum is shown in this section.

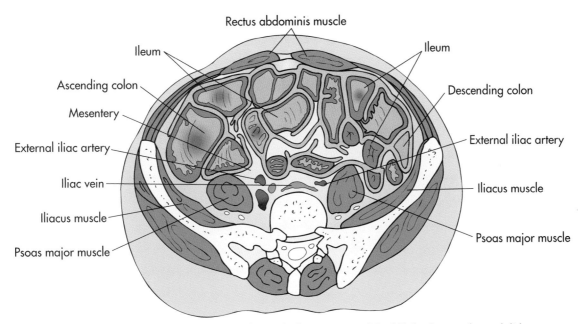

Figure 4-16 Cross section of the pelvis taken at the lower margin of the fifth lumbar vertebra and disk. The gluteus minimus muscle is shown on this section, as are the right external and internal iliac arteries. The left common iliac artery branches into the external and internal arteries. The ileum is seen throughout this level, and the mesentery terminates at this level.

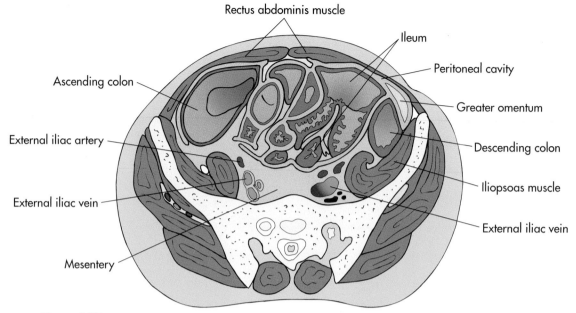

Figure 4-17 Cross section of the pelvis taken at the level of the sacrum and the anterior superior spine of the ilium. The gluteus maximus muscle appears on both sides. The internal and external iliac veins have united to form the common iliac vein. The ileum is seen throughout this section.

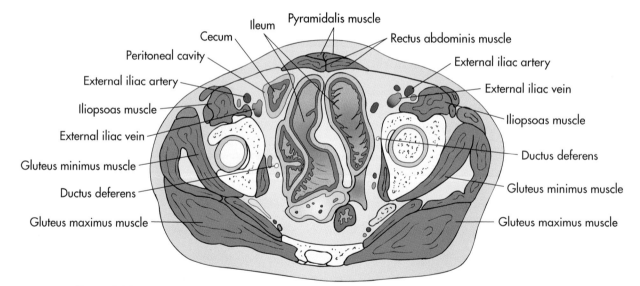

Figure 4-18 Cross section of the pelvis taken above the margins of the fifth anterior pair of sacral foramina and head of the femur. The external iliac arteries become the femoral arteries in this section. The femoral veins become the external iliac veins.

Figure 4-19 Cross section of the pelvis at the level of the coccyx, the spine of the ischium, the femur, and greater trochanter. This cross section passes through the coccyx, spine of the ischium, acetabulum, head of the femur, greater trochanter, pubic symphysis, and upper margins of the obturator foramen. The gemellus inferior and superior, coccygeus, and levator ani muscles are shown. The rectum is seen in the midline. The trigone of the bladder and the urethral orifice are well shown, and the seminal vesicles and the ampulla of the vasa deferentia can be identified. The ejaculatory ducts enter the urethra in the lower portion of this section.

Figure 4-20 Cross section of the pelvis at the tip of the coccyx, inferior ramus of the pubis, and neck of the femur. This cross section passes below the tip of the coccyx, upper portion of the tuberosity of the ischium and inferior ramus of the pubis, neck of the femur, and lower portion of the greater trochanter. The rectum, penis, and corpus cavernosum are seen.

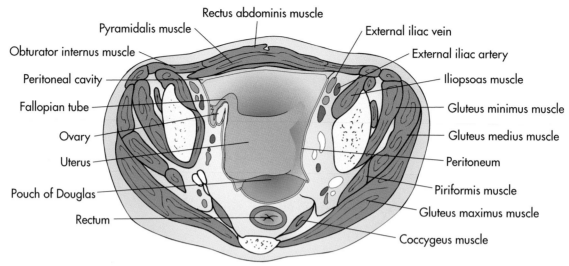

Figure 4-21 Cross section of the female pelvis just below the junction of the sacrum and coccyx. This cross section is a section through the female pelvis just below the junction of the sacrum and coccyx, through the anterior inferior spine of the ilium and the greater sciatic notch. The uterine artery and vein and the ureter are shown dissected beyond the uterine wall. The bladder is anterior to the uterus. The ovaries are cut through their midsections on this level.

Figure 4-22 Cross section of the female pelvis taken through the lower part of the coccyx and the spine of the ischium. The superior gemellus muscles and the pectineus muscle appear in this section, and the coccygeus muscle terminates here. The gluteus maximus, gluteus minimus, and gluteus medius muscles all begin their insertions in the lower part of this section. The external os of the cervix is shown. The ureters empty into the bladder at the base.

Level of the right lobe of the liver (Figure 4-23). The right lobe of the liver, diaphragm, omentum, and muscles are shown.

Level of the liver and gallbladder (Figure 4-24). The diaphragm, right lobe of the liver, gallbladder, and perirenal fat area are shown. The costodiaphragmatic recess is seen superior to the diaphragm.

Level of the liver, gallbladder, and right kidney (Figure 4-25). The diaphragm, right lobe of the liver, gallbladder, and right kidney are seen. The perirenal fat and fascia are shown sur-

rounding the kidney. The caudate lobe of the liver is beginning to show.

Level of the liver, caudate lobe, and psoas muscle (Figure 4-26). The diaphragm, right lobe of the liver, caudate lobe, and neck of the gallbladder are seen. **Morison's pouch** is found anterior to the kidney and posterior to the inferior right lobe of the liver.

Level of the liver, duodenum, and pancreas (Figure 4-27). The portal vein and cystic duct are shown. The duodenum wraps around the head of the pancreas.

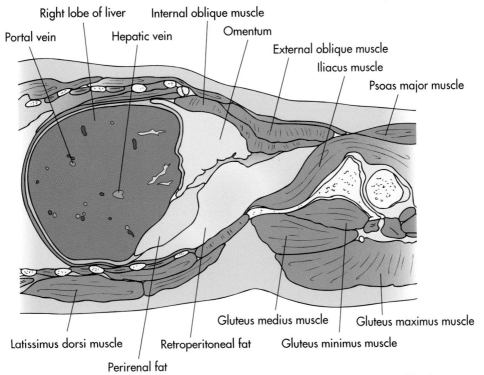

Figure 4-23   Sagittal section of the abdomen taken along the right abdominal border.

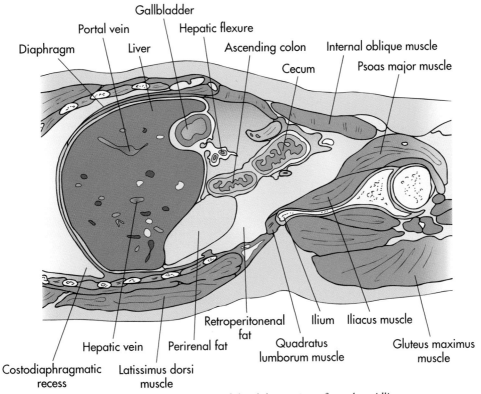

Figure 4-24   Sagittal section of the abdomen 8 cm from the midline.

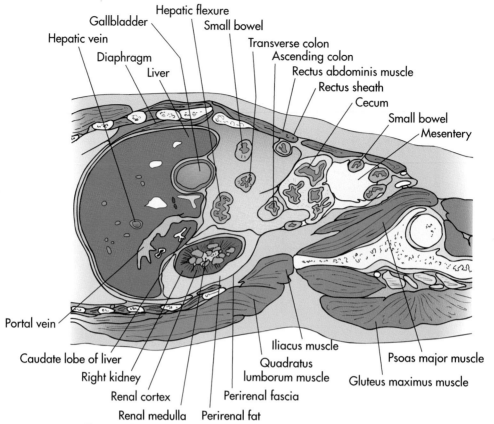

Figure 4-25 Sagittal section of the abdomen 7 cm from the midline.

Hepatic flexure
Gallbladder
Small bowel
Hepatic vein
Diaphragm
Transverse colon
Liver
Ascending colon
Rectus abdominis muscle
Rectus sheath
Cecum
Small bowel
Mesentery

Portal vein

Caudate lobe of liver
Right kidney
Renal cortex
Renal medulla
Perirenal fat
Perirenal fascia
Quadratus lumborum muscle
Iliacus muscle
Psoas major muscle
Gluteus maximus muscle

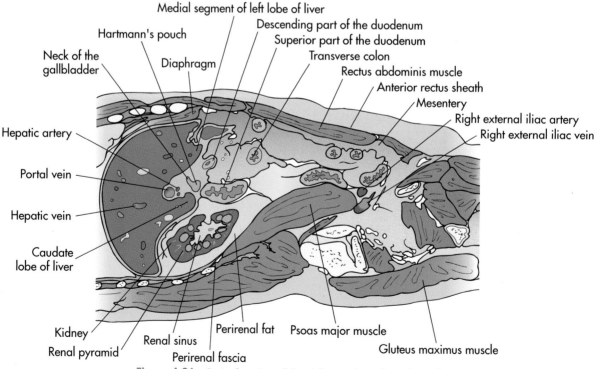

Figure 4-26 Sagittal section of the abdomen 6 cm from the midline.

Medial segment of left lobe of liver
Hartmann's pouch
Descending part of the duodenum
Superior part of the duodenum
Neck of the gallbladder
Diaphragm
Transverse colon
Rectus abdominis muscle
Anterior rectus sheath
Mesentery
Right external iliac artery
Right external iliac vein

Hepatic artery

Portal vein

Hepatic vein

Caudate lobe of liver

Kidney
Renal pyramid
Renal sinus
Perirenal fascia
Perirenal fat
Psoas major muscle
Gluteus maximus muscle

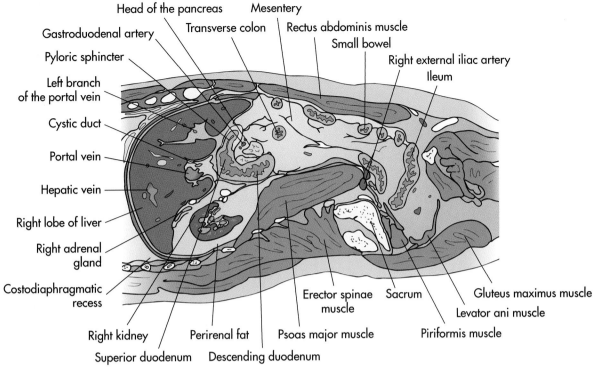

Head of the pancreas   Mesentery
Gastroduodenal artery   Transverse colon   Rectus abdominis muscle
Pyloric sphincter   Small bowel
Left branch   Right external iliac artery
of the portal vein   Ileum
Cystic duct
Portal vein
Hepatic vein
Right lobe of liver
Right adrenal
gland
Costodiaphragmatic
recess   Erector spinae   Sacrum   Gluteus maximus muscle
muscle   Levator ani muscle
Right kidney   Perirenal fat   Psoas major muscle   Piriformis muscle
Superior duodenum   Descending duodenum

Figure 4-27   Sagittal section of the abdomen 5 cm from the midline.

Level of the liver, inferior vena cava, pancreas, and gastro-duodenal artery (Figure 4-28). The gastroduodenal artery is the anterior border of the head of the pancreas. The **left portal vein** is shown to enter the left lobe of the liver.

Level of the inferior vena cava, left lobe of the liver, and pancreas (Figure 4-29). The inferior vena cava is shown along the posterior border of the liver. The pancreas lies anterior to the inferior vena cava and inferior to the portal vein.

Level of the hepatic vein and inferior vena cava, pancreas, and superior mesenteric vein (Figure 4-30). The superior mesenteric vein flows anterior to the uncinate portion of the pancreas and posterior to the body. The middle hepatic vein empties into the inferior vena cava. The falciform ligament is seen along the anterior border of the abdomen.

Level of the crus of the diaphragm and caudate lobe (Figure 4-31). The caudate lobe is seen posterior to the ligamentum venosum. The aorta is starting to come into view.

Level of the aorta and superior mesenteric artery (Figure 4-32). The **superior mesenteric artery (SMA)** arises from the anterior border of the aorta. The pancreas is seen anterior to the SMA; the splenic artery and vein form the posterior border. The left renal vein is posterior to the SMA and anterior to the aorta. The area of the lesser sac is shown.

Level of the spleen and left kidney (Figure 4-33). The spleen is shown just below the diaphragm in the left upper quadrant. The left kidney is inferior to the spleen. The tail of the pancreas lies anterior to the kidney and inferior to the **splenic hilum.**

GENERAL ABDOMINAL ULTRASOUND PROTOCOLS

It is the responsibility of the sonographer to ensure that patients are afforded the highest-quality care possible during their ultrasound procedure. This entails identifying the patient properly, ensuring confidentiality of information and patient privacy, providing proper nursing care, and maintaining clean and sanitary equipment and examination rooms.

The upper abdomen is scanned with high-resolution real-time ultrasound equipment. The transducer selected may be a sector or curved linear array or, in many cases, a combination of the two. The frequency of the transducer depends on the size, muscle, and fat composition of the patient. Generally a broad bandwidth transducer is used, with variations of 2.25 to 7.5 MHz, depending on the size of the patient and the depth of field.

TRANSVERSE SCANS

The horseshoe-shaped contour of the vertebral column should be well delineated to ensure sound penetration through the abdomen without obstruction from bowel gas interference.

The vascular structures, aorta, and inferior vena cava should be well seen anterior to the vertebral column as echo-free, or anechoic, structures.

The posterior border of the liver should be imaged as the transducer is angled in a cephalic to caudal direction from the dome of the liver to its inferior edge. This ensures that time gain compensation (TGC) is set correctly (at the posterior border of the liver). The overall gain should be adjusted to provide a smooth, homogeneous liver parenchyma

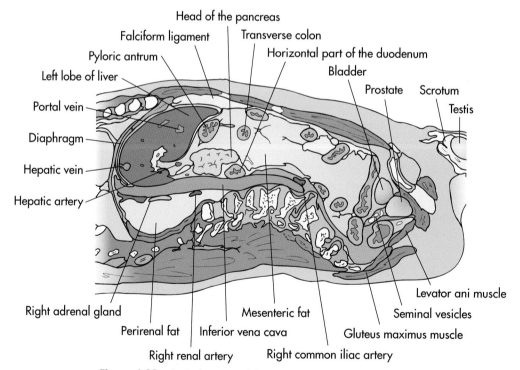

Figure 4-28   Sagittal section of the abdomen 4 cm from the midline.

Figure 4-29   Sagittal section of the abdomen 3 cm from the midline.

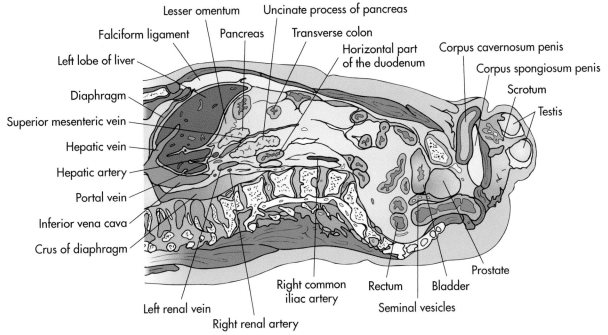

Figure 4-30   Sagittal section of the abdomen 2 cm from the midline.

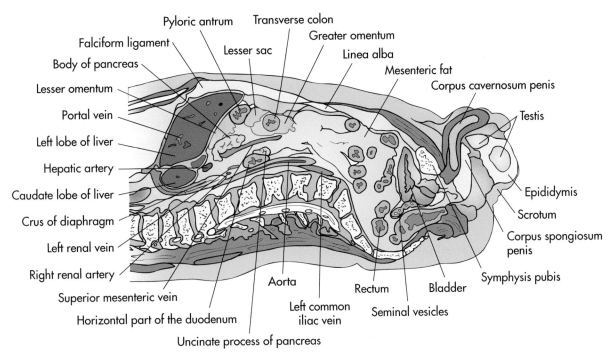

Figure 4-31   Sagittal section of the abdomen 1 cm from the midline.

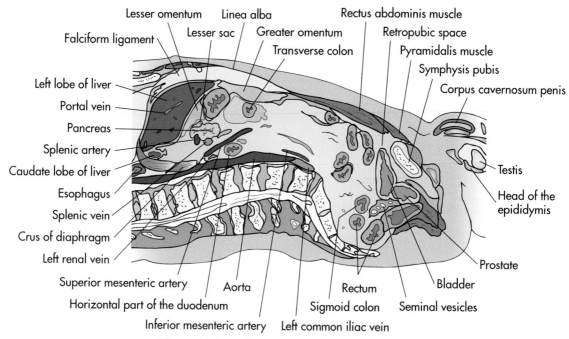

Figure 4-32   Midline sagittal section of the abdomen.

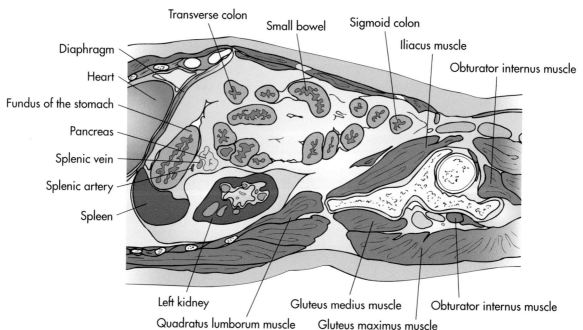

Figure 4-33   Sagittal section of the abdomen along the left abdominal border.

throughout. If there are too many echoes "outside the liver," the overall gain should be decreased. If the near gain is set too low, the anterior surface of the liver is not delineated.

LONGITUDINAL SCANS

The transducer should be angled from the diaphragm to the inferior border of the right lobe of the liver. The diaphragm should be well defined as a linear bright line superior to the dome of the liver. The liver parenchyma should be homoge-

neous and uniform throughout. If gain is maximum without good uniform penetration, a lower frequency transducer could be used to provide increased sensitivity. Vascular structures should be outlined with the patient in deep inspiration.

The baseline upper abdominal ultrasound examination includes a survey of the liver and **porta hepatis,** vascular structures, biliary system, pancreas, kidneys, spleen, and para-aortic area. If variations in anatomy or pathology are seen, multiple views are obtained over the area of interest.

LIVER AND PORTA HEPATIS PROTOCOL

The liver is examined as part of a comprehensive ultrasound evaluation of the abdomen (Figures 4-34 through 4-47) (Table 4-1). Abnormalities that can be evaluated include cirrhosis, fatty infiltration, hepatomegaly, portal hypertension, primary and metastatic tumors, abscess formation, and trauma. Pulsed and color flow Doppler are used to assess the hepatic vascular system.

TABLE 4-1	ABDOMINAL ULTRASOUND PROTOCOL: LIVER	
Organ	Scan Plane	Anatomy
Liver (Figures 4-34 to 4-47)	Trv Rt lobe/(dome) hepatic veins	Rt lobe/lung
		Lt lobe/lt portal vein
		Lt lobe/caudate lobe
		Rt lobe/portal veins (main, rt)
		Rt lobe/gallbladder/kidney
	Long	Lt lobe/aorta
		Lt lobe/caudate lobe/ IVC
		Rt lobe/dome (diaphragm)
		Rt lobe/lung
		Rt lobe/portal vein
		Rt lobe/kidney (measure Rt lobe)

Lt, Left; *IVC,* inferior vena cava; *Rt,* right; *Long,* longitudinal; *Trv,* transverse.

Figure 4-34 Transverse image at the right lobe of the liver *(L)* at the liver-lung interface.

Figure 4-35 Transverse image at the dome of the liver *(L)* in full inspiration to demonstrate the hepatic veins *(HV)* flowing into the inferior vena cava *(IVC)*.

Figure 4-36 Transverse image of the right lobe of the liver *(L)* with the right hepatic vein *(HV)*.

Figure 4-37 Transverse image of the left lobe of liver *(LLL)* and left portal vein *(arrows)*.

Figure 4-38 Transverse image of the liver, main portal vein *(MPV)*, and right portal vein with bifurcation of anterior *(ARPV)* and posterior branches *(PRPV)*.

Figure 4-39   Transverse image of liver *(L)*, gallbladder *(gb)*, and right kidney *(RK)*.

Figure 4-42   Longitudinal image of tip of left lobe of liver *(LLL)*.

Figure 4-40   Longitudinal image of left lobe of liver *(LLL)*.

Figure 4-43   Longitudinal image of left lobe of liver *(LLL)*, caudate lobe *(CL)*, ligamentum venosum *(arrow)*, and inferior vena cava *(IVC)*.

Figure 4-41   Longitudinal image of left lobe of liver *(LLL)*, aorta *(A)*, and superior mesenteric vein *(arrow)*.

Figure 4-44   Longitudinal image of left lobe of liver *(LLL)*, portal vein *(arrows)*, and inferior vena cava *(IVC)*.

1. Patient preparation: Nothing by mouth (NPO) for at least 6 hours.
2. Transducer selection: 2.5 to 4 MHz curvilinear/sector, or 3 to 5 MHz curvilinear. Lower frequency transducers are often necessary in patients with fatty infiltration or cirrhosis.
3. Patient position: Supine and decubitus as necessary.
4. Images and observations should include the following:
   - The echogenicity of the liver parenchyma should be compared with that of the renal parenchyma.

- The hepatic venous, inferior vena cava, and right and left portal structures should be imaged.
- The **ligamentum teres** should be identified in the left lobe of the liver.
- The dome of the right lobe of the liver should be surveyed with the patient in deep inspiration.
- The right hemidiaphragm and right pleural gutter should be examined.
- The main lobar fissure, as it projects from the **right portal vein (RPV)** to the neck of the gallbladder, should be imaged.

Figure 4-48   Longitudinal image of gallbladder (gb), main lobar fissure (arrow), and portal vein (curved arrow).

Figure 4-45   Longitudinal oblique image of right lobe of liver (RLL) and right portal vein (arrow).

Figure 4-49   Longitudinal image of gallbladder (gb), including neck.

Figure 4-46   Longitudinal image of right lobe of liver (RLL) and right hepatic vein (arrow). This long axis view is used to measure the long axis of the liver from the diaphragm to the tip.

- Assessment of the patency and direction of flow of the main, right, and left portal veins.
- Assessment of the patency of the right, middle, and left hepatic veins (HV).
- Assessment of the patency of the umbilical vein (recanalized umbilical vein) or other collateral vessels.
- Assessment of the patency of surgically or angiographically placed shunts.
- Performance of pulsed Doppler analysis of the hepatic artery with resistance measurements.

BILIARY SYSTEM PROTOCOL

Ultrasound examinations of the gallbladder and bile ducts are performed to determine cholelithiasis, changes secondary to acute and chronic cholecystitis, obstruction, and primary or metastatic tumor involvement. The examination is performed as part of a comprehensive general abdominal evaluation (Figures 4-48 through 4-53) (Table 4-2).

1. Patient preparation: NPO for at least 6 hours.
2. Transducer selection: 2.5 to 5 MHz curvilinear.
3. Patient position: Supine and decubitus.
4. Images and observations should include the following:
   - The fundus, body, and neck should be surveyed.
   - Gallbladder wall thickness (normal is less than 3 mm) should be recorded. If thickened, the wall should be measured in the transverse plane at the anterior wall with the transducer perpendicular to the anterior wall.

Figure 4-47   Longitudinal image of lateral segment of the right lobe of liver (RLL) and vascular structures. Diaphragm (arrows).

- Liver size in a parasagittal scan demonstrating the diaphragm and tip of the right lobe of the liver should be recorded.
- The size of any demonstrated masses should be recorded.

The presence of ascites (include the four quadrants of the abdomen) should be evaluated and recorded.

Doppler of the vascular structures in the liver if pathology is present:

Figure 4-50   Transverse image of gallbladder *(gb)*.

Figure 4-51   Transverse decubitus image of gallbladder *(gb)*, inferior vena cava *(IVC)*, and aorta *(A)*.

Figure 4-52   Longitudinal image of common bile duct *(arrow)* anterior to portal vein *(pv)* that lies anterior to the inferior vena cava *(IVC)*.

- The presence of echogenic foci (e.g., stones or polyps) within the gallbladder lumen should be evaluated. If echogenic foci are present, the sonographer should attempt to demonstrate acoustic shadowing and mobility.
- The common bile duct should be imaged in at least the oblique long-axis plane because it lies anterior to the **main portal vein (MPV)** before coursing posterior to the head of the pancreas.
- The transverse scan of the porta hepatis may help delineate the portal vein from the common duct (anterior and to the right) and hepatic artery (anterior and to the left).

Figure 4-53   Transverse image of portal triad in the center of the image: portal vein *(pv)* with common bile duct *(curved arrow)* anterior and lateral; hepatic artery *(arrow)* anterior and medial; inferior vena cava *(IVC)*; and aorta *(A)*.

TABLE 4-2	ABDOMINAL ULTRASOUND PROTOCOL: GALLBLADDER	
Organ	Scan Plane	Anatomy
GB (Supine and LLD)	Long	Body/fundus
(Figures 4-48 to 4-51)	Trv	Body/neck (measure wall)
		Body/neck
CBD	Trv	Portal triad
(Figures 4-52 and 4-53)	Long	Measure duct

CBD, Common bile duct; *GB,* gallbladder; *LLD,* left lateral decubitus; *Long,* longitudinal; *Trv,* transverse.

- Visualization of the intrahepatic ducts is not possible unless dilation is present. Ductal dilation may be seen as the liver is scanned, demonstrating right and left branches of the portal vein as the hepatic ducts follow a parallel course.
- To examine gallstones, the focal point of the transducer is placed at the region of the posterior gallbladder wall and the gain reduced. This facilitates demonstration of acoustic shadowing.

PANCREAS PROTOCOL

The pancreas is examined as part of a comprehensive general abdominal study (Figures 4-54 through 4-59) (Table 4-3). Specific indications for pancreatic scanning include abdominal pain, clinically manifested acute or chronic pancreatitis, abnormal laboratory values, cholecystitis, or obstructive jaundice. The examination determines the presence of cystic and solid masses, biliary and ductal dilation, and the presence of extrapancreatic masses and fluid collections.

1. Patient preparation: NPO for at least 6 hours; may need to give water to fill the stomach as a window to image the pancreas.
2. Transducer selection: 2.5 to 5 MHz curvilinear.
3. Patient position: Supine, decubitus, or upright.
4. Images and observations should include the following:

Figure 4-54 Transverse image of pancreas *(p)* as it lies anterior to superior mesenteric artery *(arrow)* and vein *(curved arrow)*. The aorta *(A)* and inferior vena cava *(IVC)* are anterior to the horseshoe shape of the spine.

Figure 4-57 Longitudinal image of the pancreas (posterior to the gallbladder) with the common bile duct *(arrows)* beginning to move posterior to join the pancreatic duct.

Figure 4-55 Transverse image of head *(h)*, body *(b)*, and tail *(t)* of the pancreas. The gastroduodenal artery *(curved arrow)* is the anterolateral border of the head; the common bile duct *(arrow)* is the posterior lateral border of the head.

Figure 4-58 Longitudinal image of the superior mesenteric vein *(smv)* as it flows anterior to the uncinate process *(arrow)* and posterior to the head of the pancreas *(curved arrows)*.

Figure 4-56 Transverse image of the pancreas; a sliver of splenic vein *(arrows)* lies posterior to the body and tail.

Figure 4-59 Longitudinal image of the body of the pancreas *(arrows)* anterior to the aorta *(A)*.

- The head, body, and tail should be well delineated once the celiac axis, superior mesenteric artery and vein, aorta, and inferior vena cava are identified. (Often the lie of the pancreas makes it difficult to image the gland in one plane; the tail may be seen on an image that is more superior than the head of the gland.)

- Transverse scans along the region of the splenic vein should be performed to demonstrate the body and tail of the pancreas.
- The pancreatic duct may be seen on the transverse scan as it courses through the body of the gland.

TABLE 4-3 ABDOMINAL ULTRASOUND PROTOCOL: PANCREAS

Organ	Scan Plane	Anatomy
Pancreas (Figures 4-54 to 4-59)	Trv	Head/IVC/SMV Body and tail/ SMV/ SMA
	Long	Head/portal vein/ IVC Body and tail/aorta

IVC, Inferior vena cava; *Long*, longitudinal; *SMA*, superior mesenteric artery; *SMV*, superior mesenteric vein; *Trv*, transverse.

- The longitudinal view of the pancreatic head lies anterior to the inferior vena cava and inferior to the portal vein.
- The superior mesenteric vein may be seen to course anterior to the uncinate process of the head and posterior to the body.
- The pancreatic tail may be seen as gentle but firm pressure is applied to the abdomen to display overlying gas in the antrum of the stomach or transverse colon. The tail may also be seen with the patient in a right decubitus position as the transducer is angled through the spleen and left kidney; the pancreatic tail is anterior to the left kidney.
- The presence of dilated pancreatic or biliary ducts should be assessed and their size measured.
- The presence of cystic or solid masses should be assessed.
- The presence of peripancreatic nodes should be assessed.
- The presence of peripancreatic fluid collections (e.g., pseudocysts) should be assessed.
- The presence of any pancreatic calcifications detected should be recorded.

SPLEEN PROTOCOL

Ultrasound examinations are performed to assess overall splenic architecture, to examine or detect intrasplenic masses, to examine the splenic hilum and vasculature, and to determine splenic size (Figures 4-60 and 4-61) (Table 4-4).

1. Patient preparation: NPO for at least 6 hours.
2. Transducer selection: 2.5 to 4 MHz curvilinear.
3. Patient position: Steep right lateral decubitus or right lateral.
4. Images and observations include the following:
   - Coronal scans of the long axis of the spleen should be performed.
   - The left hemidiaphragm, splenic hilus, and upper and lower borders of the spleen should be demonstrated.
   - The splenic length should be measured.
   - The texture of the spleen should be compared with that of the liver. The splenic parenchyma should be homogeneous with the liver.
   - A transverse scan of the spleen at the level of the splenic hilus should be performed. The sonographer should look for increased vascularity or splenic nodes.

TABLE 4-4 ABDOMINAL ULTRASOUND PROTOCOL: SPLEEN

Organ	Scan Plane	Anatomy
Spleen (Figures 4-60 and 4-61)	Long	Spleen/LK (measure length)
	Trv	Splenic hilum

LK, Left kidney; *Long*, longitudinal; *Trv*, transverse.

Figure 4-60   Longitudinal image of spleen *(Sp)*. The long axis is measured from the crossbars.

Figure 4-61   Transverse image of spleen *(Sp)*.

RENAL PROTOCOL

Ultrasound examinations are performed to assess overall renal architecture, examine or detect intrarenal and extrarenal masses, document hydronephrosis, detect calculi, examine renal vasculature, and determine renal size and echogenicity (Figures 4-62 through 4-73) (Table 4-5). The condition of the bladder and ureters is evaluated as part of the examination protocol.

1. Patient preparation: Patient should be hydrated, unless contraindicated.
2. Transducer selection: 2.5 to 4 MHz curvilinear.
3. Patient position: Supine or decubitus.
4. Images and observations should include the following:
   - The right kidney should be demonstrated in a supine or slightly decubitus position. The liver should be used as the acoustic window.

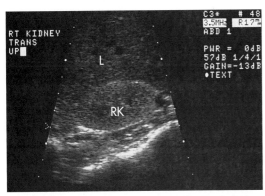

Figure 4-62   Transverse image of upper pole of right kidney (RK); liver (L).

Figure 4-65   Longitudinal image of right kidney (RK).

Figure 4-63   Transverse image of midright kidney with the renal vein (arrows).

Figure 4-66   Longitudinal image of right kidney (RK) with measurements of long axis.

Figure 4-64   Transverse image of lower pole of right kidney (RK). The psoas muscle is medial to the kidney (arrows).

Figure 4-67   Longitudinal image of right kidney (RK).

TABLE 4-5	ABDOMINAL ULTRASOUND PROTOCOL: RENAL	
Organ	Scan Plane	Anatomy
Kidneys (Figures 4-62 to 4-73)	Trv	Upper pole
		Mid (at pelvis)
		Lower pole
	Long	Mid (measure length)
		Lateral
		Medial

Long, Longitudinal; *Trv,* transverse.

Figure 4-68   Transverse image of upper pole of left kidney (LK) and spleen (Sp).

Figure 4-69   Transverse image of midleft kidney *(LK)*.

Figure 4-72   Longitudinal image of left kidney.

Figure 4-70   Transverse image of lower pole of left kidney *(LK)* and psoas muscle *(arrows)*.

Figure 4-73   Longitudinal image of left kidney *(LK)* with measurement of long axis.

Figure 4-71   Longitudinal image of left kidney *(LK)*.

- The bladder wall should be assessed for thickness or irregularities, and the presence of focal lesions recorded.
- If the bladder is large or if hydronephrosis is present, the evaluation of ureteral jets should be noted within the bladder (with color). Ureteral jets should also be examined in patients with renal calculus or hematuria.

Doppler flow analysis of the renal area:

- Image the origin of the renal arteries, measure resistive index and acceleration time of the pulsed waveform.
- All Doppler studies of the kidneys include pulsed Doppler tracings with resistance measurements taken of the main, interlobar, and arcuate arteries.
- The patency of the main renal vein should be determined.

AORTA AND ILIAC ARTERY PROTOCOL

The aorta is examined primarily to determine the presence of aneurysmal dilation (Figures 4-74 through 4-79) (Table 4-6). Aortic aneurysms are defined as those with vessel diameters greater than 3 cm or with focal dilation of the vessel. Iliac aneurysms are defined as vessels with diameters greater than 2 cm. Aneurysms above 5 cm or those with documented rapid rates of expansion have an increased risk of catastrophic rupture. The physician must be made aware of these patients before they leave the department.

- The left kidney should be surveyed with the patient in a right lateral decubitus position. The spleen should be used as the acoustic window.
- The renal cortex and medulla should be well delineated.
- Longitudinal scans should be made through the midline and lateral and medial borders. Measurement of the long axis should be made from upper to lower poles.
- Transverse scans should be made through the upper pole, middle section at the level of the renal pelvis, and lower pole.
- The bladder should be imaged in a longitudinal and transverse plane.

Figure 4-74   Longitudinal image of the proximal aorta *(A)* anterior to the spine.

Figure 4-77   Transverse image of the high abdominal aorta *(A)* at the level of the superior mesenteric artery *(arrow)*.

Figure 4-75   Longitudinal image of the aorta *(A)* with the celiac axis *(ca)* and superior mesenteric artery *(sma)*.

Figure 4-78   Transverse image of the midabdominal aorta *(A)* at the level of the renal vessels (left renal artery—one *arrow*; right renal artery—two *arrows*).

Figure 4-76   Longitudinal image of the distal aorta *(A)*.

Figure 4-79   Transverse image of the distal aorta near the bifurcation *(arrows)*.

1. Patient preparation: NPO for at least 6 hours.
2. Transducer selection: 2.5 to 4 MHz curvilinear.
3. Patient position: Supine or slightly decubitus.
4. Images and observations should include the following:
   - The aorta should be imaged in the longitudinal plane from the diaphragm to below the bifurcation at the iliac junction.
   - Transverse scans should be made at the level of the diaphragm, superior to the renal arteries, inferior to the

TABLE 4-6	ABDOMINAL ULTRASOUND PROTOCOL: AORTA		
Organ		Scan Plane	Anatomy
Aorta		Long	Prox, mid, and distal
(Figures 4-74 to 4-79)		Trv	Prox, mid, and distal

Prox, Proximal; *Long,* longitudinal; *Trv,* transverse.

renal arteries, and at the bifurcation. Scans of the iliac arteries should be made.

- Lymph adenopathy should also be evaluated because the lymph nodes lie anterior to the vessels.
- The inferior vena cava is best imaged on a longitudinal plane through the right lobe of the liver with the patient in full inspiration.
- An alternative imaging plane is the slight decubitus view. The patient rolls onto his or her left side; the transducer is longitudinal and sharply angled from the right lobe of the liver to the left iliac wing. This allows the sonographer to image the inferior vena cava "anterior" to the aorta. It usually allows the sonographer to follow the entrance and exit of the renal veins and arteries into the great vessels and provides an excellent window to perform color flow or Doppler interrogation of the renal vessels.
- Outer to outer measurements should be taken of the aorta in the longitudinal and transverse planes.

If an aneurysm is present:

- Longitudinal scans of each iliac vessel from the bifurcation to the most distal segment should be taken.
- Transverse scans of the iliacs below the bifurcation should be taken.

THYROID PROTOCOL

The role of ultrasound in evaluating the thyroid is primarily limited to differentiating cystic masses from solid masses, recording the number of masses, assessing overall echogenicity and homogeneity, and evaluating the size of the gland. It is normally performed as a result of an abnormal physical examination or to correlate with nuclear medicine scans.

1. Patient preparation: None.
2. Transducer selection: 8 to 12 MHz linear.
3. Patient position: Place a rolled sheet under the shoulders to elevate the neck.
4. Images and observations should include the following:
   - Longitudinal scans of each lobe (lateral, middle, and medial portions) should be performed. Landmarks include the carotid artery laterally and the trachea medially.
   - Transverse scans of each lobe, including the most inferior, middle, and superior portions of the gland, should be performed.
   - Transverse and longitudinal scans of the thyroid isthmus should be performed.
   - Measurements of the gland and any detected nodules should be performed.
   - If possible, split-screen images of the right and left lobes should be made for texture comparison.

PARATHYROID PROTOCOL

The role of ultrasound in evaluating the parathyroid is primarily to detect adenomas. The examination is normally performed as a result of abnormal calcium levels or an abnormal physical examination. There are normally four parathyroid glands, two on each side at the upper and lower aspects of the thyroid gland. It should be noted, however, that parathyroid adenomas can be positioned distinctly separate from the thyroid gland. Use the thyroid protocol.

BREAST PROTOCOL

The role of ultrasound in evaluating the breast is primarily to determine if a mass is a simple cyst or a complex or solid lesion. The patient generally has a palpable mass or an abnormal mammogram without a palpable mass, is pregnant, or has other complications that may prevent her from receiving a mammogram. There are multiple approaches to evaluating the breast. Please refer to the breast chapter for further delineation. This protocol is specific to evaluating a palpable breast mass.

1. Patient preparation: None.
2. Transducer selection: 8 to 12 MHz. The linear array transducer allows a larger field of view.
3. Patient position: Supine or shallow oblique is most frequently used. Steep oblique or decubitus positions are used for lesions that are more lateral.
4. Images and observations should include the following:
   - If the lesion is very superficial, an acoustically matched stand-off pad may be used with gel placed on the skin and the pad to afford adequate contact. (Standoff pad thickness should not exceed 1.0 cm because of the elevation plane focus of the transducer.)
   - All scans should be labeled in the proper zone including the clock position, distance from nipple (1,2,3), and depth to the chest (A, B, C).
   - Scans should be made in the radial and antiradial planes over the area of interest.
   - The gain should be adjusted to note the borders, through-transmission, and internal echo pattern of the lesion. Gain settings should demonstrate breast fat as medium level gray shades.
   - The size of the lesion should be measured.

SCROTAL PROTOCOL

High-resolution ultrasound imaging is the primary screening modality for most testicular pathology. Applications include inflammatory processes of the testes and epididymis, tumors, trauma, torsion, hydrocele, varicocele, hernias, spermatoceles, and undescended testes.

1. Patient preparation: None.
2. Transducer selection: 8 to 12 MHz linear array.
3. Patient position: Supine. (Valsalva maneuver or upright position to check for varicocele.)
4. Images and observations should include the following:
   - Gray scale
   - Long testicle (include medial, mid, and lateral)
   - Long epididymis
   - Anteroposterior (AP) and long measurements of above anatomy
   - Transverse scan of each testis (upper, mid, lower)
   - Transverse scan of head of epididymis

- Include AP and transverse measurement of the middle pole of the testicles
- If possible, a split-screen image should be obtained to compare the echogenicity of each testis
- Images of the extratesticular area should be obtained to determine the presence of hydrocele, hernia, or other conditions

Doppler flow analysis of the scrotal area:

- When indicated, color and pulsed Doppler analysis of intratesticular flow with resistance measurements should be obtained.
- The scanning instrument should be optimized for slow flow detection (e.g., decrease pulse repetition frequency/scale, lower filters, or increase gain or power).

ABDOMINAL DOPPLER

Doppler ultrasound has been used for many decades to evaluate cardiovascular flow patterns. As in other areas of ultrasound, there have been many improvements in the technology, such as the development of pulsed wave Doppler, spectral analysis of the returning wave form, and color flow mapping. These advances in Doppler instrumentation, combined with high-resolution imaging of the vessels, have led to "duplex scanning equipment," which combines these modalities into a single probe.

Doppler is used to ascertain the presence or absence of flow. It can be used to differentiate vessels from nonvascular structures with confusingly similar images (e.g., common duct from hepatic artery, arterial aneurysm from a cyst). The determination and direction of flow may also be of diagnostic value. Once the presence and direction of flow have been determined, spectral analysis of the flow gives further information on flow velocity and turbulence. Increased velocity and poststenotic turbulence may be seen in vascular stenoses. In postoperative patients, increased turbulence alone may be present at the site of a graft anastomosis with the native vessel. The evaluation of the shape of the waveform, with comparison of the systolic and diastolic components, may give information on increased vascular impedance, such as is seen in renal transplant rejection.

The specific Doppler patterns of the vascular system are described in Chapter 5. Only brief comments are given in this section.

DOPPLER SCANNING TECHNIQUES

The normal, routine longitudinal, transverse, coronal, and oblique scans of vascular structures are used to produce adequate images. Doppler techniques supplement the routine examination by permitting blood flow within those vessels to be detected and characterized. Flow toward the transducer is positive, or above the baseline, whereas flow away from the transducer is negative, or below the baseline. Arterial flow pulsates with the cardiac cycle and shows its maximal peak during the systolic part of the cycle. Venous flow shows no pulsatility and has lower flow than arterial structures. A phasic pattern

may be seen in the hepatic veins (near the heart) that is associated with overload of the right ventricle.

As seen in echocardiography, many of the abdominal vessels have characteristic waveforms. If the sample volume can be directed parallel to the flow, quantification of peak gradients can be estimated. However, in the tortuous course of most vascular structures, this is very difficult.

Pulsed Doppler is the most common instrumentation used to evaluate abdominal flow patterns. This equipment uses combined real-time and pulsed or continuous wave Doppler. The pulsed Doppler allows placement of the small sample volume within the vascular structure of interest by means of a trackball.

AORTA

- The Doppler flow in the pulsatile aorta demonstrates arterial signals in the patent lumen. If the vessel were occluded, no arterial signals would be recorded.
- *Aortic dissection and pseudoaneurysms:* Flow, often with two distinct patterns, can be seen in the true and false lumens by Doppler ultrasound. The development of a pseudoaneurysm as a complication of an aortic graft procedure may be difficult to determine if pulsations are present or transmitted through the aortic wall. Doppler ultrasound may be useful to detect flow within the pseudoaneurysm.

INFERIOR VENA CAVA

- Decreased velocity. The Doppler waveform recorded in the inferior vena cava shows a lower flow than is found in arterial structures. The flow is increased in the presence of thrombus formation.

PORTAL VENOUS SYSTEM

- Doppler flow patterns can be used to diagnose varices or collaterals in the **portal venous system.**
- Doppler flow patterns can be used to evaluate changes of flow patterns occurring in the course of portal hypertension.
- As liver function improves, normal hepatopetal flow is restored.
- If pressures worsen, there may be increased shunting away from the liver.
- If a shunt is present in the porta hepatis, Doppler may be useful to determine the patency of the shunt.

PORTAL HYPERTENSION

Portal hypertension is caused by increased resistance to venous flow through the liver. It is associated with cirrhosis, hepatic vein thrombosis, portal vein thrombosis, and thrombosis of the inferior vena cava. Ultrasound findings include dilation of the portal, splenic, and mesenteric veins; reversal of portal venous blood flow; and the development of **collateral vessels** (e.g., patent umbilical vein, gastric varices, or splenorenal shunting).

The protocol for portal hypertension includes:

- Performing the routine abdominal imaging protocol.
- Assessing for the presence of ascites.

- Obtaining diameter measurements of the splenic and main portal veins on inspiration and expiration.
- Assessing for the presence of collateral blood vessels (splenic hilum, porta hepatis, umbilical vein).
- Determining the flow direction of the portal veins (main, left, and right portal veins) and splenic and superior mesenteric veins.
- Assessing for the presence of splenorenal shunting.
- Assessing for patency of the umbilical vein.
- Determining the patency and direction of flow in the IVC and hepatic veins.
- Assessing and documenting the patency of surgically placed shunts.

SELECTED BIBLIOGRAPHY

Curry R, Tempkin B: *Sonography: introduction to normal structures and function,* ed 2, St. Louis, 2004, Mosby.

Kremkau F: *Diagnostic ultrasound: principles and instruments,* ed 7, Philadelphia, 2006, WB Saunders.

Mittelstaedt CA: *Abdominal ultrasound,* New York, 1987, Churchill Livingstone.

Needleman L, Rifkin M: Vascular ultrasonography: abdominal applications, *Radiol Clin North Am* 24:461, 1986.

Sanders RC: *Clinical sonography,* Boston, 1995, Little, Brown.

Swobodnik W and others: *Atlas of ultrasound anatomy,* New York, 1991, Thieme.

CHAPTER 5

The Vascular System

Sandra L. Hagen-Ansert

OBJECTIVES

- Name the three layers of the artery
- Explain the difference between an artery and a vein
- Name the five sections of the aorta
- List the major anterior and lateral branches of the aorta
- List the tributaries to the inferior vena cava
- Describe the portal system
- Describe the various types of aneurysm formation
- Name what ultrasound characteristics are important to know when evaluating an abdominal aortic aneurysm
- Name the clinical symptoms associated with abdominal aortic aneurysm
- List the types of dissection possible
- Name the factors that may cause a pulsatile abdominal mass
- Describe the appearance of tumor or thrombus in the vascular system
- Describe the normal and abnormal Doppler patterns of the vascular structures

ANATOMY OF VASCULAR STRUCTURES

AORTA
ROOT OF THE AORTA
ASCENDING AORTA
DESCENDING AORTA
ABDOMINAL AORTA
ABDOMINAL AORTIC BRANCHES
COMMON ILIAC ARTERIES
ANTERIOR BRANCHES OF THE ABDOMINAL AORTA
LATERAL BRANCHES OF THE ABDOMINAL AORTA
DORSAL AORTIC BRANCHES

INFERIOR VENA CAVA
LATERAL TRIBUTARIES TO THE INFERIOR VENA CAVA
ANTERIOR TRIBUTARIES TO THE INFERIOR VENA CAVA

PORTAL VENOUS SYSTEM
PORTAL VEIN
SPLENIC VEIN
SUPERIOR MESENTERIC VEIN
INFERIOR MESENTERIC VEIN

VASCULAR PATHOPHYSIOLOGY
AORTIC ABNORMALITIES
INFERIOR VENA CAVA ABNORMALITIES
RENAL VEIN OBSTRUCTION
RENAL VEIN THROMBOSIS

ABDOMINAL DOPPLER TECHNIQUES
BLOOD FLOW ANALYSIS
DOPPLER TECHNIQUE
DOPPLER FLOW PATTERNS IN THE ABDOMINAL VESSELS

KEY TERMS

abdominal aortic aneurysm – permanent localized dilation of an artery, with an increase in diameter of 1.5 times its normal diameter

anastomosis – a communication between two blood vessels without any intervening capillary network.

aorta (AO) – largest arterial structure in the body; arises from the left ventricle to supply blood to the head, upper and lower extremities, and abdominopelvic cavity

arteries – vascular structures that carry blood away from the heart

arteriosclerosis – a disease of the arterial vessels marked by thickening, hardening, and loss of elasticity in the arterial walls

arteriovenous fistula – communication between an artery and vein

atherosclerosis – condition in which the aortic wall becomes irregular from plaque formation

Budd-Chiari syndrome – thrombosis of the hepatic veins

capillaries – minute vessels that connect the arterial and venous systems

cavernous transformation of the portal vein – periportal collateral channels in patients with chronic portal vein obstruction

common hepatic artery – arises from the celiac trunk to supply the liver

common iliac arteries – the abdominal aorta bifurcates at the level of the umbilicus into common iliac arteries to supply blood to the lower extremities

cystic medial necrosis – weakening of the arterial wall

dissecting aneurysm – tear in the intima and/or media of the abdominal aorta

Doppler sample volume – the sonographer selects the exact site to record Doppler signals and sets the sample volume (gate) at this site

fusiform aneurysm – circumferential enlargement of a vessel with tapering at both ends

gastroduodenal artery (GDA) – branch of the common hepatic artery to supply the stomach and duodenum

hepatic veins (HV) – three large veins that drain the liver and empty into the inferior vena cava at the level of the diaphragm

hepatofugal – flow away from the liver

hepatopetal – flow toward the liver

inferior mesenteric artery (IMA) – arises from the anterior aortic wall at the level of the third or fourth lumbar vertebra to supply the left transverse colon, descending colon, sigmoid colon, and rectum

inferior mesenteric vein (IMV) – drains the left third of the colon and upper colon and joins the splenic vein

inferior vena cava (IVC) – largest venous abdominal vessel that conveys blood from the body below the diaphragm to the right atrium of the heart

left gastric artery (LGA) – arises from the celiac axis to supply the stomach and lower third of the esophagus

left hepatic artery – small branch supplying the caudate and left lobes of the liver

left renal artery (LRA) – arises from the posterolateral wall of the aorta directly into the hilus of the kidney

left renal vein (LRV) – leaves the renal hilum, travels anterior to the aorta and posterior to the superior mesenteric artery to enter the lateral wall of the inferior vena cava

Marfan's syndrome – hereditary disorder of connective tissue, bones, muscles, ligaments, and skeletal structures

nonresistive – vessels that have high diastolic component and supply organs that need constant perfusion (i.e., internal carotid artery, hepatic artery, and renal artery)

portal vein (PV) – formed by the union of the superior mesenteric vein and splenic vein near the porta hepatis of the liver

portal venous hypertension – most commonly results from intrinsic liver disease; however, it also arises from obstruction of the portal vein, hepatic veins, inferior vena cava, or prolonged congestive heart failure. May cause flow reversal to the liver, thrombosis of the portal system, or cavernous transformation of the portal vein.

pseudoaneurysm – pulsatile hematoma that results from leakage of blood into soft tissues abutting the punctured artery with fibrous encapsulation and failure of the vessel wall to heal

resistive – vessels that have little or reversed flow in diastole and supply organs that do not need a constant blood supply (e.g., external carotid artery and brachial arteries)

resistive index – peak systole minus peak diastole divided by peak systole ($S - D/S = RI$); an RI of 0.7 or less indicates good perfusion; an RI of 0.7 or higher indicates decreased perfusion

right gastric artery (RGA) – supplies the stomach

right hepatic artery (RHA) – supplies the gallbladder via the cystic artery

right renal artery (RRA) – arises from the lateral wall of the aorta, travels posterior to the inferior vena cava to supply the kidney

right renal vein (RRV) – leaves the renal hilum to enter the lateral wall of the inferior vena cava

saccular aneurysm – localized dilatation of the vessel

spectral broadening – increased turbulence is seen within the spectral tracing that indicates flow disturbance

splenic artery (SA) – arises from the celiac trunk to supply the spleen

splenic vein (SV) – drains the spleen; travels horizontally across the abdomen (posterior to the pancreas) to join the superior mesenteric vein to form the portal vein

superior mesenteric artery (SMA) – arises inferior to the celiac axis to supply the proximal half of the colon and the small intestine

superior mesenteric vein (SMV) – drains the proximal half of the colon and small intestine; travels vertically (anterior to the inferior vena cava) to join the splenic vein to form the portal veins

TIPS – transjugular intrahepatic portosystemic shunt

tunica adventitia – outer layer of the vascular system; contains the vasa vasorum

tunica intima – inner layer of the vascular system

tunica media – middle layer of the vascular system; veins have thinner tunica media than arteries

vasa vasorum – the tiny arteries and veins that supply the walls of blood vessels

veins – collapsible vascular structures that carry blood back to the heart

---

Knowing the vascular structures within the abdomen, retroperitoneum, and pelvis is extremely useful for identifying specific organ structures. To understand the origin and anatomic variation of the major arterial and venous structures, the sonographer must be able to identify the anatomy correctly on the ultrasound image.

ANATOMY OF VASCULAR STRUCTURES

The function of the circulatory system, along with the heart and lymphatics, is to transport gases, nutrient materials, and other essential substances to the tissues and subsequently transport waste products from the cells to the appropriate sites for excretion.

Blood is carried away from the heart by the arteries and returned from the tissues to the heart by the veins. Arteries divide into progressively smaller branches, the smallest of which are the arterioles. These lead into the capillaries, which are minute vessels that branch and form a network where the exchange of materials between blood and tissue fluid takes place. After the blood passes through the capillaries, it is collected in the small veins, or venules. These small vessels unite to form larger vessels that eventually return the blood to the heart for recirculation.

A typical artery in cross section consists of the following three layers (Figure 5-1):

- **Tunica intima** (inner layer), which itself consists of the following three layers: a layer of endothelial cells lining the arterial passage (lumen), a layer of delicate connective tissue, and an elastic layer made up of a network of elastic fibers
- **Tunica media** (middle layer), which consists of smooth muscle fibers with elastic and collagenous tissue
- **Tunica adventitia** (external layer), which consists of loose connective tissue with bundles of smooth muscle fibers and elastic tissue. The **vasa vasorum** comprises the tiny arteries and veins that supply the walls of blood vessels.

Specific differences exist between the arteries and the veins. The **arteries** are hollow elastic tubes that carry blood away from the heart. They are enclosed within a sheath that includes a vein and nerve. The smaller arteries contain less elastic tissue and more smooth muscles than the larger arteries. The elasticity of the larger arteries is important in maintaining a steady blood flow.

The **veins** are hollow collapsible tubes with diminished tunica media that carry blood toward the heart. The veins appear collapsed because they have little elastic tissue or muscle within their walls. Veins have a larger total diameter than the arteries, and they move blood more slowly. The veins contain special valves that prevent backflow and permit blood to flow only in one direction—toward the heart. Numerous valves are found within the extremities, especially the lower extremities, because flow must work against gravity. Venous return is also aided by muscle contraction, overflow from capillary beds, gravity, and suction from negative thoracic pressure.

The **capillaries** are minute, hair-size vessels connecting the arterial and venous systems. Their walls have only one layer. The cells and tissues of the body receive their nutrients from the fluids passing through the capillary walls; at the same time, waste products from the cells pass into the capillaries. Arteries do not always end in capillary beds; some end in anastomoses, which are end-to-end grafts between different vessels that equalize pressure over vessel length and also provide alternative flow channels.

AORTA

The **aorta** is the largest principal artery of the body. It may be divided into the following five sections: (1) root of the aorta, (2) ascending aorta, (3) descending aorta, (4) abdominal aorta and abdominal aortic branches, and (5) bifurcation of the aorta into iliac arteries (Figure 5-2).

ROOT OF THE AORTA

The systemic circulation leaves the left ventricle of the heart by way of the aorta. The root of the aorta arises from the left ventricular outflow tract in the heart. The aortic root has three semilunar cusps that prevent blood from flowing back into the left ventricle. The cusps open with ventricular systole to allow blood to be ejected into the ascending aorta; the cusps are closed during ventricular diastole. The coronary arteries arise superiorly from the right and left coronary cusps to form the right and left coronary arteries, respectively. These coronary arteries further bifurcate to supply the vasculature of the cardiac structures. After the aorta arises from the left ventricle, it ascends posterior toward the main pulmonary artery to form the ascending aorta.

ASCENDING AORTA

The ascending aorta arises a short distance from the ventricle and arches superior to form the aortic arch. Three arterial branches arise from the superior border of the aortic arch to supply the head, neck, and upper extremities: the brachiocephalic, left common carotid, and left subclavian arteries.

DESCENDING AORTA

From the aortic arch, the aorta descends posteriorly along the back wall of the heart through the thoracic cavity, where it pierces the diaphragm. The descending (thoracic) aorta enters the abdomen through the aortic opening of the diaphragm

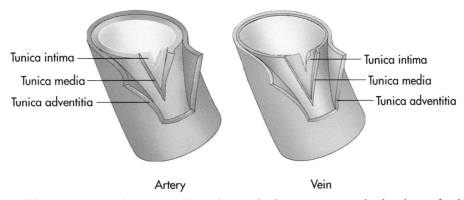

Artery   Vein

Figure 5-1   Cross section of an artery and vein showing the distinctions among the three layers of each vessel: tunica intima (inner layer), tunica media (middle layer), and tunica adventitia (external layer).

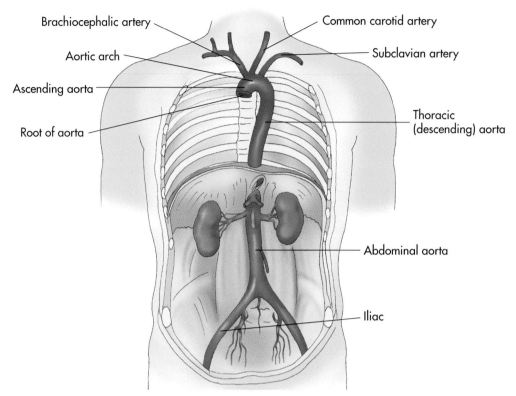

Figure 5-2   The aorta is divided into five sections: the aortic root, the ascending aorta, aortic arch (brachiocephalic artery, common carotid artery, and subclavian artery), the thoracic (descending) artery, the abdominal aorta, and the bifurcation.

anterior to the twelfth thoracic vertebra in the retroperitoneal space.

ABDOMINAL AORTA

The aorta then continues to flow in the retroperitoneal cavity anterior and slightly left of the vertebral column. The aorta lies posterior to the left lobe of the liver, the body of the pancreas, pylorus of the stomach, and splenic vein (Figure 5-3). The aorta is posterior to the superior mesenteric artery and left renal vein. Many branches arise from the abdominal aorta (i.e., celiac axis, superior mesenteric, inferior mesenteric, renal, suprarenal, and gonadal arteries). At the level of the fourth lumbar vertebra (near the umbilicus), the aorta bifurcates into the right and left common iliac arteries. The aorta has four branches that supply other visceral organs and the mesentery: the celiac trunk, the superior and inferior mesenteric arteries, and the renal arteries.

The diameter of the abdominal aorta measures approximately 2 to 3 cm, with tapering to 1.0 to 1.5 cm after it proceeds inferiorly to the bifurcation into the iliac arteries. The size of the aorta will vary slightly according to body mass index. Generally speaking, a dilatation (aneurysm) is considered when any abnormal bulging of the vessel is noted.

ABDOMINAL AORTIC BRANCHES

The small phrenic arteries arise from the lateral walls of the aorta to supply the undersurface of the diaphragm. The celiac trunk is the first anterior branch of the aorta, arising 1 to 2 cm

inferior to the diaphragm. The short celiac trunk gives rise to three smaller vessels: the splenic, hepatic, and left gastric arteries (Figure 5-4). The superior mesenteric artery is the second anterior branch, arising approximately 2 cm from the celiac trunk. The right renal artery and left renal artery are lateral branches arising just inferior to the superior mesenteric artery. The small inferior mesenteric artery arises anteriorly near the bifurcation. The distribution of these branch arteries is to the visceral organs and the mesentery.

COMMON ILIAC ARTERIES

The **common iliac arteries** arise at the bifurcation of the abdominal aorta at the fourth lumbar vertebra. These vessels further divide into the internal and external iliac arteries. The internal iliac artery enters the pelvis anterior to the sacroiliac joint, at which point it is crossed anteriorly by the ureter. It divides into anterior and posterior branches to supply the pelvic viscera, peritoneum, buttocks, and sacral canal. The external iliac artery runs along the medial border of the psoas muscle, following the pelvic brim. The inferior epigastric and deep circumflex iliac branches branch off before they pass under the inguinal ligament to become the femoral artery. The portion of the femoral artery posterior to the knee is the popliteal artery. This artery further divides into the anterior and posterior tibial arteries.

Sonographic Findings. The abdominal aorta is usually one of the easiest abdominal structures to visualize by ultrasound because of the marked change in acoustic impedance between its elastic walls and blood-filled lumen. Sonography provides the diagnostic information needed to provide an image of the entire abdominal aorta, to assess its diameter, and to visualize the presence of thrombus, calcification, or dissection within the walls.

The patient is routinely scanned in the supine position. Gas-filled or barium-filled loops of bowel may prevent adequate visualization of the aorta, but this can sometimes be overcome by applying gentle pressure with the transducer or by changing the angle of the transducer to move the gas out of the way. Other visualization problems encountered in

the abdominal aortic ultrasound may occur with increased amounts of mesenteric fat in obese patients. Patients should not be imaged 12 to 24 hours following an endoscopic evaluation as air may still be a residual impairment to adequate visualization.

Longitudinal scans should be made beginning in the midline with a slight angulation of the transducer to the left—from the xiphoid to well below the level of bifurcation (Figure 5-5). In the normal individual, the luminal dimension of the aorta gradually tapers as it proceeds distally in the abdomen. A low to medium gain should be used to demonstrate the walls

A

B

Figure 5-3   **A,** Cross section of the abdomen at the level of the eleventh thoracic disk. **B,** Cross section of the abdomen at the level of the second lumbar vertebra.   *Continued*

C

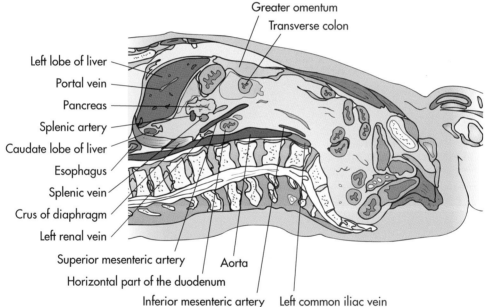

D

Figure 5-3, cont'd.   C, Cross section of the abdomen at the level of the third lumbar disk. **D,** Midline sagittal section of the abdomen.

of the aorta without "noisy" artifactual internal echoes. These weak echoes may result from increased gain, reverberation from the anterior abdominal wall fat or musculature, or poor lateral resolution. These factors result in echoes being recorded at the same level as those from soft tissue that surround the vessel lumen, particularly if the vessels are smaller in diameter than the transducer. Try to use different techniques of breath holding to eliminate these artifactual echoes. Sometimes, increased gentle pressure may help displace the bowel gas or compress the fatty tissue so that the transducer will be closer to the abdominal aorta. If the abdomen is very concave, the patient may be instructed to "extend his abdomen" ("push

the abdomen muscle out") so as to provide a better scanning plane.

Because the aorta follows the anterior course of the vertebral column, it is important that the transducer also follow a perpendicular path along the entire curvature of the spine. The anterior and posterior walls of the aorta should be easily seen as two thin parallel lines. This facilitates measuring the antero-posterior diameter of the aorta, which in most institutions is done from the leading outer edge of the anterior wall to the leading inner edge of the posterior wall.

In the transverse plane, the aorta is imaged as a circular structure anterior to the spine and slightly to the left of the

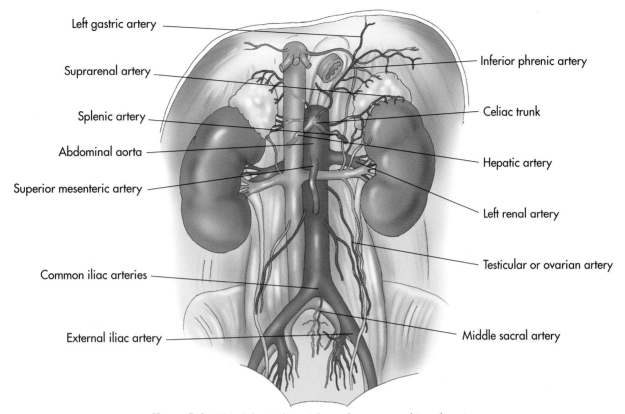

Figure 5-4   The abdominal arterial vascular system and its tributaries.

midline. In some cases the transverse diameter of the aorta differs from that found in longitudinal measurements; thus it is important to identify the vessel in two dimensions. Multiple scans should be made from the xiphoid to the bifurcation.

If the patient has a very tortuous aorta, scans may be difficult to obtain in a single sagittal plane. When scanning in the longitudinal plane, the upper portion of the abdominal aorta may be well visualized, but the lower portion may be out of the plane of view. In this case the sonographer should obtain a complete scan of the upper segment and then concentrate fully on the lower segment. In some patients, the aorta may stretch from the far right of the abdomen to the far left.

To better visualize the aortic bifurcation, use the lateral decubitus position. The patient should be examined in deep inspiration, which projects the liver and diaphragm into the abdominal cavity and provides an acoustic window to image the vascular structures. The patient should be rotated 5 to 10 degrees from the true lateral position. Slight medial to lateral angulation may be necessary to image the bifurcation in the longitudinal plane. With the patient rolled into this oblique plane, the inferior vena cava may be visualized anterior to the aorta. This view is useful to identify the renal vessels with the aid of color flow Doppler.

ANTERIOR BRANCHES OF THE ABDOMINAL AORTA

Celiac Trunk. The celiac trunk originates within the first 2 cm from the diaphragm (Figure 5-6). It is surrounded by the liver, spleen, inferior vena cava, and pancreas. After arising

from the anterior wall, it immediately branches into the following three vessels: the common hepatic, left gastric, and splenic arteries.

Common hepatic artery. The **common hepatic artery** arises from the celiac trunk and courses to the right of the abdomen at almost a 90-degree angle. At this point it branches into the proper hepatic artery and the gastroduodenal artery. The gastroduodenal artery courses along the upper border of the head of the pancreas, behind the posterior layer of the peritoneal bursa, to the upper margin of the superior part of the duodenum, which forms the lower boundary of the epiploic foramen. The duodenum and parts of the stomach are supplied by the **gastroduodenal** and the **right gastric artery** (see Figure 5-6). Along with the hepatic duct and the portal vein, the common hepatic artery then ascends into the liver (through the porta hepatis), which it divides into two branches: the right and left hepatic arteries.

Left and right hepatic arteries. The **left hepatic artery** is a small branch supplying the caudate and left lobes of the liver. The **right hepatic artery** supplies the gallbladder via the cystic artery and the liver.

Left gastric artery. The **left gastric artery** is a small branch of the celiac trunk, passing anterior, cephalic, and left to reach the esophagus and then descending along the lesser curvature of the stomach (see Figure 5-6). It supplies the lower third of the esophagus and the upper right of the stomach.

Splenic artery. The **splenic artery** is the largest of the three branches of the celiac trunk (see Figure 5-6). From its origin,

Figure 5-5 Normal aorta protocol. **A** through **C,** Longitudinal images. **D** through **F,** Transverse images at level of celiac trunk *(CT). Ao,* Aorta; *HA,* hepatic artery; *LRA,* left renal artery; *LRV,* left renal vein; *RRA,* right renal artery; *SA,* splenic artery; *SMA,* superior mesenteric artery; *SV,* splenic vein.

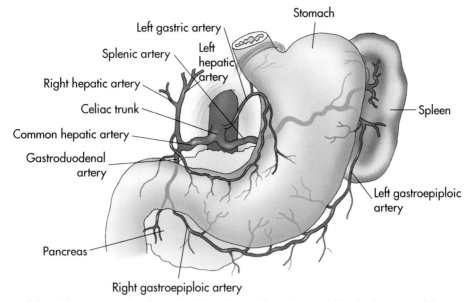

Figure 5-6 Celiac artery and its branches. The celiac trunk originates within the first 2 cm of the abdominal aorta and immediately branches into the left gastric, splenic, and common hepatic arteries.

the artery takes a somewhat tortuous course horizontally to the left as it forms the superior border of the pancreas. At a variable distance from the spleen, it divides into two branches. One of these branches, the left gastroepiploic artery, runs caudally into the greater omentum toward the right gastroepiploic artery. The other courses in a cephalic direction and divides into the short gastric artery, which supplies the fundus of the stomach, and into a number of splenic branches, which supply the spleen.

Several smaller arterial branches originate at the splenic artery as it courses through the upper border of the pancreas: the dorsal pancreatic, great pancreatic, and caudal pancreatic arteries. The dorsal or superior pancreatic artery originates from the beginning of the splenic artery or from the hepatic artery, celiac trunk, or aorta. It runs behind and within the substance of the pancreas, dividing into right and left branches. The left branch is the transverse pancreatic artery. The right branch constitutes an anastomotic vessel to the anterior pancreatic arch and also a branch to the uncinate process.

The great pancreatic artery originates from the splenic artery farther to the left and passes downward, dividing into branches that anastomose with the transverse or inferior pancreatic artery. The caudal pancreatic artery supplies the tail of the pancreas and divides into branches that anastomose with terminal branches of the transverse pancreatic artery. The transverse pancreatic artery courses behind the body and tail of the pancreas close to the lower pancreatic border. It may originate from or communicate with the superior mesenteric artery.

The distribution of the celiac trunk vessels is to the liver, spleen, stomach, pancreas, and duodenum.

Sonographic Findings. The celiac trunk may be visualized sonographically on transverse or longitudinal images (see

Figure 5-5). It is usually seen as a small vascular structure, arising anteriorly from the abdominal aorta just below the diaphragm. Because it is only 1 to 2 cm long, it is sometimes difficult to record unless the area near the midline of the aorta is carefully examined. Sometimes the celiac trunk can be seen to extend in a cephalic rather than a caudal presentation. The superior mesenteric artery is usually just inferior to the origin of the celiac trunk and may be used as a landmark in locating the celiac trunk. Transversely, one can differentiate the celiac trunk as the "wings of a seagull," arising directly anterior from the abdominal aorta (Figure 5-7).

The splenic artery may be seen to flow from the celiac trunk toward the spleen (Figure 5-8). Because it is so tortuous, it may be difficult to follow on the transverse scan. Generally, small pieces of the splenic artery are visible as the artery weaves in and out of the left upper quadrant.

The hepatic artery can be seen to branch anterior and to the right of the celiac trunk, where it then divides into the right and left hepatic arteries (Figure 5-9).

The left gastric artery has a very small diameter and often is difficult to visualize with ultrasound. It becomes difficult to separate from the splenic artery unless distinct structures are seen in the area of the celiac trunk branching to the left of the abdominal aorta.

Superior Mesenteric Artery. The superior mesenteric artery arises from the anterior abdominal aortic wall approximately 1 cm inferior to the celiac trunk (see Figure 5-5). Occasionally the SMA may have a common origin with the celiac trunk. It runs posterior to the neck of the pancreas and anterior to the uncinate process, which is anterior to the third part of the duodenum; it then branches into the mesentery and colon. The right hepatic artery is sometimes seen to arise from the superior mesenteric artery.

The superior mesenteric artery has the following five main branches (Figure 5-10): inferior pancreatic artery, duodenal artery, colic artery, ileocolic artery, and intestinal artery. These branch arteries supply the small bowel; each consists of 10 to 16 branches arising from the left side of the superior mesen-

teric trunk. They extend into the mesentery, where adjacent arteries unite with them to form loops or arcades. Their distribution is to the proximal half of the colon (cecum, ascending, and transverse) and the small intestine.

Sonographic Findings. The superior mesenteric artery is well seen on both transverse and longitudinal scans (Figure 5-11). As it arises from the anterior aortic wall, it may follow a parallel course along the abdominal aorta or branch off at a slight angle to the anterior wall of the aorta and then follow a parallel course. If the angle is severe (greater than 15 degrees), adenopathy should be considered (Figure 5-12).

Transversely the artery can be seen as a separate small, circular structure anterior to the abdominal aorta and posterior to the pancreas. Characteristically, it is surrounded by highly reflective echoes from the retroperitoneal fascia.

Inferior Mesenteric Artery. The **inferior mesenteric artery (IMA)** arises from the anterior abdominal aorta approximately at the level of the third or fourth lumbar vertebra (Figure 5-13). It proceeds to the left to distribute arterial blood to the descending colon, sigmoid colon, and rectum. It has the following three main branches: the left colic, sigmoid, and superior rectal arteries. The distribution is to the left transverse colon, descending colon, sigmoid colon, and rectum.

Sonographic Findings. The inferior mesenteric artery is more difficult to visualize using ultrasound; when it is seen, it is generally on a longitudinal scan. It is a small structure inferior to the superior mesenteric artery. On transverse scans, it is difficult to separate from small loops of bowel within the abdomen.

LATERAL BRANCHES OF THE ABDOMINAL AORTA

Phrenic Arteries. The phrenic arteries are paired small vessels that arise from the lateral wall of the aorta. They supply the undersurface of the diaphragm.

Renal Arteries. The renal arteries arise from the lateral aspect of the aorta at the level of and anterior to the first lumbar vertebra just inferior to the superior mesenteric artery

Figure 5-7 Transverse image of the celiac axis *(CT)* as it arises from the anterior aortic wall *(AO)* and branches into splenic *(SA)* and hepatic arteries *(HA)*.

Figure 5-8 Transverse image of the splenic artery *(SA)* shown posterior to the left lobe of the liver and tail of the pancreas. *AO,* Aorta; *HA,* hepatic artery.

A   **B**

Figure 5-9 **A,** The common hepatic artery *(HA)* arises from the celiac trunk *(CT)* and courses toward the liver, anterior to the portal vein. *AO,* Aorta. **B,** Oblique transverse view of the portal triad; the portal vein *(PV)* is posterior, the common duct *(CD)* anterior and lateral, and the hepatic artery *(HA)* anterior and medial.

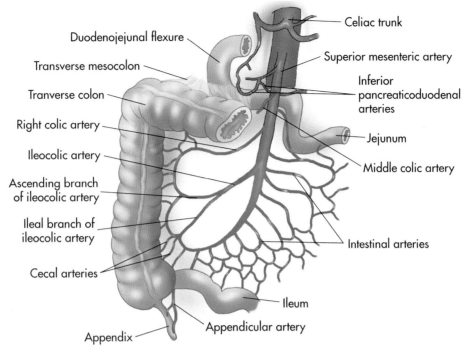

Celiac trunk

Duodenojejunal flexure

Transverse mesocolon

Superior mesenteric artery

Tranverse colon

Inferior pancreaticoduodenal arteries

Right colic artery

Jejunum

Ileocolic artery

Middle colic artery

Ascending branch of ileocolic artery

Ileal branch of ileocolic artery

Intestinal arteries

Cecal arteries

Ileum

Appendix

Appendicular artery

Figure 5-10   The superior mesenteric artery arises anteriorly from the abdominal aorta approximately 1 cm below the celiac trunk. It supplies the proximal half of the colon and small intestine.

A   **B**

Figure 5-11   Superior mesenteric artery. **A,** Longitudinal image of the abdominal aorta *(A),* celiac axis *(CA),* and superior mesenteric artery *(SMA)* arising from the anterior wall of the aorta. **B,** Transverse images show the SMA as a circle anterior to the aorta and left renal vein. The SMA is surrounded by a thick band of echogenic reflections from the mesenteric fat *(arrow).*

(Figure 5-14). Both vessels divide into the anterior and inferior suprarenal arteries. Duplication of the renal arteries is not uncommon.

Right renal artery.   The **right renal artery** is a longer vessel than the left; it courses from the aorta posterior to the inferior vena cava and anterior to the vertebral column in a posterior and slightly caudal direction to enter the hilus of the right kidney. The renal artery passes posterior to the renal vein before entering the renal hilus.

Left renal artery.   The **left renal artery** courses from the aorta directly into the hilus of the left kidney.

Sonographic Findings.   Both renal arteries are best seen on transverse sonograms (Figure 5-15). The right renal artery passes posterior to the inferior vena cava and anterior to the vertebral column in a posterior and slightly caudal direction. Occasionally, on longitudinal scans, a segment of the right renal artery is seen as a circular structure posterior to the inferior vena cava (Figures 5-16 and 5-17). The left renal artery takes a direct course from the aorta, anterior to the psoas muscle, to enter the renal sinus.

The coronal oblique scan of the aorta and inferior vena cava is excellent for demonstrating the origin of the renal arteries

Figure 5-12   If the superior mesenteric artery arises at an angle steeper than 15 degrees from the aorta, lymphadenopathy should be considered, as is shown in this image with three well-defined nodes anterior to the aorta *(Ao)*. *CT,* celiac trunk; *SMA,* superior mesenteric artery; *LN,* enlarged lymph nodes.

Figure 5-13   The inferior mesenteric artery *(arrows)* is well outlined with B-color (B-color is manufacturer-specific name for the ability to detect flow velocity by assigning gray scale interpolation to flow velocity).

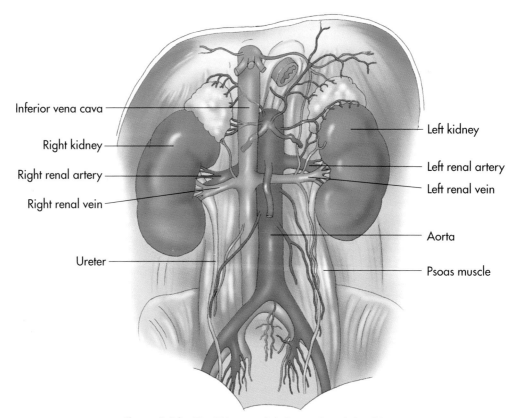

Figure 5-14   The kidneys and their vascular relationships.

and veins (see Figure 5-16). The patient is rolled into a steep decubitus position. The transducer is directed longitudinally with its axis across the inferior vena cava and aorta in efforts to see the origin of the renal vessels. The patient should be in full inspiration to dilate the venous structures for better visualization.

Gonadal Artery.   The gonadal artery arises inferior to the renal arteries and courses along the psoas muscle to the respective gonadal area.

DORSAL AORTIC BRANCHES

Lumbar Artery.   There are usually four lumbar arteries on each side of the aorta. The vessels travel lateral and posterior to supply muscle, skin, bone, and spinal cord. The midsacral artery supplies the sacrum and rectum.

INFERIOR VENA CAVA

The **inferior vena cava (IVC)** is formed by the union of the common iliac veins posterior to the right common iliac artery at the level of the fifth lumbar vertebra (Figure 5-18). The infe-

A   **B**

Figure 5-15   Renal arteries. **A,** Transverse image of both renal arteries *(LRA, RRA)* as they arise from the lateral borders of the abdominal aorta *(AO).* **B,** The right renal artery may be seen posterior to the inferior vena cava *(IVC)* on the longitudinal image.

A   **B**

Figure 5-16   Color **(A)** and gray scale **(B)** images of a patient with a duplicated right renal artery. The images are made in the right coronal oblique view.

rior vena cava ascends vertically through the retroperitoneal space on the right side of the aorta posterior to the liver, piercing the central tendon of the diaphragm at the level of the eighth thoracic vertebra to enter the right atrium of the heart. Its entrance into the lesser sac separates it from the portal vein. Caudal to the renal vein entrance, the inferior vena cava shows posterior "hammocking" through the bare area of the liver (Figure 5-19).

The tributaries of the inferior vena cava include the following:

- Three anterior hepatic veins
- Three lateral tributaries: the right suprarenal vein (the left drains into the left renal vein), the renal veins, the right testicular or ovarian vein
- Five lateral abdominal wall tributaries: the inferior phrenic vein and the four lumbar veins
- Three veins of origin: the two common iliac veins, and the median sacral vein.

The venous blood drains all organs and structures from the upper and lower abdomen and lower extremities through the system's major tributaries. The superior vena cava drains the head, neck, thoracic cavity, and upper extremities and will be discussed in Chapter 27.

Sonographic Findings. The inferior vena cava serves as a landmark for many other abdominal structures and should be routinely visualized on all examinations (Figure 5-20). The inferior vena cava is first imaged on a sagittal scan beginning at the midline, the transducer being angled slightly to the right with a slight oblique tilt until the entire vessel is seen. The patient should be instructed to hold his or her breath; this causes the patient to perform a slight Valsalva maneuver toward the end of inspiration, which dilates the inferior vena cava. The inferior vena cava may expand to 3 to 4 cm in diameter with this maneuver. The pulsatile aorta is easily differentiated from the inferior vena cava as the IVC travels in a horizontal course with its proximal portion curving slightly anterior as it pierces the diaphragm to empty into the right atrial cavity. On the contrary, the aorta follows the curvature of the spine with its distal portion lying more posterior before bifurcating into the iliac vessels.

On transverse scans, the almond-shaped inferior vena cava serves as a landmark for localizing the superior mesenteric vein, which is generally found anterior and slightly to the right of

Figure 5-17 **A** through **C,** Variations in renal arteries may be seen; this patient has a right renal artery *(RRA)* that lies anterior (instead of posterior) to the inferior vena cava *(IVC)*. Normal spectral flow is shown in the renal parenchyma.

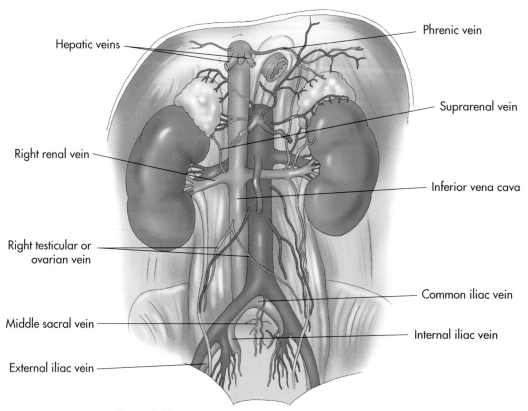

Figure 5-18 The abdominal venous system and its tributaries.

or just medial to the cava. On longitudinal scans, it serves as a landmark for the portal vein, which is located just anterior to or midway down the anterior wall of the cava. The inferior vena cava is also useful in identifying the pancreas and common bile duct. The head of the pancreas is seen just inferior to the portal vein and anterior to the inferior vena cava as it makes a slight impression or indentation on the anterior wall of the cava. The common duct is seen anterior to the portal vein as it dips posterior to enter the head of the pancreas.

Dilation of the inferior vena cava is noted in several pathologies, including right ventricular heart failure (Figure 5-21), congestive heart disease, constrictive pericarditis, tricuspid disease, and right heart obstructive tumors. In patients with hepatomegaly, the hepatic veins are dilated and increased pressure is transmitted through the sinusoids, resulting in

portal vein distention. If severe cirrhosis is present, the sinusoids may be unable to transmit pressure, and the portal veins will not distend.

Compression of the inferior vena cava may be seen in later stages of pregnancy as the enlarged uterus compresses the vena cava. This compression over time will produce edema of the ankles and feet, and temporary varicose veins. Other forms of caval compression may arise from malignant retroperitoneal tumors, hepatic neoplasm, or pancreatic mass. The presence of thrombus within the vessel should be evaluated, especially in patients with a known renal tumor.

LATERAL TRIBUTARIES TO THE INFERIOR VENA CAVA

Renal Veins. Five or six branches of the renal vein unite to form the main renal vein. The vessels arise anterior to the renal

Figure 5-19 **A,** Cross section of the abdomen at the level of the tenth intervertebral disk. **B,** Cross section of the abdomen at the first lumbar vertebra.   *Continued*

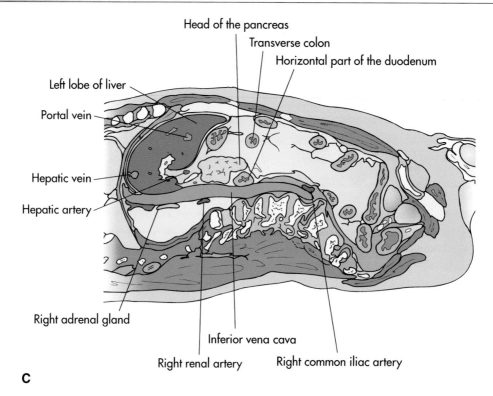

Head of the pancreas
Transverse colon
Horizontal part of the duodenum
Left lobe of liver
Portal vein
Hepatic vein
Hepatic artery
Right adrenal gland
Inferior vena cava
Right renal artery
Right common iliac artery

C

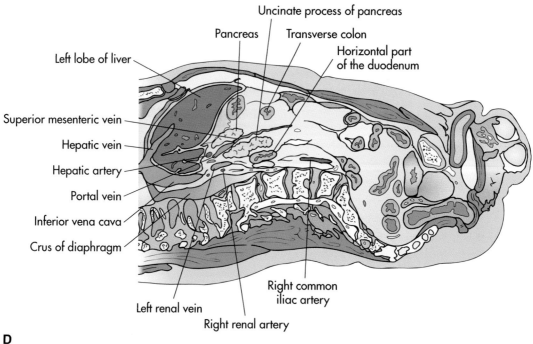

Uncinate process of pancreas
Pancreas
Transverse colon
Horizontal part of the duodenum
Left lobe of liver
Superior mesenteric vein
Hepatic vein
Hepatic artery
Portal vein
Inferior vena cava
Crus of diaphragm
Right common iliac artery
Left renal vein
Right renal artery

D

Figure 5-19, cont'd · **C,** Sagittal section of the abdomen 3 cm from the midline. **D,** Sagittal section of the abdomen 2 cm from the midline.

arteries at their respective sides of the inferior vena cava at the level of L2 (see Figure 5-18).

Left renal vein. The **left renal vein** arises medially to exit from the hilus of the kidney (Figure 5-22). It flows from the left kidney posterior to the superior mesenteric artery and anterior to the aorta to enter the lateral wall of the inferior vena cava. Above the entry of the renal veins, the inferior vena cava enlarges because of the increased volume of blood returning from the kidneys. The left renal vein is larger than the right renal vein. It accepts branches from the left adrenal, left gonadal, and lumbar veins. The left renal vein is visualized as a circular structure coursing between the SMA and aorta on the longitudinal image. On the transverse image, the LRV is an anechoic tubular structure posterior to the SMA and anterior to the aorta.

Figure 5-20 Normal inferior vena cava protocol. **A** and **B,** Longitudinal images. **A,** The hepatic vein *(HV)* drains into the inferior vena cava *(IVC)* at the diaphragm. **B,** The IVC is the posterior border of the portal vein. *HA,* Hepatic artery; *MPV,* main portal vein; *RPV,* right portal vein. **C,** Transverse image: the three hepatic veins are shown to drain into the IVC at the dome of the liver. *LHV,* Left hepatic vein. **D,** Oblique coronal image: the patient is rolled into a slight oblique position (right side up). The transducer is angled from the midclavicular line toward the midline of the abdomen to see the IVC "anterior" to the abdominal aorta *(AO).*

Right renal vein. The **right renal vein** is seen best on transverse images because it flows directly from the right kidney into the posterolateral aspect of the inferior vena cava (Figure 5-23). It seldom accepts tributaries; the right adrenal and right gonadal veins enter the cava directly.

Gonadal Veins. The gonadal veins (testicular and ovarian) course anterior to the external and internal iliac veins and continue cranially and retroperitoneally along the psoas muscle until their terminus. The left gonadal vein usually enters the left renal vein or the left adrenal vein, which empties into the inferior vena cava. The right gonadal vein enters the inferior vena cava on the anterolateral border above the entrance of the lumbar veins.

Suprarenal Veins. The right suprarenal vein arises from the suprarenal gland and usually drains directly into the inferior

vena cava. The left arises from the suprarenal gland and drains into the left renal vein.

ANTERIOR TRIBUTARIES TO THE INFERIOR VENA CAVA

Hepatic Veins. The **hepatic veins** are the largest visceral tributaries of the inferior vena cava. They originate in the liver and drain into the inferior vena cava at the level of the diaphragm (Figure 5-24). The hepatic veins return unoxygenated blood from the liver. The veins collect blood from the three minor tributaries within the liver; the right hepatic vein drains the right lobe of the liver, the middle hepatic vein drains the caudate lobe, and the left hepatic vein drains the left lobe of the liver.

Sonographic Findings. The hepatic veins are best visualized on longitudinal scans of the liver as they drain into the inferior vena cava at the level of the diaphragm. Transverse scans obtained with a cephalic angle of the transducer at the level of

Figure 5-21   Sagittal scan of the dilated inferior vena cava *(IVC)* as seen in a patient with right heart failure.

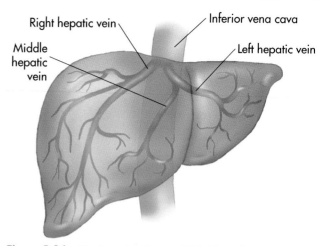

Figure 5-24   The hepatic veins are divided into three components: right, middle, and left. They all drain into the inferior vena cava at the level of the diaphragm.

Figure 5-22   The left renal vein *(LRV)* is well seen as it leaves the renal hilus, flows anterior to aorta *(A)* and posterior to the superior mesenteric artery *(SMA)* to enter the lateral wall of the inferior vena cava *(IVC)*.

Figure 5-25   Transverse images at the dome of the liver with the transducer angled in a cephalad direction show the three hepatic veins draining into the inferior vena cava.

Figure 5-23   The right renal vein is shown as it leaves the renal hilum toward the inferior vena cava.

the xiphoid often show at least two of the three veins draining into the inferior vena cava (Figure 5-25). The hepatic veins resemble the "bunny" or "reindeer" sign on the sonogram.

To distinguish hepatic veins from other vascular structures requires recognition of their anatomic patterns. Hepatic veins drain cephalad toward the diaphragm and then dorsomedially toward the inferior vena cava (Figure 5-26). Hepatic veins increase in caliber as they approach the diaphragm. Unlike portal veins, they are not surrounded by bright acoustic reflections, although a slight amount of acoustic enhancement may be seen along their posterior border.

PORTAL VENOUS SYSTEM

PORTAL VEIN

The **portal vein** is formed posterior to the pancreas by the union of the superior mesenteric vein and splenic veins at the level of L2. Its trunk is 5 to 7 cm in length (Figure 5-27). The portal vein courses posterior to the first portion of the duodenum and then between the layers of the lesser omentum to the porta hepatis, where it bifurcates into its hepatic branches. It carries blood from the intestinal tract to the liver by means of its two main branches: the right and left portal veins. It drains blood from the gastrointestinal tract, from the lower end of the esophagus to the upper end of the anal canal, from the pancreas, gallbladder, bile ducts, and spleen. The portal vein has an **anastomosis** with the esophageal veins, rectal venous plexus, and superficial abdominal veins. The portal venous blood traverses the liver and drains into the inferior vena cava via the hepatic veins.

Sonographic Findings. The portal vein is clearly seen on both transverse and sagittal scans. On transverse scans the main portal vein is a thin-walled circular structure, generally lateral and somewhat anterior to the inferior vena cava (Figure 5-28). It is often possible to record the splenic vein as it crosses the

midline of the abdomen to join the superior mesenteric vein to form the main portal trunk. Thus a long section of the splenic vein can be visualized. Often the right or left portal vein can be seen branching from the portal trunk to enter the hilum of the liver.

Portal veins become smaller as they progress into the liver from the porta hepatis. Large radicles situated near or approaching the porta hepatis are portal veins, not hepatic veins. The portal veins are characterized by high-amplitude acoustic reflections that presumably arise from the fibrous tissues surrounding the portal triad as it courses through the liver substance.

The right and left portal veins course transversely through the liver; thus transverse scans display their longest extent (Figure 5-29). The right portal vein is most consistently demonstrated on the sonogram. Anatomically, any intraparenchymal segment of the portal venous system lying to the right of the lateral aspect of the inferior vena cava is a branch of the right portal system. The left portal vein has a narrow-caliber trunk and may be seen coursing transversely through the left hepatic lobe from a posterior to an anterior position (see Figure 5-28, *B*). The main portal vein is well seen as a circular anechoic structure to the inferior vena cava. The portal radicle may have many different variations; therefore, it is important to become familiar with their patterns to be able to distinguish them from dilated biliary radicles.

SPLENIC VEIN

The **splenic vein** is a tributary of the portal circulation. It begins at the hilum of the spleen, where it is formed by the union of several veins. It is subsequently joined by the short gastric and left gastroepiploic veins (see Figure 5-27). The splenic vein runs along the posteromedial border of the pancreas. It joins the superior mesenteric vein posterior to the neck of the pancreas to form the portal vein. Additional veins from the pancreas and inferior mesenteric vein join the splenic vein. It drains blood from the stomach, spleen, and pancreas.

Figure 5-26 Longitudinal image of the hepatic vein draining the liver into the inferior vena cava. Note the thin-walled hepatic vein compared with the thicker wall of the portal vein.

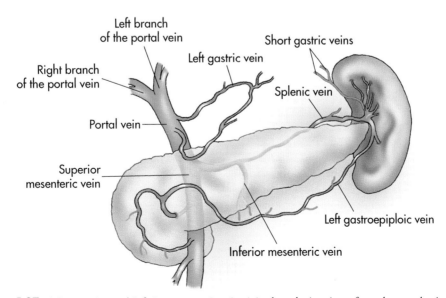

Figure 5-27 The superior and inferior mesenteric veins join the splenic vein to form the portal vein.

A   **B**

Figure 5-28 Transverse views of the portal vein. **A,** The right portal vein bifurcates into the anterior and posterior branches. **B,** The main portal vein *(MPV)* bifurcates into the right and left branches. This scan shows the left portal vein *(LPV)* as it supplies the left lobe of the liver. *AO,* Aorta; *IVC,* inferior vena cava.

Figure 5-29 Longitudinal scan of the inferior vena cava, with the main portal vein just anterior to its border.

Figure 5-30 Transverse image of the splenic vein as it leaves the splenic hilum, courses posterior to the pancreas, and anterior to the superior mesenteric artery to form the portal vein.

Sonographic Findings. The splenic vein is best visualized in the transverse plane as it crosses the upper abdomen from the hilum of the spleen to join the superior mesenteric vein to form the portal vein slightly to the right of midline (Figure 5-30). The splenic vein crosses anteriorly to the aorta and the inferior vena cava and generally relates to the medial and posterior borders of the pancreatic body and tail. Its course is variable, so small degrees of obliquity may be necessary to image the vein entirely. It is usually smaller than the superior mesenteric vein and the main portal vein.

On sagittal scans the splenic vein can be visualized posterior to the left lobe of the liver and anterior to the major vascular structures. The pancreas may be seen inferior and slightly anterior to the vein (Figure 5-31). The larger diameter of the portal vein is the result of the influx of blood from the superior mesenteric vein. An obvious widening is demonstrated at the junction of the portal and splenic veins. When splenomegaly is present, it is often possible to identify the origin of the splenic vein at the splenic hilum.

Figure 5-31 Longitudinal image of the splenic vein shown as a circular structure just anterior to the celiac axis. *AO,* aorta; *SMA,* superior mesenteric artery; *SV,* splenic vein; *SA,* splenic artery; *CT,* celiac trunk.

SUPERIOR MESENTERIC VEIN

The **superior mesenteric vein (SMV)** is also a tributary to the portal vein (see Figure 5-27). It begins at the ileocolic junction and runs cephalad along the posterior abdominal wall within the root of the mesentery of the small intestine to the right of the superior mesenteric artery. The superior mesenteric vein passes anterior to the third part of the duodenum and posterior to the neck of the pancreas, where it joins the splenic vein to form the main portal vein. It also receives tributaries that correspond to the branches of the superior mesenteric artery, where it is joined by the inferior pancreaticoduodenal vein to the right gastroepiploic vein from the right aspect of the greater curvature of the stomach. The superior mesenteric vein drains blood from several smaller veins: the middle colic vein (transverse colon), right colic vein (ascending colon), and pancreatic duodenal vein.

Sonographic Findings. The superior mesenteric vein is somewhat variable in its anatomic location. Generally it is anterior to the inferior vena cava and to the right of the superior mesenteric artery. The superior mesenteric vein drains into the main portal vein (with the splenic vein); therefore, the sonographer should not be able to demonstrate these three structures together on a single transverse scan (Figure 5-32). The superior mesenteric vein is the posterior border of the neck of the pancreas and the anterior border of the uncinate process of the pancreatic head.

On sagittal scans, the vein is seen as a long, tubular structure anterior to the inferior vena cava (Figure 5-33). With correct oblique angulation of the transducer, the path of the superior mesenteric vein can be followed as it enters the portal system.

The following points help to distinguish the superior mesenteric artery from the vein:

- The superior mesenteric vein is of larger caliber than the artery.
- Respiratory variations are seen in the vein.

- On sagittal scans, the superior mesenteric artery angles away from the aorta, whereas the vein tends to parallel the aorta or course anteriorly away from the aorta near the portal-splenic confluence.
- Real-time identification of the confluence of the superior mesenteric vein-portal vein or superior mesenteric artery is possible as the superior mesenteric artery originates from the aorta.

INFERIOR MESENTERIC VEIN

The **inferior mesenteric vein** arises from the left third of colon and upper colon and ascends retroperitoneally along the left psoas muscle. It begins midway down the anal canal as the superior rectal vein (see Figure 5-27). It runs cranial in the posterior abdominal wall on the left side of the inferior mesenteric artery and duodenojejunal junction to join the splenic vein posterior to the pancreas. It receives many tributaries

Figure 5-32 Transverse image of the superior mesenteric vein *(SMV)*, adjacent to the superior mesenteric artery *(SMA)* and anterior to the inferior vena cava *(IVC)* and aorta *(AO)*.

A   **B**

Figure 5-33 **A** and **B,** Longitudinal image of the superior mesenteric vein *(SMV)* as it lies anterior to the uncinate process of the pancreas *(P)* and posterior to the body. *IVC,* inferior vena cava; *L,* liver.

along its way, including the left colic vein. The inferior mesenteric vein drains several tributaries: the left colic vein (descending colon), sigmoid vein (sigmoid colon), and superior rectal vein (upper rectum).

Sonographic Findings. The inferior mesenteric vein is difficult to recognize on ultrasound because of its anatomic location and small diameter. It is generally covered by the small bowel and has no major vascular structures posterior to it to aid in its recognition.

VASCULAR PATHOPHYSIOLOGY

AORTIC ABNORMALITIES

Abdominal Aortic Aneurysm. An aneurysm is defined as a permanent localized dilation of an artery, with an increase in diameter of greater than 1.5 times its normal diameter. The normal diameter for an artery depends on several factors, including age, gender, and blood pressure. The diagnosis of an aneurysm depends on a comparison of the aortic diameter of the suspicious area with that of the normal area of the vessel above and below that area.

The assessment is often made by physical examination of the abdomen, which reveals a localized dilation of the aorta, most commonly encountered in the infrarenal portion of the abdominal aorta. On physical examination, a pulsatile mass slightly to the left of the midline, between the umbilicus and xiphoid process, may be palpated.

Patients at high risk to have an aneurysm develop include individuals over the age of 60 who smoke, have hypertension, or have vascular disease. Other risk factors include chronic obstructive pulmonary disease and positive family history for abdominal aortic aneurysm.

Abdominal aortic aneurysms occur in 5% to 7% of people over the age of 60 in the United States. The visualization of the abdominal aorta has traditionally been an asset in diagnosing the clinical problem. Ultrasound is very capable of demonstrating abnormalities in the diameter, length, and extent of the abdominal aortic aneurysm.

There are a number of factors that may cause the development of an aortic aneurysm:

1. Atherosclerosis
2. Trauma (following transection)
3. Congenital defects (aortic sinus, postcoarctation of the aorta, ductus diverticulum)
4. Syphilis (involving the ascending aorta and arch)
5. Mycosis (fungal dissection)
6. Cystic medial necrosis (e.g., Marfan's syndrome)
7. Inflammation of media and adventitia (e.g., rheumatic fever, polychondritis, ankylosing spondylitis, etc.)
8. Increased pressure (systemic hypertension, aortic valve stenosis)
9. Abnormal volume load (severe aortic regurgitation)

Arteriosclerosis and **atherosclerosis** are the most common causes of aneurysms (Figure 5-34). The ulcerated atheromas are seen in the aorta above the renal arteries; the lower aneurysm contains thrombi. It is found more often in late

Figure 5-34   Atherosclerotic aneurysm with severe atherosclerosis of the aorta. (From Damjanov I, Linder J: *Pathology: a color atlas,* St. Louis, 2000, Mosby.)

middle-aged men than women and involves the aorta, often with extension into the common iliac arteries. The disease sometimes involves the ascending and descending aorta.

Clinical symptoms. Symptoms may vary in the patient with an abdominal aneurysm. Approximately 75% of the patients with an abdominal aortic aneurysm are asymptomatic and the enlarged vessel is found during routine physical examination or during an unrelated radiologic or surgical procedure.

Symptoms of the aortic aneurysm may result from rupture or expansion of the vessel. The enlarged vessel may produce symptoms by impinging on adjacent structures, or it may occlude a vessel by direct pressure or thrombus with resulting embolism. The large aneurysm may rupture into the peritoneal cavity or retroperitoneum, causing intense back pain and a drop in hematocrit. Patients may present with satiety (becoming full easily) or nausea and vomiting. The abrupt onset of severe, constant pain in the abdomen, back, or flank that is unrelieved by positional changes is characteristic of rapid expansion or rupture of an aneurysm.

The patient who presents with an aneurysm most likely has many other medical problems as well. It is important that the clinician be able to examine the size of the aneurysm noninvasively and follow it sequentially over a structured time period by sonography. Aneurysms smaller than 4 cm in diameter are followed every 6 months with intervention if the patient becomes symptomatic. It is also important in these cases to mark on the films the exact location of the aneurysm and measurements so that follow-up information will be accurate. In patients with aneurysms ranging from 4 to 5 cm in diameter, surgical intervention may be suggested if the patient is in good health. Patients with aneurysms ranging from 5 to 6 cm may benefit from surgical repair, especially if they have other factors for rupture (e.g., hypertension, smoking, and chronic obstructive pulmonary disease). The highest risk patients are those with aneurysms more than 6 to 7 cm. The risk increases with age and other medical problems.

Surgical intervention also considers whether there is associated renal and iliac involvement, both with either occlusive disease or involved in the aneurysm process. The length of the infrarenal aortic neck is important to help determine the surgical approach (retroperitoneal versus transabdominal) and the location of the aortic cross clamp. Endovascular stent grafts for treatment are a less invasive approach to the repair of an aneurysm. The graft is placed through two small incisions in the abdomen.

Three primary factors are related to the growth rate of abdominal aneurysms: the initial size of the aortic aneurysm, the presence of cardiac disease, and the presence of beta-adrenergic blockade (blood pressure lowering medications) (Box 5-1).

Another important consideration is the relationship of the aneurysm to the renal arteries. Thus not only should the diameter be measured but also the longitudinal extent of the aneurysm as it relates to the origin of the renal vessels. Often bowel gas impairs adequate visualization of the renal arteries, and a more indirect method must be used to locate the origin of the superior mesenteric artery and renal arteries. Color Doppler may be useful to produce an image of arterial flow from the lateral margins of the abdominal aorta to the kidneys.

Classification of aneurysms. The aneurysm may be fusiform or saccular (Figure 5-35). It usually begins below the renal arteries (inferior to the superior mesenteric artery) and extends to the bifurcation of the aorta at the iliac arteries (Figure 5-36).

The most common presentation of an atherosclerotic aneurysm is as a **fusiform aneurysm** of the distal aorta at the aortic bifurcation (Figure 5-37). Atherosclerosis causes decreased pulsations of the aortic walls with bright echoes reflecting the degree of thickening and calcification.

Saccular aneurysms are somewhat spherical and larger (5 to 10 cm) than fusiform aneurysms. This type of aneurysm is connected to vascular lumen by a mouth that varies in size but may be as large as an aneurysm. It may be partially or completely filled with thrombus (Figure 5-38). The sonographer must carefully follow the course of such an aneurysm to differentiate it from a retroperitoneal mass or lymphadenopathy. Pulsations are usually diminished secondary to clot formation.

The aneurysm may extend into the iliac arteries. The sonographer should examine both iliac arteries in at least two planes. At the level of the bifurcation, the iliac vessels may be seen as circular, pulsatile vessels just anterior to the spine. The oblique longitudinal scan is used to produce an image of the vessel in its entire length. Normal iliac arteries do not measure more than 1 cm in diameter. If the artery becomes so enlarged, it has an increased chance of rupture.

Sonographic Findings. The normal measurement for an adult abdominal aorta is less than 3 cm, measuring from outer to outer walls (this measurement correlates with the measurement made by the surgeon). The sonographer should search for focal dilation of the abdominal aorta or lack of normal tapering distally. When an aneurysm is present, the presence of a thrombus should be evaluated. A thrombus usually occurs along an anterior or anterolateral wall. An old clot is easier to

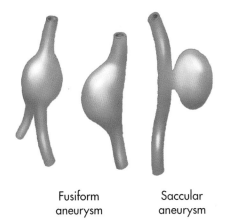

Fusiform
aneurysm

Saccular
aneurysm

Figure 5-35 Fusiform and saccular aneurysms.

BOX 5-1

GROWTH PATTERNS FOR ABDOMINAL ANEURYSMS

The normal aortic lumen diameter is less than 3 cm. With careful sonographic technique, ultrasound has a 98.8% accuracy in detecting aneurysms. Aneurysms less than 6 cm show a very slow growth pattern, so patients are followed at yearly intervals. The following information has been found on follow-up of aneurysms:

- Seventy-five percent of patients have a 1-year survival rate if the aneurysm is less than 6 cm.
- Fifty percent of patients have a 1-year survival rate if the aneurysm is more than 6 cm.
- Twenty-five percent of patients have a 1-year survival rate if the aneurysm is more than 7 cm.
- There is a 75% risk of fatal rupture if the aneurysm is more than 7 cm.
- One percent of aneurysms less than 5 cm rupture.
- Operative mortality before rupture is 5%, but with emergency surgery, mortality increases to 50%.

---

see because of calcification that appears as thick, echogenic echoes, sometimes with posterior shadowing. Thrombus within an aneurysm is shown ultrasonically as medium- to low-level echoes (Figures 5-39 and 5-40). Generally, increased sensitivity is likely to highlight the thrombus echoes. The echoes should be seen in both planes on more than one scan to be separated from low-level reverberation echoes.

If an aneurysm extends beyond the diaphragm into the thoracic aorta, it may be difficult to trace with ultrasound because of lung interference in the beam. Several attempts may be necessary to demonstrate this thoracic aneurysm. The transducer can be sharply angled from the xiphoid toward the sternal notch to visualize the lower extent of the aorta. Another technique allows the sonographer to make a longitudinal parasternal scan over the long axis of the heart. The thoracic aorta should be seen posterior to the cardiac structures. A third alternative is to scan along the patient's back with the patient sitting upright or prone. The transducer should be angled slightly

Figure 5-36 Abdominal aortic aneurysm. **A,** Longitudinal image of a large abdominal aortic aneurysm extending the entire length of the aorta. Multiple echoes within represent thrombus formation. **B** and **C,** Transverse images of the aorta show the width to measure larger than the A-P dimension. *Sp,* spine; *Th,* thrombus.

medially and placed in a sagittal plane along the left intercostal space. This is very effective if the thoracic aorta is deviated slightly to the left of the spine. Scalloped reverberations from the ribs will be recorded, with the luminal echoes of the thoracic aorta directly posterior.

Pseudoaneurysm. A **pseudoaneurysm** is a pulsatile hematoma, which results from the leakage of blood into the soft tissue abutting the punctured artery, with subsequent fibrous encapsulation and failure of the vessel wall to heal. They may occur after a cardiac catheterization or angiography procedure. Ultrasound evaluation of the pulsatile mass is made with color flow Doppler showing communication between the artery and the vein. Compression of the mass with a linear transducer at 20-minute compression intervals may allow the lesion to close if the communication is small. Sometimes it takes several compressions (20 minutes on and 20 minutes off) to completely close the communication. Color flow allows the sonographer to visually see if the communication is closed.

Pseudoaneurysms that are not closed require surgical intervention as they may become a source of emboli, site of increased chance of infection secondary to the abnormal communication of blood flow, or a cause of local pressure effects. In addition they can rupture, which may result in exsanguinations.

Aortic Dissection. A **dissecting aneurysm** may be detected by ultrasound and usually displays one or more clinical signs and symptoms. The typical patient is 40 to 60 years old and hypertensive; males predominate over females. The patient is usually known to have an aneurysm, and sudden, excruciating chest pain radiating to the back may develop because of a dissection. The sonographer should look for a dissection "flap" or recent channel with or without frank aneurysmal dilation. The dissection of blood is along the laminar planes of the aortic media with formation of a blood-filled channel within the aortic wall (Figure 5-41). Most aneurysms enlarge fairly symmetrically in the anteroposterior and lateral

Figure 5-37   Fusiform aortic aneurysm with extension into the iliac arteries.

dimensions; therefore, an irregular enlargement with scattered internal echoes may represent an aneurysm with a clot.

When the dissection develops, hemorrhage occurs between the middle and outer thirds of the media. An intimal tear is considered if the tear is found in the ascending portion of the arch. This type of dissection extends proximally toward the heart, and distally, sometimes to the iliac and femoral arteries. A small portion of dissections do not have an obvious intimal tear. Extravasation may completely encircle the aorta or extend along one segment of its circumference, or it may rupture into any of the body cavities.

Types of dissection. There are three classifications of aortic dissection according to the DeBakey model (Figure 5-42). Types I and II involve the ascending aorta and the aortic arch; Type III involves the descending aorta at the level inferior to the left subclavian artery. There is a high incidence of mortality with Types I and II dissections because of the origin of the coronary arteries and the possible obstruction of blood into the head and neck vessels. The lowest mortality rate is the Type III dissection, which begins inferior to the left subclavian artery with possible extension into the abdominal aorta.

The Type I dissection begins at the root of the aorta and may extend the entire length of the arch, descending to the aorta and into the abdominal aorta. This is the most dangerous, especially if the dissection spirals around the aorta, cutting off the blood supply to the coronaries, carotid, brachiocephalic, and subclavian vessels. The third type of dissection (Type III) begins at the lower end of the descending aorta and extends into the abdominal aorta. This may be critical if the

dissection spirals around to impede the flow of blood into the renal vessels.

Dissection of the aorta (Type II) may be secondary to **cystic medial necrosis** (weakening of the arterial wall) to the inherited disease **Marfan's syndrome** (individuals with this disorder are extremely tall, lanky, and double-jointed; a progressive stretching disorder exists in all arterial vessels, especially in the aorta, causing abnormal dilation, weakened walls, and eventual dissection, rupture, or both) or hypertension. Color flow Doppler may be used to detect flow into the false channel.

Ruptured Aortic Aneurysms. The classic symptoms of ruptured aortic aneurysm are excruciating abdominal pain, shock, and an expanding abdominal mass. The operative mortality for such ruptures may exceed 40% to 60%. The rupture may be into perirenal space with displacement of renal hilar vessels, effacement of the aortic border, and silhouetting of the lateral psoas border at the level of the kidney. The most common site is the lateral wall below the renal vessels. The hemorrhage into the posterior pararenal space accounts for a loss of visualization of the lateral psoas muscle merging inferior to the kidney and may also displace the kidney.

A large aneurysm may compress the neighboring structures (i.e., the common bile duct, causing obstruction; and the renal artery, causing hypertension; and renal ischemia). Retroperitoneal fibrosis with an aneurysm may involve the ureter.

Aortic Graft. An abdominal aortic aneurysm may be surgically repaired with a flexible graft material attached to the end of the remaining aorta. The synthetic material used for a graft produces bright echo reflections compared with those from normal aortic walls. After surgery, the attached walls may swell at the site of the attachment and form another aneurysm or pseudoaneurysm (Figures 5-43 and 5-44). Other complications of prosthetic grafts include hematoma, infection, and degeneration of graft material.

Newer surgical techniques now repair the aneurysm with an endovascular graft treatment. These grafts would be placed either within the aorta, at the level of the aorta and iliac artery, or within the femoral artery. Further development in techniques placed the grafts in the aortofemoral and juxtarenal positions. Complications of these grafts resulted in endoleak formations that were immediate, without outflow, and persistent. The type of graft used, the technique of graft insertion, and aortic anatomic features all affected the rate of endoleaks.

Other Pseudo-"Pulsatile" Abdominal Masses. Masses other than an aortic aneurysm that can simulate a pulsatile abdominal mass are retroperitoneal tumor, fibroid uterus, and para-aortic nodes. Because the mass is adjacent to the aorta, the pulsations are transmitted from the aorta to the mass. After an abdominal aneurysm, the most common cause for a pulsatile abdominal mass is enlarged retroperitoneal lymph nodes. This mass is usually the result of lymphoma in the middle-aged patient. On ultrasound, the nodes are homogeneous masses surrounding the aorta. The aortic wall may be poorly defined because of the close acoustic impedance of the

A   **B**

C

Figure 5-38   Saccular aneurysms are spherical and larger than the fusiform aneurysm. This patient had a "dumbbell" type of aneurysm, more typically seen in a patient with cystic medial necrosis. **A,** Sagittal view. **B,** Transverse at the umbilicus. **C,** Transverse at the umbilicus with caudal angulation.

Figure 5-39   Longitudinal image of a large aortic aneurysm with thrombus along the anterior and posterior walls. The true lumen is anechoic.

Figure 5-40   Transverse image of a patient with a horseshoe kidney and abdominal aortic aneurysm. The isthmus of the kidneys is shown draping anterior to the aorta.

nodes and the aorta. The sonographer should also look for splenomegaly.

Pancreatic carcinoma may appear as a hypoechoic mass and may displace the normal pancreas; biliary dilation with an enlarged gallbladder may be present. A retroperitoneal sarcoma may present as a pulsatile mass; it may extend into the root of the mesentery and give rise to a larger intraperitoneal component. The echodensity depends on the tissue type that predominates; fatty lesions are more echodense than fibrous or myomatous lesions.

Arteriovenous Fistulas. The development of an **arteriovenous fistula** is not a common finding with ultrasound. The majority of fistulas are acquired secondary to trauma. Some may develop as a complication of arteriosclerotic aortic aneurysms.

Clinical Signs. The patient may have low back and abdominal pain, progressive cardiac decompensation, a pulsatile

abdominal mass associated with a bruit, and massive swelling of the lower trunk and lower extremities. Clinical signs are explained on the basis of the altered hemodynamics produced by a high-velocity shunt leading to increased blood volume, increased venous pressure, and cardiac output with cardiac failure and cardiomegaly.

If there is lower trunk and leg edema and a dilated inferior vena cava, an arteriovenous fistula should be suspected. If the fistula is large, the vein becomes very distended. A normal inferior vena cava is less than 2.5 cm wide. Right-sided heart disease or failure can also cause inferior vena cava distention.

Renal arteriovenous fistulas can be congenital or acquired. Congenital arteriovenous fistulas may be of the cirsoid type or the aneurysmal type. Acquired fistulas are secondary to trauma, surgery, or inflammation or are associated with a neoplasm, such as renal cell carcinoma.

The sonographer will find multiple anechoic tubular structures feeding the malformation with an enlarged renal artery and vein, confirming increased blood flow to the kidney. It may look like hydronephrosis or a parapelvic cyst in association with a dilated inferior vena cava. The diagnosis is made by identifying one or more channels that enter the mass,

Figure 5-41 Dissecting aneurysm of the thoracic aorta. The blood has filled the space formed by the separation of intima and media of the aorta. (From Damjanov I, Linder J: *Pathology: a color atlas,* St. Louis, 2000, Mosby.)

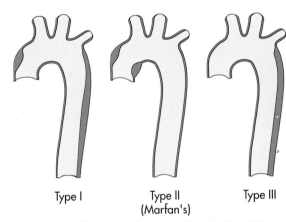

Type I   Type II   Type III
                (Marfan's)

Figure 5-42 Aortic dissection: Types I, II, and III.

Figure 5-43 Complications of graft repair of aneurysms may result in new aneurysm formation (**A**) or pseudoaneurysm formation (**B**).

Figure 5-44 **A** through **C,** Images of a postoperative patient with an aortic graft stent in place *(g).*

suggesting that the lesion is related to the renal vasculature. The sonographer should look for pulsations. The fistula has a characteristic ultrasound appearance of a cluster of tubular anechoic structures within the kidney; it is supplied by an enlarged renal artery and drained by a dilated renal vein. In the aneurysmal type of fistula, a vascular lesion should be suspected when the presence of a thrombus is noted in the periphery of a mass with a tubular anechoic lumen with pulsations. Occasionally, renal cell carcinoma is associated with arteriovenous shunting, resulting from invasion of larger arteries and venous structures.

INFERIOR VENA CAVA ABNORMALITIES

Congenital Abnormalities. The inferior vena cava is formed by three pairs of cardinal veins in the retroperitoneum; these veins undergo sequential development and regression. The posterior cardinal veins appear at 6 weeks and form no part of the cava, but may be part of the anomalies. The subcardinal veins appear at 7 weeks to produce the prerenal segment of the inferior vena cava. The supracardinal system at 8 weeks produces the postrenal segment of the inferior vena cava. The supracardinals form the azygos and hemiazygos system above the diaphragm. The anastomosis between the subcardinal and supracardinal systems forms the renal veins. The normal left cardinal system involutes, and the right con-

sists of the posterior infrarenal vein, supracardinal vein, renal segment, anterior suprarenal subcardinal vein, and the confluence of hepatic veins.

Double Inferior Vena Cava. Double inferior vena cava has an incidence of under 3%. The size of the two vessels can be the same or vary, depending on the dominant side. In the most common type the left inferior vena cava joins the left renal vein, which crosses the midline at its normal level to join the right inferior vena cava. There is no continuation of the left inferior vena cava above the left renal vein. Less commonly, the right inferior vena cava joins the left inferior vena cava to join the hemiazygos.

Infrahepatic interruption of the inferior vena cava. This condition is the failure of union of the hepatic veins and the right subcardinal vein, in which there can be azygos or, less commonly, hemiazygos continuation. The azygos veins consist of the main azygos vein, the inferior hemiazygos vein, and the superior hemiazygos vein (Figure 5-45). They drain blood from the posterior parts of the intercostal spaces, the posterior abdominal wall, the pericardium, the diaphragm, the bronchi, and the esophagus. The interruption of the inferior vena cava connection to the heart is associated with acyanotic and cyanotic congenital heart disease, abnormalities of cardiac position, and abdominal situs with asplenia and polysplenia.

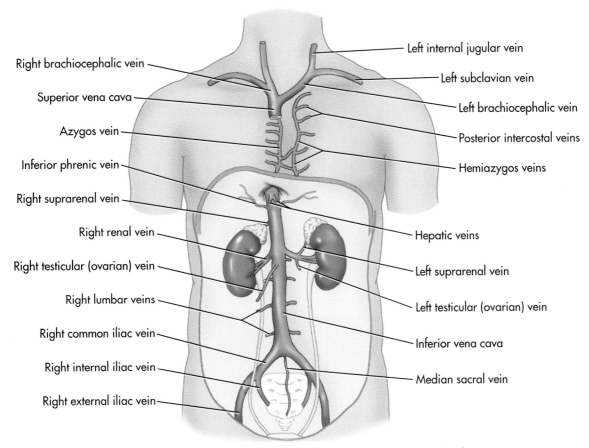

Right brachiocephalic vein

Superior vena cava

Azygos vein

Inferior phrenic vein

Right suprarenal vein

Right renal vein

Right testicular (ovarian) vein

Right lumbar veins

Right common iliac vein

Right internal iliac vein

Right external iliac vein

Left internal jugular vein

Left subclavian vein

Left brachiocephalic vein

Posterior intercostal veins

Hemiazygos veins

Hepatic veins

Left suprarenal vein

Left testicular (ovarian) vein

Inferior vena cava

Median sacral vein

Figure 5-45   Illustration of the relationship of the azygos vein to the superior and inferior vena cava.

Sonographic Findings. In patients with an interruption of the inferior vena cava, the azygos vein continuation is identical to or larger than the inferior vena cava, which passes along the aorta medial to the right crus of the diaphragm. The hepatic veins drain into an independent confluence that passes through the diaphragm to enter the right atrium. A membranous obstruction of the inferior vena cava may simulate infrahepatic interruption of the cava with azygos continuation. A web or membrane obstructs the inferior vena cava at the level of the diaphragm and leads to chronic congestion of the liver with centrilobular and periportal fibrosis.
The following three types of obstruction occur:

- A thin membrane at the level of the entrance to the right atrium
- An absent segment of the inferior vena cava without characteristic conical narrowing
- Complete obstruction secondary to thrombosis

Clinically, patients present in their third to fourth decade of life with portal hypertension. Ultrasound shows obstruction at the diaphragm and dilation of the azygos system. On longitudinal scans it is very difficult to identify the presence of the inferior vena cava. The azygos system is dilated on the right side of the midline, "acting" as the inferior vena cava.

Inferior Vena Cava Dilation. In patients with right ventricular failure, the inferior vena cava does not collapse with

expiration. This may be because of atherosclerosis, pulmonary hypertension, pericardial tamponade, constrictive pericarditis, or atrial tumor (Figure 5-46).

Inferior Vena Cava Tumor. It is important for the sonographer to identify the entire inferior vena cava; bowel gas can make the distal cava difficult to identify.

Hepatic portion of inferior vena cava. Masses posterior to the hepatic portion of the inferior vena cava are the right adrenal, neurogenic, and hepatic. With enlargement of the liver, the cava is compressed rather than displaced. A localized liver mass would produce posterior, lateral, or medial displacement of the inferior vena cava, whereas a mass in the posterior caudate lobe and right lobe may elevate the cava.

Middle, or pancreatic, portion of the inferior vena cava. The middle or pancreatic portion of the inferior vena cava may elevate the cava from abnormalities of the right renal artery, right kidney, lumbar spine, or lymph node masses.

Lower, or small bowel, segment. Lumbar spine abnormalities or lymph nodes would elevate the inferior vena cava.

Sonographic Findings. The inferior vena cava may become obstructed by tumor formation. The ultrasound appearance of tumor is of a single or multiple echogenic nodules along the wall. The cava may be distended and filled with a tumor. The most common tumor is renal cell carcinoma, usually from the right kidney. Wilms' tumor is also seen extending into the inferior vena cava and right atrium. Other less common

Figure 5-46 Transverse and sagittal scans of a patient in right ventricular heart failure show a dilated inferior vena cava *(IVC)* and hepatic veins *(HV)*.

Figure 5-47 **A,** Longitudinal image of the inferior vena cava with a tumor lying along the posterior wall *(arrows)*. **B,** Color flow Doppler will delineate the patency of the inferior vena cava in the event of tumor or thrombus formation.

tumors are retroperitoneal liposarcoma, leiomyosarcoma, pheochromocytoma, osteosarcoma, and rhabdomyosarcoma. Benign tumors, such as angiomyolipoma, can have venous involvement.

Inferior Vena Cava Thrombosis. Complete thrombosis of the inferior vena cava is life-threatening. Patients present with leg edema, low back pain, pelvic pain, gastrointestinal complaints, and renal and liver abnormalities (Figures 5-47 and 5-48). Thrombosis within the inferior vena cava appears as a homogeneous echo mass. Color Doppler is useful to determine if the vessel is occluded.

Inferior Vena Cava Filters. The most common origin of pulmonary emboli is venous thrombosis from the lower extremities. Surgical and angiographic placement of transvenous filters into the cava has been used to prevent recurrent

embolization in patients who cannot tolerate anticoagulants (Figure 5-49). The preferred location of the filter is in the iliac bifurcation below the renal veins. The filter is a tubular wire mesh that is implanted into the IVC to trap small emboli that may cause problems in the heart or the lungs. Some filters, after placement, can migrate cranially or caudally and perforate the cava, producing a retroperitoneal bleed. Filters can also perforate the duodenum, aorta, ureter, and hepatic vein.

RENAL VEIN OBSTRUCTION

Renal vein obstruction is seen in the dehydrated or septic infant. It may also be seen in adults with multiple renal abnormalities (nephrotic syndrome, shock, renal tumor, kidney transplant, or trauma). Left renal vein obstruction may result from the spread of such nonrenal malignancies as carcinoma of the pancreas or lung, or lymphoma. A retroperitoneal tumor

Figure 5-48   A, Longitudinal image of thrombus near the distal end of the inferior vena cava *(IVC).* **B,** The spectral Doppler shows flow is still patent.

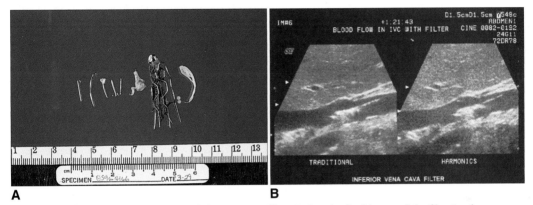

Figure 5-49   A, Surgical specimen of the vena cava filter. **B,** Longitudinal image of the filter in place within the inferior vena cava.

Figure 5-50   Hydronephrosis of the right kidney.

can occlude the left renal vein by direct extension into the vein lumen or compression of the lumen by a contiguous mass.

Clinical Signs. The patient presents with flank pain, hematuria, flank mass, and proteinuria. The condition may be associated with maternal diabetes and transient high blood pressure.

Sonographic Findings. Ultrasound can be used to confirm that a palpable flank mass is kidney and to exclude hydronephrosis and multicystic kidney as causes of a nonfunctioning kidney (Figure 5-50). In infants with renal vein obstruction, enlarged kidneys without cysts are seen. Medium echoes or "clumps" of echoes may be randomly scattered within the kidney, with surrounding echo-free spaces. The parenchymal anechoic areas are the result of hemorrhage and infarcts. The renal pattern progresses to atrophy over 2 months. Late findings are increased parenchymal echoes, loss of corticomedullary junction, and decreased renal size.

RENAL VEIN THROMBOSIS

If the following are present on ultrasound, renal vein thrombosis can be diagnosed.

1. Direct visualization of thrombi in the renal vein and inferior vena cava
2. Demonstrated renal vein dilation proximal to the point of occlusion
3. Loss of normal renal structure
4. Increased renal size (acute phase)
5. Decreased flow or no flow shown on Doppler

Clinical Signs. The patient presents with pain, nephromegaly, hematuria, or thromboembolic phenomena elsewhere in the body. A variety of lesions may be associated with this abnormality.

ABDOMINAL DOPPLER TECHNIQUES

Doppler ultrasound is a useful clinical tool for diagnosing many disease processes. The following paragraphs present an overview of abdominal applications that have been used with color flow detection and pulsed Doppler techniques. Doppler has helped detect the presence or absence of blood flow, the direction of blood flow, and flow-disturbance patterns. It has also been used in tissue characterization and waveform analysis.

BLOOD FLOW ANALYSIS

Presence or Absence of Flow. Doppler ultrasound frequently is used to differentiate vessels from nonvascular structures. For example, to distinguish the common bile duct from the hepatic artery, look for absence of flow in the common duct; to distinguish the hepatic artery from the splenic artery, look for direction of flow; to differentiate an aneurysm from a pancreatic pseudocyst, look for slow flow in the aneurysm; to differentiate dilated intrahepatic bile ducts and prominent hepatic artery, again look for absence of flow in the bile duct.

Direction of Flow. In patients who develop **portal venous hypertension,** the portal blood flow becomes **hepatofugal** (away from the liver) instead of **hepatopetal** (toward the liver). This may be secondary to portal venous shunts or varices. The sonographer detects a high-velocity flow pattern at the site of the shunt with a turbulent flow pattern on color Doppler.

Disturbance of Flow. A flow disturbance (increased velocity or obstruction of flow) may result from the formation of an atheroma, AV fistula, pseudoaneurysm, or aneurysmal dilation.

Tissue Characterization. Research is currently under way in the area of tissue characterization. Doppler is thought to be capable of characterizing tissue because of the specific perfusion patterns characteristic of some tissues or states of tissue activity. Hepatocellular carcinomas of the liver appear to have a specific pattern. Pseudoaneurysms of peripancreatic arteries have turbulent flow patterns. Pancreatic tumors may have specific flow patterns.

Doppler Waveform Analysis. The shape of the waveform provides information on the vascular impedance of the organ the vessel supplies. Spectral analysis tells the velocity and turbulence of blood flow.

Nonresistive versus resistive. **Nonresistive** vessels have a high diastolic component and supply organs that need constant perfusion, such as the internal carotid artery, the hepatic artery, and the renal artery. **Resistive** vessels have very little or even reversed flow in diastole and supply organs that do not need a constant blood supply, such as the external carotid and the iliac and brachial arteries.

Peak systole is compared with minimum diastole to quantify a vessel's impedance. This ratio is the **resistive index.**

Spectral display shows us the following:
x = Time is depicted on the horizontal axis.
y = Doppler shift frequency (velocity) is on the vertical axis (flow toward the transducer equals positive shift, or above baseline; flow away from transducer equals negative shift, or below baseline).
z = Gray scale indicates the quantity of blood flowing at a given velocity. More red blood cells produce a brighter gray scale assignment.

Plug flow is a pattern of blood flow, typically seen in large arteries, in which most cells are moving at the same velocity across the entire diameter of the vessel. In other vessels the different velocities are the result of friction between the cells and arterial walls. A "clear window" under systole is typical of plug flow. When plug flow is present, the volume of blood flow can be calculated.

DOPPLER TECHNIQUE

Unlike visualization of the heart, in which high-velocity flows are present, visualization of abdominal vessels requires very sensitive Doppler instrumentation. Abdominal vessels generally have low velocity and flow.

Methods. Doppler is performed as part of the routine real-time examination. The patient should be fasting and suspend respirations for the best color and pulsed **Doppler sample volume** to be obtained. The Doppler sample volume (sometimes referred to as the Doppler "gate") should be adjusted to encompass but not exceed the diameter of the vessel. If the sample volume exceeds the diameter, noise and ghost echoes may appear. This is because too wide of a Doppler gate causes interference from the surrounding vessels and structures.

The sonographer has the ability to control the velocity of the returning echoes to prevent the alias pattern by using a lower frequency transducer or changing from pulse wave to continuous wave. Another feature of Doppler is that the beam only records accurate velocity patterns when the beam is parallel to the flow (the angle of flow can be changed up to 60 degrees and still be accurate). The more perpendicular the beam is to the flow, the less signal is recorded; it falls to zero velocity when the beam is directly perpendicular to flow. Thus Doppler causes the sonographer to be creative in attempting to record accurate velocity flow patterns. The patient must be rolled into various obliquities with different angulations of the transducer to be parallel to many vascular structures.

Color Doppler is a relatively new and exciting modality that makes it easier to localize and identify smaller vessels from the biliary tree, or lymphadenopathy or other pathology. The colors are arbitrarily assigned on all equipment and refer to the direction of flow. If red is assigned as a positive flow signal, all the flow toward the transducer is coded in various shades of red, depending on their returning velocity. If blue is assigned a negative flow signal, the flow away from the transducer is coded in various shades of blue. The sonographer may select the particular color scheme to be used; some laboratories choose to code all positive-flow patterns red and negative-flow patterns blue. Other laboratories code all arterial flows red and venous flows blue.

DOPPLER FLOW PATTERNS IN THE ABDOMINAL VESSELS

Box 5-2 lists Doppler flow patterns in the abdominal arteries.

Aorta. The patient should be scanned in the longitudinal plane (Figure 5-51). The flow pattern of the proximal abdominal aorta above the renal arteries shows a high systolic peak

---

BOX 5-2   DOPPLER FLOW PATTERNS IN ABDOMINAL ARTERIES

AORTA
- Flow varies at different levels
- Proximal aorta has high systolic/low diastolic flow
- Distal demonstrates triphasic flow

CELIAC AXIS
- Some spectral broadening
- Unchanged after meals

HEPATIC ARTERY
- Spectral broadening
- Crucial in heart transplants

SPLENIC ARTERY
- Very turbulent flow pattern
- Very prone to aneurysm

SUPERIOR MESENTERIC ARTERY
- Highly resistive in fasting patient
- Nonresistive in nonfasting patient

RENAL ARTERY
- Nonresistive
- Spectral broadening

---

and a relatively low diastolic component. There is little **spectral broadening.** A clear window under systole means there is plug flow.

The distal abdominal aorta below the renal arteries shows flow with a small reversed component present during diastole. The closer the sonographer approaches to the common iliac vessels, the greater the reverse component becomes. This is because of the high impedance of the peripheral circulation in the leg as it becomes triphasic, crossing the baseline three times.

Celiac Axis. The sonographer should scan transversely to search for the seagull sign, celiac trunk, hepatic artery, and splenic artery. If they cannot be seen, the sonographer should scan longitudinally. Typically the spectral analysis of the celiac trunk shows some window under systole with spectral broadening (turbulence) in diastole. There is no change in the flow pattern after meals.

Hepatic Artery. The hepatic artery is the most variable of all abdominal arteries. It has been reported that 12% of the population has a replaced hepatic artery arising from the superior mesenteric artery (Figure 5-52, *A*). Two thirds of the patients have a right hepatic artery that crosses posterior to the common bile duct or right hepatic duct, whereas the left hepatic artery crosses anterior to the left hepatic duct. Flow in diastole persists because of the low vascular impedance of the liver. Similar waveforms are seen in the main hepatic and intrahepatic arteries. Typically, there is more spectral broadening during both systole and diastole.

In a patient with a heart transplant, the sonographer should always document flow in the hepatic artery. Occlusion is one of the most dangerous complications, potentially resulting in death.

Splenic Artery. This splenic artery shows the most turbulence of all the celiac branches (probably because of its tortuosity). Aneurysms of the celiac branches have been described most commonly in the splenic branch. Patients with chronic pancreatitis are particularly prone to these. The sonographer should always apply Doppler to pancreatic pseudocysts; their appearance is very similar to that of vascular aneurysms.

Superior Mesenteric Artery. Typically the **superior mesenteric artery (SMA)** is a highly resistive vessel (with decreased diastolic flow) in the fasting state, with little or no flow in diastole (see Figure 5-52, *B*). However, after a meal the pattern of the superior mesenteric artery changes to a low-resistive waveform demonstrating enhanced diastolic flow. Doppler analysis of the superior mesenteric artery has the potential to diagnose mesenteric arterial occlusion and abdominal angina.

Renal Artery. The main renal artery has a low impedance (nonresistive) pattern with significant diastolic flow—usually 30% to 50% of peak systole (Figure 5-53). The continuous diastolic flow provides continuous perfusion of the kidneys. There is spectral broadening in systole and diastole. The

Figure 5-51   A and **B,** Sagittal scans of the normal flow in the abdominal aorta. The flow pattern of the proximal aorta above the renal arteries shows a high systolic peak and a relatively low diastolic component. **C,** Transverse view.

Figure 5-52   A, Transverse view of the hepatic artery flow. More spectral broadening is seen during systole and diastole. **B,** Sagittal scan of the superior mesenteric artery flow. This vessel has high resistance in the fasting state with little flow in diastole.

Figure 5-53   **A** and **B,** Transverse scans of the left renal artery flow. The main renal artery has a low impedance (nonresistive) pattern with significant diastolic flow, usually 30% to 50% of peak systole. **C,** Transverse scan of the right renal artery. In this view it is much more difficult to obtain an adequate Doppler flow because the beam is perpendicular to the flow pattern. As a result, decreased velocities are obtained.

segmental, interlobar, and arcuate arteries demonstrate a pattern similar to that of the main renal artery. However, the flow is progressively dampened in the periphery and shows reduced velocity patterns.

Renal artery stenosis. Box 5-3 lists Doppler flow patterns observed in renal disease.

It is very hard to demonstrate renal artery stenosis in a native kidney because of the difficulty in seeing the vessel at its origin and in its entirety (Figure 5-54). Renal artery occlusion can only be declared when the artery is unquestionably imaged. The sonographer should be careful because with complete obstruction of the native artery, collaterals may be mistaken for a patent renal artery. At least 30% of the population has multiple renal arteries, which makes it more difficult to rule out obstruction.

Renal hydronephrosis. When there is even minimal separation of the renal pelvis, the sonographer should use Doppler to image the area (Figure 5-55). Surprisingly, no hydronephrosis may be found, just prominent renal vessels in the renal pelvis.

> **BOX 5-3**   **DOPPLER FLOW PATTERNS IN RENAL DISEASE**
>
> **RENAL ARTERY STENOSIS**
> * Stenoses difficult to demonstrate
> * Collaterals may form
>
> **RENAL HYDRONEPHROSIS**
> * Doppler needed to rule out prominent vessels
>
> **RENAL TRANSPLANTS**
> * Turbulence near the anastomosis
> * Renal artery stenosis develops in only 12% of renal transplants
> * Occlusion easier to diagnose than in native kidney
>
> **RENAL TRANSPLANT REJECTION**
> * Normal flow = 30% to 50% of diastolic flow
> * Impedance increases with rejection

Figure 5-54 **A,** High-velocity jet shown in the right renal artery. **B,** Spectral waveform shows increased velocity of more than 4 m/sec, representing renal artery stenosis. **C,** With color Doppler, flow analysis may be made out to the peripheral renal arteries.

Figure 5-55 Doppler energy may be useful to show adequate renal artery flow in the postoperative renal transplant patient.

Renal transplants. In the main renal artery, there is turbulence near the anastomosis. Only 12% of patients has renal artery stenosis develop after transplantation; it is characterized by a high-velocity jet with distal turbulence. Renal artery occlusion is easier to diagnose in transplanted kidneys than in native kidneys because there is no flow throughout the entire transplant.

Rejection. Normal transplants have a diastolic flow that is 30% to 50% that of systole. During rejection, the vascular impedance increases, resulting in a decrease or even reversal of the diastolic flow. There are a few methods to quantify the Doppler signals.

A resistive index (RI) is the most popular method in use. An RI of 0.7 or less indicates good perfusion, whereas an RI of 0.7 to 0.9 indicates possible rejection and greater than 0.9 indicates probable rejection.

Renal Vein. Box 5-4 lists Doppler flow patterns in abdominal veins and their related conditions.

The renal vein shows variable flow like that of the inferior vena cava (Figure 5-56). The sonographer should closely examine the renal veins in any patient with a suspected tumor or renal obstructive lesion because they may be invaded by tumor or clot (Figure 5-57). In renal transplant patients, the sonographer should always look for a patent renal vein. An occlusion backs up the whole blood supply, and the kidney acts like it is in rejection (with elevated blood, urea, nitrogen, creatinine, and protein).

Inferior Vena Cava and Hepatic Veins. The inferior vena cava and hepatic veins present a complex waveform, which flows above and below the baseline, reflecting the reflux of

Figure 5-56 **A** and **B,** Transverse scans of right renal vein flow show variable flow similar to the pattern of the inferior vena cava.

Figure 5-57 Color Doppler demonstrates the renal vascular anatomy. **A,** Duplicated left renal vein crossing anterior and posterior to the aorta; right renal artery leaving the lateral wall of the aorta toward the right kidney. **B,** Spectral Doppler shows increased turbulence in the posterior left renal vein. **C,** Coronal view of the association of the renal veins to the aorta.

blood from the right atrium during systole and variations with the respiratory cycle (Figure 5-58). The sonographer should always look at the cava and renal veins for tumor invasion when a renal cell carcinoma is observed.

Budd-Chiari syndrome. A thrombosis of hepatic veins is called *Budd-Chiari syndrome.* Duplex Doppler is an effective

method for screening patients suspected of having Budd-Chiari syndrome. Sonographically, hepatic veins appear reduced in size and may contain echogenic thrombotic material. The presence of "typical" blood flow in the hepatic veins permits the exclusion of Budd-Chiari syndrome. Budd-Chiari syndrome is a rare disease; 30% of cases are idiopathic. It is

Figure 5-58   The inferior vena cava and hepatic veins show a complex waveform flowing above and below the baseline. This reflects the reflux of blood from the right atrium during systole and variations with the respiratory cycle. **A,** Sagittal. **B,** Transverse. **C,** Transverse scan of the middle hepatic vein flow shows normal flow patterns. **D,** Sagittal scan shows the complex waveform above and below the baseline.

associated with hematologic disorders, oral contraceptives, collagen disease, echinococcus, and the periods before or after pregnancy.

Portal Vein.   In the normal superior mesenteric vein and splenic vein, flow is hepatopetal (toward the liver) (Figures 5-59 and 5-60). The portal vein shows a relatively continuous flow at low velocities, which may vary slightly with respirations. Portal vein thrombosis can be easily diagnosed with sonography. A direct sign is visualization of a thrombus. Indirect signs are the loss of normal portal venous landmarks, dilation of the superior mesenteric vein and splenic vein, and venous collaterals in the porta hepatis (cavernous transformation of the portal vein).

Pulsed Doppler adds to these findings; lack of Doppler signals from the lumen indicates absence of blood flow. In cirrhotic patients, thrombosis is often suspected when ascites suddenly worsens. Consequently, in these patients, special attention must be paid to the portal vein to identify a thrombus. It is often difficult to visualize the portal vein in such patients.

Cavernous transformation of the portal vein.   Cavernous transformation of the portal vein demonstrates periportal collateral channels in patients with chronic portal vein obstruction. The Doppler analysis of the tubular structures is characteristic of portal venous flow hepatopetal (toward the liver) with continuous low velocity flow. Diagnosis can be made sonographically based on the following indications:

1. Extrahepatic portal vein is not visualized.
2. High-level echoes produced by fibrosis are present in the porta hepatis.
3. Multiple tubular structures are present in the porta hepatis, representing periportal collaterals.

Portal venous hypertension.   The majority of portal venous hypertension is the result of intrinsic liver disease. Portal hypertension is also caused by obstruction of the portal vein, hepatic vein, inferior vena cava, or prolonged congestive heart failure. Doppler techniques can determine whether portal flow is hepatopetal (toward) or hepatofugal (away). In portal venous hypertension, portal blood is diverted in a hepatofugal direction via various collateral venous pathways,

A   **B**

Figure 5-59   **A,** Transverse scan of the main portal vein shows positive flow as it proceeds into the liver (hepatopetal). **B,** Transverse scan of the superior mesenteric vein–portal vein flow.

BOX 5-4   DOPPLER FLOW PATTERNS IN ABDOMINAL VEINS

RENAL VEIN
• Variable flow much like the inferior vena cava
• Evaluate with transplants

INFERIOR VENA CAVA AND HEPATIC VEINS
• Varies with respiration
• Flow above and below the baseline, reflux from right atrium

BUDD-CHIARI SYNDROME
• Thrombosis of hepatic veins
• Hepatic veins are small, with echogenic material
• Presence of normal flow excludes Budd-Chiari syndrome

PORTAL VEIN
• Hepatopetal flow
• Continuous flow pattern; varies slightly with respirations

CAVERNOUS TRANSFORMATION OF THE PORTAL VEIN
• Seen in patients with chronic portal vein obstruction
• Extrahepatic portal vein not visualized
• Echogenic area present in porta hepatis
• Periportal collaterals

PORTAL VENOUS HYPERTENSION
• Determine hepatopetal versus hepatofugal flow
• Low velocity in portal vein
• Patent umbilical vein
• Loss of respiratory variation

Figure 5-60   Color Doppler of the portal flow within the liver.

• The condition is most frequently caused by cirrhosis and obstruction of portal venous radicles by fibrosis and regenerating nodules.
• The condition is less frequently caused by portal venous thrombosis or other obstruction.
• Respiratory variation of vessels is usually lost in portal hypertension (there is no collapse of veins).

Sonographic findings in portal hypertension include the following:

• Dilated portal, splenic, superior mesenteric vein
• Patent paraumbilical vein
• Varices
• Splenomegaly with dilated splenic radicles
• Diminished response to respiration in portal system
• Dilated hepatic and splenic arteries
• Ascites
• Small liver with irregular surface or large liver with abnormal texture

In patients with portal hypertension, the blood flow may take one of several pathways through coronary-esophageal varices, splenic varices, splenorenal shunts, a recanalized umbilical vein, or surgical shunts.

with the formation of multiple portosystemic anastomoses (Figure 5-61). Doppler findings include the following:

• The portal vein shows low velocity.
• A patent paraumbilical vein is the definitive diagnosis.
• Typical portal hypertensive venous flow varies.

Figure 5-61   **A,** Bidirectional flow within the main portal vein. **B,** Spectral Doppler shows flow above and below the baseline. **C,** Flow is reversed in the splenic vein, going away from the liver.

With splenic varices, flow in the main, right, and left portal veins is reversed (hepatofugal), as is the flow in the splenic vein, and flow in the superior mesenteric vein is normal.

With splenorenal shunts, all portal flows are reversed, as are flows in the splenic vein. The superior mesenteric vein is normal.

With a recanalized umbilical vein, the main portal vein and the left portal vein show normal flow, but the flow is reversed in the right portal vein. The superior mesenteric vein and splenic veins are normal.

Spontaneous Shunting. Spontaneous shunting occurs at the following four main sites:

1. *Coronary-gastroesophageal:* (most common) Lower esophageal varices occur where esophageal branches of the left gastric vein form anastomoses with branches of the azygos and hemiazygos veins in the submucosa of the lower esophagus.
2. *Paraumbilical vein:* This appears as a continuation of the left portal vein and extends down the anterior abdominal wall to the umbilicus.
3. *Hemorrhoidal anastomoses:* These occur between the superior and middle hemorrhoidal veins.
4. *Retroperitoneal anastomoses:* Vascular structures within the lesser omentum may cause thickening of the omentum (especially in children). Small vessels may be seen around the pancreas. Doppler is useful in distinguishing these vessels from nodes.

Once a portosystemic shunt has been performed, shunt patency can be directly identified with Doppler. This is usually easier with direct portacaval shunts (portal vein drains into inferior vena cava) than with mesocaval (superior mesenteric vein and inferior vena cava) shunts or splenorenal (splenic vein to renal vein) shunts. If the portacaval shunt itself cannot be identified, the demonstration of hepatofugal flow in the intrahepatic portal veins and hepatopetal flows in the superior mesenteric vein and splenic veins is a reliable indication of shunt patency. In long-term follow-up after implantation of a **transjugular intrahepatic portosystemic shunt (TIPS),** the intrashunt and portal venous Doppler velocities alone do not accurately predict elevation of the portosystemic gradient. This will be further discussed in Chapter 6.

SELECTED BIBLIOGRAPHY

Allen KS and others: Renal allografts: prospective analysis of Doppler sonography, *Radiology* 169:371, 1988.

Anderson LA. Abdominal aortic aneurysm, *J Cardiovasc Nurs* 15:1-14, 2001.

Barakat M and others: Intrasplenic venous flow patterns demonstrated by Doppler ultrasound in patients with portal hypertension, *Br J Radiol* 71:384, 1998.

Becker CD, Cooperberg PL: Sonography of the hepatic vascular system, *Am J Roentgenol* 150:999, 1988.

Ebaugh JL, Garcia ND, Matsumura JS. Screening and surveillance for abdominal aortic aneurysm: who needs it and when, *Semin Vasc Surg* 14:193-199, 2001.

Englund R and others: Expansion rates of small abdominal aortic aneurysms, Aust *N Z J Surg* 68:21, 1998.

Erbel R et al: Diagnosis and management of aortic dissection. *Eur Heart J* 22:1642-1681, 2001.

Flachskampf FA, Daniel WG: Aortic dissection, *Cardiol Clin* 18:807-817, 2000.

Goyal AK, Pokharna DS, Sharma SK: Ultrasonic measurements of portal vasculature in diagnosis of portal hypertension: a controversial subject reviewed, *J Ultrasound Med* 9:45, 1990.

Grant EG, Perrella RR: Wishing won't make it so: duplex Doppler sonography in the evaluation of renal transplant dysfunction, *Am J Roentgenol* 155:538, 1990.

Han DC, Feliciano DV: The clinical complexity of splenic vein thrombosis, *Am Surg* 64:558, 1998.

Kelcz F and others: Pyramidal appearance and resistive index: insensitive and nonspecific sonographic indicators of renal transplant rejection, *Am J Roentgenol* 155:531, 1990.

Kronzon I and others: Ultrasound evaluation of endovascular repair of abdominal aortic aneurysms, *J Am Soc Echocardiogr* 11:377, 1998.

Michielsen PP, Duysburgh IK, Pelckmans PA: Ultrasound and duplex Doppler in the diagnosis and follow up of portal hypertension, *ACTA Gastroenterol Belg* 58:409, 1995.

Powell JT, Brown LC: The natural history of abdominal aortic aneurysms and their risk of rupture. *Acta Chir Belg* 101:11-16, 2001.

Singh K et al: Prevalence of and risk factors for abdominal aortic aneurysms in a population-based study. *Am J Epidemiol* 154:236-244, 2001.

Spaulding KA and others: 3-D gray scale ultrasonographic imaging of the celiac axis, *J Ultrasound Med* 17:239, 1998.

Tullis MJ and others: Clinical evidence of contralateral renal parenchymal injury in patients with unilateral atherosclerotic renal artery stenosis, *Ann Vasc Surg* 12:122, 1998.

Wachsberg RH and others: Echogenicity of hepatic versus portal vein walls revisited with histologic correlation, *J Ultrasound Med* 16:807, 1997.

Wain RA and others: Endoleaks after endovascular graft treatment of aortic aneurysms: classification, risk factors, and outcome, *J Vasc Surg* 27:69, 1998.

Watson CJ and others: What is the long-term outcome for patients with very small abdominal aortic aneurysms? *Eur J Vasc Endovasc Surg* 14:299, 1997.

CHAPTER 6

The Liver

Sandra L. Hagen-Ansert

OBJECTIVES

- Describe the location and size of the liver
- Define the relational landmarks of the liver
- List the four fossae of the liver
- Describe the vascular supply to the liver
- Illustrate the surface and internal anatomy of the liver and adjacent structures
- List the functions of the liver
- Describe the liver function tests and their relevance to hepatic disease
- List the clinical signs, sonographic features, and differentials for normal liver parenchyma, diffuse disease, focal anomalies, cystic lesions, congenital lesions, infection and inflammatory lesions, benign neoplasms, malignant neoplasms, traumatic lesions, and vascular anomalies of the liver
- Differentiate between the sonographic appearances of intrahepatic and extrahepatic biliary obstruction

ANATOMY OF THE LIVER
NORMAL ANATOMY
VASCULAR SUPPLY

PHYSIOLOGY AND LABORATORY DATA OF THE HEPATOBILIARY SYSTEM
HEPATIC PHYSIOLOGY
HEPATIC VERSUS OBSTRUCTIVE DISEASE
HEPATIC METABOLIC FUNCTIONS
HEPATIC DETOXIFICATION FUNCTIONS
BILE
LIVER FUNCTION TESTS

SONOGRAPHIC EVALUATION OF THE LIVER
SAGITTAL PLANE
TRANSVERSE PLANE
LATERAL DECUBITUS PLANE

PATHOLOGY OF THE LIVER
DIFFUSE DISEASE
DIFFUSE ABNORMALITIES OF THE LIVER PARENCHYMA
FOCAL HEPATIC DISEASE
HEPATIC TUMORS
HEPATIC TRAUMA
LIVER TRANSPLANTATION
HEPATIC VASCULAR FLOW ABNORMALITIES

KEY TERMS

alkaline phosphatase – enzyme of the liver

ALT – alanine aminotransferase – enzyme of the liver

AST – aspartase aminotransferase – enzyme of the liver

bare area – area superior to the liver that is not covered by peritoneum so that inferior vena cava may enter the chest

bilirubin – broken down product of hemoglobin; excreted by the liver and stored in the gallbladder

bull's eye (target) lesion – hypoechoic mass with an echogenic central core (abscess, metastases)

BUN – blood urea nitrogen

caudate lobe – small lobe of the liver situated on the posterosuperior surface of the left lobe; the ligamentum venosum is the anterior border

collateral circulation – develops when normal venous channels become obstructed

diffuse hepatocellular disease – affects hepatocytes and interferes with liver function

epigastrium – area between the right and left hypochondrium that contains part of the liver, duodenum, and pancreas

extrahepatic – outside the liver

falciform ligament – extends from the umbilicus to the diaphragm in a sagittal plane and contains the ligamentum teres

hepatocellular disease – refers to liver cells or hepatocytes as primary problem

hepatocyte – a parenchymal liver cell that performs all functions ascribed to the liver

hepatofugal – flow away from the liver

hepatopetal – flow toward the liver

hyperglycemia – uncontrolled increase in glucose

hypoglycemia – deficiency of glucose

intrahepatic – within the liver

left hypochondrium – left upper quadrant of the abdomen that contains the left lobe of the liver, spleen, and stomach

left lobe of the liver – lies in the epigastrium and left hypochondrium

left portal vein – supplies the left lobe of the liver

ligamentum teres – appears as bright echogenic foci on transverse image; along with falciform ligament, it divides medial and lateral segments of left lobe of the liver

ligamentum venosum – separates left lobe from caudate lobe; shown as echogenic line on the transverse and sagittal images

liver function tests – specific laboratory tests that look at liver function (aspartate or alanine aminotransferase, lactic acid dehydrogenase, alkaline phosphatase, and bilirubin)

main lobar fissure – boundary between the right and left lobes of the liver; seen as hyperechoic line on the sagittal image extending from the portal vein to the neck of the gallbladder

main portal vein – enters the liver at the porta hepatis

metastatic disease – most common form of neoplasm of the liver; primary sites are colon, breast, and lung

neoplasm – refers to any new growth (benign or malignant)

obstructive disease – refers to bile excretion blocked within the liver or biliary system

pyogenic abscess – pus-forming collection of fluid

right hypochondrium – right upper quadrant of the abdomen that contains the liver and gallbladder

right lobe of the liver – largest of the lobes of the liver

right portal vein – supplies the right lobe of the liver; branches into anterior and posterior segments.

The liver is the largest organ in the body and is quite accessible to sonographic evaluation. The parenchyma of the normal liver is used to evaluate other organs and glands in the body (e.g., the kidneys are equally echogenic or less echogenic than the liver, the spleen is about the same echogenicity, and the pancreas is about as echogenic or slightly more echogenic than the liver). The size and shape of the liver determine the quality of the sonographic examination performed. For example, the prominent left lobe of the liver facilitates visualization of the pancreas, which is situated just inferior to the border of the left lobe, whereas if the right lobe extends just below the costal margin, it may facilitate visualization of the gallbladder and right kidney.

ANATOMY OF THE LIVER

NORMAL ANATOMY

The liver occupies almost all of the **right hypochondrium,** the greater part of the **epigastrium,** and the **left hypochondrium** as far as the mammillary line. The contour and shape of the liver vary according to the patient's habitus and lie. Its shape is also influenced by the lateral segment of the left lobe and the length of the right lobe of the liver. The liver lies inferior to the diaphragm. The ribs cover the greater part of the right lobe (usually a small part of the right lobe is in contact with the abdominal wall). In the epigastric region, the liver extends

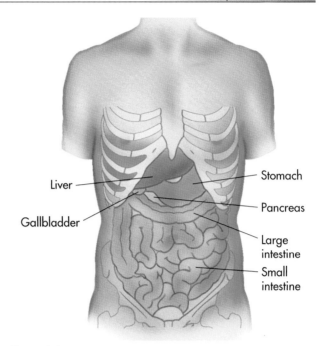

Figure 6-1 AP view of the abdomen shows the right lobe of the liver covered by the ribs. The left lobe of the liver lies in the midline just posterior to the tip of the sternum. The stomach lies posterior and lateral to the left lobe of the liver.

several centimeters below the xiphoid process. Most of the left lobe is covered by the rib cage.

The fundus of the stomach lies posterior and lateral to the left lobe of the liver and may frequently be seen on transverse sonograms (Figure 6-1). The remainder of the stomach lies inferior to the liver and is best visualized on sagittal sonograms. The duodenum lies adjacent to the right lobe and medial segment of the left lobe of the liver. The body of the pancreas is usually seen just inferior to the left lobe of the liver. The posterior border of the liver contacts the right kidney, inferior vena cava, and aorta. The diaphragm covers the superior border of the liver (Figure 6-2). The liver is suspended from the diaphragm and anterior abdominal wall by the falciform ligament and from the diaphragm by the reflections of the peritoneum.

Most of the liver is covered by peritoneum, but a large area rests directly on the diaphragm; this is called the **bare area** (Figure 6-3). The subphrenic space between the liver (or spleen) and the diaphragm is a common site for abscess formation. The right posterior subphrenic space lies between the right lobe of the liver, the right kidney, and the right colic flexure. The lesser sac is an enclosed portion of the peritoneal space posterior to the liver and stomach. This sac communicates with the rest of the peritoneal space at a point near the head of the pancreas. It also may be a site for abscess formation. The right subhepatic space is located inferior to the right lobe of the liver and includes Morison's pouch, which lies between the posterior aspect of the right lobe and the upper pole of the right kidney.

Projections of the liver may be altered by some disease states. Inferior displacement is often caused by tumor infiltration,

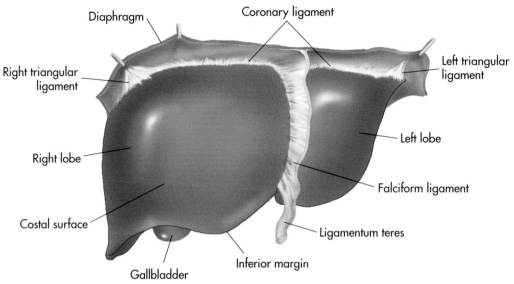

Figure 6-2   Anterior view of the liver. The right lobe is the largest of the four lobes of the liver.

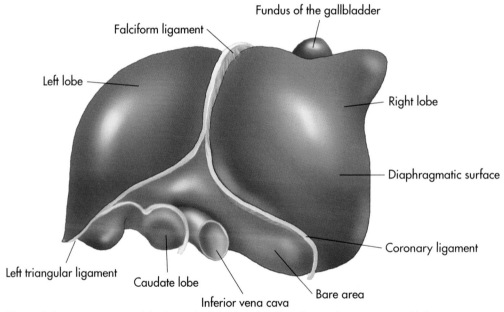

Figure 6-3   Superior view of the liver. The left lobe of the liver lies in the epigastric and left hypochondriac regions.

cirrhosis, or a subphrenic abscess, whereas ascites, excessive dilation of the colon, or abdominal tumors can elevate the liver. Retroperitoneal tumors may move the liver slightly anterior.

LOBES OF THE LIVER

Right lobe.   The **right lobe of the liver** is the largest of the liver's three lobes (see Figure 6-2). It exceeds the left lobe by a ratio of 6 : 1. It occupies the right hypochondrium and is bordered on its upper surface by the falciform ligament, on its posterior surface by the left sagittal fossa, and in front by the umbilical notch. Its inferior and posterior surfaces are marked by three fossae: the porta hepatis, the gallbladder fossa, and the inferior vena cava fossa. A congenital variant, Riedel's lobe, can

sometimes be seen as an anterior projection of the liver and may extend to the iliac crest.

Left lobe.   The **left lobe of the liver** lies in the epigastric and left hypochondriac regions (see Figure 6-3). Its upper surface is convex and molded onto the diaphragm. Its undersurface includes the gastric impression and omental tuberosity. The medial segment of the left lobe is oblong and situated on the posteroinferior surface of the left lobe (Figure 6-4). In front it is bounded by the anterior margin of the liver, behind by the porta hepatis, on the right by the fossa for the gallbladder, and on the left by the fossa for the umbilical vein. The size of the left lobe of the liver varies considerably; the more prominent left lobe will allow the sonographer to image the pancreas and vascular structures anterior to the spine.

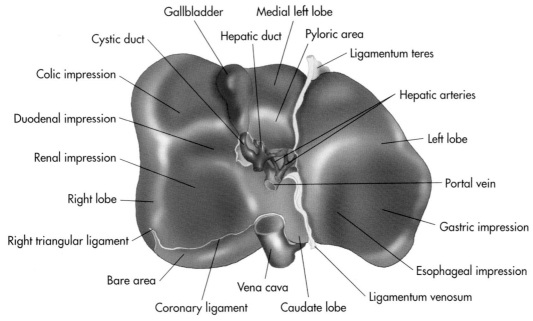

Figure 6-4   Inferior view of the visceral surface of the liver.

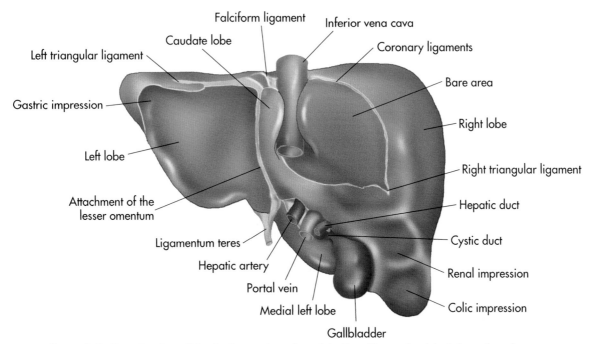

Figure 6-5   Posterior view of the diaphragmatic surface of the liver. The caudate lobe is located on the posterosuperior surface of the right lobe, opposite the tenth and eleventh thoracic vertebrae.

Caudate lobe. The **caudate lobe** is a small lobe situated on the posterosuperior surface of the left lobe opposite the tenth and eleventh thoracic vertebrae (Figure 6-5). It is bounded below by the porta hepatis, on the right by the fossa for the inferior vena cava, and on the left by the fossa for the ductus venosus.

Hepatic Nomenclature. Couinaud's system of hepatic nomenclature (Box 6-1) provides the anatomic basis for

hepatic surgical resections. By using this system, the radiologist may be able to precisely isolate the location of a lesion for the surgical team. The description of the liver segments is based on the portal and hepatic venous segments. There are eight segments (Figure 6-6). The right, middle, and left hepatic veins divide the liver longitudinally into four sections. Each of these sections is further divided transversely by an invisible plane through the right and left portal veins. The caudate lobe (segment I) may receive branches of both the right and left

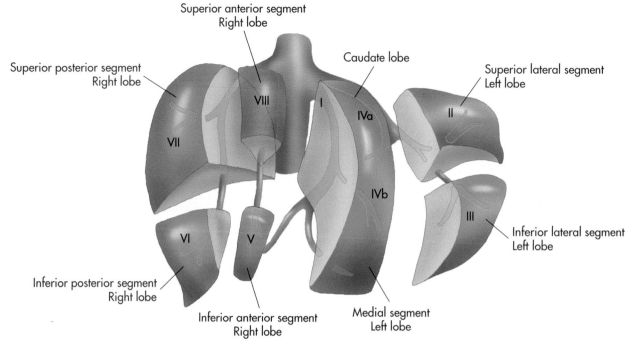

Superior anterior segment
Right lobe

Caudate lobe

Superior lateral segment
Left lobe

Superior posterior segment
Right lobe

VIII

I

IVa

II

VII

IVb

Inferior lateral segment
Left lobe

VI

V

III

Inferior posterior segment
Right lobe

Inferior anterior segment
Right lobe

Medial segment
Left lobe

Figure 6-6 Couinaud's hepatic segments divide the liver into eight segments. The three hepatic veins are the longitudinal boundaries. The transverse plane is defined by the right and left portal pedicles. The caudate lobe (segment I) is situated posteriorly. Segment I includes the caudate lobe. Segments II and III include the left superior and inferior lateral segments. Segments IVa and IVb include the medial segment of the left lobe. Segments V and VI are caudal to the transverse plane. Segmebts VII and VIII are cephalad to the transverse plane.

BOX 6-1 HEPATIC SEGMENTAL ANATOMY

Segment I: Caudate lobe
Segments II and III: Left superior and inferior lateral segments
Segments IVa and IVb: Medial segments of the left lobe
Segments V and VI: Caudal to the transverse plane
Segments VII and VIII: Cephalad to the transverse plane

portal veins and may have one or more hepatic veins draining into the inferior vena cava.

Ligaments and Fissures. There are several important ligaments and fissures to remember in the liver: Glisson's capsule, main lobar fissure, falciform ligament, ligamentum teres (round ligament), and ligamentum venosum. These ligaments and fissures appear echogenic or hyperechoic because of the presence of collagen and fat within and around the structures.

The liver is covered by a thin connective tissue layer called Glisson's capsule. This capsule completely surrounds the liver and is thickest around the inferior vena cava and portal hepatis. At the porta hepatis, the main portal vein, the proper hepatic artery, and the common duct are contained within the hepatoduodenal ligament.

The **main lobar fissure** is the boundary between the right and left lobes of the liver. On the longitudinal scan, it may be seen as a hyperechoic line extending from the portal vein to

the neck of the gallbladder (Figure 6-7, *A*). The sonographer uses this ligament to find the gallbladder on the longitudinal scan, especially when it is packed with stones and not well imaged.

The **falciform ligament** extends from the umbilicus to the diaphragm in a parasagittal plane and contains the ligamentum teres (see Figure 6-7, *B*). In the anteroposterior axis, the falciform ligament extends from the right rectus muscle to the bare area of the liver, where its echogenic reflections separate to contribute to the hepatic coronary ligament and attach to the undersurface of the diaphragm.

The **ligamentum teres** appears as a bright echogenic focus on the sonogram and is seen as the rounded termination of the falciform ligament (see Figure 6-7, *C*). Both the falciform ligament and the ligamentum teres divide the medial and lateral segments of the left lobe of the liver.

The fissure for the **ligamentum venosum** separates the left lobe from the caudate lobe (Figure 6-8). On ultrasound, it may be seen just inferior to the dome of the liver as a linear horizontal line just anterior to the caudate lobe and inferior vena cava. The caudate lobe, ligamentum venosum, portal vein, and left lobe of the liver may be seen on the longitudinal plane over the area of the inferior vena cava.

VASCULAR SUPPLY

Portal Venous System. The portal venous system is a reliable indicator of various ultrasonic tomographic planes throughout the liver (Figure 6-9).

Figure 6-7 **A,** Main lobar fissure *(MLF)* extends between the long axis neck of the gallbladder *(GB)* and the main portal vein *(PV)* on the longitudinal image. **B,** Falciform ligament extends from the umbilicus to the diaphragm in a longitudinal plane. **C,** Ligamentum teres *(LT, arrows)* appears as a bright echogenic focus in the left lobe of the liver on a transverse image.

Figure 6-8 Ligamentum venosum. **A,** Transverse image high in the liver shows the spine *(S)*, aorta *(AO)*, and inferior vena cava *(IVC)*. The caudate lobe *(CL)* is anterior to the inferior vena cava *(IVC)* and is separated from the left lobe of the liver *(LLL)* by the ligamentum venosum *(arrow)*. **B,** Longitudinal image through the right lobe of the liver *(RLL)* shows the ligamentum venosum *(arrow)* and caudate lobe *(CL)*.

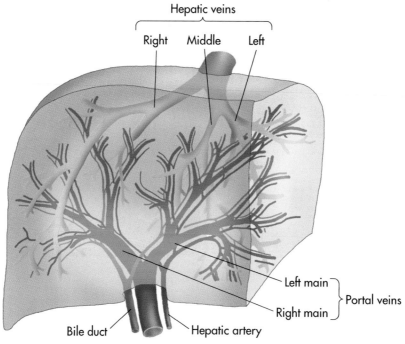

Figure 6-9   Vascular system of the liver.

Main portal vein. The **main portal vein** approaches the porta hepatis in a rightward, cephalic, and slightly posterior direction within the hepatoduodenal ligament. It comes in contact with the anterior surface of the inferior vena cava near the porta hepatis and serves to locate the liver hilum (Figure 6-10). It then divides into two branches: the right and left portal veins.

Right portal vein. The **right portal vein** is the larger of the two branches and requires a more posterior and more caudal transducer approach. It usually is possible to identify the anterior and posterior divisions of the right portal vein on sonography (Figure 6-11). The anterior division closely parallels the anterior abdominal wall.

Left portal vein. The **left portal vein** lies more anterior and cranial than the right portal vein. The main portal vein is seen to elongate at the origin of the left portal vein (Figure 6-12). The vessel lies within a canal containing large amounts of connective tissue, which results in the visualization of an echogenic linear band coursing through the central portion of the lateral segment of the left lobe.

Hepatic Veins. The hepatic veins are divided into three components: right, middle, and left (Figure 6-13). The right hepatic vein is the largest and enters the right lateral aspect of the inferior vena cava. The middle hepatic vein enters the anterior or right anterior surface of the inferior vena cava. The left hepatic vein, which is the smallest, enters the left anterior surface of the inferior vena cava. Often it is possible to identify a long horizontal branch of the right hepatic vein coursing between the anterior and posterior divisions of the right portal vein.

Distinguishing Characteristics of Portal and Hepatic Veins. The best way to distinguish the hepatic from the portal

vessels is to trace their points of entry to the liver. The hepatic vessels flow into the inferior vena cava, whereas the splenic vein and superior mesenteric vein join together to form the portal venous system. Real-time sector scanning allows the sonographer to make this assessment within a few seconds (Figure 6-14). Hepatic veins course between the hepatic lobes and segments. Hepatic veins are larger as they drain into the inferior vena cava before entering the right atrium; the portal veins are larger at their origin as they emanate from the porta hepatis. Portal veins have more echogenic borders than the hepatic veins because they have a thicker collagenous sheath.

Intrahepatic Vessels and Ducts. The portal veins carry blood from the bowel to the liver, whereas the hepatic veins drain the blood from the liver into the inferior vena cava (see Figure 6-9). The hepatic arteries carry oxygenated blood from the aorta to the liver (Figure 6-15). The bile ducts transport bile, manufactured in the liver, to the duodenum.

PHYSIOLOGY AND LABORATORY DATA OF THE HEPATOBILIARY SYSTEM

The liver, bile ducts, and gallbladder constitute the hepatobiliary system, which performs metabolic and excretory functions essential to physical well-being. Sonography is an important method for detecting anatomic changes associated with hepatobiliary disease; but accurate ultrasound evaluation can be accomplished only when other diagnostic information (e.g., signs, symptoms, and laboratory results) are considered with the sonographic findings.

The task of correlating these clinical and ultrasound data falls primarily to the sonologist. However, the sonographer

Figure 6-10 Main portal vein. **A,** Transverse image of the main portal vein *(MPV)* as it enters the liver. *IVC,* Inferior vena cava. **B,** Transverse image of the main portal vein *(MPV)* as it bifurcates into right *(RPV)* and left *(LPV)* branches. *AO,* Aorta; *IVC,* inferior vena cava; *S,* spine. **C,** Longitudinal image just to the right of midline shows the inferior vena cava *(IVC)*, main portal vein *(MPV)*, and left portal vein *(LPV)*.

Figure 6-11 Right portal vein. **A,** Transverse image of the right portal vein as it bifurcates into the anterior *(ARPV)* and posterior *(PRPV)* branches. **B,** Transverse image of the main portal vein *(MPV)* as it bifurcates into right *(RPV)* and left *(LPV)* branches.

Figure 6-12   Left portal vein. **A,** Transverse image of the right portal vein branching into the left portal vein *(LPV)* as it flows into the left lobe of the liver. **B,** Longitudinal image just to the right of midline shows the inferior vena cava *(IVC)*, the main portal vein *(MPV)*, and the left portal vein *(LPV)*.

Figure 6-13   Hepatic veins. **A,** Transverse image at the dome of the liver shows the hepatic veins as they empty into the inferior vena cava *(IVC)*. **B,** Longitudinal image through the right lobe of the liver shows the right hepatic vein *(RHV)* as it empties into the inferior vena cava *(IVC)*. **C,** Longitudinal image just to the right of midline shows the middle hepatic vein *(MHV)* heading towards the inferior vena cava *(IVC)*.

must also understand the entire clinical picture to be able to plan and properly perform the ultrasound examination. It is necessary therefore that the sonographer be aware of the normal and abnormal physiology of the hepatobiliary system. This section is intended as a primer of hepatobiliary physiology, with particular attention to physiologic alterations that commonly occur in hepatobiliary disease.

HEPATIC PHYSIOLOGY

The liver has many functions, including metabolism, digestion, storage, and detoxification (Box 6-2). The liver is a major center of metabolism, which may be defined as the physical and chemical process whereby foodstuffs are synthesized into complex elements, complex substances are transformed into simple ones, and energy is made available for use by the organism. Through the process of digestion, the liver expels these waste products from the body via its excretory product, bile,

which also plays an important role in fat absorption. **Bilirubin** is a pigment released when the red blood cells are broken down. The liver is a storage site for several compounds used in a variety of physiologic activities throughout the body. In hepatobiliary disease, each of these functions may be altered, leading to abnormal physical, laboratory, and sonographic findings. Finally, the liver is also a center for detoxification of the waste products of metabolism accumulated from other sources in the body and foreign chemicals (usually drugs) that enter the body.

Figure 6-14 Portal versus hepatic veins. The portal veins *(PV)* have more echogenic borders than the hepatic veins *(HV)*. *IVC,* Inferior vena cava.

BOX 6-2   PRIMARY FUNCTIONS OF THE LIVER

METABOLISM
- Carbohydrate: The liver converts glucose to glycogen and stores it; when glucose is needed, it breaks down the glycogen and releases glucose into the blood.
- Protein: The liver performs many important functions in metabolism of proteins, fats, and carbohydrates. It manufactures many of the plasma proteins found in the blood. The liver converts excess amino acids to fatty acids and urea. It also removes nutrients from the blood and phagocytizes bacteria and worn-out red blood cells.

DIGESTION
The liver secretes bile, which is important in the digestion of fats. Bilirubin, a pigment released when red blood cells are broken down, is excreted in the bile.

STORAGE
The liver stores iron and certain vitamins.

DETOXIFICATION
The liver detoxifies many drugs and poisons that enter the body.

Figure 6-15 Hepatic artery *(HA)* may be seen anterior and medial to the portal vein on a oblique transverse image; this is known as the *portal triad. Arrow,* Hepatic artery; *CBD,* common bile duct; *PV,* portal vein.

HEPATIC VERSUS OBSTRUCTIVE DISEASE

Diseases affecting the liver may be classified as *hepatocellular*, when the liver cells or **hepatocytes** are the immediate problem; or *obstructive* when bile excretion is blocked.

Viral hepatitis is an example in which the virus attacks liver cells and damages or destroys them, resulting in an alteration of liver function. In obstructive disorders, the flow of bile from the liver is blocked at some point and secondarily results in liver malfunction.

The differentiation between **hepatocellular disease** and **obstructive disease** is of considerable importance clinically. Hepatocellular diseases are treated medically with supportive measures and drugs; obstructive disorders are usually relieved by surgery. In some cases the distinction between hepatocellular and obstructive disease can be made through clinical laboratory tests, but often the laboratory findings are equivocal. Sonography has been of great benefit because it allows the physician to accurately separate hepatocellular and obstructive causes of liver disease.

HEPATIC METABOLIC FUNCTIONS

Raw materials in the form of carbohydrates (sugars), fats, and amino acids (the basic components of proteins) are absorbed from the intestine and transported to the liver via the circulatory system. In the liver, these substances are converted chemically to other compounds or are processed for storage or energy production. The following paragraphs are a brief discussion of the metabolic functions of the liver and basic disturbances in these functions that result from liver disease.

Carbohydrates. Sugars may be absorbed from the blood in several forms, but only glucose can be used by cells throughout the body as a source of energy.

The liver functions as a major site for conversion of dietary sugars into glucose, which is released into the bloodstream for general use. The body requires only a certain amount of glucose at any one time, however. Excess sugar is converted by the liver to glycogen (a starch), which may be stored in the liver cells or transported in the blood to distant storage sites. When dietary sugar is unavailable, the liver converts glycogen released from stores into glucose; it can also manufacture glucose directly from other compounds, including proteins or fats, when other sources of glucose have been depleted. Thus the liver helps to maintain a steady state of glucose in the bloodstream.

In very severe liver disease, unless glucose is administered intravenously, the body may become glucose deficient (**hypoglycemia**), with profound effects on the function of the brain and other organs. Uncontrolled increases in blood glucose (**hyperglycemia**) may occur in severe liver disease if a large dose of glucose is administered because the liver fails to convert the excess glucose to glycogen.

Fats. The liver is also a principal site for metabolism of fats, which are absorbed from the intestine in the form of monoglycerides and diglycerides.

Dietary fats are converted in the hepatocytes to lipoproteins, in which form fats are transported throughout the body to sites where they are stored or used by other organs. Conversely, stored fats may be transported to the liver and converted into energy, yielding glucose or other substances, such as cholesterol.

In severe liver disease, abnormally low blood levels of cholesterol may be noted because the liver is the principal site for cholesterol synthesis. Furthermore, failure of hepatic conversion of fat to glucose in liver disease may contribute to hypoglycemia. A striking histologic manifestation of many forms of hepatocellular disease is the so-called fatty liver. On gross pathologic examination, the fatty liver has a yellow color and feels greasy to the touch; on microscopic study, globules of fat (primarily triglycerides) crowd the hepatocytes. The cause of fat accumulation in the liver cells is poorly understood, but it is believed to result from failure of the hepatocytes to manufacture special proteins, called lipoproteins, that coat small quantities of fat, making the fat soluble in plasma and allowing for its release into the bloodstream. Fatty liver is a nonspecific finding that may be seen in a variety of conditions including viral hepatitis, alcoholic liver disease, obesity, diabetes, pregnancy, and exposure to toxic chemicals.

Proteins. The liver produces a variety of proteins, either indirectly from amino acids absorbed from the gut or directly from raw materials stored within the body.

Albumin, in particular, is produced in great quantities. In the bloodstream, it functions as a transport medium for some kinds of molecules. Because it is nonionic, it also functions to draw water into the vascular system from tissue spaces; stated more technically, it helps to maintain oncotic pressure within the vascular system. When the liver is chronically diseased, clinical laboratory results may reveal a significant lowering of the serum albumin (hypoalbuminemia). The accompanying loss of oncotic pressure in the vascular system allows fluid to migrate into the interstitial space, resulting in edema (swelling) in dependent areas, such as the lower extremities. In patients with severe liver disease, especially advanced cirrhosis, ascites also develop. Hypoalbuminemia may account in part for the ascites, but the development of ascites is principally caused by portal hypertension.

In addition to being the primary source of albumin synthesis, the liver is the principal source of proteins necessary for blood coagulation, including fibrinogen (factor I), prothrombin (factor II), and factors V, VII, IX, and X. In liver disease, decreased production of these proteins may lead to inadequate blood coagulation and uncontrollable hemorrhage. Commonly such hemorrhages occur into the bowel after rupture of a dilated vein or development of an ulcer. These hemorrhages are often the immediate or contributing cause of death. Deficiencies of clotting factors II, VII, IX, and X also may result from failure of intestinal absorption of vitamin K, which is a precursor (raw material) required for synthesis of these factors. Vitamin K is a fat-soluble vitamin (as are vitamins D, A, and E) and is absorbed only from the intestine in solution with fat.

Fat absorption is severely limited in cases of bile duct obstruction because of the absence of bile salts (discussed later), and absorption of fat-soluble vitamins is therefore severely reduced. Ultimately the deficiency of vitamin K lowers the amount of the previously mentioned factors and coagulation is retarded. Deficiency of prothrombin and other vitamin K-dependent factors can be corrected in cases of obstruction through parenteral administration of vitamin K.

In hepatocellular disease, administration of vitamin K may improve the coagulopathy but frequently does not restore normal clotting function because the primary problem is hepatocyte dysfunction.

Clotting deficiencies related to liver disease may be detected with several laboratory tests. Of particular interest are the prothrombin time (pro-time) and partial thromboplastin time (PTT) tests. The results of these tests are presented as percentages of the time required for certain coagulation steps to occur in the patient's blood compared with normal blood. Longer periods (lower percentages) indicate greater degrees of abnormality in each of these tests.

Hepatic Enzymes. Enzymes are protein catalysts used throughout the body in all metabolic processes. Because the liver is a major center of metabolism, large quantities of enzymes are present in hepatocytes, and these leak into the bloodstream when the liver cells are damaged or destroyed by disease. The presence of increased quantities of enzymes in the blood is a very sensitive indicator of a hepatocellular disorder.

In hepatobiliary disease the enzymes **aspartase aminotransferase (AST), alanine aminotransferase (ALT),** and **alkaline phosphatase** are of particular interest. Serum levels of all three of these enzymes are increased in both hepatocellular disease and biliary obstruction, but the patterns of elevation may help differentiate hepatocellular from obstructive causes (Table 6-1). In biliary obstruction, elevation of AST and ALT is usually mild (serum levels typically do not exceed 300 units). However, in severe hepatocellular destruction, such as acute viral or toxic hepatitis, a striking elevation of AST and ALT may be seen (levels frequently exceed 1000 units).

Marked elevation of alkaline phosphatase, on the other hand, is typically associated with biliary obstruction or the presence of mass lesions in the liver (e.g., metastatic disease or abscesses). Low levels of alkaline phosphatase are very unusual in obstruction, and high levels (greater than 15 Bodansky units) are uncommon in hepatocellular disorders. Alkaline phosphatase is such a sensitive indicator of obstruction that it may become elevated before the serum bilirubin in cases of acute obstruction. Hence a disproportional increase of alkaline phosphatase relative to bilirubin always suggests obstruction.

Elevation of serum alkaline phosphatase may be the only abnormal laboratory finding in metastatic disease.

Whereas the pattern of enzyme abnormality may strongly suggest hepatocellular disease or obstruction in some cases, it may not allow this distinction to be made in others because obstruction may be superimposed on preexisting hepatocellular disease or unrelieved obstruction may cause hepatocellular damage. Confusion in interpretation of serum enzyme abnormalities may also occur when AST, ALT, or alkaline phosphatase is released from diseased tissues other than the liver. For example, AST and ALT are increased with damage to heart and skeletal muscle, and alkaline phosphatase is elevated in bone disease and in normal pregnancies. ALT is somewhat more specific for liver disease than AST; therefore elevation of ALT above AST suggests a hepatic cause.

HEPATIC DETOXIFICATION FUNCTIONS

The liver is a major location for detoxification of waste products of energy production and other metabolic activities occurring throughout the body. It is also the principal site of breakdown of foreign chemicals, such as drugs. Although these functions fall under the general definition of metabolism and could therefore be grouped in the preceding section, it is useful for instructional purposes to think of these functions as separate categories of hepatic activity.

Ammonium, a toxic product of nitrogen metabolism, is converted to nontoxic urea in the liver, which is practically the only site where this conversion occurs. Urea is subsequently eliminated from the body by the kidneys. The level of urea in the blood is measured as the **blood urea nitrogen (BUN),** and in severe liver disease (acute or chronic) the BUN may be abnormally low because of falloff of urea production. The exhaled breath of patients with severe liver disease may have a fruity or pungent odor (known as *fetor hepaticus*) because of ammonium (NH_4) accumulation. More important, the concentration of NH_4 in the blood may rise to toxic levels and cause brain dysfunction (including confusion, coordination disturbances, tremor, and coma).

Gastrointestinal hemorrhage frequently leads to the accumulation of toxic levels of NH_4 in the blood. Blood lost into the intestine is broken down by bacteria into nitrogen-containing substances, which are absorbed into the bloodstream. The failing liver may therefore be presented with a large amount of NH_4 that it cannot detoxify; coma may result and is frequently a precursor to death if the patient does not succumb to the direct effects of blood loss. Thus failure of

TABLE 6-1	COMPARISON OF LABORATORY ABNORMALITIES IN HEPATOCELLULAR DISEASE AND BILIARY OBSTRUCTION				
Condition	Bilirubin	Serum Albumin	AST (SGOT)	ALT (SGPT)	Alkaline Phosphatase
Hepatocellular disease	Minimal to severe increase	Decreased	Moderate to severe increase	Moderate to severe increase	Minimal to moderate increase
Obstruction	Severe increase	Normal	Mild increase	Mild increase	Severe increase

ammonium detoxification is a serious consequence of liver failure.

Bilirubin Detoxification. Bilirubin, the breakdown product of hemoglobin, is also an important substance detoxified in the liver. Along with detoxification, the liver also excretes bilirubin into the gut via the biliary tree.

Red blood cells survive an average of 120 days in the circulatory system; they are then trapped and broken down by reticuloendothelial cells, primarily within the spleen. Hemoglobin released from the red cells is converted to bilirubin within the reticuloendothelial system and is then released into the bloodstream. The bilirubin molecules become attached to albumin in the blood and are transported to the liver, where the following metabolic steps take place in the hepatocytes:

1. *Uptake:* The bilirubin is separated from albumin, probably at the cell membrane, and is taken within the hepatocytes.
2. *Conjugation:* The bilirubin molecule is combined with two glucuronide molecules, forming bilirubin diglucuronide.
3. *Excretion:* The bilirubin molecule is actively transported across the cell membrane into the bile canaliculi, which are the microscopic "headwaters" of the biliary system. Bilirubin released from the hepatocytes passes through the bile ducts with other components of bile and is delivered to the bowel, where most bilirubin diglucuronide is excreted into the feces (a small portion is broken down into urobilinogen by intestinal bacteria, absorbed into the portal system, and reexcreted by the liver).

Measurement of the concentration of bilirubin in the blood is a standard laboratory test for hepatocellular disease. The following two fractions of bilirubin are measured: the direct-acting fraction, which reacts chemically in an aqueous medium and consists of conjugated bilirubin, and the indirect-acting fraction, which consists of unconjugated bilirubin released from the reticuloendothelial system. Indirect bilirubin reacts only in a nonaqueous (alcohol) medium. The total bilirubin is the sum of the direct-acting and the indirect-acting fractions and normally does not exceed 1 mg/100 ml of serum. In hematologic diseases associated with abrupt breakdown of large numbers of red blood cells (hemolytic anemias, transfusion reactions), the liver may receive more bilirubin from the reticuloendothelial system than it can detoxify. The level of indirect, or unconjugated, bilirubin therefore is elevated.

In biliary obstruction, the hepatocytes pick up bilirubin and conjugate it with glucuronide molecules but cannot dispose of it. The conjugated form is then regurgitated into the bloodstream, with resultant elevation of the direct-acting bilirubin fraction. The indirect-acting bilirubin may also rise slightly in biliary obstruction, but the direct bilirubin predominates.

The direct, or conjugated, form also predominates in hepatocellular disease. Excretion of bilirubin is the step most readily affected when the hepatocytes are damaged; therefore, the diseased hepatocytes continue to take in and conjugate bilirubin but are unable to excrete it. As in biliary obstruction, the accumulated conjugated bilirubin is regurgitated into the blood.

	TABLE 6-2	**DIRECT AND INDIRECT PATTERNS OF BILIRUBIN**	
Condition		Direct Bilirubin Predominates	Indirect Bilirubin Predominates
Hemolysis			X
Hepatocellular disease		X	
Biliary obstruction		X	

The direct and indirect patterns may be summarized as in Table 6-2.

Elevation of serum bilirubin results in jaundice, which is a yellow coloration of the skin, sclerae, and body secretions. Jaundice is a nonspecific finding seen in massive blood breakdown, hepatocellular disease, or biliary obstruction. Chemical separation of bilirubin into direct and indirect fractions helps to specify a hepatocellular or hematologic cause for jaundice. Furthermore, if jaundice results from liver disease, the level of bilirubin may help to separate hepatocellular disease from obstruction because it is uncommon for the total bilirubin to rise above 35 mg/100 ml of serum with obstruction.

Hormone and Drug Detoxification. The liver breaks down several hormones that otherwise would accumulate in the body. For example, failure to metabolize estrogen in men with chronic hepatocellular disease, such as cirrhosis, causes gynecomastia (breast enlargement), testicular atrophy, and changes in body-hair patterns. Reduced detoxification of the hormone glucagon, which is an insulin antagonist, occurs in liver disease and may contribute to the fluctuations in blood sugar levels seen in severe hepatic disorders. The liver is also the primary location for breakdown of medications and other foreign chemicals administered orally or parenterally. It is of particular concern that doses of medications be reduced to compensate for the loss of this function in patients with severe liver disease; otherwise, accumulation of drugs may lead to overdosage.

BILE

Bile is the excretory product of the liver. It is formed continuously by the hepatocytes, collects in the bile canaliculi adjacent to these cells, and is transported to the gut via the bile ducts (Figure 6-16). The principal components of bile are water, bile salts, and bile pigments (primarily bilirubin diglucuronide). Other components include cholesterol, lecithin, and protein. The primary functions of bile are the emulsification of intestinal fat and the removal of waste products excreted by the liver.

Fats are absorbed into the portal blood and intestinal lymphatics in the form of monoglycerides and triglycerides by the action of the intestinal mucosa, but efficient absorption occurs only when the fat molecules are suspended in solution through the emulsifying action of bile salts. As emulsifiers, bile salts act like nonionic detergents to suspend fats in solution within the watery medium of the intestinal contents. Both hepatocellular

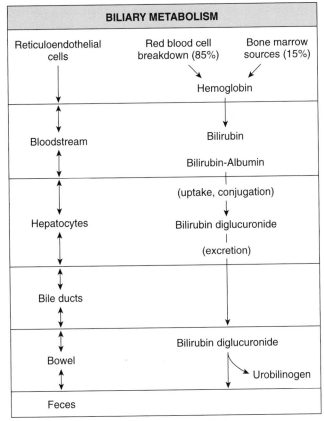

BILIARY METABOLISM		
Reticuloendothelial cells	Red blood cell breakdown (85%)	Bone marrow sources (15%)
	Hemoglobin	
Bloodstream	Bilirubin	
	Bilirubin-Albumin	
	(uptake, conjugation)	
Hepatocytes	Bilirubin diglucuronide	
	(excretion)	
Bile ducts		
Bowel	Bilirubin diglucuronide	
	Urobilinogen	
Feces		

Figure 6-16　Biliary metabolism.

disease and biliary obstruction affect the amount of bile salts available for fat absorption, but obstruction generally has the more profound effect. Absence of bile salts may lead to steatorrhea (fatty stools), but a more important effect is failure of absorption of the fat-soluble vitamins (D, A, K, and E). As previously noted, vitamin K is an essential precursor for hepatic production of several clotting factors; the absence of this vitamin leads to bleeding tendencies in patients with hepatobiliary disease.

Bile Pigments. Bile pigments are the principal cause of ultrasonic scattering in echogenic bile, although cholesterol crystals may also contribute to this finding. The presence of echogenic bile indicates stasis, but this stasis is not always pathologic and may simply result from prolonged fasting.

LIVER FUNCTION TESTS

The term **liver function tests** refers to a group of laboratory tests established to analyze how the liver is performing under normal and diseased conditions.

In patients with known liver disease, a number of laboratory tests are used to help in the diagnosis, including the following:

- Aspartate aminotransferase (AST, formerly SGOT)
- Alanine aminotransferase (ALT, formerly SGPT)
- Lactic acid dehydrogenase (LDH)
- Alkaline phosphatase (alk phos)
- Bilirubin (indirect, direct, and total)

- Prothrombin time
- Albumin and globulins

Aspartate Aminotransferase. Aspartate aminotransferase (AST, formerly SGOT) is an enzyme present in tissues that have a high rate of metabolic activity, one of which is the liver. As a result of death or injury to the producing cells, the enzyme is released into the bloodstream in abnormally high levels. Any disease that injures the cells causes an elevation in AST levels. This enzyme is also produced in other high-metabolic tissues, so an elevation does not always mean liver disease is present. Significant elevations are characteristic of acute hepatitis and cirrhosis. The level is also elevated in patients with hepatic necrosis, acute hepatitis, and infectious mononucleosis.

Alanine Aminotransferase. Alanine aminotransferase (ALT or SGPT) is more specific than AST for evaluating liver function. This enzyme is slightly elevated in acute cirrhosis, hepatic metastasis, and pancreatitis. There is a mild to moderate increase in obstructive jaundice. Hepatocellular disease and infectious or toxic hepatitis produce moderate to highly increased levels. In alcoholic hepatitis, AST is higher.

Lactic Acid Dehydrogenase. Lactic acid dehydrogenase is found in the tissues of several systems including the kidneys, heart, skeletal muscle, brain, liver, and lungs. Cellular injury and death cause this enzyme to increase. This test is moderately increased in infectious mononucleosis and mildly elevated in hepatitis, cirrhosis, and obstructive jaundice. Its primary use is in detection of myocardial or pulmonary infarction.

Alkaline Phosphatase. Alkaline phosphatase is produced by the liver, bone, intestines, and placenta. It may be a good indicator of intrahepatic or extrahepatic obstruction, hepatic carcinoma, abscess, or cirrhosis. In hepatitis and cirrhosis the enzyme is moderately elevated.

Bilirubin. Bilirubin is a product of the breakdown of hemoglobin in tired red blood cells. The liver converts these by-products into bile pigments, which, along with other factors, are secreted as bile by the liver cells into the bile ducts. The following are three ways this cycle can be disturbed:

- An excessive amount of red blood cell destruction
- Malfunction of liver cells
- Blockage of ducts leading from cells

These disturbances cause a rise in serum bilirubin, which leaks into the tissues and thus gives the skin a jaundice, or yellow, coloration.

Indirect bilirubin is unconjugated bilirubin. Elevation of this test result is seen with increased red blood cell destruction (anemias, trauma from a hematoma, or hemorrhagic pulmonary infarct).

Direct bilirubin is conjugated bilirubin. This product circulates in the blood and is excreted into the bile after it reaches the liver and is conjugated with glucuronide. Elevation of direct bilirubin is usually related to obstructive jaundice (from stones or neoplasm).

Specific liver diseases may cause an elevation of both direct and indirect bilirubin levels, but the increase in the direct level is more marked. These diseases are hepatic metastasis, hepatitis, lymphoma, cholestasis secondary to drugs, and cirrhosis.

Prothrombin Time. Prothrombin is a liver enzyme that is part of the blood clotting mechanism. The production of prothrombin depends on adequate intake and use of vitamin K. The prothrombin time is increased in the presence of liver disease with cellular damage. Cirrhosis and metastatic disease are examples of disorders that cause prolonged prothrombin time.

Albumin and Globulins. Assessment of depressed synthesis of proteins, especially serum albumin and the plasma coagulation factors, is a sensitive test for metabolic derangement of the liver. In patients with hepatocellular damage, a low serum albumin suggests decreased protein synthesis. A prolonged prothrombin time indicates a poor prognosis. Chronic liver diseases commonly show an elevation of gamma globulins.

SONOGRAPHIC EVALUATION OF THE LIVER

Evaluation of the hepatic structures is one of the most important procedures in sonography for many reasons. The normal, basically homogeneous parenchyma of the liver allows imaging of the neighboring anatomic structures in the upper abdomen. Echo amplitude, attenuation, and transmission and parenchymal textures may be physically assessed with proper evaluation of the hepatic structures.

Within the homogeneous parenchyma lie the thin-walled hepatic veins, the brightly reflective portal veins, the hepatic arteries, and the hepatic duct (Figure 6-17). Color flow Doppler imaging is useful in determining the direction of flow of the portal and hepatic veins. The portal flow is shown to be hepatopetal (toward the liver), whereas the hepatic venous flow is **hepatofugal** (away from the liver). The portal vein serves as the landmark to locate the smaller hepatic duct and artery. Near the porta hepatis, the hepatic duct can be seen along the anterior lateral border of the portal vein, whereas the hepatic artery can be seen along the anterior medial border (Figure 6-18). With color Doppler, the hepatic artery would show flow toward the liver, whereas the ductal system would show no flow.

The system gain should be adjusted to adequately penetrate the entire right lobe of the liver as a smooth, homogeneous echo-texture pattern (Figure 6-19, *A* and *B*). Adequate sensitivity (gain) must be present to image the normal smooth liver parenchyma. If too much gain is used, the electronic "noise" or "snow" is produced that appears as low-level echoes in the background of the image (e.g., outside of the liver parenchyma, above the diaphragm, or within the vascular structures). The ultrasound manufacturers have made it possible to preselect various preprocessing and postprocessing controls to allow the sonographer to emphasize or highlight various aspects of the liver parenchyma. This setting will automatically be seen on the monitor once the equipment is turned on or the "reset" button is depressed.

The time gain compensation should be adjusted to balance the far-gain and the near-gain echo signals. The easiest way to do this is to hold the transducer over a deep segment of the right lobe of the liver. The far time-gain control pods should gradually be increased with a smooth motion of the index finger until the posterior aspect of the liver is well seen. The near-field, time-gain controls should be adjusted (usually decreased) to image the anterior wall and musculature, the anterior hepatic capsule, and the near field of the hepatic parenchyma.

The depth should be adjusted so the posterior right lobe is positioned at the lower border of the screen (Figure 6-19, *C* and *D*). The electronic focus on the equipment is positioned near the posterior border of the liver, or the multiple focus points may be positioned equidistant throughout the liver to further enhance the hepatic parenchyma.

A   **B**

Figure 6-17   **A,** Sagittal image of the right lobe of liver shows a homogeneous texture with hepatic and portal veins scattered throughout the parenchyma. **B,** Color flow demonstrates the low flow pattern in the hepatic and portal veins.

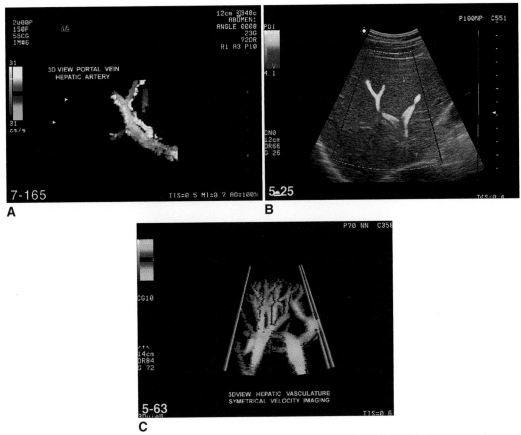

Figure 6-18 **A,** Color of the portal vein and hepatic artery shows the close relationship (anterior and medial) of the hepatic artery, seen in yellow, to the portal vein. **B,** Color of the portal system within the liver in a transverse image. **C,** Three-dimensional view of the hepatic vasculature in the liver.

The multifocal technique causes the frame rate to decrease and thus causes a "slower sweep" of the real-time image (Figure 6-20). If the patient cannot take a deep breath, the sonographer may choose not to use the multiple-frequency focus with decreased frame rate. In most patients who can suspend their respiration for a variable amount of time, this multifocal technique works very well because the liver is a nondynamic organ and does not need a high frame rate to obtain a quality image.

The appropriate transducer depends on the patient's body habitus and the clinical request for the ultrasound examination. The transducer frequency depends on the body habitus and size. The average adult abdomen usually requires at least a broad band 2.5- to 5-MHz frequency, whereas the more obese adult may require a lower frequency 2.25-MHz transducer. Slender adults and young children may require above a 5- to 7-MHz frequency, and the neonate may need an even higher frequency, 7.5- to 12-MHz transducer.

Generally, a wider "pie" sector or curved linear array transducer is the most appropriate to optimally image the near field of the abdomen (Figure 6-21). This transducer is especially useful in detecting liver abscesses or metastases. To image the far field better, a sector or annular array transducer with a longer focal zone is used. Often the transducers are interchanged throughout the examination to obtain the ideal image pattern.

Adequate scanning technique demands that each patient be examined with the following criteria assessment (Figures 6-22 and 6-23):

1. The size of the liver in the longitudinal plane
2. The attenuation of the liver parenchyma
3. Liver texture
4. The presence of hepatic vascular structures, ligaments, and fissures

The basic instrumentation should be adjusted in the following parameters:

1. Time gain compensation
2. Overall gain
3. Transducer frequency and type
4. Depth and focus

SAGITTAL PLANE

The sagittal plane offers an excellent window to visualize the hepatic structures (Figure 6-24). With the patient in full inspiration, the transducer may be swept under the costal margin (with slight to medium pressure) to record the liver parenchyma from the anterior abdominal wall to the diaphragm.

Scan I. The initial scan should be made slightly to the left of the midline to record the left lobe of the liver and

Text continued on p. 164

Figure 6-19   A, Longitudinal image of the liver shows equal distribution of echoes from anterior to posterior, which means the gain and time gain compensation settings are correct. **B,** Incorrect gain settings show the lack of echoes in the distal portion of the liver. **C,** Depth of field at 24 cm. **D,** Depth of field at 15 cm.

Figure 6-20 **A** through **C,** Examples of incorrect focal zone settings (look at the line to the right of the image). The focal zone should be set to encompass the total area of interest, or to "clean up" the far field echoes to increase sharpness.

Figure 6-21 Curved array **(A)** versus sector **(B)** changes the near field of field and the focal zone in the far field.

Figure 6-22   Longitudinal images of the right lobe of the liver are used to determine adequate gain settings and also to measure the liver from the diaphragm to its inferior border. The inferior border may be difficult to image at the same time as the diaphragm, depending on the size of the liver.

Figure 6-23   Transverse images should show adequate gain, time gain compensation, depth, and landmarks within the liver (ligaments, vascular structures, and spine).

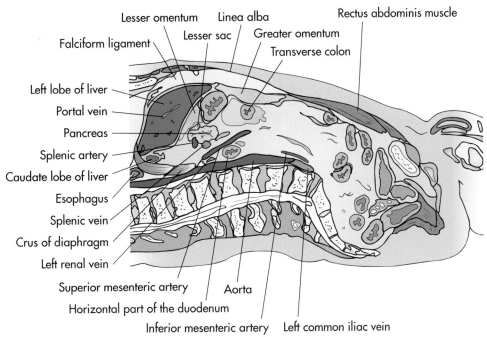

Lesser omentum   Linea alba   Rectus abdominis muscle
Falciform ligament   Lesser sac   Greater omentum
Transverse colon

Left lobe of liver

Portal vein

Pancreas

Splenic artery

Caudate lobe of liver

Esophagus

Splenic vein

Crus of diaphragm

Left renal vein

Superior mesenteric artery   Aorta

Horizontal part of the duodenum

Inferior mesenteric artery   Left common iliac vein

A

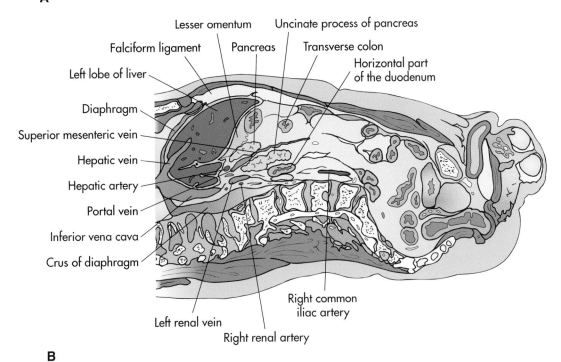

Lesser omentum   Uncinate process of pancreas
Falciform ligament   Pancreas   Transverse colon
Left lobe of liver   Horizontal part
of the duodenum

Diaphragm

Superior mesenteric vein

Hepatic vein

Hepatic artery

Portal vein

Inferior vena cava

Crus of diaphragm

Right common
iliac artery

Left renal vein

Right renal artery

B

Figure 6-24 Longitudinal plane. **A,** Midline sagittal section of the abdomen. **B,** Sagittal section of the abdomen. *Continued*

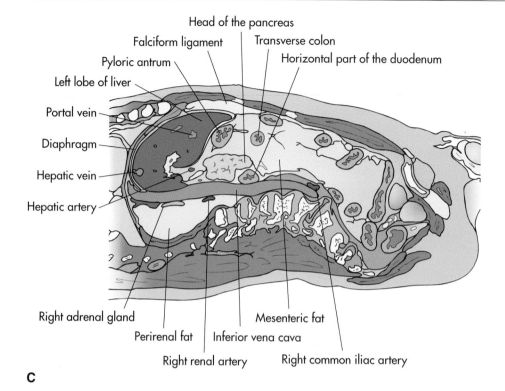

Head of the pancreas
Falciform ligament
Pyloric antrum
Left lobe of liver
Portal vein
Diaphragm
Hepatic vein
Hepatic artery

Transverse colon
Horizontal part of the duodenum

Right adrenal gland
Perirenal fat
Right renal artery

Mesenteric fat
Inferior vena cava
Right common iliac artery

C

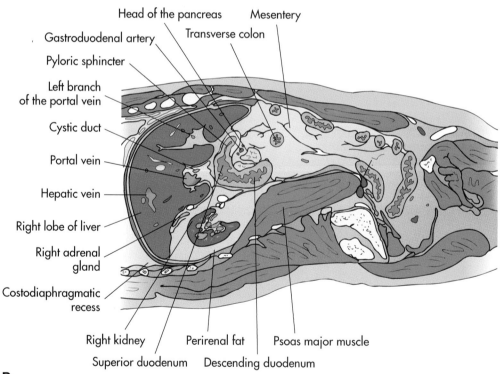

Head of the pancreas
Gastroduodenal artery
Pyloric sphincter
Left branch of the portal vein
Cystic duct
Portal vein
Hepatic vein
Right lobe of liver
Right adrenal gland
Costodiaphragmatic recess

Mesentery
Transverse colon

Right kidney
Superior duodenum

Perirenal fat
Descending duodenum

Psoas major muscle

D

Figure 6-24, cont'd   C, Sagittal section of the abdomen 3 cm from the midline. **D,** Sagittal section of the abdomen 5 cm from the midline.

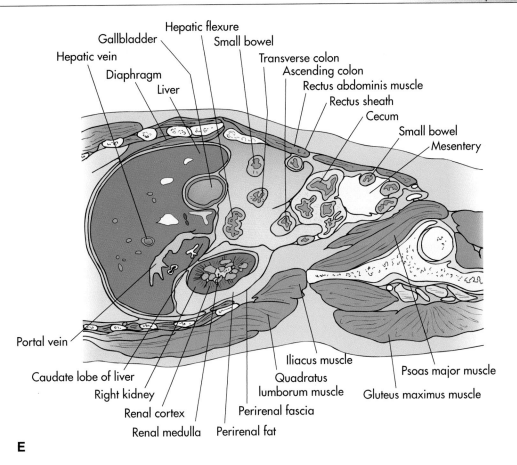

Hepatic flexure
Gallbladder
Small bowel
Hepatic vein
Diaphragm
Transverse colon
Ascending colon
Liver
Rectus abdominis muscle
Rectus sheath
Cecum
Small bowel
Mesentery

Portal vein
Iliacus muscle
Psoas major muscle
Caudate lobe of liver
Quadratus lumborum muscle
Gluteus maximus muscle
Right kidney
Renal cortex
Perirenal fascia
Renal medulla
Perirenal fat

E

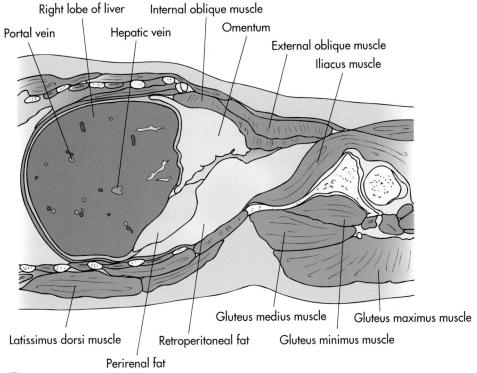

Right lobe of liver
Internal oblique muscle
Omentum
Portal vein
Hepatic vein
External oblique muscle
Iliacus muscle

Gluteus medius muscle
Gluteus maximus muscle
Latissimus dorsi muscle
Retroperitoneal fat
Gluteus minimus muscle
Perirenal fat

F

Figure 6-24, cont'd   E, Sagittal section of the abdomen 7 cm from the midline. **F,** Sagittal section of the abdomen taken along the right abdominal border.

Figure 6-25 Longitudinal images. **A,** *Scan I:* left lobe liver, aorta. **B,** *Scan II:* left lobe liver, inferior vena cava, portal vein, caudate lobe. **C,** *Scan III:* right lobe liver, right kidney. **D,** *Scan IV:* right lobe liver, right kidney. **E,** *Scan V:* right lobe liver, portal vein, hepatic veins.

the abdominal aorta. The left hepatic and portal veins may be seen as small circular structures in this view (Figure 6-25, *A*).

Scan II. As the sonographer scans at midline or slightly to the right of midline, a larger segment of the left lobe and the inferior vena cava may be seen posteriorly. In this view, it is useful to record the inferior vena cava as it is dilated near the end of inspiration. The left or middle hepatic vein may be imaged as it drains into the inferior vena cava near the level of

the diaphragm. The area of the porta hepatis is shown anterior to the inferior vena cava as the superior mesenteric vein and splenic vein converge to form the main portal vein. The common bile duct may be seen just anterior to the main portal vein. The head of the pancreas may be seen just inferior to the right lobe of the liver and main portal vein and anterior to the inferior vena cava (see Figure 6-25, *B*).

Scan III. The next image should be made slightly lateral to this sagittal plane to record part of the right portal vein and right lobe of the liver. The caudate lobe is often seen in this view (see Figure 6-25, *B*).

Scans IV, V, and VI. The next three scans should be made in small increments through the right lobe of the liver (Figure 6-25, *C, D,* and *E*). The last scan is usually made to show the right kidney and lateral segment of the right lobe of the liver. The liver texture is compared with the renal parenchyma. The normal liver parenchyma should have a softer, more homogeneous texture than the dense medulla and hypoechoic renal cortex. Liver size may be measured from the tip of the liver to the diaphragm. Generally this measurement is less than 15 cm, with 15 to 20 cm representing the upper limits of normal.

Hepatomegaly is present when the liver measurement exceeds 20 cm.

TRANSVERSE PLANE

Multiple transverse scans are made across the upper abdomen to record specific areas of the liver (Figure 6-26). The transducer should be angled in a steep cephalic direction to be as parallel to the diaphragm as possible. The patient should be in full inspiration to maintain detail of the liver parenchyma, vascular architecture, and ductal structures.

Scan I. The initial transverse image is made with the transducer under the costal margin at a steep angle perpendicular

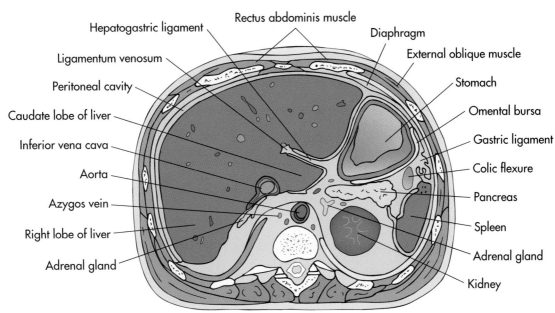

Figure 6-26   Transverse plane. **A,** Cross-section of the abdomen at the level of the tenth intervertebral disk. **B,** Cross-section of the abdomen at the level of the eleventh thoracic disk.   *Continued*

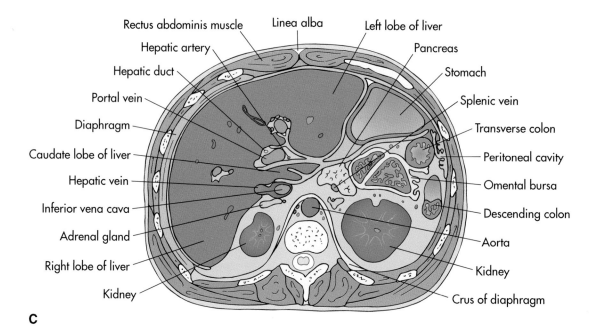

Rectus abdominis muscle
Hepatic artery
Hepatic duct
Portal vein
Diaphragm
Caudate lobe of liver
Hepatic vein
Inferior vena cava
Adrenal gland
Right lobe of liver
Kidney

Linea alba

Left lobe of liver
Pancreas
Stomach
Splenic vein
Transverse colon
Peritoneal cavity
Omental bursa
Descending colon
Aorta
Kidney
Crus of diaphragm

C

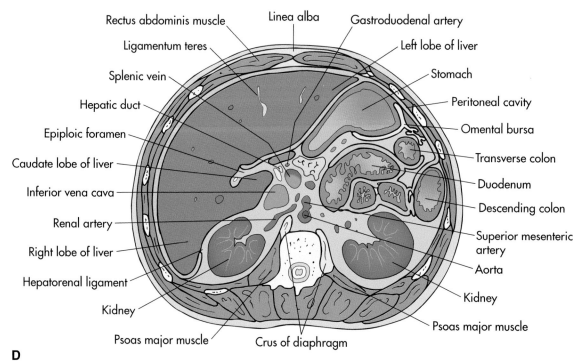

Rectus abdominis muscle
Ligamentum teres
Splenic vein
Hepatic duct
Epiploic foramen
Caudate lobe of liver
Inferior vena cava
Renal artery
Right lobe of liver
Hepatorenal ligament
Kidney
Psoas major muscle

Linea alba

Gastroduodenal artery
Left lobe of liver
Stomach
Peritoneal cavity
Omental bursa
Transverse colon
Duodenum
Descending colon
Superior mesenteric artery
Aorta
Kidney
Psoas major muscle

Crus of diaphragm

D

Figure 6-26, cont'd   C, Cross section of the abdomen at the level of the twelfth thoracic vertebra.
D, Cross-section of the abdomen at the first lumbar vertebra.

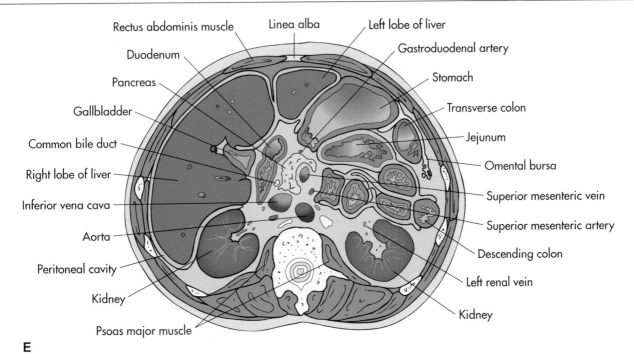

Rectus abdominis muscle
Linea alba
Left lobe of liver
Gastroduodenal artery
Duodenum
Stomach
Pancreas
Transverse colon
Gallbladder
Jejunum
Common bile duct
Omental bursa
Right lobe of liver
Superior mesenteric vein
Inferior vena cava
Superior mesenteric artery
Aorta
Descending colon
Peritoneal cavity
Left renal vein
Kidney
Kidney
Psoas major muscle

E

Rectus abdominis muscle
Linea alba
Rectus abdominis muscle
Parietal peritoneum
Hepatocolic ligament
Transverse colon
Gallbladder
Transverse mesocolon
Superior mesenteric artery
Peritoneal cavity
Duodenum
Jejunum
Inferior vena cava
Greater omentum
Aorta
Splenic vein
Kidney
Descending colon
Kidney
Psoas major muscle
Psoas major muscle

F

Figure 6-26, cont'd   E, Cross-section of the abdomen at the level of the second lumbar vertebra. **F,** Cross-section of the abdomen at the level of the third lumbar vertebra.

to the diaphragm (Figure 6-27, *A*). The patient should be in deep inspiration to adequately record the dome of the liver. The sonographer should identify the inferior vena cava and three hepatic veins as they drain into the cava. This pattern has sometimes been referred to as the "reindeer sign" or "Playboy bunny" sign.

Scan II. The transducer is then directed slightly inferior to the point described in scan I to record the left portal vein as it flows into the left lobe of the liver (see Figure 6-27, *B*).

Scan III. The porta hepatis is seen as a tubular structure within the central part of the liver. Sometimes the left or right portal vein can be identified. The caudate lobe may be seen just superior to the porta hepatis; thus, depending on the angle, either the caudate lobe is shown anterior to the inferior vena cava, or, as the transducer moves inferior, the porta hepatis is identified anterior to the inferior vena cava (see Figure 6-27, *C*).

Scan IV. The fourth scan should show the right portal vein as it divides into the anterior and posterior segments of the

Figure 6-27   Transverse images. **A,** *Scan I:* right lobe liver *(RL),* hepatic veins *(arrows),* inferior vena cava *(IVC).* **B,** *Scan II:* left lobe liver, left portal vein *(arrow),* ligamentum venosum *(arrows),* caudate lobe *(CL).* **C,** *Scan III:* caudate lobe *(CL),* left lobe *(LL),* right lobe *(RL)* of liver, left and right portal veins, IVC, and aorta *(Ao).* **D,** *Scan IV:* right lobe liver *(RL),* main portal vein *(MPV),* right portal vein with branches *(RPV),* and IVC. **E,** *Scan V:* right lobe liver *(RL).* **F,** *Scan VI:* right lobe liver *(RL)* and right kidney *(RK).*

right lobe of the liver. The gallbladder may be seen in this scan as an anechoic structure medial to the right lobe and anterior to the right kidney (see Figure 6-27, *D*).

Scans V and VI. These two scans are made through the lower segment of the right lobe of the liver. The right kidney is the posterior border (Figure 6-27, *E*). Usually intrahepatic vascular structures are not identified in these views (see Figure 6-27, *F*).

LATERAL DECUBITUS PLANE

Left Posterior Oblique. The left posterior oblique image requires that the patient roll slightly to the left. A 45-degree

sponge or pillow may be placed under the right hip to support the patient (Figure 6-28). This view allows better visualization of the lower right lobe of the liver, usually displacing the duodenum and transverse colon to the midline of the abdomen, out of the field of view. Transverse, oblique, or longitudinal scans may be made in this position.

Left Lateral Decubitus. If the previously described scans do not allow adequate visualization of the liver and vascular structures, the lateral decubitus position may be used. If the body habitus allows the transducer to image between the intercostal spaces, additional views may be obtained of the dome of the liver and medial segment of the left lobe of the liver.

Figure 6-28   Oblique scans. The patient may be rolled from a supine (**A**) position into the anterior oblique position (**B**). Note the change in position of the inferior vena cava *(arrows)* as the patient is rotated.

PATHOLOGY OF THE LIVER

Evaluation of the liver parenchyma includes the assessment of its size, configuration, homogeneity, and contour. Liver volume can be determined from serial scans in an effort to detect subtle increases in size or hepatomegaly. The development and clinical utility of three-dimensional ultrasound in determining organ volumes is currently under clinical investigation in many academic institutions.

As in other organ systems, the hepatic parenchymal pattern changes with disease processes. Hepatocellular disease affects the hepatocytes and interferes with liver function enzymes. Cirrhosis, ascites, or fatty liver patterns may be detected with the ultrasound examination. In an effort to provide a differential diagnosis for the clinician, intrahepatic, extrahepatic, subhepatic, and subdiaphragmatic masses may be outlined and their internal composition recognized as specific echo patterns.

Subsequent sections discuss the pathology of liver disease in the following categories: diffuse disease, functional disease, abscess formation, hepatic trauma and transplantation, benign disease, malignant disease, and vascular problems.

DIFFUSE DISEASE

Diffuse hepatocellular disease both affects the hepatocytes and interferes with liver function. The **hepatocyte** is a parenchymal liver cell that performs all the functions ascribed to the liver. This abnormality is measured through the series of liver function tests. The hepatic enzyme levels are elevated with cell necrosis. With cholestasis (i.e., interruption in the flow of bile through any part of the biliary system, from the liver to the duodenum), the alkaline phosphatase and direct bilirubin levels increase. Likewise, when there are defects in protein synthesis, there may be elevated serum bilirubin levels and decreased serum albumin and clotting factor levels.

Figure 6-29   Gross appearance of the fatty liver. (From Damjanov I, Linder J: *Pathology: a color atlas,* St. Louis, 2000, Mosby.)

There are many subcategories of diffuse parenchymal disease, including fatty infiltration, acute and chronic hepatitis, early alcoholic liver disease, and acute and chronic cirrhosis. See Table 6-3 for clinical findings, sonographic findings, and differential considerations for diffuse hepatic disease.

Fatty Infiltration. Fatty infiltration implies increased lipid accumulation in the hepatocytes and results from major injury to the liver or a systemic disorder leading to impaired or excessive metabolism of fat (Figure 6-29). Fatty infiltration is a benign process and may be reversible. The patient is usually asymptomatic; however, some patients may present with jaundice, nausea and vomiting, and abdominal tenderness or pain. Common causes of fatty liver are alcoholic liver disease, diabetes mellitus, obesity, pregnancy, severe hepatitis, chronic illness, and steroids.

Sonographic Findings. Moderate to severe fatty infiltration shows increased echogenicity on ultrasound. Enlargement of the lobe affected by fatty infiltration is evident. The portal vein structures may be difficult to visualize because of the increased

TABLE 6-3 LIVER FINDINGS: DIFFUSE DISEASE

Clinical Findings	Sonographic Findings	Differential Considerations
Fatty Infiltration		
Normal to ↑ hepatic enzymes ↑ Alk phos ↑ Direct bilirubin	↑ Echogenicity ↑ Attenuation Impaired visualization of borders of portal/hepatic structures (secondary to increased attenuation) Hepatomegaly May be patchy, inhomogeneous Focal sparing	Hepatitis Cirrhosis Metastases
Acute Hepatitis		
↑ AST, ALT ↑ Bilirubin Leukopenia	Nonspecific and variable Normal to slightly ↑ Echogenicity ↑ Brightness of portal vein borders Hepatosplenomegaly ↑ Thickness of gallbladder wall	Fatty liver
Chronic Hepatitis		
↑ AST, ALT ↑ Bilirubin Leukopenia	Coarse hepatic parenchyma ↑ Echogenicity ↓ Visualization brightness of portal triad Fibrosis may produce soft shadowing	Cirrhosis Fatty liver
Cirrhosis		
↑ Alk phos ↑ Direct bilirubin ↑ AST, ALT Leukopenia	Coarse liver parenchyma with nodularity ↑ Echogenicity ↑ Attenuation ↓ Vascular markings with acute cirrhosis Hepatosplenomegaly with ascites Shrunken liver with chronic cirrhosis (also ↑ nodularity) Regeneration of hepatic nodules Portal hypertension	Fatty liver Hepatitis
Glycogen Storage Disease		
Disturbance of acid-base balance	Hepatomegaly ↑ Echogenicity ↑ Attenuation von Gierke's adenoma (round, homogeneous)	Focal nodular hyperplasia Fatty liver
Hemochromatosis		
↑ Iron levels in blood	↑ Echogenicity throughout liver	Cirrhosis

Alk phos, Alkaline phosphatase; *ALT,* alanine aminotransferase; *AST,* aspartame aminotransferase.

attenuation of the ultrasound. The increased attenuation also causes a decrease in penetration of the sound beam, which may be a clue for the sonographer to think of fatty liver disease (the liver is so dense that "typical" gain settings do not allow penetration to the posterior border of the liver). Thus it becomes more difficult to see the outline of the portal vein and hepatic vein borders. Authors have stated that this increase in echo texture may result from increased collagen content of the liver or increases in lipid accumulation. The following three grades of liver texture have been defined in sonography for classification of fatty infiltration:

- *Grade 1:* A slight diffuse increase in fine echoes in the hepatic parenchyma with normal visualization of the diaphragm and intrahepatic vessel borders (Figure 6-30, *A*).

- *Grade 2:* A moderate diffuse increase in fine echoes with slightly impaired visualization of the intrahepatic vessels and diaphragm (see Figure 6-30, *B*).

- *Grade 3:* A marked increase in fine echoes with poor or no visualization of the intrahepatic vessel borders, diaphragm, and posterior portion of the right lobe of the liver (see Figure 6-30, *C*).

Fatty infiltration is not always uniform throughout the liver parenchyma. It is not uncommon to see patchy distribution of fat, especially in the right lobe of the liver. The fat does not displace normal vascular architecture.

The other characteristic of fatty infiltration is focal sparing. This condition should be suspected in patients who have masslike hypoechoic areas in typical locations in a liver that is

Figure 6-30   Fatty infiltration. **A,** Grade I. **B,** Grade II. **C,** Grade III.

Figure 6-31   Focal sparing of the caudate lobe.

otherwise increased in echogenicity. The most common areas are anterior to the gallbladder or the portal vein and the posterior portion of the left lobe of the liver (Figure 6-31).

Hepatitis. Hepatitis is the general name for inflammatory and infectious disease of the liver, of which there are many causes. The disease may result from a local infection (viral hepatitis), from an infection elsewhere in the body (e.g., infectious mononucleosis or amebiasis), or from chemical or drug toxicity. Mild inflammation impairs hepatocyte function, whereas more severe inflammation and necrosis may lead to obstruction of blood and bile flow in the liver and impaired liver cell function.

Hepatitis is considered to result from infection by a group of viruses that specifically target the hepatocytes. These include hepatitis A virus (HAV), hepatitis B virus (HBV), hepatitis C virus (HCV), hepatitis D virus (HDV), and hepatitis E virus (HEV). In the United States, about 60% of acute viral hepatitis is type B, about 20% is type A, and about 20% is other types. Type A hepatitis is spread primarily by fecal contamination, because the virus lives in the alimentary tract. Hepatitis B is caused by the type B virus, which exists in the bloodstream and can be spread by transfusions of infected blood or plasma or through the use of contaminated needles. Hepatitis B is of the greatest risk to health care workers because of the nature of transmission. This virus is also found in body fluids, such as saliva and semen, and may be spread by sexual contact. Patients with acute and chronic hepatitis may initially present with flulike and gastrointestinal symptoms, including loss of appetite, nausea, vomiting, and fatigue.

Acute hepatitis. In acute hepatitis, damage to the liver may range from mild disease to massive necrosis and liver failure. The pathologic changes seen include the following: (1) liver cell injury, swelling of the hepatocytes, and hepatocyte degeneration, which may lead to cell necrosis; (2) reticuloendothelial and lymphocytic response with Kupffer cells enlarging; and (3) regeneration.

Sonographic Findings. On ultrasound examination the liver texture may appear normal or the sonographer may note that the portal vein borders are more prominent than usual and the liver parenchyma is slightly more echogenic than normal; attenuation may be present. Hepatosplenomegaly is present, and the gallbladder wall is thickened.

Chronic hepatitis. Chronic hepatitis exists when there is clinical or biochemical evidence of hepatic inflammation for at least 3 to 6 months. Causes include viral, metabolic, autoimmune, or drug induced. In chronic active hepatitis there are more extensive changes than in chronic persistent hepatitis, with inflammation extending across the limiting plate, spreading out in a perilobular fashion, and causing piecemeal necrosis, which is frequently accompanied by fibrosis. Patients may present with nausea, anorexia, weight loss, tremors, jaundice, dark urine, fatigue, and varicosities. Chronic persistent hepatitis is a benign, self-limiting process. Chronic active hepatitis usually progresses to cirrhosis and liver failure.

Sonographic Findings. On ultrasound examination the liver parenchyma is coarse with decreased brightness of the portal triads, but the degree of attenuation is not as great as is seen in fatty infiltration (Figure 6-32). The liver does not increase in size with chronic hepatitis. Fibrosis may be evident, which may produce "soft shadowing" posteriorly.

Cirrhosis. Cirrhosis is a chronic degenerative disease of the liver in which the lobes are covered with fibrous tissue, the parenchyma degenerates, and the lobules are infiltrated with fat. The essential feature is simultaneous parenchymal necro-

sis, regeneration, and diffuse fibrosis resulting in disorganization of lobular architecture (Figure 6-33). The process is chronic and progressive, with liver cell failure and portal hypertension as the end stage. Cirrhosis is most commonly the result of chronic alcohol abuse, but can be the result of nutritional deprivation or hepatitis or other infection. There are several types of cirrhosis: biliary cirrhosis, fatty cirrhosis, and posthepatic cirrhosis. Patients with acute cirrhosis may seem asymptomatic or may have symptoms that include nausea, flatulence, ascites, light-colored stools, weakness, abdominal pain, varicosities, and spider angiomas. Chronic cirrhosis patient symptoms include nausea, anorexia, weight loss, jaundice, dark urine, fatigue, or varicosities. Chronic cirrhosis may progress to liver failure and portal hypertension.

Sonographic Findings. The diagnosis of cirrhosis by ultrasound may be difficult. Specific findings may include coarsening of the liver parenchyma secondary to fibrosis and nodularity (Figure 6-34). Increased attenuation may be present, with decreased vascular markings. Hepatosplenomegaly may be present with ascites surrounding the liver. The caudate lobe and left lateral lobe may be hypertrophied, with the caudate to right lobe ratio exceeding 0.65. In addition, there may be atrophy of the right and left medial lobes of the liver. Chronic cirrhosis may show nodularity of the liver edge, especially if ascites is present. The hepatic fissures may be accentuated. The isoechoic regenerating nodules may be seen throughout the liver parenchyma. Portal hypertension may be present with or without abnormal Doppler flow patterns. Patients who have cirrhosis have an increased incidence of hepatoma tumors within the liver parenchyma.

Glycogen Storage Disease. There are six categories of glycogen storage disease, which are divided on the basis of clinical symptoms and specific enzymatic defects. The most common is type I, or von Gierke's disease. This is a form of glycogen storage disease in which abnormally large amounts of glycogen are deposited in the liver and kidneys.

Sonographic Findings. On ultrasound, patients with glycogen storage disease present with hepatomegaly, increased echogenicity, and slightly increased attenuation. The disease is associated with hepatic adenomas, focal nodular hyperplasia, and hepatomegaly (Figure 6-35). The adenomas present as round, homogeneous, echogenic tumors (Figure 6-36). If the tumor is large, it may be slightly inhomogeneous.

Hemochromatosis. Hemochromatosis is a rare disease of iron metabolism characterized by excess iron deposits throughout the body. This disorder may lead to cirrhosis and portal hypertension.

Sonographic Findings. Ultrasound does not show specific findings other than hepatomegaly and cirrhotic changes. Some increased echogenicity may be seen uniformly throughout the hepatic parenchyma.

DIFFUSE ABNORMALITIES OF THE LIVER PARENCHYMA
Abnormalities—such as biliary obstruction, common duct stones and stricture, extrahepatic mass, and passive hepatic

Figure 6-32 Hepatitis. On ultrasound examination, the liver parenchyma is coarse with increased brightness of the portal triad.

Figure 6-33 **A,** Gross pathology of alcoholic cirrhosis with high degree of fat content. **B,** Biliary cirrhosis (liver is nodular). **C,** Micronodular cirrhosis (nodules are small with uniform size). **D,** Macronodular cirrhosis. (From Damjanov I, Linder J: *Pathology: a color atlas,* St. Louis, 2000, Mosby.)

congestion—are discussed as each lesion is seen on the ultrasound. See Table 6-4 for clinical findings, sonographic findings, and differential considerations of diffuse abnormalities of the liver parenchyma.

Biliary Obstruction: Proximal. Biliary obstruction proximal to the cystic duct can be caused by gallstones, carcinoma of the common bile duct, or metastatic tumor invasion of the porta hepatis (Figure 6-37). Clinically the patient may be jaundiced and have pruritus (itching). Liver function tests show an elevation in the direct bilirubin and alkaline phosphatase levels.

Sonographic Findings. Sonographically, carcinoma of the common duct shows as a tubular branching with dilated intrahepatic ducts best seen in the periphery of the liver (Figure 6-38). It may be difficult to image a discrete mass lesion. The gallbladder is of normal size, even after a fatty meal is administered.

Biliary Obstruction: Distal. A biliary obstruction distal to the cystic duct may be caused by stones in the common duct (Figure 6-39), an extrahepatic mass in the porta hepatis, or stricture of the common duct. Clinically, common duct stones cause right upper quadrant pain, jaundice, and pruritus, as well as an increase in direct bilirubin and alkaline phosphatase.

Sonographic Findings. On ultrasound examination, the dilated intrahepatic ducts are seen in the periphery of the liver (Figure 6-40). The gallbladder size is variable, usually small. Gallstones are often present and appear as hyperechoic lesions along the posterior floor of the gallbladder, with a sharp posterior acoustic shadow. Careful evaluation of the common duct may show shadowing stones within the dilated duct.

Extrahepatic Mass. An extrahepatic mass in the area of the porta hepatis causes the same clinical signs as seen in biliary obstruction.

Sonographic Findings. On ultrasound examination, an irregular, ill-defined, hypoechoic, and inhomogeneous mass lesion may be seen in the area of the porta hepatis. There is intrahepatic ductal dilation, with a hydropic gallbladder. The lesion may arise from the lymph nodes, pancreatitis, pseudocyst, or carcinoma in the head of the pancreas.

Common Duct Stricture. Clinically the patient is jaundiced and has had a previous cholecystectomy. Laboratory values show an increase in the direct bilirubin and alkaline phosphatase levels.

Figure 6-34 Diffuse liver disease. **A,** Fatty infiltration secondary to cystic fibrosis. **B,** Early stages cirrhosis: hepatomegaly, decreased vasculature. **C,** Cirrhotic liver with ascites. **D,** Advanced cirrhosis with attenuation. **E,** Late-stage cirrhosis with shrunken liver, ascites. **F,** Late-stage cirrhosis with thick gallbladder wall, ascites, shrunken liver.

Sonographic Findings. On ultrasound examination, common duct stricture presents as dilated intrahepatic ducts with absence of a mass in the porta hepatis.

Passive Hepatic Congestion. Passive hepatic congestion develops secondary to congestive heart failure with signs of hepatomegaly. Laboratory data indicate normal to slightly elevated liver function tests.

Sonographic Findings. On ultrasound examination, dilation of the inferior vena cava, superior mesenteric, hepatic,

portal, and splenic veins is noted. The venous structures may decrease in size with expiration and increase with inspiration.

Focal Hepatic Disease

Very few hepatic lesions have specific sonographic features. Therefore, it is important to know the patient's clinical history and the sonographic patterns associated with various lesions. The knowledge of laboratory values in liver function tests also helps determine the hepatic lesions. The differential diagnosis

TABLE 6-4 LIVER FINDINGS: DIFFUSE ABNORMALITIES OF THE LIVER PARENCHYMA

Clinical Findings	Sonographic Findings	Differential Considerations
Biliary Obstruction: Proximal		
↑ Direct bilirubin ↑ Alk phos	Carcinoma of common bile duct shows tubular branching with dilated intrahepatic ducts Gallbladder small to normal size; gallstones	Obstruction to distal duct Extrahepatic metastases
Biliary Obstruction: Distal		
↑ Direct bilirubin ↑ Alk phos	Carcinoma of common bile duct shows tubular branching with dilated intrahepatic ducts Gallbladder small; gallstones and common duct stones	Obstruction to proximal duct Extrahepatic metastases
Extrahepatic Mass		
↑ Direct bilirubin ↑ Alk phos	Irregular, ill-defined hypoechoic, heterogeneous lesion in area of porta hepatis Intrahepatic ductal dilation Hydropic gallbladder	Proximal or distal obstruction to the cystic duct Metastases
Common Duct Stricture		
↑ Direct bilirubin ↑ Alk phos Previous cholecystectomy	Dilated intrahepatic ducts Absence of mass in porta hepatis	Extrahepatic mass Passive hepatic congestion
Passive Hepatic Congestion		
↑ LFT	↑ IVC, HV, PV	N/A

Alk phos, Alkaline phosphatase; *IVC,* inferior vena cava; *HV,* hepatic vein; *LFT,* liver function test; *N/A,* not applicable; *PV,* portal vein.

Figure 6-35 Gross pathology of hepatic adenoma with hemorrhage. (From Damjanov I, Linder J: *Pathology: a color atlas,* St. Louis, 2000, Mosby.)

for focal diseases of the liver includes cysts, abscess, hematoma, primary tumor, and metastases. See Table 6-5 for clinical findings, sonographic findings, and differential considerations for focal hepatic disease.

The sonographer should be able to differentiate whether the mass is **extrahepatic** or **intrahepatic.** Intrahepatic masses may

cause the following findings on ultrasound: displacement of the hepatic vascular radicles, external bulging of the liver capsule, or a posterior shift of the inferior vena cava. An extrahepatic mass may show internal invagination or discontinuity of the liver capsule, formation of a triangular fat wedge, anteromedial shift of the inferior vena cava, or anterior displacement of the right kidney.

Cystic Lesions. *Hepatic cyst* usually refers to a solitary non-parasitic cyst of the liver. The cyst may be congenital or acquired, solitary or multiple. Patients are often asymptomatic and require no treatment. When the cysts become large, pain may develop as the lesion compresses the hepatic vasculature or ductal system.

Cystic lesions within the liver include the following: simple or congenital hepatic cysts, traumatic cysts, parasitic cysts, inflammatory cysts, polycystic disease, and pseudocysts.

Simple hepatic cysts. The sonographic finding of a simple hepatic cyst is usually incidental because most patients are asymptomatic. As the cyst grows, it may cause pain or a mass effect to suggest a more serious condition, such as infection, abscess, or necrotic lesion. Hepatic cysts occur more often in females than in males.

Sonographic Findings. On ultrasound examination, the cyst walls are thin, with well-defined borders, and anechoic, with distal posterior enhancement (Figure 6-41). Infrequently, cysts contain fine linear internal septa. Complications, such as

Figure 6-36   Hepatic adenoma. **A,** Patient with von Gierke's disease: hepatic adenoma is seen within the caudate lobe. **B,** A 31-year-old female with a hepatic adenoma *(arrows)* in the right lobe.

Figure 6-37   Gross pathology of gallstones in the hepatic duct. (From Damjanov I, Linder J: *Pathology: a color atlas,* St. Louis, 2000, Mosby.)

Figure 6-39   Obstruction distal to cystic duct may be caused by stones in the common duct. The distal cystic duct is enlarged and obstructed by a stone at the distal end. The inferior vena cava is posterior to the duct.

Figure 6-38   Obstruction proximal to cystic duct may be secondary to pancreatic carcinoma or tumor invasion to the porta hepatis. Dilated intrahepatic ducts will result from this obstruction.

hemorrhage, may occur and cause pain (Figure 6-42). Calcification may be seen within the cyst wall and may cause shadowing.

Congenital hepatic cysts.   A solitary congenital cyst of the liver is rare and usually is an incidental lesion. This abnormality arises from developmental defects in the formation of bile ducts.

Sonographic Findings. The mass is usually solitary and may vary in size from tiny to as large as 20 cm (Figure 6-43). The cyst is usually found on the anterior undersurface of the liver. It usually does not cause liver enlargement and is found in the right lobe of the liver more often than the left lobe.

Polycystic liver disease.   Polycystic liver disease is autosomal dominant and affects 1 person in 500. At least 25% to

A   B

Figure 6-40   **A,** Sagittal scan of the dilated common duct. **B,** Sagittal scan of a mass in the porta hepatis.

Figure 6-41   Solitary hepatic cyst in the left lobe of the liver shows increased through-transmission and well-defined borders.

50% of patients with polycystic renal disease have one to several hepatic cysts. Of patients with polycystic liver disease, 60% have associated polycystic renal disease. The cysts are small, less than 2 to 3 cm, and multiple throughout the hepatic parenchyma (Figure 6-44). Cysts within the porta hepatis may enlarge and cause biliary obstruction. Histologically, they appear similar to simple hepatic cysts. It may be very difficult to assess an abscess formation or neoplastic lesion in a patient with polycystic liver disease.

Sonographic Findings. On ultrasound examination, the cysts generally present as anechoic, well-defined borders with acoustic enhancement (Figure 6-45). The differential diagnosis for a cystic lesion includes the following: necrotic metastasis, echinococcal cyst, hematoma, hepatic cystadenocarcinoma, and abscess. Ultrasound may be used to direct the needle if

percutaneous aspiration is necessary to obtain specific diagnostic information.

Inflammatory Disease of the Liver. Hepatic abscesses occur most often as complications of biliary tract disease, surgery, or trauma. The following three basic types of abscess formation occur in the liver: intrahepatic, subhepatic, and subphrenic.

Generally, the patient presents with fever, elevated white cell counts, and right upper quadrant pain. The search for an abscess must be made to locate solitary or multiple lesions within the liver or to search for abnormal fluid collections in Morison's pouch or in the subdiaphragmatic or subphrenic space. The following infectious processes are discussed: pyogenic abscess, hepatic candidiasis, chronic granulomatous disease, amebic abscess, and echinococcal disease.

Pyogenic abscess. A **pyogenic abscess** is a "pus-forming" abscess. There are many routes for bacteria to gain access to the liver—through the biliary tree, the portal vein, or the hepatic artery; through a direct extension from a contiguous infection; and, rarely, through hepatic trauma. Sources of infection include cholangitis; portal pyemia secondary to appendicitis, diverticulitis, inflammatory disease, or colitis; direct spread from another organ; trauma with direct contamination; or infarction after embolization or from sickle cell anemia.

Clinically the patient presents with fever, pain, pleuritis, nausea, vomiting, and diarrhea. Elevated liver function tests, leukocytosis, and anemia are present. The abscess formation is multiple in 50% to 67% of patients. The most frequent organisms are *Escherichia coli* and anaerobes.

Sonographic Findings. The ultrasound appearance of a pyogenic abscess may be variable, depending on the internal consistency of the mass. The size varies from 1 cm to very large. The right central lobe of the liver is the most common site for abscess development. The abscess may be hypoechoic with

TABLE 6-5 LIVER FINDINGS: FOCAL DISEASE

Clinical Findings	Sonographic Findings	Differential Considerations
Simple Hepatic Cysts		
N/A	Anechoic Thin walls Well-defined borders Distal posterior enhancement May have calcification	Congenital Hematoma Necrotic tumor
Polycystic Liver Disease		
Autosomal dominant 25%–50% of patients with polycystic kidney disease have hepatic cysts 60% of patients with polycystic liver disease have associated PKD	Anechoic Well-defined borders ↑ Acoustic enhancement Multiple cysts throughout liver parenchyma	Necrotic metastasis Echinococcal cyst Hematoma Abscess Hepatic cystadenocarcinoma
Pyogenic Abscess		
↑ White cell count Abnormal LFT Anemia	Variable appearance Right central lobe most common site Hypoechoic to complex to hyperechoic when fluid level present Round to oval or irregular Complex	Amebic abscess Echinococcal cyst Hepatic candidiasis
Hepatic Candidiasis		
↑ WBC Fever	Multiple small hypoechoic masses with echogenic central core "bulls-eye" lesions "Wheel-within-wheel" pattern	Abscess Echinococcal cyst Metastases
Chronic Granulomatous Disease		
N/A	Poorly marginated Hypoechoic Posterior enhancement May have calcification/shadowing	Abscess
Amebic Abscess		
↑ Leukocytes Low fever Abdominal pain and diarrhea	Mass is variable Round or oval; lack notable borders Hypoechoic with debris	Pyogenic abscess Echinococcal cyst Hepatic candidiasis
Echinococcal Cyst		
↑ WBC History of sheep-farming exposure	Simple to complex cysts Acoustic enhancement Oval or spherical Calcification Honeycomb appearance/"water lily" sign	Polycystic liver disease Amebic abscess Pyogenic abscess

LFT, Liver function test; *N/A,* not applicable; *PKD,* polycystic kidney disease.

round or ovoid margins and acoustic enhancement, or it may be complex, with some debris along the posterior margin and irregular walls (Figure 6-46). It may have a fluid level; if gas is present, it can be hyperechoic with dirty shadowing.

Hepatic candidiasis. Hepatic candidiasis is caused by a species of *Candida.* It usually occurs in immunocompromised hosts, such as patients undergoing chemotherapy, organ transplant recipients, or individuals with human immunodeficiency infection (HIV). The candidal fungus invades the bloodstream

and may affect any organ, with the more perfused kidneys, brain, and heart affected the most.

Clinically the patient may present with nonspecific findings, such as fever and localized pain.

Sonographic Findings. On ultrasound examination, candidiasis within the liver may present as multiple small hypoechoic masses with echogenic central cores, referred to as **bull's-eye** or **target lesions.** Other sonographic patterns have been described as "wheel-within-wheel" patterns, or multiple

Figure 6-42 Simple hepatic cyst. A simple liver cyst may appear anechoic with conventional settings *(left)* and appear with low-level echoes with harmonics *(right)*.

Figure 6-43 Simple hepatic cyst shows smooth, uniform borders and no internal echoes (anechoic).

small hypoechoic lesions. Specific diagnosis can only be made with fine-needle aspiration.

Chronic granulomatous disease. Chronic granulomatous disease is a recessive trait related to a congenital defect in the leukocytes that is able to ingest but not kill certain bacteria. This occurs mostly in children, with a more frequent occurrence in girls. A pediatric patient may have recurrent respiratory infections.

Sonographic Findings. On ultrasound, a poorly marginated, hypoechoic mass is seen with posterior enhancement. Calcification may be present with posterior shadowing. Aspiration is necessary to specifically classify the mass as granulomatous disease.

Amebic abscess. Amebic abscess is a collection of pus formed by disintegrated tissue in a cavity, usually in the liver, caused by the protozoan parasite *Entamoeba histolytica* (Figure 6-47). The infection is primarily a disease of the colon, but it can also spread to the liver, lungs, and brain. The parasites

Figure 6-44 Gross pathology of polycystic liver disease. There are numerous large cysts throughout the liver parenchyma. (From Damjanov I, Linder J: *Pathology: a color atlas,* St. Louis, 2000, Mosby.)

reach the liver parenchyma via the portal vein. Amebiasis is contracted by ingesting the cysts in contaminated water and food. The ameba usually affects the colon and cecum, and the organism remains within the gastrointestinal tract. If the organism invades the colonic mucosa, it may travel to the liver via the portal venous system.

Patients may be asymptomatic or may show the gastrointestinal symptoms of abdominal pain, diarrhea, leukocytosis, and low fever.

Figure 6-45 **A** to **C,** Polycystic liver disease shows multiple cysts throughout the liver and kidney.

Figure 6-46 Pyogenic abscess is shown as a complex mass in the right lobe of the liver in a patient with cirrhosis, abdominal pain, and fever. The mass is irregular with slightly increased through-transmission.

Sonographic Findings. The ultrasound appearance of amebic abscess is variable and nonspecific. The abscess may be round or oval and lack notable defined wall echoes. The lesion is hypoechoic compared with normal liver parenchyma, with low-level echoes at higher sensitivity. There may be some internal echoes along the posterior margin secondary to debris (Figure 6-48). Distal enhancement may be seen beyond the mass lesion. Some organisms may rupture through the diaphragm into the hepatic capsule.

Echinococcal cyst. Hepatic echinococcosis is an infectious cystic disease common in sheep-herding areas of the world, but seldom encountered within the United States. The echinococcus is a tapeworm that infects humans as the intermediate host. The worm resides in the small intestine of dogs. The ova from the adult worm are shed through canine feces into the environment, where the intermediate hosts ingest the eggs. After entering the proximal portion of the small intestine in humans, the larvae burrow through the mucosa, enter the portal circulation, and travel to the liver.

The echinococcal cyst has two layers: the inner layer and outer, or inflammatory reaction, layer. The smaller, daughter cysts may develop from the inner layer. The cysts may enlarge and rupture. The cysts may also impinge on the blood vessels and lead to vascular thrombosis and infarction.

Sonographic Findings. On ultrasound, several patterns may occur, from a simple cyst to a complex mass with acoustic enhancement. The shape may be oval or spherical, with regularity of the walls. Calcifications may occur. Septations are very frequent and include honeycomb appearance with fluid collections; "water lily" sign, which shows a detachment and collapse

Figure 6-47 Gross pathology of an amebic abscess. The cavitary lesion is filled with yellow necrotic material and does not contain pus. (From Damjanov I, Linder J: *Pathology: a color atlas,* St. Louis, 2000, Mosby.)

of the germinal layer; or "cyst within a cyst." Sometimes the liver contains multiple parent cysts in both lobes of the liver; the cyst with the thick walls occupies a different part of the liver (Figure 6-49). The tissue between the cysts indicates that each cyst is a separate parent cyst and not a daughter cyst. If a daughter cyst is found, it is specific for echinococcal disease.

HEPATIC TUMORS

A **neoplasm** is any new growth of new tissue, either benign or malignant. A benign growth occurs locally but does not spread or invade surrounding structures. It may push surrounding structures aside or adhere to them. A malignant mass is uncontrolled and is prone to metastasize to nearby or distant structures via the bloodstream and lymph nodes. Thus it is important not only to recognize the tumor mass itself but also to appreciate which structures the malignancy may invade. See Table 6-6 for clinical findings, sonographic findings, and differential considerations for hepatic tumors.

Benign Hepatic Tumors

Cavernous hemangioma. A hemangioma is a benign, congenital tumor consisting of large, blood-filled cystic spaces. Cavernous hemangioma is the most common benign tumor of the liver. The tumor is found more frequently in females. Patients are usually asymptomatic, although a small percentage may bleed, causing right upper quadrant pain. Hemangiomas enlarge slowly and undergo degeneration, fibrosis, and calcification. They are found in the subcapsular hepatic parenchyma or in the posterior right lobe more than the left lobe of the liver.

Sonographic Findings. The ultrasound appearance is typically hyperechoic with acoustic enhancement (Figures 6-50 and 6-51). Many authors have speculated that the echo-dense

Figure 6-48 Amebic abscess is a complex lesion, usually in the right lobe of the liver. This patient recently returned from a vacation in Mexico and presented with right upper quadrant pain and fever for 2 weeks.

Figure 6-49   Echinococcal cyst. This complex mass found in the right lobe of the liver shows fluid and debris components.

pattern results from the multiple interfaces between the walls of the cavernous sinuses and blood within them. They are round, oval, or lobulated with well-defined borders. The larger hemangiomas may have a mixed pattern resulting from necrosis (Figure 6-52). Hemangiomas may become more heterogeneous as they undergo degeneration and fibrous replacement. They may also project with calcifications or a complex or anechoic echo pattern (Figure 6-53). The differential considerations for hemangioma should include metastases, hepatoma, focal nodular hyperplasia, and adenoma.

Liver cell adenoma.   An adenoma is a tumor of the glandular epithelium in which the cells of the tumor are arranged in a recognizable glandular structure. The liver cell adenoma consists of normal or slightly atypical hepatocytes, frequently containing areas of bile stasis and focal hemorrhage or necrosis. The lesion is found more commonly in women and has been related to oral contraceptive usage. Patients may present

Figure 6-50   Cavernous hemangioma was found in a 43-year-old asymptomatic male. The mass is irregular and echogenic secondary to the vascular component of the lesion.

Figure 6-51   Cavernous hemangioma in this patient shows a well-defined echogenic lesion in the dome of the right lobe of the liver. Color flow is seen within the lesion.

TABLE 6-6 LIVER FINDINGS: TUMORS

Clinical Findings	Sonographic Findings	Differential Considerations
Cavernous Hemangioma		
Small percentage may bleed; RUQ pain More frequent in women	Most are hyperechoic with enhancement Round or oval, well defined Larger masses may show necrosis, degeneration, calcification	Metastasis Hepatoma (HCC) Adenoma Focal nodular hyperplasia
Liver Cell Adenoma		
RUQ pain when mass bleeds	Hyperechoic with central echogenic area caused by hemorrhage Solitary or multiple Fluid may be present	Hemangioma Focal nodular hyperplasia Hepatoma (HCC)
Focal Nodular Hyperplasia		
More frequent in women <40	Multiple, well defined with hyperechoic to isoechoic patterns Frequently found in right lobe of liver	Hemangiomas Hepatoma (HCC) Metastases Adenoma
Hepatocellular Carcinoma		
70% of patients have ↑ alpha-fetoprotein level Abnormalities in liver function tests, with the indications of cirrhosis	Solitary, multiple Infiltrative, diffuse Hypoechoic, isoechoic, or hyperechoic May invade hepatic veins Thrombus	Hemangioma Metastases
Metastatic Disease		
Abnormal LFTs Jaundice Hepatomegaly Weight loss Decreased appetite	Hypoechoic or echogenic mass Diffuse distortion of bull's eye pattern Solitary or multiple Well to ill-defined	Abscess Hemangioma Hepatoma (HCC) Adenoma
Lymphoma		
Abnormal LFT	Hypoechoic or diffuse patterns Target or echogenic lesions Intrahepatic and lucent multiple small, discrete solid lesions without enhancement	Hemangioma HCC Metastases

HCC, Hepatocellular carcinoma; *LFT,* liver function test; *N/A,* not applicable.

Figure 6-52 Cavernous hemangioma was found in a 62-year-old male with a palpable abdominal mass. The lesion has a complex pattern secondary to necrosis and degeneration.

with right upper quadrant pain secondary to rupture with bleeding into the tumor. The incidence is increased in patients with type I glycogen storage disease or von Gierke's disease.

Sonographic Findings. On ultrasound examination, the mass can look similar to focal nodular hyperplasia. It is hyperechoic with a central hypoechoic area caused by hemorrhage (Figure 6-54). The lesion may be solitary or multiple (Figure 6-55). If the lesion ruptures, fluid should be found in the peritoneal cavity.

Hepatic cystadenoma. Hepatic cystadenoma contains cystic structures within the lesion. This adenoma is a rare neoplasm occurring in middle-aged women. Most have a palpable abdominal mass.

Sonographic Findings. On ultrasound examination, the lesions may be multilocular with mucinous fluid.

Focal nodular hyperplasia. Focal nodular hyperplasia is the second most common benign liver mass after hemangioma. It is found in women under 40 years of age. The mass is

Figure 6-53   Cavernous hemangioma with calcifications and shadowing.

Figure 6-54   Hepatic adenoma appears as a well-defined lesion with a central hyperechoic area surrounded by a halo.

thought to arise from developmental hyperplastic lesions related to an area of congenital vascular formation. The patient is asymptomatic. The lesions occur more in the right lobe of the liver. There may be more than one mass; many are located along the subcapsular area of the liver, some are pedunculated, and many have a central scar (Figure 6-56). The lesion consists of normal hepatocytes, Kupffer cells, bile duct elements, and fibrous connective tissue. The multiple nodules are separated by bands of fibrous tissue. There may be increased bleeding within the tumors in these patients.

Sonographic Findings. On ultrasound examination, the lesions appear well defined with hyperechoic to isoechoic patterns compared with the liver (Figure 6-57). The internal linear echoes may be seen within the lesions if multiple nodules occur together.

Malignant Disease. Primary malignant tumors are relatively rare in the liver. The most common tumor is hepatocel-

lular carcinoma, developing in cirrhotic livers. Cirrhosis may be secondary to metabolic disorders or hepatitis. Tumors may also result from prolonged exposure to carcinogenic chemicals. Ultrasound has the advantage over other imaging modalities in defining liver texture in many different planes. This technique is especially useful in the diagnosis of malignant hepatic disease. A comparison of the different liver textures and patterns is shown in Figure 6-58.

The clinical signs of liver cancer are mild and general—similar to those of other hepatocellular diseases. These symptoms include nausea and vomiting, fatigue, weight loss, and hepatomegaly. Portal hypertension and splenomegaly are common.

Hepatocellular carcinoma. As noted, hepatocellular carcinoma (HCC) is the most common primary malignant neoplasm. The prevalence varies, depending on predisposing factors such as hepatitis B and aflatoxin exposure, which contributes to the high incidence of hepatocellular carcinoma

Figure 6-55   Three-dimensional imaging of a hepatic mass that appears to be well defined in the dome of the right lobe of the liver. Three-D allows one to record the image from multiple directions without moving the transducer. This most likely represents a hepatic adenoma.

Figure 6-56   Gross pathology of focal nodular hyperplasia with a lobular mass with a central fibrotic scar. (From Damjanov I, Linder J: *Pathology: a color atlas,* St. Louis, 2000, Mosby.)

Figure 6-57   Focal nodular hyperplasia appears as a well-defined lesion with a hyperechoic internal texture.

in Africa and Southeast Asia. The incidence of HCC in the United States is low, occurring in 5 of 100,000 of the population.

The pathogenesis of hepatocellular carcinoma is related to cirrhosis (80% of patients with preexisting cirrhosis develop hepatocellular carcinoma), chronic hepatitis B virus infection, and hepatocarcinogens in foods. The tumor occurs more frequently in men. Clinically, patients with HCC usually present with a previous history of cirrhosis, a palpable mass, hepatomegaly, appetite disorder, and fever.

The carcinoma may present in one of three patterns: solitary massive tumor, multiple nodules throughout the liver, or diffuse infiltrative masses in the liver. Pathologically the tumor may present as a focal lesion, an invasive lesion with necrosis and hemorrhage, or a poorly defined lesion (Figure 6-59). The carcinoma can be very invasive and has been known to invade

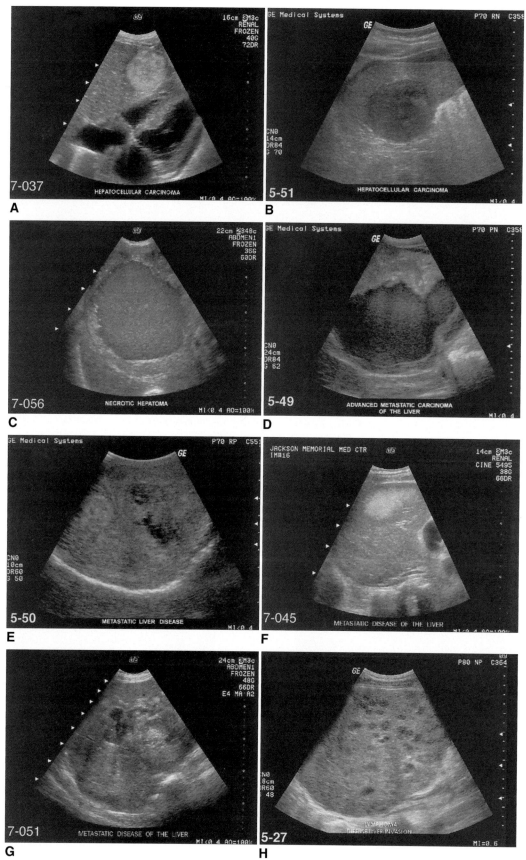

Figure 6-58 Malignant hepatic disease. **A,** Hepatocellular carcinoma: well-defined hyperechoic lesion. **B,** Hepatocellular carcinoma: well-defined hypoechoic lesion. **C,** Necrotic hepatoma: necrotic isoechoic lesion. **D,** Advanced metastases: large hypoechoic lesion. **E,** Metastases: ill-defined complex necrotic lesion. **F,** Metastases: well-defined hyperechoic lesion. **G,** Metastases: large isoechoic lesions in right lobe. **H,** Lymphoma: diffuse hypoechoic lesions.

A   **B**

Figure 6-59   Gross pathology of hepatocellular carcinoma. **A,** The cirrhotic liver contains a solitary malignant nodule. **B,** The huge tumor is poorly demarcated from the remaining liver. (From Damjanov I, Linder J: *Pathology: a color atlas,* St. Louis, 2000, Mosby.)

Figure 6-60   Hepatocellular carcinoma shows a discrete hypoechoic lesion in the right lobe of the liver.

A

B

Figure 6-61   Transverse **(A)** and sagittal **(B)** images of the upper right quadrant show a large hepatocellular carcinoma in the right lobe of the liver.

the hepatic veins to produce Budd-Chiari syndrome. The portal venous system may also be invaded with tumor or thrombosis. Hepatocellular carcinoma has a tendency to destroy the portal venous radicle walls, with invasion into the lumen of the vessel.

Sonographic Findings. On ultrasound examination, a variable appearance is noted with discrete lesions, either solitary or multiple, that are usually hypoechoic or hyperechoic. Sometimes the lesions may be isoechoic, and a halo may surround the lesion (Figure 6-60). Another pattern presents as diffuse parenchymal involvement with inhomogeneity throughout the liver without distinct masses (Figure 6-61). The last pattern is a combination of discrete and diffuse echoes (Figure 6-62). Hepatocellular carcinoma cannot be differentiated from metastases on ultrasound.

Internal echoes within the portal veins, hepatic veins, or inferior vena cava indicate tumor invasion or thrombosis within the vessel. The evaluation of the vascular structures with

A

B

Figure 6-62 Hepatocellular carcinoma in a 58-year-old male shows hepatomegaly with diffuse abnormal lesions throughout the liver parenchyma. **A,** Transverse; **B,** longitudinal.

Figure 6-63 Metastatic carcinoma. The liver contains numerous spherical nodules, many of which show central indentation corresponding to the areas of necrosis. (From Damjanov I, Linder J: *Pathology: a color atlas,* St. Louis, 2000, Mosby.)

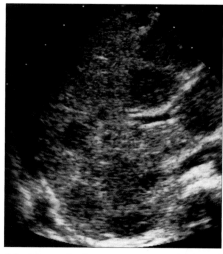

Figure 6-64 Metastatic disease appears as multiple, well-defined hypoechoic lesions throughout the liver.

color Doppler helps to rule out the presence of clot or tumor invasion. Hepatic flow is abnormal if an obstruction is present.

Metastatic disease. The most common form of neoplastic involvement of the liver is metastatic disease. The primary sites are the colon, breast, and lung. The majority of metastases arise from a primary colonic malignancy or a hepatoma. Metastatic spread to the liver occurs as the tumor erodes the wall and travels through the lymphatic system or through the bloodstream to the portal vein or hepatic artery to the liver.

Sonographic Findings. The ultrasound patterns of metastatic tumor involvement in the liver vary. It is typical to have multiple nodes throughout both lobes of the liver (Figure 6-63). The following three specific patterns have been described: (1) a well-defined hypoechoic mass (Figure 6-64); (2) a well-defined echogenic mass (Figure 6-65); and (3) diffuse distortion of the normal homogeneous parenchymal pattern without a focal mass (Figure 6-66). The hypovascular lesions produce hypoechoic patterns in the liver because of necrosis and ischemic areas from neoplastic thrombosis. Most cases of hypervascular lesions correspond to hyperechoic patterns.

The common primary masses include renal cell carcinoma, carcinoid, choriocarcinoma, transitional cell carcinoma, islet cell carcinoma, and hepatocellular carcinoma. The echogenic lesions are common with primary colonic tumors and may present with calcification. Target types of metastases or bull's-

eye patterns are the result of edema around the tumor or necrosis or hemorrhage within the tumor. As the nodules increase rapidly in size and outgrow their blood supply, central necrosis and hemorrhage may result.

Various combinations of these patterns can be seen simultaneously in a patient with metastatic liver disease. The first abnormality is hepatomegaly or alterations in contour, especially on the lateral segment of the left lobe. The lesions may be solitary or multiple, be variable in size and shape, and have sharp or ill-defined margins. Metastases may be extensive or localized to produce an inhomogeneous parenchymal pattern.

Ultrasound may be useful to follow patients after surgery. After a baseline hepatic ultrasound has been performed, the sonographer can assess any regression or progression of tumor and change in parenchymal pattern.

Lymphoma. Lymphomas are malignant neoplasms involving lymphocyte proliferation in the lymph nodes. The two main disorders, Hodgkin's lymphoma and non-Hodgkin's lymphoma, are differentiated by lymph node biopsy. No specific

Figure 6-65   Metastatic disease may appear as well-defined hyperechoic lesions throughout the liver.

Figure 6-66   Metastatic disease appears as diffuse hypoechoic small lesions throughout the liver parenchyma.

Figure 6-67   Lymphoma was found in this elderly male with hepatomegaly. Multiple isoechoic lesions were found throughout the liver.

cause is known. Patients with lymphoma have hepatomegaly with a normal or diffuse alteration of parenchymal echoes. A focal hypoechoic mass is sometimes seen. The patient may present with enlarged, nontender lymph nodes, fever, fatigue, night sweats, weight loss, bone pain, or an abdominal mass. The presence of splenomegaly or retroperitoneal nodes may help confirm the diagnosis of lymphadenopathy.

Sonographic Findings. Hodgkin's lymphoma shows up as diffuse parenchymal changes in the liver. Non-Hodgkin's lymphoma may appear with target hypoechoic mass lesions. Burkitt's lymphoma lesions may appear intrahepatic and lucent. Patients with leukemia have multiple small, discrete hepatic masses that are solid with no acoustic enhancement (Figure 6-67). A bull's-eye appearance with a dense central core may be present as a result of tumor necrosis.

In the pediatric population, the most common malignancies are neuroblastomas, Wilms' tumor, and leukemia. The neuroblastoma presents as a densely reflective echo pattern

with liver involvement similar to that of a hepatoma. In patients with a Wilms' tumor, metastases generally invade the lung; however, the liver may be a secondary site. These lesions present as a densely reflective pattern with lucencies resulting from necrosis.

HEPATIC TRAUMA

The liver is the third most common organ injured in the abdomen after the spleen and kidney. Laceration of the liver occurs in 3% of trauma patients and is frequently associated with other injured organs. The need for surgery is determined by the size of the laceration, the amount of hemoperitoneum, and the patient's clinical status. The right lobe is affected more often than the left. The degree of trauma can vary, with a small laceration, large laceration with a hematoma, subcapsular hematoma, or capsular disruption.

Sonographic Findings. Computerized tomography is used more often than ultrasound to localize the extent of the laceration within the liver and surrounding areas. Ultrasound does not clearly distinguish small lacerations in the dome of the right lobe of the liver. Intraperitoneal fluid should be assessed along the flanks and into the pelvis. Intrahepatic hematomas are hyperechoic in the first 24 hours and hypoechoic and sonolucent thereafter because of the resolution of the blood within the area. Septations and internal echoes develop 1 to 4 weeks after the trauma (Figure 6-68). A subcapsular hematoma may appear as anechoic, hypoechoic, septated lenticular, or curvilinear. It may be differentiated from ascitic fluid in that it occurs unilaterally, along the area of laceration. The degree of homogenicity depends on the age of the laceration.

LIVER TRANSPLANTATION

Liver transplantation is performed to eliminate irreversible disease when more conservative medical and surgical treat-

ments have failed. The most common indications for transplantation in adults are cirrhosis (especially secondary to chronic active hepatitis), fulminant active hepatitis, congenital metabolic disorders, sclerosing cholangitis, Budd-Chiari syndrome, and unresectable hepatoma.

The surgical procedure of the recipient includes hepatectomy, revascularization of the new liver (hepatic artery, hepatic veins, portal venous system, and inferior vena cava), hemostasis, and biliary reconstruction. Complications of transplantation include rejection, thrombosis or leak, biliary stricture or leak, infection, and neoplasia. Rejection is the most common cause of hepatic dysfunction that is confirmed by clinical diagnosis and liver biopsy. Vascular complications include thrombosis, stricture, and arterial anastomotic pseudoaneurysms. Vascular thrombosis may affect the hepatic artery, the portal

Figure 6-68   Hepatic trauma. **A** and **B,** A complex mass was found in the right lobe of the liver in a patient who had been in a car accident. **C,** Computed tomographic scan of the 54-year-old female shows a collection of blood in the right lateral border of the liver.

vein, or, less commonly, the inferior vena cava (more common in Budd-Chiari patients) and aorta. Biliary complications, stricture, and leakage affect a small percentage of transplant patients. Since the hepatic artery is the sole supply of blood to the bile ducts in transplant patients, identification of a stricture of the bile duct is an indication for assessment of hepatic artery patency. Hepatic arterial occlusion, pretransplant primary sclerosing cholangitis, choledochojejunostomy, cholangitis at liver biopsy, and young age are greatly associated with biliary strictures.

Sonographic Findings. Ultrasound can play an important role in the preoperative and postoperative evaluation of hepatic transplantation. The primary function of the ultrasound examination is to evaluate the portal venous system, the hepatic artery, the inferior vena cava, and the liver parenchymal pattern. The vascular structures should be assessed for size and patency in the preoperative evaluation. The liver parenchyma should be examined to rule out the presence of hepatic architecture disruption. The sonographer should also evaluate the biliary system, to look for dilation, and the portosystemic collateral vessels.

In the pediatric patient the most common reason for liver transplantation is biliary atresia and associated anomalies of the spleen, hepatic vasculature, and kidneys. Therefore, in addition to the examination described above, both kidneys and the spleen must be examined.

In the postoperative period, hepatic artery thrombosis is the most serious complication of liver transplantation. The hepatic artery is examined with Doppler and color flow ultrasound in the area of the porta hepatis. The normal hepatic artery flow produces a low-resistance arterial signal. Thrombosis may be detected when this signal is absent. In the adult patient, collateral vessels in the region of the hepatic artery have not developed. However, collateral hepatic arterial circulation may have developed in children. Thus the scans should be made within 24 hours after surgery, 48 hours after surgery, and weekly thereafter to assess for changes in the velocity flow pattern.

The development of anastomotic stenoses is another problem in the transplant patient. This flow pattern is a turbulent, high-velocity signal indicative of hepatic arterial stenosis. Portal vein thrombosis may also occur in the postoperative period (Figure 6-69). Air in the portal vein may be seen as brightly echogenic moving targets within the portal venous system. Compromise of the inferior vena cava is another complication of transplantation. A fatal complication is hepatic necrosis associated with thrombosis of the hepatic artery or portal vein. Massive necrosis produces gangrene of the liver and air in the hepatic parenchyma.

Figure 6-69 Liver transplantation. **A,** Ascites may be seen as a postoperative finding in a liver transplant patient. **B,** Color can define the site of the piggyback anastomosis of the suprahepatic inferior vena cava (IVC) to the intrahepatic IVC. **C,** Patency of the portal vein can be assessed by gray scale and color Doppler.

HEPATIC VASCULAR FLOW ABNORMALITIES

Portal Venous Hypertension. Portal hypertension is defined as an increase in portal venous pressure or hepatic venous gradient. It exists when the portal venous pressure is above 10 mm Hg or the hepatic venous gradient is more than 5 mm Hg. The development of increased pressure in the portal-splenic venous system is the cause of portal hypertension. Acute or chronic hepatocellular disease can block the flow of blood throughout the liver, causing it to back up into the hepatic portal circulation. This causes the blood pressure in the hepatic circulation to increase, thus the development of portal hypertension. In an effort to relieve the pressure, collateral veins are formed that connect to the systemic veins. These are known as varicose veins and occur most frequently in the area of the esophagus, stomach, and rectum. Rupture of these veins can cause massive bleeding that may result in death.

Portal hypertension may also develop when hepatopetal flow (toward the liver) is impeded by thrombus or tumor invasion. The blood becomes obstructed as it passes through the liver to the hepatic veins and is diverted to collateral pathways in the upper abdomen. Box 6-3 lists the indications for portal hypertension.

Portal hypertension may develop along two pathways. One entails increased resistance to flow, and the other entails increased portal blood flow. The most common mechanism for increased resistance to flow occurs in patients with cirrhosis (Figures 6-70 and 6-71). The disease process of cirrhosis produces areas of micronodular and macronodular regeneration, atrophy, and fatty infiltration, which make it difficult for the blood to perfuse. This condition may be found in patients with liver disease or diseases of the cardiovascular system. Patients who present with increased portal blood flow may have an arteriovenous fistula or splenomegaly secondary to a hematologic disorder.

Collateral circulation develops when the normal venous channels become obstructed. This diverted blood flow causes embryologic channels to reopen; blood flows hepatofugally (away from the liver) and is diverted into collateral vessels. The collateral channels may be into the gastric veins (coronary veins), esophageal veins, recanalized umbilical vein, or splenorenal, gastrorenal, retroperitoneal, hemorrhoidal, or intestinal veins (Figure 6-72). The most common collateral pathways are through the coronary and esophageal veins, as occurs in 80% to 90% of patients with portal hypertension. Varices, tortuous dilations of veins, may develop because of increased pressure in the portal vein, usually secondary to cirrhosis. Bleeding from the varices occurs with increased pressure.

The most definitive way to diagnose portal hypertension is with arteriography. Ultrasound may be very useful in these patients to define the presence of ascites, hepatosplenomegaly, and collateral circulation; the cause of jaundice; and the patency of hepatic vascular channels. See Table 6-7 for clinical findings, sonographic findings, and differential considerations for portal venous hypertension.

Patient preparation and positioning. A history should be obtained from the patient to focus on the risk factors, signs, and symptoms of hepatocellular disease. Any previous medical history relating to hepatocellular disease should be noted. Likewise, any recent surgical intervention or shunt placement within the portal venous system should be documented in the patient history worksheet. The patient is placed initially in the supine position; the patient may also be rolled into a slight left lateral decubitus position to obtain a better intercostal window. The images and Doppler evaluation may be obtained

---

> **BOX 6-3   INDICATIONS FOR PORTAL HYPERTENSION**
>
> - Suspected portal hypertension secondary to liver disease
> - Portal vein compression or thrombosis
> - Acute onset of hepatic vein occlusion (Budd-Chiari syndrome), constrictive pericarditis, or congestive heart failure with tricuspid regurgitation
> - Congenital, traumatic, or neoplastic arterioportal fistula

A   **B**

Figure 6-70   Portal hypertension. **A,** Transverse image of hepatosplenomegaly in a patient with advanced cirrhosis, decreased vasculature, and ascites. **B,** Transverse image of the thickened gallbladder wall, accentuated by the ascitic fluid.

Figure 6-71   Portal hypertension. **A,** Hepatofugal flow in the splenic vein. **B,** Hepatofugal flow in the left portal vein. **C,** Recanalization of the paraumbilical vein. **D,** Thrombosis of the main portal vein with reduced flow. **E,** Patency of the middle hepatic vein into the inferior vena cava (IVC). **F,** Reduced flow in the IVC secondary to thrombosis.

in the longitudinal, coronal, oblique, or transverse plane. Breath holding is very important in obtaining good Doppler color and spectral waveforms. Initially scan the patient in shallow respiration to set up your controls and depth. Then instruct the patient to stop breathing or take in a deep breath and hold it while you obtain the Doppler images. You can watch the image on the screen to see which technique works the best to obtain the clearest images. It is helpful to remember that a vein diameter of greater than or equal to 12.5 mm has been associated with portal hypertension.

Keep in mind these important technical points:

- Place ultrasound gel on the abdomen to ensure good transducer-to-skin contact during the abdominal Doppler imaging examination.
- The transducer's orientation marker should be pointing toward the patient's right side during the examination when a transverse scan is performed; the orientation marker is directed toward the patient's head when a longitudinal scan is performed.

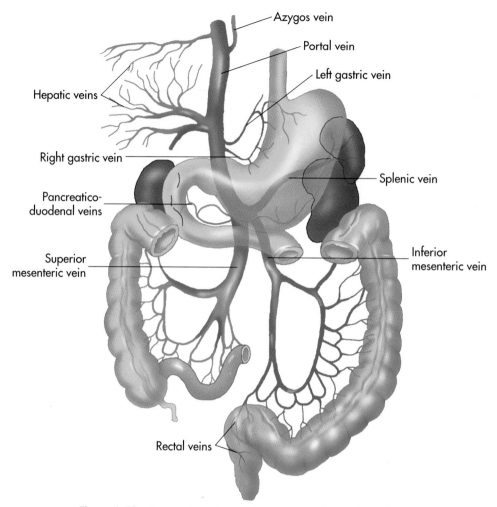

Azygos vein

Portal vein

Left gastric vein

Hepatic veins

Right gastric vein

Pancreatico-
duodenal veins

Splenic vein

Superior
mesenteric vein

Inferior
mesenteric vein

Rectal veins

Figure 6-72   Collateral circulation of the extrahepatic portal circulation.

TABLE 6-7	LIVER FINDINGS: PORTAL VENOUS HYPERTENSION	
Clinical Findings	Sonographic Findings	Differential Considerations
↑ Liver enzymes	Collateral circulation/ reversal of flow	Occlusion of vessels
Gastrointestinal bleeding	Ascites	
Jaundice Hematemesis	Hepatosplenomegaly	

- The examination is performed with both gray scale and Doppler evaluation of the portal system, the hepatic veins, and the hepatic arteries.
- Remember, the transducer must be PARALLEL to the vessel; the Doppler angle should be less than 60 degrees to obtain the maximum peak systolic velocity.
- The evaluation of the portal venous system, hepatic veins, and hepatic artery is performed during the Doppler imaging examination.

- A liver Doppler examination should also evaluate flow in the extra–hepatic-portal venous system and the inferior vena cava, as well as the size of the common bile duct, liver, kidneys, and spleen.
- The pelvic cavity, flanks, and lower quadrants should be evaluated for the presence of free fluid.

Doppler technique. Box 6-4 summarizes Doppler technique for abdominal exams.

Color Doppler evaluation of collateral circulation. On ultrasound examination, the dilated venous structures near the superior mesenteric-splenic vein confluence, the main portal vein, and the gastric veins should be evaluated (Figure 6-73). As the sonographer scans in the longitudinal plane, medial to the superior mesenteric and splenic vein confluence, the right and left gastric veins may be seen as collateral circulation. If the gastric veins are serving as collateral circulation, their diameter should be enlarged to 4 to 5 mm. Remember, the Doppler signals should be obtained from the imaging plane that allows the beam to be as parallel to the vessel as possible.

The umbilical vein may become recanalized secondary to portal hypertension. This vessel is best seen on the longitudinal plane near the midline, as a tubular structure coursing pos-

BOX 6-4 DOPPLER TECHNIQUE

- The pulse repetition frequency (PRF) allows one to record lower velocities as the PRF is lowered; as the PRF is increased, the lower velocities are filtered out to record only the higher velocity signal.
- The PRF may be changed with the scale control on the Doppler panel (look at the color bar on the left side of the monitor; the PRF will change as the "scale" on the Doppler control is changed).
- The PRF increases as imaging depth increases and decreases as depth decreases. Flow within the normal hepatic venous system is low; therefore, a lower PRF is necessary to record the flow pattern. As the flow increases beyond 40 cm/sec, the PRF should be increased to prevent aliasing. (Aliasing may also be reduced by scanning at a lower frequency.)
- The Doppler sample volume should be smaller than the diameter of the lumen. If you have difficulty finding the vessel, increase the width of the sample volume to locate the flow, and then reduce the volume width to clear up the spectral waveform.
- The Doppler angle correction should be less than 60 degrees to display the peak spectral velocity.
- Wall filters help to eliminate "noise" or low-level Doppler shifts seen within the vessel.
- Pulse wave Doppler provides quantitative information from a selected location.
- Color Doppler velocity is dependent on the direction of flow, velocity, and angle to flow. A positive Doppler shift is towards the transducer; negative shows flow away from the transducer. The laminar flow is distinguished from turbulent flow by varying the shades of color on the color map.
- Doppler measurements:

Peak systolic velocity (calculated highest velocity in cm/sec)
   Resistive Index (RI): subtract the end diastolic velocity from the peak systolic velocity and divide by the peak systolic velocity. Normal or low resistive RI measures <0.7.

terior to the medial surface of the left lobe of the liver (Figure 6-74). On transverse scans a bull's-eye is seen within the ligamentum teres as the enlarged umbilical vein. Color Doppler helps the sonographer identify this vascular structure. Table 6-8 summarizes hepatic vasculature technique.

Other vessels that may become collaterals include the esophageal vessels, which are best seen in the midline transverse plane as the transducer is angled in a cephalic direction through the left lobe of the liver. The dilated gastrorenal, splenorenal, and short gastric veins are seen in the transverse and longitudinal planes near the splenic hilum.

As discussed earlier, the normal portal venous blood flows toward the liver, with the main portal vein flowing in a hepatopetal direction into the liver. Color Doppler will show this flow as a red or positive color pattern. The portal branches running posteriorly, or away, will appear as blue, or negative, flow. Thus the right portal vein will appear blue and the left portal vein will appear red. The normal portal vein waveform is monophasic with low velocity. There should be little change with the patient's respiration and cardiac motion. The flow should be smooth and laminar. The normal diameter of the portal vein is 1.0 to 1.6 cm. The superior mesenteric vein and splenic vein are more influenced by respiration and patient position; thus, if they appear larger, it may not be as a result of portal hypertension. Flow reversal is seen both with spectral waveform patterns below the baseline in the main portal vein and with reversed color direction. Obstruction of the portal venous system is recognized by turbulence within the vessel. Table 6-9 summarizes observations important to abdominal Doppler exams.

Doppler interrogation. The hepatic vessels should be imaged at four anatomical locations:

1. Midline, beneath the xiphoid at the LHV, LHA, and LPV
2. Midclavicular and intercostals at the portal hepatis for the MHA and MPV
3. Lateral and intercostals at the right lobe for the RHA and RPV
4. Subcostal and midclavicular for the RHV and MHV

A   **B**

Figure 6-73 Hepatofugal flow in portal vein. **A,** Flow reversal is shown in the main portal vein. **B,** Spectral Doppler shows flow below the baseline in the main portal vein.

Figure 6-74   Hepatopetal flow in portal vein and paraumbilical vein. **A,** Main portal vein with normal forward flow. **B,** Portal hypertension with recanalization of the paraumbilical vein.

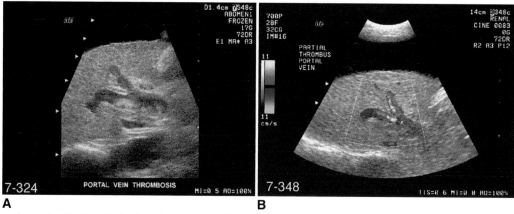

Figure 6-75   Portal vein thrombosis. **A,** Low-level echoes are seen along the posterior border of the main portal vein. **B,** Color Doppler shows some patency of the main portal vein.

Portal hypertension secondary to portal vein thrombosis. The invasion of the portal system with tumor or thrombosis may cause portal hypertension if the vessel is significantly occluded so that blood cannot flow into the liver. The clinical symptoms are very different from those of intrahepatic disease; ascites is the primary complaint. The patient does not have jaundice or a tender, enlarged liver. Splenomegaly and bleeding varices may be present.

Portal vein thrombosis may develop secondary to trauma, sepsis, cirrhosis, or hepatocellular carcinoma (Figure 6-75). The definitive diagnosis is made with a liver biopsy and positive findings of portal hypertension.

Sonographic Findings. On ultrasound examination, portal flow is absent and the vessel may be filled with hypoechoic thrombus.

Portal vein hypertension and portal caval shunts. If portal hypertension becomes extensive, the portal system can be decompressed by shunting blood to the systemic venous system. Basically, the three types of shunts are portacaval, mesocaval, and splenorenal. It is the responsibility of the sono-

grapher to know specifically which type of shunt the patient has in place to image the flow patterns correctly.

The portacaval shunt attaches the main portal vein at the superior mesenteric vein-splenic vein confluence to the anterior aspect of the inferior vena cava (Figure 6-76). The mesocaval shunt attaches the middistal superior mesenteric vein to the inferior vena cava. This shunt may be difficult to image if overlying bowel gas is present. The splenorenal shunt attaches the splenic vein to the left renal vein. The shunt and connecting vessel should be documented with real-time pulsed Doppler and color Doppler to determine flow patterns and patency.

Intrahepatic shunts are created percutaneously with the use of metallic expandable stents, which can be seen on ultrasound. This type of shunt is the transjugular intrahepatic portosystemic shunt (TIPS) (Figure 6-77). The TIPS shunt is easy to evaluate for patency because the liver provides an acoustic window to image the shunt. Baseline studies are performed with color and spectral Doppler so variations in flow patterns may be monitored before clinical symptoms are apparent. Stenosis may occur at the hepatic vein level or within the shunt.

TABLE 6-8   HEPATIC VASCULATURE TECHNIQUE

Vessel	Image Plane	Technique
LHV (left hepatic vein)	Transverse/longitudinal	• Locate the left lobe of the liver. • Identify the IVC and angle steeply towards the diaphragm. • The LHV and MHV should be seen as they drain into the IVC.
LPV (left porta vein)	Transverse, coronal, intercostal, decubitus	• Locate horizontal segment of PLV, adjust transducer to obtain steepest angle for Doppler (parallel to the vessel), and zoom in on the LPV.
LHA (left hepatic artery)	Transverse	• Usually found posterior to horizontal segment of LPV. • After interrogating the LPV, look for LHA with color Doppler (expand color box to cover the LPV and adjacent liver tissue). • Place PW cursor/sample volume in area of LHA (suspend respiration); watch for "flashing" of signal as it comes in and out of view with respiration. • Look for LHA on deep inspiration. • If you cannot get the signal in the periphery of the liver, move to another location closer to the main portal vein.
Common HA (common hepatic artery)	Longitudinal—porta hepatis	• Use same technique as described for LHA. • Transplant recipient patients: usually only able to Doppler HA at the porta hepatis. • Include extrahepatic and intrahepatic segments of HA. • Difficult to image site of anastomosis.
MPV (main portal vein)	Longitudinal—porta hepatis	• If shunt is present, anastomosis site easier to identify (more prone to thrombosis); be sure to investigate the MPV proximal, within, and distal to anastomosis.
IVC (inferior vena cava)	Longitudinal, coronal— slightly to right of midline; suspend breath. Angle transducer in cephalad to caudal sweep to record flow.	• May be difficult to obtain good angle because of horizontal location on transverse plane. • If shunt is present, evaluate site of anastomosis carefully (proximal, within, and distal). • Look carefully for presence of internal echoes that represent thrombosis. • If you suspect thrombus is present, and the Doppler signal is very "choppy" with high velocity and little phasicity, the likelihood of thrombus is good. • Be sure to follow the IVC all the way into the right atrium of the heart.
SV (splenic vein)	Transverse	• Examine SV from the splenic hilum to the portal-splenic confluence.
RHA (right hepatic artery)	Transverse, anterior to right posterior portal branch	• Use same techniques as mentioned to Doppler the RPV and RHA. • If you are unable to locate the RHA in the periphery of the liver, move closer to the trunk of the adjacent PV. • If you cannot find the RHA at the right posterior portal branch, try looking for it at the level of the right anterior PV branch.
RPV (right portal vein)	Anterior, intercostal approach; one rib space away from window for porta hepatis	• To locate the right posterior branch of RPV, begin with the MPV at the porta hepatis. • Follow the MPV into the liver until you see the RPV. • The posterior branch extends posteriorly into the right lobe. It is easier to obtain a good Doppler angle if you use a more anterior intercostal approach.
RHV (right hepatic vein)	Transverse, subcostal	• Place the probe just below the level of the xiphoid with a steep angulation toward the diaphragm. • Locate the IVC; the RHV will be seen in the right lobe of the liver in a horizontal plane as it empties into the IVC.
MHV (middle hepatic vein)	Transverse, subcostal	• Place the probe just below the level of the xiphoid with a steep angulation toward the diaphragm. • Locate the IVC; the MHV will be seen in a vertical plane as it separates the right lobe from the left lobe of the liver as it empties into the IVC.

Budd-Chiari Syndrome. Budd-Chiari syndrome is an uncommon, often dramatic illness caused by thrombosis of the hepatic veins or inferior vena cava. It was first described by Budd in 1846 and by Chiari in 1899. Budd-Chiari syndrome has a poor prognosis and is characterized by abdominal pain, massive ascites, and hepatomegaly. It may present acutely or as a chronic illness lasting from a few weeks to several years. Extensive hepatic vein occlusion is usually fatal within weeks or months of the onset of symptoms.

Budd-Chiari syndrome may be classified as primary or secondary on the basis of its pathophysiology. The primary type is caused by congenital obstruction of the hepatic veins or inferior vena cava by membranous webs across the upper vena cava at or just above the entrance of the left and middle hepatic veins. This lesion has been found to be most common in Asia.

The secondary type results from thrombosis in the hepatic veins or inferior vena cava. It often occurs in patients with predisposing conditions, such as polycythemia rubra vera,

TABLE 6-9   DOPPLER OBSERVATIONS

Hepatic Artery

• Left hepatic artery—LHA • Right hepatic artery—RHA • Common hepatic artery—CHA	• Low resistance waveform; forward flow in diastolic above baseline. • Vessel is tortuous; flow may appear to move toward and away from the transducer. • Systolic window with narrow bandwidth with parabolic flow profile. • Spectral fill-in of systolic window because of small vessel diameter. • High-resistance waveforms may indicate venoocclusive disease.

Portal Venous System

• Left portal vein—LPV • Right portal vein—RPV • Main portal vein—MPV	• Continuous, low-velocity phasic signal (phasic means that the velocity increases and decreases with respiration, giving the signal a smooth wavelike appearance). • Normal flow is termed *hepatopetal* (toward the liver). • Reversed flow is *hepatofugal* (away from the liver). • Portal venous thrombosis or postoperative anastomosis from a liver transplant can cause an abnormal portal vein signal. This results from decreased vessel lumen size, which reduces the pressure and consequently increases the velocity of flow through the narrowed region giving a "choppy" appearance as a result of increased velocities. NOTE: The hepatic artery and portal vein flow should be in the same direction, since the hepatic artery runs parallel with the portal vein.

Hepatic Venous System

• Left hepatic vein—LHV • Right hepatic vein—RHV • Middle hepatic vein—MHV	• Multiphasic pulsatile flow pattern secondary to proximity of the right atrium with flow above and below the baseline caused by close proximity to the right atrium, which results in hemodynamic changes. • Right-sided heart failure may cause the hepatic veins to become pulsatile and dilated. • Increased intrahepatic pressure or venous obstruction demonstrates a more continuous or monophasic signal.

Inferior Vena Cava

	• Continuous waveform with respiratory variations; becomes more pulsatile as it empties into the right atrium. • Best imaged with a slight cranial-caudal sweep in the longitudinal plane with the patient in deep inspiration. • Anastomosis from surgical transplantation may alter the normal flow into the inferior vena cava. • Thrombosis can cause the inferior vena cava waveform to appear monophasic with high velocities ("choppy" appearance). Examine for thrombus in the renal veins as well. • If a surgical shunt is present, be sure to check the patient's history to find out if the specific type of shunt (portal/cava or mesenteric/cava) is in place.

Figure 6-76   Mesocaval shunt. The mesocaval shunt attaches the mid-distal superior mesenteric vein to the inferior vena cava. This patient had thrombus at the distal end with to-and-fro flow reversal.

paroxysmal nocturnal hemoglobinuria, prolonged use of oral contraceptives, pregnancy tumors (hepatocellular carcinoma, renal cell carcinoma, adrenal carcinoma, leiomyosarcoma of the inferior vena cava), infections, and in rare cases trauma. In approximately 25% to 30% of all cases the exact cause is never determined.

Ascites is the most characteristic clinical feature of this disease. Other symptoms are abdominal pain, hepatosplenomegaly, jaundice, vomiting, and diarrhea. Rarely, patients present with acute illness with abdominal pain, hepatomegaly, and shock. This condition often occurs in patients with an underlying disease, such as renal cell carcinoma, primary cancer of the liver, thrombophlebitis migrans, or polycythemia. More commonly, patients have a vague illness and abdominal distress weeks or months in duration, followed by the appearance of ascites and hepatomegaly. Jaundice is mild or absent. As portal hypertension increases, the spleen becomes palpable. When thrombus is found in the inferior vena cava, edema of the legs is gross and there is venous distention over the abdomen, flanks, and back. Albuminuria may be found.

CHAPTER 7

The Gallbladder and the Biliary System

Sandra L. Hagen-Ansert

OBJECTIVES

- Describe the internal, surface, and relational anatomies of the gallbladder
- Describe the normal sonographic pattern of the gallbladder, cystic duct, hepatic ducts, and common bile duct
- Differentiate the sectional anatomy of the hepatobiliary system and adjacent structures
- Describe the congenital anomalies that affect the biliary system
- Explain the function of the gallbladder
- Differentiate the sonographic appearances of jaundice, cholelithiasis, cholecystitis, cholesterosis, benign tumors, carcinoma, gangrenous cholecystitis, wall changes, sludge, polyps, emphysematous cholecystitis, porcelain gallbladder, sclerosing cholangitis, and cholangiocarcinoma (Klatskin's tumor)
- Describe the sonographic appearance of dilated intrahepatic ducts

WALL THICKNESS
CHOLECYSTITIS
CHOLELITHIASIS
CHOLEDOCHAL CYSTS
HYPERPLASTIC CHOLECYSTITIS
PORCELAIN GALLBLADDER
GALLBLADDER CARCINOMA
DILATED BILIARY DUCTS
BILIARY OBSTRUCTION
INTRAHEPATIC BILIARY NEOPLASMS
CHOLANGITIS
CHOLEDOCHOLITHIASIS
CAROLI'S DISEASE

KEY TERMS

adenomyomatosis – small polypoid projections from the gallbladder wall

ampulla of Vater – small opening in the duodenum in which the pancreatic and common bile duct enter to release secretions

bilirubin – yellow pigment in bile formed by the breakdown of red blood cells

cholangitis – inflammation of the bile duct

cholecystectomy – removal of the gallbladder

cholecystitis – inflammation of the gallbladder; may be acute or chronic

cholecystokinin – hormone secreted into the blood by the mucosa of the upper small intestine; stimulates contraction of the gallbladder and pancreatic secretion of enzymes

choledochal cyst – dilation of the common duct that may cause obstruction

choledocholithiasis – stones in the bile duct

cholelithiasis – gallstones in the gallbladder

cholesterosis – variant of adenomyomatosis; cholesterol polyps

common bile duct – extends from the point where the common hepatic duct meets the cystic duct; drains into the duodenum after it joins with the main pancreatic duct

common duct – refers to common bile or hepatic ducts when cystic duct is not seen

common hepatic duct – bile duct system that drains the liver into the common bile duct

cystic duct – connects the gallbladder to the common hepatic duct

gallbladder (GB) – storage pouch for bile

ANATOMY OF THE BILIARY SYSTEM
NORMAL ANATOMY
VASCULAR SUPPLY

PHYSIOLOGY AND LABORATORY DATA OF THE GALLBLADDER AND BILIARY SYSTEM
REMOVAL OF THE GALLBLADDER

SONOGRAPHIC EVALUATION OF THE BILIARY SYSTEM
GALLBLADDER
BILE DUCTS

PATHOLOGY OF THE GALLBLADDER AND BILIARY SYSTEM
CLINICAL SYMPTOMS OF GALLBLADDER DISEASE
SLUDGE

Hartmann's pouch – small part of the gallbladder that lies near the cystic duct where stones may collect

Heister's valve – tiny valves found within the cystic duct

hydrops – massive enlargement of the gallbladder

jaundice – excessive bilirubin accumulation causes yellow pigmentation of the skin; first seen in the whites of the eyes

junctional fold – small septum within the gallbladder, usually arising from the posterior wall

Klatskin's tumor – cancer at the bifurcation of the hepatic ducts; may cause asymmetric obstruction of the biliary tree

Murphy's sign – positive sign implies exquisite tenderness over the area of the gallbladder upon palpation

pancreatic duct – travels horizontally through the pancreas to join the common bile duct at the ampulla of Vater

Phrygian cap – gallbladder variant in which part of the fundus is bent back on itself

polyp – small, well-defined soft tissue projection from the gallbladder wall

porcelain gallbladder – calcification of the gallbladder wall

porta hepatis – central area of the liver where the portal vein, common duct, and hepatic artery enter

sludge – low-level echoes found along the posterior margin of the gallbladder; move with change in position

sphincter of Oddi – small muscle that guards the ampulla of Vater

wall echo shadow (WES) sign – sonographic pattern found when the gallbladder is packed with stones

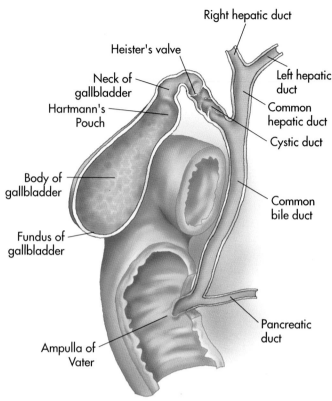

Figure 7-1   Gallbladder and biliary system.

Together with the liver and pancreas, the biliary system plays a role in the digestive process. The gallbladder serves as a reservoir for bile that is drained from the hepatic ducts in the liver. Ultrasonic evaluation of the gallbladder and biliary system is used as a primary diagnostic tool and has proven to be effective in diagnosing various types of gallbladder disease, including the more common problems of cholelithiasis, cholecystitis, and dilation of the ductal system.

ANATOMY OF THE BILIARY SYSTEM

NORMAL ANATOMY

The biliary apparatus consists of the right and left hepatic ducts, the common hepatic duct, the common bile duct, the gallbladder, and the cystic duct (Figure 7-1).

Hepatic Ducts. The right and left hepatic ducts emerge from the right lobe of the liver in the **porta hepatis** and unite to form the common hepatic duct, which then passes caudally and medially. The hepatic duct runs parallel with the portal vein. Each duct is formed by the union of bile canaliculi from the liver lobules.

The common hepatic duct is approximately 4 mm in diameter and descends within the edge of the lesser omentum. It is joined by the cystic duct to form the common bile duct. The **common hepatic duct** is the bile duct system that drains the liver into the common bile duct.

Common Bile Duct. The normal **common bile duct** has a diameter of up to 6 mm. The first part of the duct lies in the right free edge of the lesser omentum (Figure 7-2). The second part of the duct is situated posterior to the first part of the duodenum. The third part lies in a groove on the posterior surface of the head of the pancreas. It ends by piercing the medial wall of the second part of the duodenum about halfway down the duodenal length. There the common bile duct is joined by the main pancreatic duct, and together they open through a small ampulla (the **ampulla of Vater**) into the duodenal wall. The end parts of both ducts (common bile duct and main **pancreatic duct**) and the ampulla are surrounded by circular muscle fibers known as the **sphincter of Oddi.**

The proximal portion of the common bile duct is lateral to the hepatic artery and anterior to the portal vein. The duct moves more posterior after it descends behind the duodenal bulb and enters the pancreas. The distal duct lies parallel to the anterior wall of the vena cava.

Within the liver parenchyma, the bile ducts follow the same course as the portal venous and hepatic arterial branches. The hepatic and bile ducts are encased in a common collagenous sheath, forming the portal triad.

Cystic Duct. The **cystic duct** is about 4 cm long and connects the neck of the gallbladder with the common hepatic duct to form the common bile duct. It is usually somewhat S-shaped and descends for a variable distance in the right free edge of the lesser omentum.

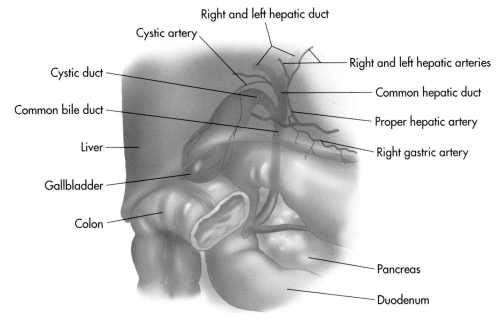

Figure 7-2   Relationships within the porta hepatis.

Gallbladder. The **gallbladder** is a pear-shaped sac in the anterior aspect of the right upper quadrant, closely related to the visceral surface of the liver. It is divided into the fundus, body, and neck. Representative transverse (Figure 7-3) and sagittal (Figure 7-4) anatomy demonstrates the relational anatomy to the gallbladder and biliary system. The rounded fundus usually projects below the inferior margin of the liver, where it comes into contact with the anterior abdominal wall at the level of the ninth right costal cartilage. The body generally lies in contact with the visceral surface of the liver and is directed upward, backward, and to the left. The neck becomes continuous with the cystic duct, which turns into the lesser omentum to join the right side of the common hepatic duct to form the common bile duct.

The neck of the gallbladder is oriented posteromedially toward the porta hepatis. The fundus is situated lateral, caudal, and anterior to the neck. Occasionally the gallbladder lies in an intrahepatic, or other anomalous location, and it may be difficult to detect by sonography if the entire upper abdomen is not examined.

The size and shape of the gallbladder are variable. Generally the normal gallbladder measures about 2.5 to 4 cm in diameter and 7 to 10 cm in length. The walls are less than 3 mm thick. Dilation of the gallbladder is known as **hydrops**.

Several anatomic variations may occur within the gallbladder to give rise to its internal echo pattern on the sonogram. The gallbladder may fold back on itself at the neck, forming **Hartmann's pouch** (see Figure 7-1). Other anomalies include partial septation, complete septation (double gallbladder), and folding of the fundus (**Phrygian cap**) (Figure 7-5).

With a capacity of 50 ml, the gallbladder serves as a reservoir for bile. It also has the ability to concentrate the bile. To aid this process, its mucous membrane contains folds that unite with each other, giving the surface a honeycomb appear-

ance. **Heister's valve** in the neck of the gallbladder helps to prevent kinking of the duct (see Figure 7-1).

VASCULAR SUPPLY

The arterial supply of the gallbladder is from the cystic artery, which is a branch of the right hepatic artery. The cystic vein drains directly into the portal vein. Smaller arteries and veins run between the liver and the gallbladder.

PHYSIOLOGY AND LABORATORY DATA OF THE GALLBLADDER AND BILIARY SYSTEM

The primary functions of the extrahepatic biliary tract are (1) the transportation of bile from the liver to the intestine and (2) the regulation of its flow. Because the liver secretes approximately 1 to 2 liters of bile per day, this is an important function.

When the gallbladder and bile ducts are functioning normally, they respond in a fairly uniform manner in various phases of digestion. Concentration of bile in the gallbladder occurs during a state of fasting. It is forced into the gallbladder by an increased pressure within the common bile duct, which is produced by the action of the sphincter of Oddi at the distal end of the gallbladder.

During the fasting state, very little bile flows into the duodenum. Stimulation produced by the influence of food causes the gallbladder to contract, resulting in an outpouring of bile into the duodenum. When the stomach is emptied, duodenal peristalsis diminishes, the gallbladder relaxes, the tonus of the sphincter of Oddi increases slightly, and thus very little bile passes into the duodenum. Small amounts of bile secreted by the liver are retained in the **common duct** and forced into the gallbladder.

Text continued on p. 210

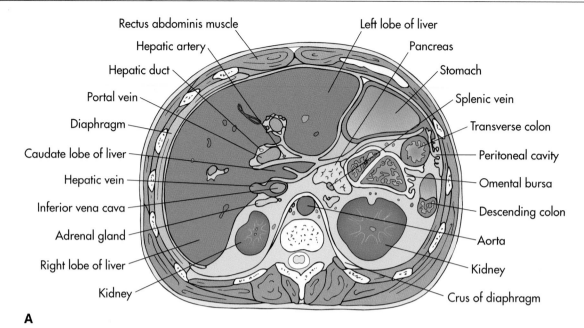

A

B

Figure 7-3   Transverse views of the right upper quadrant to include the biliary system, beginning at the level of the caudate lobe and proceeding in a caudal direction. **A,** Cross-section of the abdomen at the level of the twelfth thoracic vertebra. **B,** Cross-section of the abdomen at the first lumbar vertebra. Transverse views of the right upper quadrant to include the biliary system, beginning at the level of the caudate lobe and proceeding in a caudal direction.

C

D

Figure 7-3, cont'd   **C,** Cross-section of the abdomen at the level of the second lumbar vertebra. **D,** Cross-section of the abdomen at the level of the third lumbar vertebra.

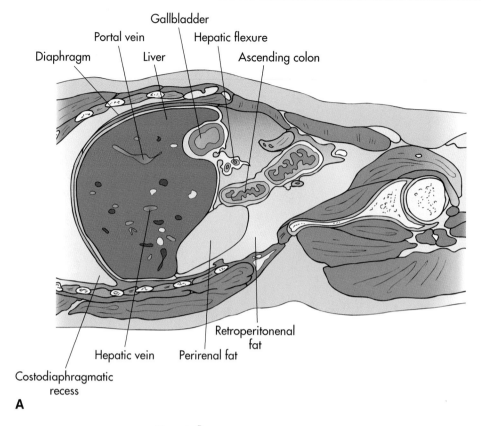

Gallbladder

Portal vein   Hepatic flexure

Diaphragm   Liver   Ascending colon

Retroperitonenal
fat

Hepatic vein   Perirenal fat

Costodiaphragmatic
recess

A

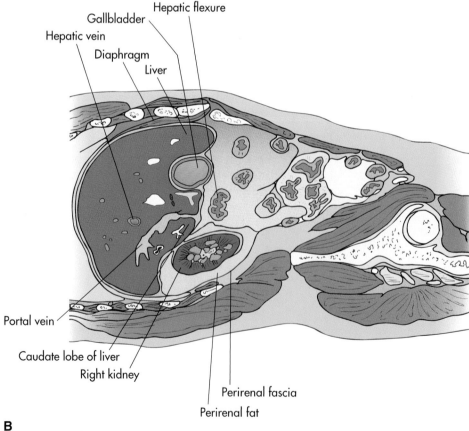

Hepatic flexure

Gallbladder

Hepatic vein

Diaphragm

Liver

Portal vein

Caudate lobe of liver

Right kidney

Perirenal fascia

Perirenal fat

B

Figure 7-4   Sagittal views of the right upper quadrant to include the biliary system beginning near the midclavicular line and moving toward the midline. **A,** Sagittal section of the abdomen 8 cm from the midline. **B,** Sagittal section of the abdomen 7 cm from the midline. Sagittal views of the right upper quadrant to include the biliary system beginning near the midclavicular line and moving toward the midline.

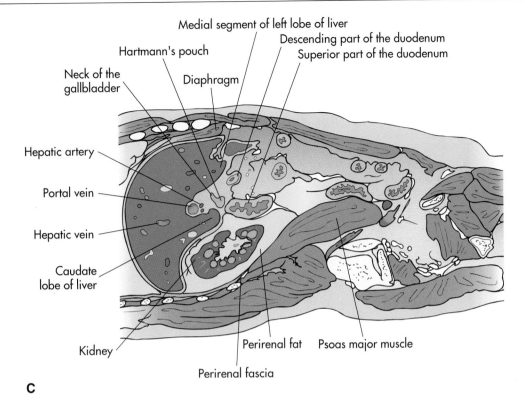

Medial segment of left lobe of liver
Hartmann's pouch
Descending part of the duodenum
Superior part of the duodenum
Neck of the gallbladder
Diaphragm
Hepatic artery
Portal vein
Hepatic vein
Caudate lobe of liver
Kidney
Perirenal fat
Psoas major muscle
Perirenal fascia

C

Head of the pancreas
Mesentery
Gastroduodenal artery
Transverse colon
Pyloric sphincter
Left branch of the portal vein
Cystic duct
Portal vein
Hepatic vein
Right lobe of liver
Right adrenal gland
Costodiaphragmatic recess
Right kidney
Perirenal fat
Superior duodenum
Descending duodenum

D

Figure 7-4, cont'd   **C,** Sagittal section of the abdomen 6 cm from the midline. **D,** Sagittal section of the abdomen 5 cm from the midline.

REMOVAL OF THE GALLBLADDER

When the gallbladder is removed, the sphincter of Oddi loses tonus, and pressure within the common bile duct drops to that of intraabdominal pressure. Bile is no longer retained in the bile ducts, but is free to flow into the duodenum during fasting and digestive phases. Dilation of the extrahepatic bile ducts (usually less than 1 cm) occurs after **cholecystectomy.**

Secretion is largely caused by a bile salt–dependent mechanism, and ductal flow is controlled by secretion. Bile salts form micelles, solubilize triglyceride fat, and assist in its absorption and that of calcium, cholesterol, and fat-soluble vitamins from the intestine.

Bile is the principal medium for excretion of **bilirubin** and cholesterol. The products of steroid hormones are also excreted in the bile, as are drugs and poisons (e.g., salts of heavy metals). The bile salts from the intestine stimulate the liver to make more bile. Bile salts activate intestinal and pancreatic enzymes.

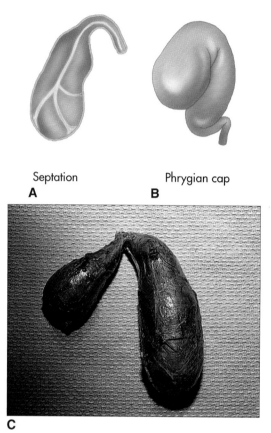

Septation   Phrygian cap
A   **B**

C

Figure 7-5 A, Septations may be found in the gallbladder. Changes in patient position will show the septation to remain in the same position in the gallbladder. **B,** A Phrygian cap is a variant in which part of the fundus of the gallbladder is bent back on itself. **C,** The double gallbladder is seen infrequently; the recognition of two distinct sacs will confirm the diagnosis.

SONOGRAPHIC EVALUATION OF THE BILIARY SYSTEM

GALLBLADDER

To ensure maximum dilation of the gallbladder, the patient should be given nothing to eat for at least 8 to 12 hours before the ultrasound examination. The patient is initially examined with ultrasound in full inspiration. Transverse (Figure 7-6), sagittal (Figure 7-7), and oblique (Figure 7-8) scans are made over the upper abdomen to identify the gallbladder, biliary system, liver, right kidney, and head of the pancreas. The patient should also be rolled into a steep decubitus or upright position (to ensure there are no stones within the gallbladder) in an attempt to separate small stones from the gallbladder wall or cystic duct.

The gallbladder may be identified as a sonolucent oblong structure located anterior to the right kidney, lateral to the head of the pancreas and duodenum. The gallbladder fossa shows a slight indentation on the posterior surface of the medial aspect of the right lobe of the liver (Figure 7-9). The sagittal scans show the right kidney posterior to the gallbladder. The fundus is generally oriented slightly more anterior and, on sagittal scans, often reaches the anterior abdominal wall. Box 7-1 lists the sonographic characteristics of the normal gallbladder.

A bright linear echo within the liver connecting the gallbladder and the right or main portal vein is common

A   **B**

Figure 7-6 A and **B,** Transverse images of the gallbladder as it lies anterior to the kidney within the right lobe of the liver.

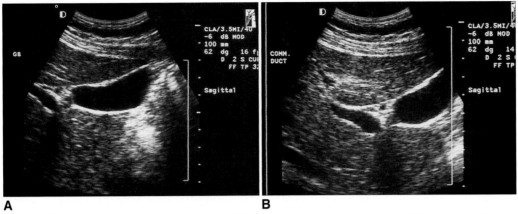

Figure 7-7 **A** and **B,** Sagittal images of the gallbladder from the neck to the fundus. The portal vein is seen off the neck of the gallbladder.

Figure 7-8 **A** and **B,** As the patient is rolled into a slight decubitus position and the transducer angled toward the midline of the abdomen, the gallbladder is seen anterior to the inferior vena cava and aorta in the sagittal plane. **C,** Transverse image of the gallbladder in the decubitus position.

(Figure 7-10). The neck of the gallbladder usually comes into contact with the main segment of the portal vein near the origin of the left portal vein. The gallbladder commonly resides in a fossa on the medial aspect of the liver. Because of fat or fibrous tissue within the main lobar fissure of the liver (which lies between the gallbladder and the right portal vein), this bright linear reflector is a reliable indicator of the location of the gallbladder. The gallbladder lies in the posterior and caudal

aspect of the fissure. The caudal aspect of the linear echo "points" directly to the gallbladder.

A small echogenic fold has been reported to occur along the posterior wall of the gallbladder at the junction of the body and infundibulum. It may be very small (3 to 5 mm), but may give rise to an acoustic shadow in the supine position. It is not duplicated in the oblique position. The causes for such a **junctional fold** are the incisurae between the body and

Figure 7-9 The gallbladder *(GB)* is identified as a sonolucent oblong structure located anterior to the right kidney *(RK)* and inferior vena cava *(IVC)*, lateral to the head of the pancreas (P) and duodenum, and indenting the inferior to medial aspect of the right lobe of the liver *(L)*.

Figure 7-10 The main lobar fissure *(MLF)* is seen as an echogenic linear echo within the liver *(L)* connecting the right portal vein *(PV)* to the neck of the gallbladder *(GB)*.

> **BOX 7-1   SONOGRAPHIC CHARACTERISTICS OF THE NORMAL GALLBLADDER**
>
> - Size: ≤4 cm transverse; ≤10 cm longitudinal
> - Wall thickness: <3 mm
> - Lumen: anechoic
> - Landmarks: right upper quadrant, between right and left lobes of liver, right kidney, main lobar fissure, and portal vein

---

infundibulum or Heister's valve, which is a spiral fold beginning in the neck of the gallbladder and lining the cystic duct (see Figure 7-1).

A prominent gallbladder may be normal in some individuals because of their fasting state (Figure 7-11). A large gallbladder has been detected in patients with diabetes, patients bedridden with protracted illness or pancreatitis, and patients taking anticholinergic drugs. A large gallbladder may even fail to contract after a fatty meal or intravenous **cholecystokinin;** other studies may be needed before making a diagnosis of obstruction.

If a gallbladder appears too large, a fatty meal may be administered and further sonographic evaluation made to detect whether the enlargement is abnormal or normal. If the gallbladder fails to contract during the examination, the pan-

creatic area should be investigated further. Courvoisier's sign indicates an extrahepatic mass compressing the common bile duct, which can produce an enlarged gallbladder (Figure 7-12). In addition, the liver should be carefully examined for the presence of dilated bile ducts.

In a well-contracted gallbladder, the wall changes from a single to a double concentric structure with the following three components: (1) a strongly reflective outer contour, (2) a poorly reflective inner contour, and (3) a sonolucent area between both reflecting structures.

BILE DUCTS

Sonographically, the common duct lies anterior and to the right of the portal vein in the region of the porta hepatis and gastrohepatic ligament. The hepatic artery lies anterior and to the left of the portal vein. On a transverse scan, the common duct, hepatic artery, and portal vein have been referred to as the "Mickey Mouse sign" (Figure 7-13). The portal vein serves as Mickey's face, with the right ear the common duct and the

A   **B**

Figure 7-11   **A,** Transverse and **B,** longitudinal scans of the distended gallbladder. The gallbladder size may be quite variable from patient to patient. A good rule of thumb is to compare the size of the gallbladder with the transverse view of the right kidney. The width should always be smaller, ≤4 cm.

Figure 7-12   A 33-year-old patient presented with jaundice and a palpable abdominal mass in the right upper quadrant. A pancreatic mass was found in the head of the gland, causing obstruction of the common bile duct with distention (hydrops) of the gallbladder known as Courvoisier's sign.

left ear the hepatic artery. To obtain such a cross-section, the transducer must be directed in a slightly oblique path from the left shoulder to the right hip.

On sagittal scans, the right branch of the hepatic artery usually passes posterior to the common duct (Figure 7-14). The common duct is seen just anterior to the portal vein before it dips posteriorly to enter the head of the pancreas. The patient may be rotated into a slight (45-degree) or steep (90-degree) right anterior oblique position, with the beam directed posteromedially to visualize the duct. This enables the examiner to avoid cumbersome bowel gas and to use the liver as an acoustic window.

When the right subcostal approach is used, the main portal vein may be seen as it bifurcates into the right and left branches. As the right branch continues into the right lobe of the liver, it can be followed laterally in a longitudinal plane. The portal vein appears as an almond-shaped sonolucent struc-

A

B

Figure 7-13   Transverse (**A**) and sagittal (**B**) views of the common bile duct. The transverse view shows the portal triad with the portal vein posterior, the common duct anterior and lateral, and the hepatic artery anterior and medial. The sagittal view shows the common duct anterior to the main portal vein.

Figure 7-14   On this sagittal image, the hepatic artery *(HA)* is shown anterior to the common duct *(CD)*. The portal vein *(PV)* is anterior to the inferior vena cava *(IVC)*. GB, Gallbladder.

Figure 7-15   The cystic duct is sometimes seen to arise from the neck of the gallbladder *(arrows)*. This coronal decubitus view shows the aorta *(AO)*, inferior vena cava *(IVC)*, gallbladder *(GB)*, portal vein *(PV)*, and liver *(L)*.

ture anterior to the inferior vena cava. The common hepatic duct is seen as a tubular structure anterior to the portal vein. The right branch of the hepatic artery can be seen between the duct and the portal vein as a small circular structure.

The small cystic duct is generally not identified. Because this landmark is necessary to distinguish the common hepatic duct from the common bile duct, the more general term **common duct** is used to refer to these structures (Figure 7-15).

PATHOLOGY OF THE GALLBLADDER AND BILIARY SYSTEM

See Table 7-1 for clinical findings, sonographic findings, and differential considerations for gallbladder and biliary diseases and conditions.

CLINICAL SYMPTOMS OF GALLBLADDER DISEASE

Pain. The most classic symptom of gallbladder disease is right upper quadrant abdominal pain, usually occurring after ingestion of greasy foods. Nausea and vomiting sometimes occur and may indicate the presence of a stone in the common bile duct. A gallbladder attack may cause pain in the right shoulder, with inflammation of the gallbladder often causing referred pain in the right shoulder blade.

Jaundice. Jaundice is characterized by the presence of bile in the tissues with resulting yellow-green color of the skin. It may develop when a tiny gallstone blocks the bile ducts between the gallbladder and the intestines, producing pressure on the liver and forcing bile into the blood.

SLUDGE

Sludge, or thickened bile, frequently occurs from bile stasis. This may be seen in patients with prolonged fasting or hyperalimentation therapy and with obstruction of the gallbladder. Some gallbladders may be so packed with this thickened bile that the gallbladder is isoechoic and difficult to separate from the liver parenchyma. Occasionally sludge is also found in the common duct. Sludge is gravity dependent. With alterations in a patient's position, the sonographer may be able to separate sludge from occasional artifactual echoes found in the gallbladder. Sludge should be considered an abnormal finding because either a functional or a pathologic abnormality exists when calcium bilirubin or cholesterol precipitates in bile.

Sonographic Findings. Occasionally a patient presents sonographically with a prominent gallbladder containing low-level internal echoes, which may be attributed to thick or inspissated bile. The source of echoes in biliary sludge is thought to be particulate matter (predominantly pigment granules with lesser amounts of cholesterol crystals). The viscosity does not appear to be important in the generation of internal echoes in fluids. The particles can be small and still produce perceptible echoes (Figure 7-16). Sludge may also be seen in combination with cholelithiasis, cholecystitis, and other biliary diseases.

WALL THICKNESS

The normal wall thickness of the gallbladder is less than 3 mm. Biliary causes of gallbladder wall thickening include cholecystitis, adenomyomatosis, cancer, acquired immunodeficiency syndrome, cholangiopathy, and sclerosing cholangitis (Box 7-2). Nonbiliary causes include diffuse liver disease (cirrhosis and hepatitis), pancreatitis, portal hypertension, and heart failure. A thickened wall is a nonspecific sign and is not necessarily related to gallbladder disease. It may also be found in the following conditions, along with those previously discussed: hepatitis, gallbladder tumor, or severe hypoalbuminemic states.

Sonographic Findings. The gallbladder wall thickness would be measured when the transducer is perpendicular to the anterior gallbladder wall. This is usually done in the transverse plane, but in some cases the longitudinal plane allows a better measurement. The gain should be reduced to clearly demarcate the anterior wall. The anterior wall is measured

TABLE 7-1   THE GALLBLADDER AND THE BILIARY SYSTEM

Clinical Findings	Sonographic Findings	Differential Considerations	Clinical Findings	Sonographic Findings	Differential Considerations
Sludge			**Choledochal Cysts**		

• May be asymptomatic	• Low-level internal echoes layering in dependent part of GB
	• Prominent gallbladder size
	• Changes with patient position
		• Pseudosludge
		• Empyema of GB
		• Hemobilia
		• Neoplasm
			• Jaundice
			• Possibly increased bilirubin
				True cysts in RUQ with or without communication with biliary system.
				• Classified by anatomy:
				  1. Localized dilated cystic CBD
				  2. Diverticulum of CBD
				  3. Invagination of CBD into duodenum
				  4. Dilated CBD and CHD
					• Hepatic cyst
					• Hepatic artery aneurysm
					• Pancreatic pseudocyst

Acute Cholecystitis					
• ↑ Serum amylase • Abnormal LFTs	• Dilation and rounding of GB • + Murphy's sign • Thick GB wall with irregular wall (edema) • Stones • Pericholecystic fluid	• Chronic cholecystitis • Nonfasting GB • Acute pancreatitis • GB carcinoma	**Adenoma of the Gallbladder**		
				• Occur as flat elevations located in the body of the GB, almost always near the fundus • Does not change with position • No shadow produced	• Adenomyomatosis
Chronic Cholecystitis					
• ↑ Serum amylase • Abnormal LFTs • RUQ pain – transient	• Contraction of GB • Stones • WES sign	• Cholelithiasis • Nonfasting GB • Acute pancreatitis • GB carcinoma	**Adenomyomatosis of the Gallbladder**		
				• Papillomas may occur singly or in groups and may be scattered over a large part of the mucosal surface of the GB • Does not move with position changes. • "Comet tail" artifact	• Adenoma
Acalculous Cholecystitis					
• ↑ Serum amylase • Abnormal LFTs	• Dilation of GB • + Murphy's sign • Thick GB wall with irregular wall (edema) • Sludge • Pericholecystic fluid • Subserosal edema	• Chronic cholecystitis • Nonfasting GB • Acute pancreatitis • GB carcinoma	**Porcelain Gallbladder**		
			• Female predominance • Found in patients over 60	• Gallbladder wall is thickly calcified with shadowing	• Gallstones with emphysematous cholecystitis
Emphysematous Cholecystitis					
• Gas-forming bacteria in GB • Abnormal LFTs	• Bright echo in area of GB with ring down or comet tail artifact • May appear as WES	• Chronic cholecystitis • GB carcinoma	**Choledocholithiasis**		
Gangrenous Cholecystitis			• Increased direct bilirubin • Abnormal liver enzymes • Leukocytosis • Increased alkaline phosphatase	• Echogenic structure in extrahepatic duct • Dilated biliary tree	• Surgical clips • Artifact from right hepatic artery • Cystic duct remnant
• Abnormal LFTs	• Medium to coarse echogenic densities that fill GB lumen in absence of duct obstruction • No shadow • Not gravity dependent • Does not layer	• GB carcinoma			
Cholelithiasis					
• Check bilirubin levels • Acute ↑ amylase • Abnormal LFTs (increased alkaline phosphatase); AST and ALT may be normal	• Dilated GB with thick wall • Hyperechoic intraluminal echoes with posterior acoustic shadowing • WES sign • Gravity dependent calcifications in GB	• Duodenal gas • Porcelain GB • Sludge			

Figure 7-16   A through **F,** Multiple patterns of sludge within the gallbladder.

<table>
<tr><td colspan="2">BOX 7-2   COMMON CAUSES OF THICKENING
OF THE GALLBLADDER WALL (≥3 MM)</td></tr>
<tr><td>Intrinsic</td><td>Extrinsic</td></tr>
<tr><td>Cholecystitis</td><td>Hepatitis/cirrhosis</td></tr>
<tr><td>Gallbladder perforation</td><td>Hypoalbuminemia</td></tr>
<tr><td>Sepsis</td><td>Renal failure</td></tr>
<tr><td>Hyperplastic cholecystosis</td><td>Right heart failure</td></tr>
<tr><td>Gallbladder carcinoma</td><td>Ascites</td></tr>
<tr><td>AIDS cholangiography</td><td>Multiple myeloma</td></tr>
<tr><td>Sclerosing cholangitis</td><td>Portal node lymphatic
obstruction</td></tr>
</table>

from outer to outer margins. Sonographically the gallbladder wall may be underestimated when the wall has extensive fibrosis or is surrounded by fat (Figure 7-17).

CHOLECYSTITIS

Cholecystitis is an inflammation of the gallbladder that may have one of several forms: acute or chronic, acalculous, emphysematous, or gangrenous.

Acute Cholecystitis. The most common cause of acute cholecystitis is cholelithiasis that creates a cystic duct obstruction (Figure 7-18). In the majority of patients obstructed with an impacted stone, the stone will spontaneously disimpact.

Figure 7-17 **A,** The gallbladder wall should be measured on the transverse image at the anterior wall that is perpendicular to the transducer (see markings). **B,** The sagittal image of the gallbladder is often at an angle to the transducer and may be used to measure the wall thickness when the sonographer can achieve a perpendicular angle.

Figure 7-18 Gross pathology of acute cholecystitis. The gallbladder contained stones. The gallbladder wall was thick and swollen. (From Damjanov I, Linder J: *Pathology: a color atlas,* St. Louis, 2000, Mosby.)

This condition is found more frequently in females. Clinically the patient with acute cholecystitis presents with acute right upper quadrant pain (positive **Murphy's sign**—inspiratory arrest upon palpation of gallbladder area; may be false positive in small percentage of patients), fever, and leukocytosis. Complications of acute cholecystitis may be serious to include empyema, emphysematous or gangrenous cholecystitis, and perforation.

Sonographic Findings. The sonographic appearance of acute cholecystitis has been identified as a gallbladder with an irregular outline of a thickened wall (Figure 7-19). A sonolucent area probably caused by edema has been found within the thickened wall. Thick gallbladder walls often indicate disease.

Some walls will be thicker because of a pericholecystic abscess. Occasionally a thickened gallbladder wall is seen in

normal individuals. It seems to be related to the degree of contraction of a normal gallbladder (Figure 7-20). If the thickened wall is localized and irregular, an abscess, cholecystosis, or carcinoma of the gallbladder should be considered. Other sonographic findings include an enlarged gallbladder (hydrops), sludge, positive Murphy's sign, and the presence or absence of pericholecystic fluid (Figure 7-21).

Chronic Cholecystitis. Chronic cholecystitis is the most common form of gallbladder inflammation. This is the result of numerous attacks of acute cholecystitis with subsequent fibrosis of the gallbladder wall (Figure 7-22). Clinically the patients may have some transient right upper quadrant pain, but not the tenderness as experienced with acute cholecystitis.

Sonographic Findings. **Cholelithiasis,** or gallstones in the gallbladder, is frequently found in a contracted gallbladder with very coarse gallbladder wall thickening. The WES sign (Wall, Echo, Shadow) is described as a contracted bright gallbladder with posterior shadowing caused by a packed bag of stones (Figure 7-23).

Acalculous Cholecystitis. This uncommon condition is an acute inflammation of the gallbladder in the absence of cholelithiasis. It is most likely caused by decreased blood flow through the cystic artery. Conditions that produce depressed motility (e.g., trauma, burns, postoperative patients, etc.) may prelude the development of acalculous cholecystitis. Extrinsic compression of the cystic duct by a mass or lymphadenopathy may also cause this condition. Clinically the patient has a positive Murphy's sign.

Sonographic Findings. The gallbladder wall is extremely thickened (greater than 4 to 5 mm), and echogenic sludge is seen within a dilated gallbladder. Look for the presence of pericholecystic fluid within ascites and/or subserosal edema.

Figure 7-19   **A** through **F,** Multiple patterns of acute cholecystitis.

Emphysematous Cholecystitis. This is a fairly rare complication of acute cholecystitis associated with the presence of gas-forming bacteria in the gallbladder wall and lumen with extension into the biliary ducts. As many as 50% of patients with emphysematous cholecystitis have diabetes, and less than 50% have gallstones. Gangrene with associated perforation is a complication. This condition is a surgical emergency.

Sonographic Findings. If the gas is intraluminal, the sonographer should look for a prominent bright echo along the anterior wall with ring down or comet-tail artifact directly posterior to the echogenic structure. If a large amount of gas is present, the appearance may simulate a packed bag or WES

sign with a curvilinear echogenic area with complete posterior fuzzy shadowing.

Gangrenous Cholecystitis. Another serious painful complication of acute cholecystitis that may lead to perforation is gangrenous cholecystitis. The gallbladder wall may be thickened and edematous, with focal areas of exudate, hemorrhage, and necrosis (Figure 7-24). In addition, there may be ulcerations and perforations resulting in pericholecystic abscesses or peritonitis. Gallstones or fine gravel occur in 80% to 95% of patients.

Sonographic Findings. The common echo features of gangrene are the presence of diffuse medium to coarse echogenic

Figure 7-20   Other fluid collections in the right upper quadrant should be observed by the sonographer for signs of change, or peristalsis, as illustrated in these images. The large collection of fluid was in the antrum and duodenum; with time, the fluid collection changed shape and distinct peristaltic movement could be seen with real-time imaging. *GB,* Gallbladder.

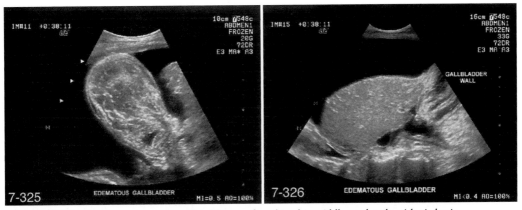

Figure 7-21   Swollen, edematous gallbladder was found in this middle-aged male with cirrhosis and ascites.

densities filling the gallbladder lumen in the absence of bile duct obstruction. This echogenic material has the following three characteristics: (1) it does not cause shadowing, (2) it is not gravity dependent, and (3) it does not show a layering effect. The lack of layering is attributed to increased viscosity of the bile. Pericholecystic fluid may be present.

CHOLELITHIASIS

Cholelithiasis is the most common disease of the gallbladder. In cholelithiasis there may be a single large gallstone or hundreds of tiny ones (Figure 7-25). The tiny stones are the most dangerous because they can enter the bile ducts and obstruct the outflow of bile. After a fatty meal, the gallbladder contracts to release bile; if the outflow tract is blocked by gallstones, pain results. As the bile is being stored in the gallbladder, small crystals of bile salts precipitate and may form gallstones varying from pinhead size to the size of the organ itself. Gallstones may also consist of cholesterol.

Clinically the patient falls under the five "Fs:" fat, female, forty, fertile, and fair. In addition, many other factors lead to the development of gallstones that include pregnancy, diabetes, oral contraceptive use, hemolytic diseases, diet-induced weight loss, and total parenteral nutrition. Patients may be asymptomatic until a stone lodges in the cystic or common duct. Right upper quadrant pain with radiation to the shoulder after a high-fat meal is a typical presentation for cholelithiasis. Epigastric pain, nausea, and vomiting are present when the symptoms become acute.

Figure 7-22   Gross pathology of chronic active cholecystitis. (From Damjanov I, Linder J: *Pathology: a color atlas*, St. Louis, 2000, Mosby.)

Sonographic Findings. The evaluation of gallstones with real-time has proven to be an extremely useful procedure in patients who show symptoms of cholelithiasis. The gallbladder is evaluated for increased size, wall thickness, presence of internal reflections within the lumen, and posterior acoustic shadowing. Frequently, patients with gallstones have a dilated gallbladder. Stones that are less than 1 to 2 mm may be difficult to separate from one another by ultrasound evaluation and thus are reported as gallstones without comment on the specific number that may have been seen on the scan (Figures 7-26 to 7-31). If a broad-band transducer is not used, a higher frequency transducer should be used to better delineate the stones and their shadowing characteristics.

When the gallbladder is completely packed full of stones, the sonographer will only be able to image the anterior border of the gallbladder, with the stones casting a distinct acoustic shadow known as the **wall echo shadow (WES) sign.**

The patient's position should be shifted during the procedure to demonstrate the presence of movement of the stones. Patients should be scanned in the left decubitus, right lateral, or upright position. The stones should shift to the most dependent area of the gallbladder. In some cases the bile has a thick consistency and the stones remain near the top of the gallbladder. Thus the density of the stones and the shadow posterior will be the sonographic evidence for stones.

With regard to acoustic shadowing, scattered reflections do not affect shadowing as much as specular reflections. The factors that produce a shadow are attributed to acoustic impedance of the gallstones; refraction through them or diffraction around them; their size, central or peripheral location, and position in relation to the focus of the beam; and the intensity of the beam.

All stones cast acoustic shadows regardless of the specific properties of the stones. The size of the stone is important. Stones greater than 3 mm always cast a shadow, and those smaller than 3 mm sometimes do not. It has been shown that

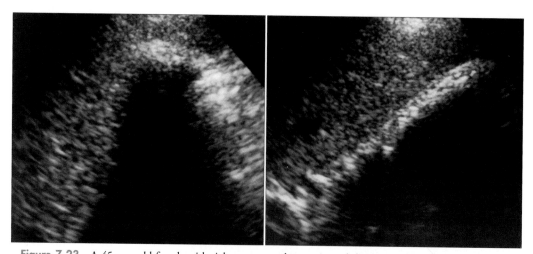

Figure 7-23   A 45-year-old female with right upper quadrant pain and distention. The "wall echo shadow" (WES) sign was visualized and indicated that the gallbladder was a packed bag. Note the sharp posterior shadow. This appearance is different from that of the porcelain gallbladder because the anterior wall is not as bright or echogenic.

Figure 7-24 A 52-year-old female presented with fever and right upper quadrant pain for the previous 2 weeks. At surgery, the patient was found to have gangrenous cholecystitis. Multiple tiny gas pockets are seen within the gallbladder, causing posterior shadowing.

any stone scanned two or more times with the same transducer and machine settings may or may not generate a shadow even when the scans are made within seconds of each other. The shadow is highly dependent on the relationship between the stone and the acoustic beam. If the central beam is at or near the stone, a shadow can be seen. Thus some critical ratio between the stone diameter and the beam width must be achieved before shadowing is seen.

Some stones are seen to float ("floating gallstones") when contrast material from an oral cholecystogram is present because the contrast material has a higher specific gravity than the bile. The gallstones seek a level at which their specific gravity equals that of the mixture of bile and contrast material (Figure 7-32).

CHOLEDOCHAL CYSTS

Choledochal cysts may be the result of pancreatic juices refluxing into the bile duct because of an anomalous junction of the pancreatic duct into the distal common bile duct, causing duct wall abnormality, weakness, and outpouching of

Figure 7-25 Gross pathology of multiple gallstones within the gallbladder. (From Damjanov I, Linder J: *Pathology: a color atlas,* St. Louis, 2000, Mosby.)

Figure 7-26 Single small stone along the posterior floor of the gallbladder casts a sharp posterior shadow.

Figure 7-27 A 45-year-old female with right upper quadrant pain and increased bilirubin. Large echogenic calculus *(St)* is seen in the dependent neck of the gallbladder *(GB)*. Acoustic shadowing *(Sh)* is present beyond the stone.

Figure 7-28 **A,** Multiple small stones are layered along the posterior wall of the gallbladder. These bright echogenic foci give acoustic shadowing beyond. **B,** A higher frequency transducer would outline the stones and the shadowing even more clearly.

Figure 7-29 Multiple images of various sizes of gallstones causing shadowing posterior to the gallbladder.

Figure 7-30 Gallstones may take several different shapes and sizes. This patient presented with a large gallstone measuring more than 3 cm.

Figure 7-31 A 55-year-old male with several episodes of right upper quadrant pain radiating to his right shoulder. Multiple echogenic foci were seen within the gallbladder. The common bile duct *(crossbars)* was normal in size. The gallbladder wall was in the upper range of normal in size.

Figure 7-32 Longitudinal and transverse scans of the gallbladder *(GB)*, with a layer of stones "floating" *(arrow)* along the thick bile layer of sludge *(Sl)*.

Figure 7-33   Transverse and longitudinal scan of a young patient with a choledochal cyst *(Ccy)* in the right upper quadrant. *IVC,* Inferior vena cava; *L,* liver; *P,* pancreas.

the ductal walls. These cysts are rare; the incidence is more common in females than males (4:1), with an increased incidence in infants (the condition may occur in adults). Choledochal cysts may be associated with gallstones, pancreatitis, or cirrhosis. The patient presents with an abdominal mass, pain, fever, or jaundice. The diagnosis may be confirmed with a nuclear medicine hepatobiliary scan. The majority of cases are thought to be congenital and result from bile reflux. The mass presents as a cystic dilation of the biliary system.

Sonographic Findings. Choledochal cysts appear as true cysts in the right upper quadrant with or without an apparent communication with the biliary system (Figure 7-33). The cysts are classified by anatomy as follows:

- Localized cystic dilation of the common bile duct
- Diverticulum from the common bile duct
- Invagination of the common bile duct into the duodenum
- Dilation of the entire common bile duct and the common hepatic duct

HYPERPLASTIC CHOLECYSTITIS

Hyperplastic cholecystitis is represented by a variety of degenerative and proliferative changes of the gallbladder characterized by hyperconcentration, hyperexcitability, and hyperexcretion. The incidence is found in 30% to 50% of all cholecystectomy specimens and is found more commonly in females. Cholesterolosis and adenomyomatosis of the gallbladder are two types of this condition.

Cholesterolosis. Cholesterolosis is a condition in which cholesterol is deposited within the lamina propria of the gallbladder. The disease process is associated with cholesterol stones in 50% to 70% of patients (although these stones are not demonstrable on radiography). It is often referred to as a "strawberry gallbladder" because the mucosa resembles the surface of a strawberry.

Most patients with cholesterolosis do not show thickening of the gallbladder wall on imaging studies; a small percentage of patients with this condition will show cholesterol polyps, which may be detected with ultrasound. **Polyps** are small, well-

defined soft tissue projections from the gallbladder wall. The cholesterol polyp is a small structure covered with a single layer of epithelium and is attached to the gallbladder with a delicate stalk. These polyps usually are found in the middle third of the gallbladder and are less than 10 mm in diameter.

Cholesterol polyp is the most common pseudotumor of the gallbladder. Other masses that occur are mucosal hyperplasia, inflammatory polyps, mucous cysts, and granulomata (resulting from parasitic infections).

Sonographic Findings. Cholesterol polyps are small, smooth wall projections seen to arise from the gallbladder wall (Figure 7-34). The polyps usually are multiple, do not shadow, and remain fixed to the wall with changes in patient position. The comet-tail artifact may be present, emanating from the cholesterol polyps, and this may be indistinguishable from adenomyomatosis.

Adenoma. Adenomas are benign neoplasms of the gallbladder with a premalignant potential much lower than colonic adenomas. This condition usually occurs as a solitary lesion. The smaller lesions are pedunculated, while the larger lesions may contain foci of malignant transformation. The adenomas tend to be homogeneously hyperechoic but become more heterogeneous as they grow in size. If the gallbladder wall is thickened adjacent to the adenoma then malignancy should be suspected.

Adenomyomatosis. A hyperplastic change in the gallbladder wall is called *adenomyomatosis.* Papillomas may occur singly or in groups and may be scattered over a large part of the mucosal surface of the gallbladder. These papillomas are not precursors to cancer.

On the oral cholecystogram, the tumor is better seen after partial contraction of the gallbladder. Various patient positions and compression show the lesion to be immobile within the gallbladder (Figure 7-35).

Sonographic Findings. Benign tumors appear as small elevations in the gallbladder lumen. These elevations maintain their initial location during positional changes and are the

Figure 7-34 **A** and **B,** Transverse image of a gallbladder polyp attached to the anterior wall. **C,** Sagittal image of another patient with a polyp on the posterior wall.

Figure 7-35 Adenomyomatosis is a hyperplastic change in the gallbladder wall. Multiple papillomas are seen along the anterior wall of the gallbladder, causing a "ring down" of echoes to occur.

cause for a "comet tail." No acoustic shadow is seen posterior to this papillomatous elevation.

Porcelain Gallbladder

A **porcelain gallbladder** is a rare occurrence that is defined as calcium incrustation of the gallbladder wall. It is associated with gallstones in the majority of patients. The patient is generally asymptomatic and the diagnosis is generally made as an incidental finding or when a mass is found on physical examination. A finding of porcelain gallbladder is significant in that 25% of those patients will develop cancer on the gallbladder wall.

Sonographic Findings. On ultrasound examination, a bright echogenic echo is seen in the region of the gallbladder with shadowing posterior. The differential will include a packed bag or WES sign. A small percentage of these patients with a porcelain gallbladder may go on to develop carcinoma of the gallbladder.

Gallbladder Carcinoma

Primary carcinoma of the gallbladder is rare and is nearly always a rapidly progressive disease, with a mortality rate approaching 100%. It is associated with cholelithiasis in about 80% to 90% of cases (although there is no direct proof that gallstones are the carcinogenic agent). Patients with a porcelain gallbladder have an increased incidence of gallbladder cancer. It is twice as common as cancer of the bile ducts and occurs most frequently in women 60 years of age and older.

The tumor arises in the body of the gallbladder or rarely in the cystic duct (Figures 7-36). The tumor infiltrates the gallbladder locally or diffusely and causes thickening and rigidity of the wall. The adjacent liver is often invaded by direct continuity extending through tissue spaces, the ducts of Luschka, the lymph channels, or some combination of these.

Obstruction of the cystic duct results from direct extension of the tumor or extrinsic compression by involved lymph nodes (this obstruction occurs early).

The gallbladder tumor is usually columnar cell adenocarcinoma, sometimes mucinous in type. Squamous cell carcinoma occurs but is unusual. Metastatic carcinoma in the gallbladder may occur secondary to melanoma. It usually is accompanied by liver metastases. Most patients have no symptoms that relate to the gallbladder unless there is complicating acute cholecystitis.

Sonographic Findings. The global shape of malignant gallbladder masses is similar to that of the gallbladder. The mass has a heterogeneous solid or semisolid echo texture. The gallbladder wall is markedly abnormal and thickened (Figures 7-37 and 7-38). The adjacent liver tissue, in the hilar area, is often heterogeneous because of direct tumoral spread. There may be dilated biliary ducts within the liver parenchyma, causing the "shotgun" sign (a "double barrel" appearance of portal veins and dilated ducts) (Figure 7-39).

Carcinoma of the gallbladder is almost never detected at a resectable stage. Obstruction of the cystic duct by the tumor or lymph nodes occurs early in the course of the disease and causes nonvisualization of the gallbladder on oral cholecystogram.

Dilated Biliary Ducts

The small size of the intrahepatic bile ducts implies that sonography cannot image the ducts routinely until their size dilates to greater than 4 mm. Evaluation of the portal structures will allow the sonographer to search for the dilated ducts as they parallel the course of the portal veins. The common hepatic duct has an internal diameter of less than 4 mm. A duct diameter of 5 mm is borderline and 6 mm requires further investigation. A patient may have a normal-size hepatic duct and still have distal obstruction. The distal duct is often obscured by gas in the duodenal loop. The common bile duct has an internal diameter slightly greater than that of the hepatic duct. Generally a duct more than 6 mm in diameter is considered borderline and more than 10 mm is dilated (Figure 7-40).

Biliary Obstruction

The most common cause of biliary ductal system obstruction is the presence of a tumor or thrombus within the ductal

Figure 7-36 Carcinoma of the gallbladder shows the gallbladder partially filled and infiltrated with neoplastic tissue. (From Damjanov I, Linder J: *Pathology: a color atlas,* St. Louis, 2000, Mosby.)

Figure 7-37 Sagittal image of a patient with adenocarcinoma of the gallbladder shows invasion of the gallbladder wall with the tumor.

Figure 7-38   The most frequent sonographic finding in gallbladder *(GB)* carcinoma is a large, irregular, fungating mass that contains low-intensity echoes within the gallbladder, causing obscurity of the gallbladder wall.

Figure 7-39   Carcinoma of the gallbladder may extend into the cystic duct either by direct extension of the tumor or extrinsic compression by the involved lymph nodes. **A,** A transverse scan of the liver shows dilated ducts with an inhomogeneous liver parenchyma. **B,** A transverse scan of the inhomogeneous liver parenchyma. **C,** A transverse scan of the dilated ducts within the liver.

system. The process may be found in the extrahepatic or intrahepatic ductal pathway. Obstruction of the biliary ductal system is diagnosed by ultrasound when the sonographer finds the presence of ductal dilation. This finding has been termed "too many tubes" or "shotgun" sign when intrahepatic ducts are dilated.

Bile ducts expand centrifugally from the point of obstruction. Therefore, extrahepatic dilation occurs before intrahepatic dilation. In patients with obstructive jaundice, isolated dilation of the extrahepatic duct may be present. Fibrosed or

infiltrative disease of the liver may prevent intrahepatic dilation because of lack of compliance of the hepatic parenchyma.

Extrahepatic Biliary Obstruction. The job of the sonographer is to localize the level and cause of the obstruction. There are three primary areas for obstruction to occur: (1) intrapancreatic, (2) suprapancreatic, and (3) porta hepatic (Figure 7-41).

Intrapancreatic obstruction. There are three important conditions that cause the majority of biliary obstruction at the level of the distal duct and cause the extrahepatic duct to be entirely dilated: (1) pancreatic carcinoma, (2) choledocholithiasis, and (3) chronic pancreatitis with stricture formation.

Suprapancreatic obstruction. This obstruction originates between the pancreas and the porta hepatis. The head of the pancreas, the intrapancreatic duct, and pancreatic duct are normal with ultrasound. The most common cause for this obstruction is malignancy or adenopathy at this level.

Porta hepatic obstruction. This area of obstruction is usually due to a neoplasm. In patients with obstruction at the level of the porta hepatis, ultrasound will show intrahepatic ductal dilation and a normal common duct. Hydrops of the gallbladder may be present.

Other causes of obstruction. Cholangiocarcinoma is a rare malignancy that originates within the larger bile ducts (usually the common duct or common hepatic duct) (Figure 7-42). A **Klatskin's tumor** is a specific type of cholangiocarcinoma that can occur at the bifurcation of the common

Figure 7-40   Sagittal scan of a prominent common bile duct *(Cd)* as it runs anterior to the portal vein *(PV)* and posterior to the head of the pancreas. *L,* Liver.

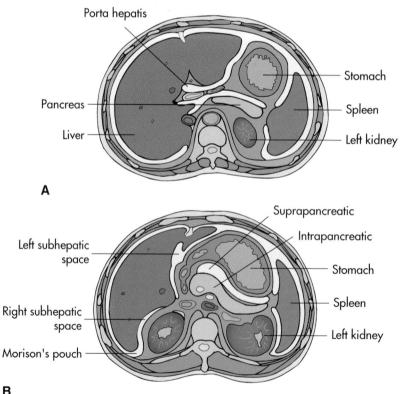

Figure 7-41   Levels of obstruction. **A,** Porta hepatic. **B,** Intrapancreatic and suprapancreatic.

hepatic duct, with involvement of both the central left and right duct. The most suggestive sonographic feature to indicate cholangiocarcinoma is isolated intrahepatic duct dilation. Even though the obstructing mass may not be imaged, a nonunion of the right and left ducts is characteristic for a Klatskin's tumor.

Mirizzi syndrome is an uncommon cause for extrahepatic biliary obstruction due to an impacted stone in the cystic duct, which creates extrinsic mechanical compression of the common hepatic duct. This stone may penetrate into the common hepatic duct or the gut, which results in a cholecystobiliary or cholecystenteric fistula. In this case, the cystic duct inserts unusually low into the common hepatic duct, and thus the two ducts have parallel alignment, which allows for the development of this syndrome. Using ultrasound, an intrahepatic ductal dilation is seen with a normal-size common duct and a large stone in the neck of the gallbladder or cystic duct.

Tumors arising from the common bile duct and ampullar carcinoma have the same ultrasonic features as pancreatic tumors. A specific pattern exists when the ampulloma bulges inside a dilated common bile duct. Cancer of the biliary convergence or of the hepatic duct usually infiltrates the ductal wall without bulging outside. It may be difficult to image these tumors; the diagnosis is indirect and based on biliary dilation above the tumor.

Sonographic Findings. Minimal dilation may be seen in nonjaundiced patients with gallstones or pancreatitis or in jaundiced patients with a common duct stone or tumor (Figures 7-43 and 7-44). However, a diameter of more than 11 mm suggests obstruction by stone or tumor of the duct or pancreas or some other source (Figure 7-45). One study reported measurement of the common duct at 7.7 mm in nonjaundiced patients who had undergone cholecystectomy.

Dilated ducts may also be found in the absence of jaundice. The patient may have biliary obstruction involving one hepatic duct, an early obstruction secondary to carcinoma, or gallstones causing intermittent obstruction resulting from a ball-valve effect (Figures 7-46 and 7-47).

The following five characteristics traditionally distinguish bile ducts from other intrahepatic structures (parasagittal scans provided the best visualization of the ducts):

- Alteration in the anatomic pattern adjacent to the main (right) portal vein segment and the bifurcation. This is more pronounced in individuals who display greater degrees of dilation of the intrahepatic bile ducts.

Figure 7-42   Gross pathology of cholangiocellular carcinoma. (From Damjanov I, Linder J: *Pathology: a color atlas,* St. Louis, 2000, Mosby.)

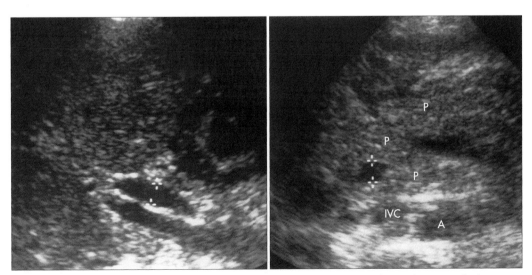

Figure 7-43   Inflammation of the pancreas may cause the common duct to dilate. This patient had acute pancreatitis *(P)* and dilation of the common duct *(crossbars)*. A, Aorta; *IVC,* inferior vena cava.

Figure 7-44   Stones within the common duct are seen if the duct is dilated. The small echogenic focus *(arrows)* is well seen within the duct in this transverse view. *IVC,* Inferior vena cava; *P,* pancreas.

Figure 7-45   Carcinoma of the head of the pancreas with obstruction of the common bile duct *(CBD).*

Figure 7-46   Dilated intrahepatic ducts secondary to a mass in the area of the porta hepatis.

Figure 7-47   A 60-year-old female with a history of cholecystectomy several years ago. The patient was known to have had previous hepatic calculi and now has right upper quadrant pain. Moderate diffuse dilation of the right and left intrahepatic ducts is present. Echogenic ovoid structures seen in the distal right hepatic and left hepatic ducts represent calculi or sludge balls. The intrahepatic duct was minimally dilated.

- Irregular walls of dilated bile ducts. As the intrahepatic biliary system dilates, the course and caliber of ducts become increasingly tortuous and irregular.
- Stellate confluence of dilated ducts. This is noted at the points where the ducts converge. Dilated ducts look like spokes of a wheel.
- Acoustic enhancement by dilated bile ducts. Both portal veins and ducts are surrounded by high-amplitude reflections.
- Peripheral duct dilation. It is normally unusual to visualize hepatic ducts in the liver periphery, whereas dilated bile ducts may be observed.

INTRAHEPATIC BILIARY NEOPLASMS

Changes in the intrahepatic biliary ducts occur secondary to extrahepatic bile duct obstruction in most cases. Occasionally intrahepatic lesions are responsible for the changes in the duct.

Intrahepatic biliary tumors are rare and are primarily limited to cystadenoma and cystadenocarcinoma. The tumors are more frequently found in middle-aged women who clinically present with abdominal pain or mass and/or jaundice (if the mass is near the porta hepatis). The sonographic appearance is a cystic mass with multiple septa and papillary excrescences. The mass may show variations in this pattern and present as unilocular, calcified, or multiple. The lesion may be associated with dilation of the intrahepatic ducts. The differential includes a hemorrhagic cyst or infection, echinococcal cyst, abscess, or cystic metastasis.

CHOLANGITIS

Cholangitis is an inflammation of the bile ducts (Figure 7-48). Clinically the patient presents with malaise and fever, followed by sweating and shivering. In severe cases the patient is lethargic, prostrate, and in shock. Cholangitis may be identified as *Oriental sclerosing cholangitis* (seen more frequently in the United States with immigration). Other forms of cholangitis include *AIDS cholangitis* and *acute obstructive suppurative cholangitis*. The cause of cholangitis is dependent on the type of disease, but may include ductal strictures, parasitic infestation, bacterial infection, stones, or neoplasm.

Cholangitis causes increasing pressure in the biliary tree with pus accumulation. Decompression of the common bile duct is necessary. More than one-half the patients with sclerosing cholangitis have ulcerative colitis. Liver function tests show increased levels of alkaline phosphatase and bilirubin. Both sclerosing and AIDS cholangitis can have intrahepatic biliary changes that are nearly identical on ultrasound.

Sonographic Findings. The common bile duct wall may show a smooth or irregular wall thickening (Figures 7-49). The ductal wall may be so thickened that it is difficult to recognize on sonography without careful evaluation. Cholangitis usually involves the bile duct in a more generalized manner.

CHOLEDOCHOLITHIASIS

Choledocholithiasis is stones in the bile duct. The majority of stones in the common bile duct have migrated from the gallbladder. Common duct stones are usually associated with calculous cholecystitis (Figure 7-50).

Sonographic Findings. Stones tend to become impacted in the ampulla of Vater and may project into the duodenum. This

is the reason it is important for the surgeons to check the common bile duct when removing the gallbladder.

Other Causes of Shadowing. The sonographer should be aware that structures or conditions other than stones may lead to attenuation of the ultrasound beam or shadowing. Calcifications of the small vascular structures within the right upper quadrant may cause shadowing to occur in the area of the gallbladder and be misinterpreted as stones. Air or gas within the duodenum may also give rise to a dirty shadow in the right upper quadrant. Intrabiliary gas is sometimes difficult to separate from stones, although the gas usually produces a brighter reflection with a ring down artifact and dirtier shadow versus the clean sharp shadow from a stone.

Sonographic Findings. Another cause of shadowing in the right upper quadrant is gas in the biliary tree. This is a spontaneous occurrence resulting from the formation of a biliary enteric fistula in chronic gallbladder disease (Figure 7-51).

CAROLI'S DISEASE

Caroli's disease is a congenital abnormality that is most likely inherited in an autosomal recessive fashion. This condition is a communicating cavernous ectasia of intrahepatic ducts characterized by congenital segmental saccular cystic dilation of major intrahepatic bile ducts. It is found in the younger adult or pediatric population and may be associated with renal disease or congenital hepatic fibrosis. Patient symptoms include recurrent cramplike upper abdominal pain.

Sonographic Findings. On ultrasound examination, multiple cystic structures in the area of the ductal system converge toward the porta hepatis. These masses may be seen as localized or diffusely scattered cysts that communicate with the bile ducts. The differential will include polycystic liver disease. In addition to the abnormality in the porta hepatis, the ducts may show a beaded appearance as they extend into the periphery of the liver. Ectasia of the extrahepatic and common bile ducts may be present. In addition, sludge or calculi may reside in the dilated ducts.

Figure 7-48 Gross pathology of bacterial cholangitis with pus in the bile ducts. (From Damjanov I, Linder J: *Pathology: a color atlas,* St. Louis, 2000, Mosby.)

Figure 7-49 Sclerosing cholangitis appears as dilated ducts with thickened walls. This may be seen in patients with severe or prolonged infections, such as acquired immunodeficiency syndrome (AIDS).

C

Figure 7-50   In patients with choledocholithiasis, the majority of stones have migrated from the gallbladder. **A,** Transverse: gallstones *(arrow)*. *GB,* gallbladder. **B,** Longitudinal. *Arrows,* stone; *Cd,* common duct; *Sh,* shadow; *single arrow,* gallstone. **C,** Longitudinal: dilated common duct with stone *(arrows)*.

Figure 7-51   Gas in the right upper quadrant may cause shadowing in the area of the gallbladder *(GB, arrows)*.

SELECTED BIBLIOGRAPHY

Ahrendt AS, Nakeeb A, Pitt HA: Cholangiocarcinoma, *Clin Liver Dis* 5:191-218, 2001.

Bloom RA, Libson E, Lebensart PD: The ultrasound spectrum of emphysematous cholecystitis, *J Clin Ultrasound* 17:251, 1989.

Bressler EL and others: Sonographic parallel channel sign: a reappraisal, *Radiology* 164:343, 1987.

Bret PM and others: Intrahepatic bile duct and portal vein anatomy revisited, *Radiology* 169:405, 1988.

Collett JA and others: Gallbladder polyps: prospective study, *J Ultrasound Med* 17:207, 1998.

Dobbins JM, Rao PM, Novelline RA: Posttraumatic hemobilia, *Emerg Radiol* 4:180, 1997.

Frezza EE, Mezghebe H: Gallbladder carcinoma: a 28 year experience, *Int Surg* 82:295, 1997.

Gates J, Kane RA, Hartnell GG: Primary biliary tract malignant melanoma, *Abdom Imaging* 21:453, 1996.

Graham MF and others: The size of the normal common hepatic duct following cholecystectomy: an ultrasonic study, *Radiology* 135:137, 1980.

Hann LE and others: Cholangiocarcinoma at the hepatic hilus: sonographic findings, *Am J Roentgenol* 168:985, 1997.

Henningsen C: *Clinical guide to ultrasonography,* St. Louis, 2005, Mosby.

Kane RA: Ultrasonographic diagnosis of gangrenous cholecystitis and empyema of the gallbladder, *Radiology* 134:191, 1980.

Klatskin G: Adenocarcinoma of the hepatic duct at its bifurcation within the porta hepatis: an unusual tumor with distinctive clinical and pathologic features, *Am J Med* 38:241, 1965.

Kurtz AB, Middleton WD: *The gallbladder in ultrasound: the requisites,* St Louis, 2004, Mosby.

Laing FC: Ultrasound diagnosis of choledocholithiasis, *Sem Ultrasound, CT MR* 8:103, 1987.

Laing FC, Jeffrey RB Jr, Wing VW: Biliary dilatation: defining the level and cause by real-time ultrasound, *Radiology* 160:39, 1986.

Laing FC and others: Sonographic appearances in the gallbladder and biliary tree with emphasis on intracholecystic blood, *J Ultrasound Med* 16:537, 1997.

Lim JH and others: Anatomic relationship of intrahepatic bile ducts to portal veins, *J Ultrasound Med* 9:137, 1990.

Mitchell DG and others: Gas containing gallstones: the sonographic "double echo sign," *J Ultrasound Med* 7:39, 1988.

Mittelstaedt CA: Ultrasound of the bile ducts, *Semin Roentgenol* 32:161, 1997.

Naganuma S and others: Sonographic findings of anomalous position of the gallbladder, *Abdom Imaging* 23:67, 1998.

Nemcek AA Jr and others: The effervescent gallbladder: a sonographic sign of emphysematous cholecystitis, *Am J Roentgenol* 150:575, 1988.

Pandey M at al: Carcinoma of the gallbladder: role of sonography in the diagnosis and staging, *J Clin Ultrasound* 28: 227-232, 2000.

Ralls PW and others: The use of color Doppler sonography to distinguish dilated intrahepatic ducts from vascular structures, *Am J Roentgenol* 152:291, 1988.

Romano AJ and others: Gallbladder and bile duct abnormalities in AIDS: sonographic findings in eight patients, *Am J Roentgenol* 150:123, 1988.

Simeone JF and others: The sonographic diagnosis of acute gangrenous cholecystitis: importance of the Murphy sign, *Am J Roentgenol* 152:289, 1989.

Simmons MZ: Pitfalls in ultrasound of the gallbladder and biliary tract, *Ultrasound Q* 14:2, 1998.

Soyer P and others: Color velocity imaging and power Doppler sonography of the gallbladder wall, *Am J Roentgenol* 171:183, 1998.

Watanabe Y and others: Usefulness of intraductal ultrasonography in gallbladder disease, *J Ultrasound Med* 17:33, 1998.

Wilkinson LS and others: Biliary sludge: can ultrasound reliably detect the presence of crystals in bile? *Eur J Gastroenterol Hepatol* 8:999, 1996.

Yassa NA, Stain S, Ralls PW: Recurrent pyogenic cholangitis, *Ultrasound Q* 14:41, 1998.

Yeh HC, Goodman J, Rabinowitz JG: Floating gallstones in bile without added contrast material, *Am J Roentgenol* 146:49, 1986.

CHAPTER 8

The Pancreas

Sandra L. Hagen-Ansert

OBJECTIVES

- Describe the normal anatomy and relational landmarks of the pancreas
- Name the exocrine and endocrine functions of the pancreas
- Describe the laboratory tests used to detect pancreatic disease
- Describe the sonographic technique and patterns of the normal pancreas
- Define the clinical signs and symptoms of pancreatic disease
- Name the congenital anomalies of the pancreas
- List the sonographic findings and differential diagnoses of the following diseases: pancreatitis, pancreatic cyst, pancreatic tumors

KEY TERMS

acini cells – cells that perform exocrine function

amylase – enzyme secreted by the pancreas to aid in the digestion of carbohydrates

body of the pancreas – lies in the midepigastrium anterior to the superior mesenteric artery and vein, aorta, and inferior vena cava

caudal pancreatic artery – branch of the splenic artery that supplies the tail of the pancreas

C-loop of the duodenum – forms the lateral border of the head of the pancreas

common hepatic artery – forms the right superior border of the body and head of the gland and gives rise to the gastroduodenal artery

Courvoisier's gallbladder – enlargement of the gallbladder caused by a slow progressive obstruction of the distal common bile duct from an external mass (such as adenocarcinoma of the pancreatic head)

cystic fibrosis – a hereditary disease that causes excessive production of thick mucus by the endocrine glands; identified as fatty replacement of the glands

dorsal pancreatic artery – branch of the splenic artery that supplies the body of the pancreas

duct of Santorini – small accessory duct of the pancreas found in the head of the pancreas

duct of Wirsung – largest duct of the pancreas that drains the tail, body, and head of the gland; it joins the common bile duct to enter the duodenum through the ampulla of Vater

endocrine – the endocrine function is production of the hormone insulin

exocrine – production and digestion of pancreatic juice; primary function of the pancreas

glucagon – stimulates the liver to convert glycogen to glucose; produced by alpha cells

head of the pancreas – lies in the C-loop of the duodenum; the gastroduodenal artery is the anterolateral border and the common bile duct is the posterolateral border

ANATOMY OF THE PANCREAS
NORMAL ANATOMY
SIZE OF THE PANCREAS
VASCULAR SUPPLY
VASCULAR AND DUCTAL LANDMARKS TO THE PANCREAS
CONGENITAL ANOMALIES

PHYSIOLOGY AND LABORATORY DATA OF THE PANCREAS
PHYSIOLOGY
LABORATORY TESTS

SONOGRAPHIC EVALUATION OF THE PANCREAS
NORMAL PANCREATIC TEXTURE
ULTRASOUND SCAN TECHNIQUE

PATHOLOGY OF THE PANCREAS
PANCREATITIS
INFLAMMATORY AND INFECTIOUS PANCREATIC LESIONS
CYSTIC LESIONS OF THE PANCREAS

hypercalcemia – elevated levels of calcium in the blood

hyperlipidemia – congenital condition in which elevated fat levels cause pancreatitis

ileus – dilated loops of bowel without peristalsis; associated with various abdominal problems, including pancreatitis, sickle cell crisis, and bowel obstruction

insulin – hormone that causes glycogen formation from glucose in the liver and allows cells within insulin receptors to take up glucose to decrease blood sugar

islets of Langerhans – small cells that comprise the endocrine portion of the pancreas for the production of insulin, glucagon, and somatostatin

leukocytosis – an abnormal increase in white blood cells caused by infections

lipase – pancreatic enzyme that breaks down fats; enzyme is elevated in pancreatitis and remains increased longer than amylase

lymphoma – a malignant neoplasm that rises from the lymphoid tissues

neck of the pancreas – small area of the pancreas between the head and the body; anterior to the superior mesenteric vein

obstructive jaundice – excessive bilirubin in the bloodstream caused by an obstruction of bile from the liver; characterized by a yellow discoloration of the sclera of the eye, skin, and mucous membranes

pancreatic ascites – occurs when the pancreatic pseudocyst ruptures into the abdomen; free-floating pancreatic enzymes are very dangerous to surrounding structures

pancreatic pseudocyst – "sterile abscess" collection of pancreatic enzymes that accumulate in the available space in the abdomen (usually in or near the pancreas)

pancreaticoduodenal arteries – help supply blood to the pancreas along with the splenic artery

pancreatitis – inflammation of the pancreas; may be acute or chronic

portal-splenic confluence – junction of the splenic and main portal vein; posterior border of the body of the pancreas

pseudocyst – a space or cavity that contains fluid but has no true endothelial lining membrane

serum amylase – pancreatic enzyme that is elevated during pancreatitis

superior mesenteric artery – serves as the posterior border to the body of the pancreas

superior mesenteric vein – lies posterior to the neck/body of the pancreas and anterior to the uncinate process of the gland

tail of the pancreas – tapered end of the pancreas that lies in the left hypochondrium near the hilus of the spleen and upper pole of the left kidney

uncinate process – small, curved tip of the pancreatic head that lies posterior to the superior mesenteric vein

---

The pancreas continues to be a technical challenge for the sonographer because this gland is located in the retroperitoneal cavity posterior to the stomach, duodenum, and prox-

imal jejunum of the small bowel. In addition, the transverse colon may obstruct visualization of the pancreas because it runs horizontally across the abdominal cavity.

Other noninvasive procedures were unsuccessful in visualization of the pancreas before the development of computed tomography (CT), magnetic resonance imaging (MRI), and ultrasound. Plain film of the abdomen can diagnosis pancreatitis if calcification is visible in the pancreatic area, but calcification does not occur in all cases. Localized **ileus,** dilated loops of bowel without peristalsis ("paralyzed gut") caused by gas and fluid accumulation near the area of inflammation, may be shown on the plain radiograph in patients with pancreatitis. The upper gastrointestinal test series provides indirect information about the pancreas when the widened duodenal loops are visualized. Other diagnostic methods, such as hypotonic duodenography, isotope examination, arteriography, fiber optic gastroscopy, and intravenous cholangiography, all provide indirect information about the pancreas or prove limited in their diagnostic ability.

CT and MRI have become the primary modalities to image the patient with pancreatic disease because of their improved resolution of the retroperitoneal structures. However, the normal pancreas can be visualized in the majority of gas-free patients with ultrasound by using the neighboring organs and vascular landmarks to aid in localization. The gland appears sonographically isoechoic to more hyperechoic than the hepatic parenchyma. Variations in patient positioning or ingestion of water to fill the stomach (to serve as a window to image the pancreas) are used routinely in many laboratories to further aid in visualizing the entire gland. In addition, clinicians performing the endoscopic retrograde cholangiopancreatography (ERCP) examination of the pancreatic duct are incorporating endoscopic ultrasound as an aid in visualizing the detailed anatomy of the pancreatic area.

ANATOMY OF THE PANCREAS

NORMAL ANATOMY

The pancreas lies anterior to the first and second lumbar bodies located deep in the epigastrium and left hypochondrium, behind the lesser omental sac (Figure 8-1). The major posterior vascular landmarks of the pancreas are the aorta and inferior vena cava. The pancreas most commonly extends in a horizontal oblique lie from the second portion of the duodenum to the splenic hilum. Other variations in the lie of the pancreas include: transverse, horseshoe, sigmoid, *L*-shaped, and inverted *V*. When this occurs, it may be more difficult to obtain a single image of the pancreatic gland as the tail will be in a different plane than the body and the head.

It may be surprising that the majority of the pancreas lies within the retroperitoneal cavity, with the exception of a small portion of the head that is surrounded by peritoneum (Figure 8-2). The gland occupies the anterior pararenal space and lies obliquely between the C-loop of the duodenum and splenic hilum. Posterior to the pancreas are the connective prevertebral tissues, the portal-splenic confluence, the superior mesenteric vessels, the aorta, the inferior vena cava, and the lower

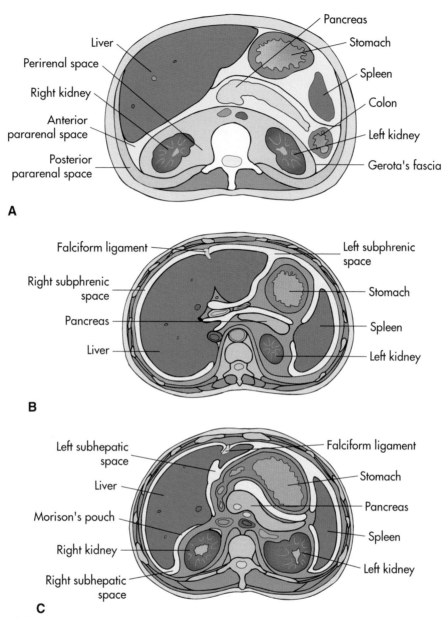

Figure 8-1 **A,** The pancreas lies in the anterior pararenal space. **B,** The stomach is anterior to the body and tail of the gland, whereas the aorta and inferior vena cava, superior mesenteric artery, and vein lie posterior to the gland. **C,** The head of the pancreas lies in the lap of the duodenum.

border of the diaphragm. The stomach, duodenum, and transverse colon form the superior and lateral borders of the pancreas, which makes visualization of the pancreas by ultrasound difficult (air and gas interference).

The pancreas is divided into the following four areas: head, neck, body, and tail (see Figure 8-2). Each area is discussed as it relates to its surrounding anatomy. The reader is referred to the multiple cross-sectional drawings (Figures 8-3 through 8-4) to gain a relational understanding of the adjacent anatomy to the pancreas.

Head. The **head of the pancreas** is the most inferior portion of the gland. It lies anterior to the inferior vena cava, to the right of the portal-splenic confluence, inferior to the

main portal vein and caudate lobe of the liver, and medial to the duodenum as it "lies in the lap" of the **C-loop of the duodenum** (see Figure 8-2). The splenic vein drains the spleen and forms the posterior medial border of the pancreas, where it is joined by the **superior mesenteric vein** (that drains the small bowel and proximal colon) to form the main portal vein, thus forming the **portal-splenic confluence** (Figure 8-5). The superior mesenteric vein crosses anterior to the uncinate process of the head of the gland and posterior to the neck and body of the pancreas. The **uncinate process** is the small, curved tip at the end of the head of the pancreas. It lies anterior to the inferior vena cava and posterior to the superior mesenteric vein. In Figure 8-6, the common bile duct passes through the first part of the duodenum and courses through a

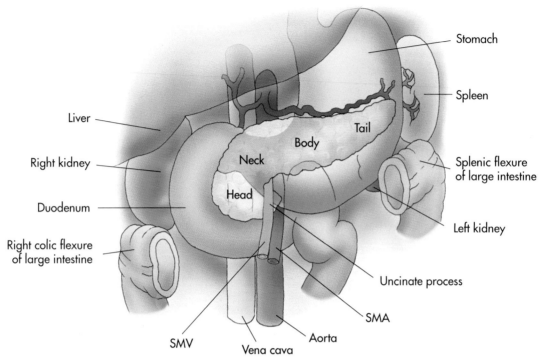

Figure 8-2 The aorta and inferior vena cava are the posterior landmarks of the pancreas; the stomach is the anterior border. The tail of the pancreas is directed toward the upper pole of the left kidney and hilum of the spleen. The body and head lie anterior to the prevertebral vessels. The four major areas of the pancreas are the head (with the uncinate process), the neck, the body, and the tail. The superior mesenteric vein *(SMV)* is anterior to the uncinate process. The superior mesenteric artery *(SMA)* is posterior to the neck/body.

groove posterior to the pancreatic head, whereas the gastro-duodenal artery (a branch of the hepatic artery rising from the celiac axis) forms the anterolateral border.

Neck. The **neck of the pancreas** is found directly anterior to the portal-splenic confluence or superior mesenteric vein. The portal vein is formed posterior to the neck by the junction of the superior mesenteric vein and the splenic vein (see Figure 8-5). The neck is located between the pancreatic head and body, and often is included as "part of the body" of the gland.

Body. The **body of the pancreas** is the largest section of the pancreas. It lies anterior to the aorta and celiac axia (superior mesenteric, common hepatic, and left gastric arteries), left renal vein, adrenal gland, and kidney. The tortuous splenic artery is the superior border of the gland (see Figure 8-4). The anterior border is the posterior wall of the antrum of the stomach. The neck of the pancreas forms the right lateral border. The splenic vein courses across the posteromedial surface of the pancreas to join the main portal vein.

Tail. The **tail of the pancreas** is more difficult to image because it lies anterior to the left kidney and posterior to the left colic flexure and transverse colon. The tail begins to the left of the lateral border of the aorta and extends toward the splenic hilum (see Figure 8-5). The splenic vein is the posterior border of the body and tail. The splenic artery forms the superior border of the tail, whereas the stomach is the anterior border.

Pancreatic Duct. Two ducts are seen within the pancreas, the duct of Wirsung and the duct of Santorini. To aid in the transport of pancreatic fluid, the ducts have smooth muscle surrounding them. The **duct of Wirsung** is a primary duct extending the entire length of the gland (see Figure 8-6). It receives tributaries from lobules at right angles and enters the medial second part of the duodenum with the common bile duct at the ampulla of Vater (guarded by the sphincter of Oddi). The **duct of Santorini** is a secondary duct that drains the upper anterior head. It enters the duodenum at the minor papilla about 2 cm proximal to the ampulla of Vater.

The duct of Wirsung is easier to visualize as it courses through the midline of the body of the gland. It appears as an echogenic line or lucency bordered by two echogenic lines. The duct should measure less than 2 mm, with tapering as it reaches the tail. Color Doppler imaging may help distinguish the dilated pancreatic duct from the vascular structures (splenic vein and artery) in the area.

SIZE OF THE PANCREAS

The normal length of the pancreas (head to tail) is about 15 cm, with the range extending between 12 and 18 cm. The head is the thickest part of the gland, measuring 2.0 to 3.0 cm

Text continues on p. 245

A

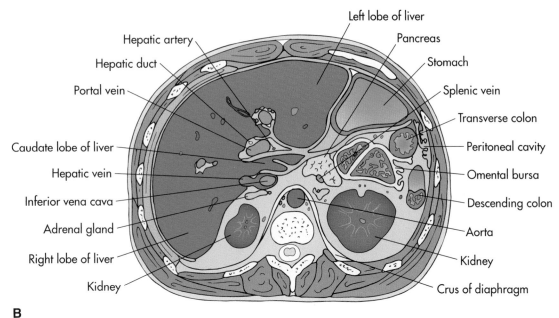

B

Figure 8-3 Transverse planes of the pancreas. **A,** Note the relationship of the tail of the pancreas to the spleen, left kidney and adrenal gland, stomach, and colic flexure. **B,** The body of the pancreas is adjacent to the left lobe of the liver, the stomach, the omental bursa, and the left kidney. *Continued*

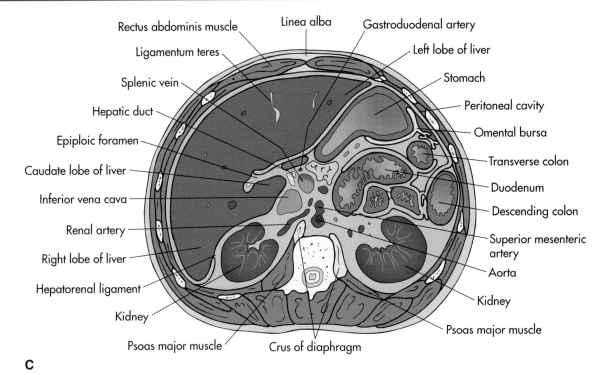

C

D

Figure 8-3, cont'd   **C,** The size of the left lobe of the liver helps to push the stomach away from the pancreatic area for better visualization. **D,** The head of the pancreas is adjacent to the duodenum, superior mesenteric vessels, inferior vena cava, and aorta.

A

B

Figure 8-4   Sagittal planes of the pancreas. **A,** The head of the pancreas lies in the lap of the duodenum. The gastroduodenal artery is the anterior lateral border of the head. **B,** The head of the pancreas may be obscured by mesenteric fat and air in the duodenum.   *Continued*

C

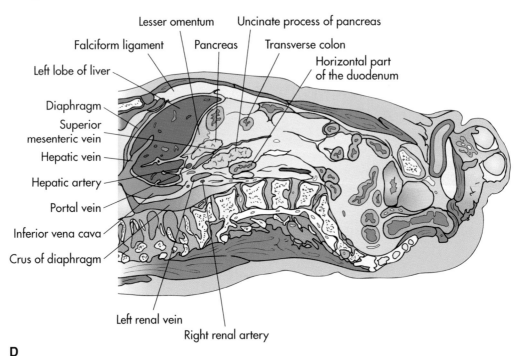

D

Figure 8-4, cont'd   **C,** The head of the pancreas lies anterior to the inferior vena cava and inferior to the portal vein. **D,** Note the adjacent relationship of the lesser omentum to the pancreas. The superior mesenteric vein is posterior to the neck and anterior to the uncinate process.

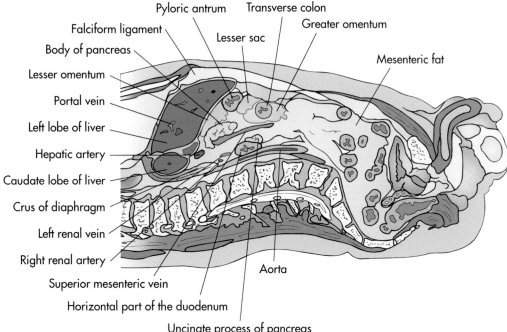

Pyloric antrum
Transverse colon
Falciform ligament
Greater omentum
Lesser sac
Body of pancreas
Mesenteric fat
Lesser omentum
Portal vein
Left lobe of liver
Hepatic artery
Caudate lobe of liver
Crus of diaphragm
Left renal vein
Right renal artery
Superior mesenteric vein
Aorta
Horizontal part of the duodenum
Uncinate process of pancreas

E

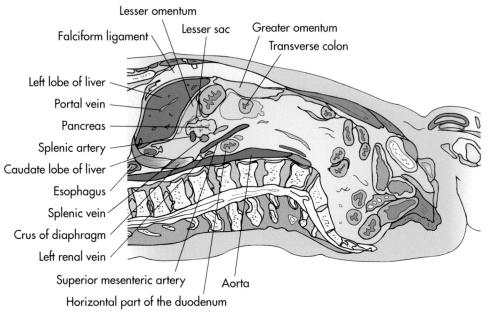

Lesser omentum
Falciform ligament
Lesser sac
Greater omentum
Transverse colon
Left lobe of liver
Portal vein
Pancreas
Splenic artery
Caudate lobe of liver
Esophagus
Splenic vein
Crus of diaphragm
Left renal vein
Superior mesenteric artery
Aorta
Horizontal part of the duodenum

F

Figure 8-4, cont'd   E, Note the relationship of the lesser omentum, pyloric antrum, lesser sac, transverse colon, and superior mesenteric vein to the body of the pancreas. **F,** Note the intimate relationship of the splenic vein and artery, superior mesenteric artery, aorta, and left lobe of the liver to the pancreas.

Continued

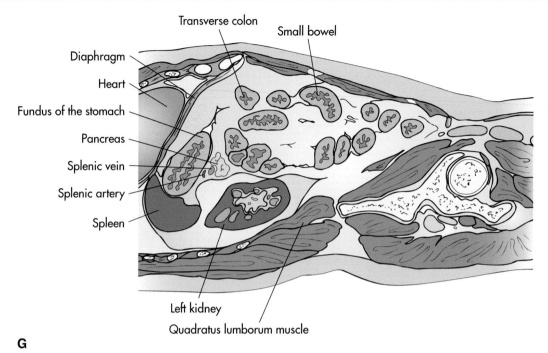

G

Figure 8-4, cont'd **G,** The tail of the pancreas is more difficult to image on the sagittal plane secondary to adjacent colon and small bowel. Occasionally a fluid-filled stomach, prominent spleen, or left kidney may help to localize the tail of the pancreas.

Figure 8-5 The portal venous system is the posterior border of the pancreas. The splenic vein lies along the posterior border, the superior mesenteric vein crosses anterior to the uncinate process and posterior to the neck, and the main portal vein is the posterior border to the head of the pancreas. The tortuous splenic artery is the superior border to the body and tail of the pancreas. The hepatic artery gives rise to the gastroduodenal artery, which serves as the anterolateral border to the head of the pancreas. The splenic artery branches into the great pancreatic artery and dorsal pancreatic artery. The celiac axis rises from the anterior abdominal aorta just below the diaphragm and serves as the superior border of the pancreas.

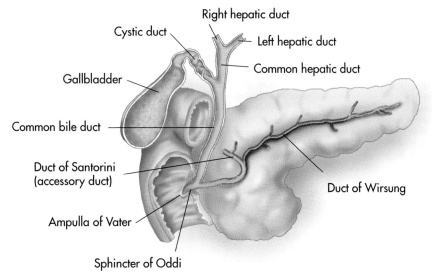

Figure 8-6   The head of the pancreas lies in the C-loop of the duodenum. The common bile duct passes through the first part of the duodenum and courses through a groove posterior to the pancreatic head, where it meets the pancreatic duct to enter the duodenum through the ampulla of Vater. This opening is guarded by the sphincter of Oddi.

in its anterior to posterior dimension. The neck measures 1.5 to 2.5 cm, the body measures 2.0 to 2.5 cm, and the tail measures 1.0 to 2.0 cm. The sonographer should evaluate the total size, contour, and texture of the gland to determine enlargement. The gland appears larger or thicker in children than in adults and decreases in size with advancing age.

VASCULAR SUPPLY

The blood supply for the pancreas is the splenic artery and **pancreaticoduodenal arteries** (see Figure 8-5). The anterior and inferior pancreaticoduodenal arteries supply the head and part of the duodenum. The splenic artery supplies the body and tail of the pancreas through four smaller branches: (1) suprapancreatic (rises from celiac axis/splenic artery), (2) pancreatic, (3) prepancreatic (before leaving the pancreas), (4) prehilar (before leaving the spleen) and hepatic artery (gastroduodenal artery). The **dorsal pancreatic artery** rises from the suprapancreatic section; the pancreatica magna artery rises from the pancreatic section; and the **caudal pancreatic artery** rises from the prepancreatic or prehilar section.

Venous drainage is through tributaries of the splenic and superior mesenteric veins.

VASCULAR AND DUCTAL LANDMARKS TO THE PANCREAS

Celiac Axis and Branches. The celiac axis originates from the anterior abdominal aorta and serves as the superior border of the pancreas. It gives rise to three branches: the left gastric, common hepatic, and splenic arteries (see Figure 8-5).

Splenic artery. The splenic artery follows a tortuous course along the superior border of the pancreatic body and tail as it crosses horizontally toward the splenic hilum.

Common hepatic artery. The common hepatic artery rises from the celiac axis and courses along the superior margin of

the first portion of the duodenum to divide into the proper hepatic artery and gastroduodenal artery, usually when it crosses anterior to the portal vein. The **common hepatic artery** forms the right superior border of the body and head of the gland and gives rise to the gastroduodenal artery. In some patients the right hepatic artery rises from the superior mesenteric artery and courses posterior to the medial portion of the splenic vein.

Gastroduodenal artery. The gastroduodenal artery is seen along the anterolateral border of the pancreas as it travels a short distance along the anterior aspect of the pancreatic head just to the right of the neck before it divides into the superior pancreaticoduodenal branches; they join with the inferior pancreaticoduodenal branches, which rise from the superior mesenteric artery.

Superior Mesenteric Artery. The **superior mesenteric artery** rises from the aorta inferior to the celiac axis and posterior to the lower portion of the pancreatic body and courses anterior to the third portion of the duodenum to enter the small bowel mesentery (see Figure 8-5).

Portal Vein and Tributaries. The main portal vein is formed posterior to the neck of the pancreas by the junction of the superior mesenteric vein and splenic vein (see Figure 8-5).

Splenic vein. The splenic vein runs from the splenic hilum along the posterior aspect of the pancreas.

Superior mesenteric vein. The superior mesenteric vein runs posterior to the neck of the pancreas and anterior to the uncinate process, which forms the small, curved tip of the pancreatic head.

Common Bile Duct. The common bile duct crosses the anterior aspect of the portal vein to the right of the proper hepatic artery. The portal vein is anterior to the inferior vena cava. The duct passes along the anterior border of the portal vein and travels posterior to the first portion of the duodenum to course inferior and somewhat posterior in the parenchyma of the head of the pancreas (see Figure 8-6). It joins the pancreatic duct close to the ampulla of Vater.

CONGENITAL ANOMALIES

Congenital abnormalities of the pancreas are uncommon. The following abnormalities are presented: ectopic pancreatic tissue, annular pancreas, fibrocystic disease, and congenital cysts.

Ectopic Pancreatic Tissue. Ectopic pancreatic tissue is the most common pancreatic anomaly, usually in the form of intramural nodules. The ectopic tissue may be found in various places in the gastrointestinal tract. Frequent sites are the stomach, duodenum, small bowel, and large bowel. On palpation these lesions may seem polypoid, and they characteristically have a central dimple. They consist of elements of the pancreas, usually the acinar and ductal structures and less frequently the islets of Langerhans. They are generally small (0.5 to 2 cm), and acute pancreatitis or tumor may occur within these elements.

Annular Pancreas. Annular pancreas is a rare anomaly in which the head of the pancreas surrounds the second portion of the duodenum (Figure 8-7). It is more common in males than in females, and all grades (from an overlapping of the posterior duodenal wall to a complete ring) may be found. It may be associated with complete or partial atresia of the duodenum and is susceptible to any of the diseases of the pancreas.

Fibrocystic Disease of the Pancreas. Fibrocystic disease of the pancreas is a hereditary disorder of the exocrine glands seen frequently in children and young adults. The pancreas is usually firm and of normal size. Cysts are very small but may be present in the advanced stages. The acini and ducts are dilated. The acini are usually atrophic and may be totally replaced by fibrous tissue in many of the lobules. Nausea and vomiting may also occur, leading to malnourishment. The pancreatic secretion is gradually lost. With advancing pancreatic fibrosis, jaundice may develop from common duct obstruction. Diabetes is a late manifestation. Grossly the pancreas is found to be somewhat nodular and firm. There may be edema and fat necrosis, but gradually fibrous replacement will occur throughout the parenchyma. The pancreatic duct may enlarge and contain calculi.

Congenital Cysts. Congenital cysts of the pancreas result from the anomalous development of the pancreatic ducts. They are usually multiple in number and range from small to 3 to 5 cm in size (Figure 8-8).

PHYSIOLOGY AND LABORATORY DATA OF THE PANCREAS

PHYSIOLOGY

The pancreas is both a digestive (**exocrine**) and hormonal (**endocrine**) gland. The primary function, exocrine, is to produce pancreatic juice, which enters the duodenum together with bile. The exocrine secretions of the pancreas and those of the liver, which are delivered into the duodenum through duct systems, are essential for normal intestinal digestion and absorption of food. Pancreatic secretion is under the control of the vagus nerve and two hormonal agents, secretin and pancreozymin, that are released when food enters the duodenum. The endocrine function controls the secretion of glucagons and insulin into the blood. Failure of the pancreas to furnish sufficient insulin leads to diabetes mellitus.

Exocrine Function. Exocrine function is performed by **acini cells** of the pancreas, which can produce up to 2 L of pancreatic juice per day. These cells are arranged in saclike clusters (acini) connected by small intercalated ducts to larger excretory ducts. The excretory ducts converge into one or two main ducts, which deliver the exocrine secretion of the pancreas into the duodenum. The enzymes of the pancreatic juice that aid in digestion include: **lipase,** which digests fats; **amylase,** which digests carbohydrates; carboxypeptidase, trypsin, and chymotrypsinogen, which digest proteins; and nucleases, which digest nucleic acids (Table 8-1).

Figure 8-7 Gross pathology of the annular pancreas in which the head surrounds the second portion of the duodenum. (From Damjanov I, Linder J: *Pathology: a color atlas,* St. Louis, 2000, Mosby.)

Figure 8-8 Gross pathology of a small congenital cyst of the pancreas. (From Damjanov I, Linder J: *Pathology: a color atlas,* St. Louis, 2000, Mosby.)

TABLE 8-1	PANCREATIC EXOCRINE FUNCTION	
Enzymes of Pancreatic Juice		Digestive Action
Lipase		Fats
Amylase		Carbohydrates
Trypsin, chymotrypsin, carboxypeptidase		Proteins
Nucleases		Nucleic acids
Sodium bicarbonate		Hydrochloric acid

TABLE 8-2	PANCREATIC ENDOCRINE FUNCTION	
Pancreatic Hormone	Cell Type	Action
Insulin	Beta	Glucose to glycogen
Glucagon	Alpha	Glycogen to glucose
Somatostatin	Delta	Alpha and beta inhibitor

TABLE 8-3	LABORATORY VALUES FOR PANCREATIC DISEASE	
Condition		Amylase Level
Amylase Levels in Disease		
Acute pancreatitis		Twice normal
Chronic pancreatitis		No change
Mumps, ischemic bowel disease, pelvic inflammatory disease		↑
Condition		Lipase Level
Lipase Levels in Disease		
Acute pancreatitis		↑
Carcinoma of the pancreas		↑
Condition		Blood Glucose Level
Blood Glucose Levels In Disease		
Severe diabetes		↑
Chronic liver disease		↑
Overactive endocrine glands		↑
Tumor in islet of Langerhans		↓

↑, Increased; ↓, decreased.

Pancreatic juice is the most versatile and active of the digestive secretions. Its enzymes are capable of nearly completing the digestion of food in the absence of all other digestive secretions. Because the digestive enzymes that are secreted into the lumen of the small intestine require an almost neutral pH for best activity, the acidity of the contents entering the duodenum must be reduced. Thus the pancreatic juice contains a relatively high concentration of sodium bicarbonate, and this alkaline salt is largely responsible for the neutralization of gastric acid.

The nervous secretion of pancreatic juice is thick and rich in enzymes and proteins. The chemical secretion, resulting from pancreozymin activity, also is thick, watery, and rich in enzymes. Pancreatic juice is alkaline and becomes more so with increasing rates of secretion. This is because of a simultaneous increase in bicarbonates and decrease in chloride concentration.

The proteolytic enzyme trypsin may hydrolyze protein molecules to polypeptides. Chymotrypsinogen is activated by trypsin. Amylase causes hydrolysis of starch with the production of maltose, which is further hydrolyzed to glucose. Lipase is capable of hydrolyzing some fats to monoglycerides and some to glycerol and fatty acids. Although lipases are also secreted by the small intestine, what is secreted by the pancreas accounts for 80% of all fat digestion. Thus impaired fat digestion is an important indicator of pancreatic dysfunction.

Partially digested food, or chyme, in the duodenum stimulates the release of hormones that act on pancreatic juice formation. These hormones include gastrin, cholecystokinin, acetylcholine (all digestive enzymes), and secretin (stimulates production of sodium bicarbonate).

The pancreatic juice enters the duodenum through the duct of Wirsung. This duct joins the common bile duct as it drains bile from the liver and both enter the duodenum through the ampulla of Vater. The sphincter of Oddi is a muscle surrounding the ampulla of Vater that relaxes to allow pancreatic juice and bile to empty into the duodenum.

Endocrine Function. The endocrine function is located in the **islets of Langerhans** in the pancreas. Specialized cells within the islets are called *alpha, beta,* and *delta* cells. The beta cells are most prevalent and produce **insulin,** a hormone that causes glycogen formation from glucose in the liver. It also enables cells within insulin receptors to take up glucose (to decrease blood sugar). Alpha cells produce **glucagon,** a hormone that causes the cells to release glucose to meet the energy needs of the body. Glucagon stimulates the liver to

convert glycogen to glucose to increase sugar levels. Delta cells are the smallest composition of endocrine tissue and produce somatostatin. This hormone inhibits the production of both insulin and glucagon. All the hormones are released into the bloodstream (Table 8-2).

LABORATORY TESTS

There are specific enzymes of the pancreas that may become altered in pancreatic disease, namely amylase and lipase. Increased glucose levels may indicate abnormalities of the pancreas (Table 8-3).

Amylase. Amylase is a digestive enzyme for carbohydrates. It is secreted by the pancreas, parotid glands, gynecologic system, and bowel. In certain types of pancreatic disease, the digestive enzymes of the pancreas escape into the surrounding tissue, producing necrosis with severe pain and inflammation. Under these circumstances there is an increase in **serum amylase.** A serum amylase level of twice normal usually indicates acute pancreatitis.

Other conditions that may cause an increase in amylase include chronic pancreatitis, obstruction of the pancreatic duct, perforated peptic ulcer, acute cholecystitis, and alcohol poisoning. Less common conditions include mumps, ischemic bowel disease, and pelvic inflammatory disease.

Urine Amylase. Urine amylase may be elevated in pancreatitis. Diseases not affecting the pancreas may cause the elevation of serum amylase without elevation of urine amylase.

Lipase. Lipase is an enzyme that is excreted specifically by the pancreas and that parallels the elevation in amylase levels. The lipase test is performed to assess damage to the pancreas. Lipase is secreted by the pancreas, and small amounts pass into the blood. The lipase level rises in acute pancreatitis and in carcinoma of the pancreas. Both amylase and lipase rise at the same rate, but the elevation in lipase concentration persists for a longer period. Lipase may also be elevated with obstruction of the pancreatic duct, pancreatic carcinoma, and acute cholecystitis.

Glucose. Glucose controls the blood sugar level in the body. The glucose tolerance test is performed to discover whether there is a disorder of glucose metabolism. An increased blood glucose level is found in severe diabetes, chronic liver disease, and overactivity of several of the endocrine glands. There may be a decreased blood sugar level in tumors of the islets of Langerhans in the pancreas.

SONOGRAPHIC EVALUATION OF THE PANCREAS

The pancreas is one of the most difficult abdominal organs to image with ultrasound because it lies posterior to the stomach and sometimes the transverse colon. To help visualize the pancreas, the patient should fast 8 to 12 hours; this decreases the amount of air and fluid in the stomach and colon that may impede visualization. It also promotes dilation of the gallbladder and ducts. If fluid is administered to better visualize the gland, real-time visualization of peristaltic movement of food particles within the duodenum and stomach can be a useful landmark to help outline the head, body, and tail of the pancreas. This will be discussed in more detail later in the chapter.

NORMAL PANCREATIC TEXTURE

The echogenicity of the pancreas is discussed in terms of how it relates to the liver's homogeneous soft echo pattern. The normal pancreas has an echo pattern that is slightly more echogenic and finer in texture than that of the surrounding retroperitoneum. The echo intensity of the pancreas is usually slightly less than that of surrounding soft tissue and slightly greater than that of the liver.

The parenchymal texture of the pancreas depends on the amount of fat between the lobules and to a lesser extent on the interlobular fibrous tissue. The internal echoes of pancreas consist of closely spaced elements of the same intensity with uniform distribution throughout the gland.

Fat is strongly echogenic, and the extensive fatty infiltrations of the pancreas are difficult to visualize by ultrasound because the pancreas blends in with the surrounding retroperitoneal fat. A lesser degree of fatty infiltration may not render

---

BOX 8-1 NORMAL CHARACTERISTICS OF THE PANCREAS

Size: Head ≤3 cm; neck ≤2.5 cm; body ≤2.5 cm; tail ≤2.0 cm
Echogenicity: >liver </> spleen (depends on fatty/fibrous texture)
Echotexture: Homogeneous
Surface: Smooth to slightly lobular (islets of Langerhans)

BOX 8-2 NORMAL PANCREATIC LANDMARKS

Head: Anterior to inferior vena cava, lateral to duodenum; gastroduodenal artery is anterolateral border; common bile duct is posterior medial border. On sagittal plane, portal vein is superior to head of the pancreas.
Uncinate process: Anterior to inferior vena cava, posterior to superior mesenteric vein.
Body: Anterior to superior mesenteric artery and vein, aorta, splenic vein; posterior to stomach, inferior to splenic artery.
Tail: Medial to hilum of spleen; superior to left kidney.
Pancreatic duct: Runs through mid portion of body of pancreas.

---

the pancreas invisible, but may raise the amplitude of returning pancreatic echoes, resulting in the clinical observation that the pancreas returns stronger echoes than the liver. Fibrous tissue may also account for the portion of increased echogenicity. Box 8-1 lists the sonographic characteristics of the normal pancreas.

ULTRASOUND SCAN TECHNIQUE

The patient is usually examined in the supine, oblique, or upright positions. Ultrasound techniques vary according to the patient's body habitus. For adult patients, use at least 3- to 5-megahertz (MHz) broad band transducer with a midfocal zone; for pediatric patients, use at least a 5- to 7.5-MHz transducer. The curved linear array transducer allows for a better near field of view than the sector transducer allows. The time gain compensation and overall gain should be adjusted so that the pancreatic tissue has the same echo brightness or slightly greater than the normal liver. The texture of the pancreas will appear coarser than the liver reflective upon the amount of fibrous/fatty tissue interfaces within the gland. The younger pediatric patients tend to have less echogenicity of the pancreas than the older patients do (i.e., more fatty interfaces in the gland of the older patient). The diabetic patient may be challenging to image through the fatty liver texture. A lower frequency transducer may be useful. Gentle transducer pressure on the abdomen allows the sonographer to get as close as possible to the pancreatic tissue to improve visualization.

Box 8-2 summarizes the normal pancreatic landmarks. The sonographer should identify the head, neck, body, and tail in

Figure 8-9 Transverse images of the pancreas *(P)*. **A,** Body and tail of the pancreas drape anterior to the aorta (A). **B,** Head, body, and tail of the pancreas shown anterior to aorta, superior mesenteric vein *(SMV)*, and inferior vena cava *(IVC)*. **C,** The superior mesenteric artery (SMA), aorta *(A)*, and inferior vena cava *(IVC)* are posterior borders to the pancreas. **D,** The splenic vein outlines the posterior border of the tail of the pancreas *(arrows)*. **E,** The SMA and splenic vein *(arrows)* outline the posterior border of the tail of the pancreas.

the transverse and longitudinal planes (Figures 8-9 and 8-10). The sonographer should evaluate the shape, contour, lie, and texture of the pancreas (as compared with the liver parenchyma). The oblique or upright position of the patient may improve visualization of the pancreas and peripancreatic region. The following surrounding structures should be identified: superior mesenteric artery and vein, portal and splenic veins, aorta and inferior vena cava, common bile duct, gastroduodenal artery, left renal vein, duodenal bulb, posterior wall of the stomach, and pancreatic duct.

Windows for Visualization. Difficulties in visualization of the pancreas may result from bowel gas, a transverse stomach obscuring the anatomy, or a small left lobe of the liver (Figure 8-11). A left lobe measuring 2 to 2.5 cm makes an excellent sonic window for imaging the pancreatic area. This subcostal view can be used with a slight caudal angle of the transducer (15 to 20 degrees) as the transducer is directed from the midabdomen (at the level of the xiphoid process), through the left lobe of the liver, and angled through the pancreatic area with the prevertebral vessels demarcating its posterior border.

Figure 8-10 Sagittal images of the pancreas *(P)*. **A,** The pancreas lies inferior to the portal vein *(PV)* and anterior to the inferior vena cava *(IVC)*. **B,** The stomach *(ST)* is anterior to the pancreas. The aorta *(A)* is the posterior border. **C,** A small segment of the superior mesenteric vein *(arrows)* is seen along the posterior border of the neck of the pancreas.

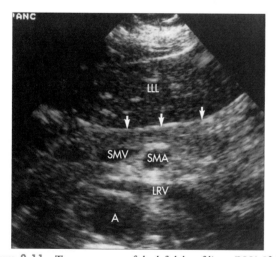

Figure 8-11 Transverse scan of the left lobe of liver *(LLL)*. If the left lobe measures at least 2 to 3 cm, it may serve as an ideal window to visualize the pancreas posterior *(arrows)*. *A,* Aorta; *LRV,* left renal vein; *SMA,* superior mesenteric artery; *SMV,* superior mesenteric vein.

The patient should be in full inspiration to image the pancreas well. This causes the liver to be inferiorly displaced and provides a better scanning window. If the patient has a concave abdomen, ask the patient to take in a deep breath and push out the abdomen to provide a better scanning window.

If the sonographer is unable to image the pancreas, the water ingestion technique may be an effective window to image the gland. The initial scans of the biliary system should be made before asking the patient to drink 32 to 300 ml of fluid through a straw (to prevent swallowing of air) in the erect or right lateral decubitus position. In the upright position, the stomach can be used as a window; if the patient is unable to sit up, the examination can be done in the decubitus position. This water method fills the body and antrum of the stomach initially to help outline the body and tail of the pancreas (Figure 8-12). The fluid then fills the duodenal cap to outline the lateral margin of the head of the pancreas. The upright position allows the air to move from the gastric antrum to the fundus of the stomach and causes the upper viscera to move downward for a better sonic window. The upright position also results in distention of the venous structures, which further aids in the localization of the pancreas (see Box 8-2).

A   **B**

Figure 8-12   **A,** To better visualize the pancreas, the patient should drink more than 16 ounces of water and be imaged in the semi-upright position. **B,** Gross anatomy of the midepigastrium at the level of the SMA. The body of the pancreas is clearly seen anterior to the SMA and posterior to the stomach.

Figure 8-13   The tortuous splenic artery *(arrows)* rises from the celiac axis. The pancreas is usually inferior to the splenic artery; however, in this patient the gland is shown anterior to the vessel. *A,* Aorta; *IVC,* inferior vena cava; *P,* pancreas.

Figure 8-14   Transverse scan of the normal pancreas and its vascular landmarks. *A,* Aorta; *IVC,* inferior vena cava; *P,* pancreas; *SMA,* superior mesenteric artery; *SV,* splenic vein.

Transverse Plane.   Generally the pancreas is imaged first in the transverse plane. The patient should be in full inspiration to distend the venous structures that serve as posterior landmarks to visualize the pancreas. As previously mentioned, the sonographer should use the left lobe of the liver at the level of the xiphoid and angle the transducer slightly toward the feet to image the aorta and celiac axis. This is near the superior border of the pancreas (remember that the tortuous splenic artery may be seen rising from the celiac axis to demarcate the superior border of the pancreas) (Figure 8-13). The body and tail of the gland should be imaged as the transducer is slowly

angled inferiorly from the celiac axis. Visualization of the superior mesenteric vessels, left renal vein, and inferior vena cava also helps delineate the borders of the body of the pancreas (Figure 8-14). The stomach may be seen as the walls are collapsed because it lies anterior to the pancreas (Figure 8-15). The duodenum, gastroduodenal artery, and common bile duct are useful landmarks in identifying the lateral margin of the pancreatic head (Figure 8-16). The sonographer may watch for peristalsis or fluid to pass through the second part of the

A   **B**

Figure 8-15 **A,** The collapsed wall of the stomach *(arrows)* may be seen as two parallel lines anterior to the body of the pancreas. **B,** The fluid-filled duodenum *(Du)* marks the lateral border of the head of the pancreas *(P)*. *A,* Aorta; *IVC,* inferior vena cava.

Figure 8-16 The small gastroduodenal artery *(Gda)* is the anterolateral border of the head of the pancreas. *A,* Aorta.

Figure 8-17 Sagittal oblique scan of the dilated inferior vena cava *(IVC)* as it demarcates the posterior border of the pancreas *(P)*. The gallbladder *(GB)* is seen anterior.

duodenum as it forms the C-loop around the lateral border of the head.

Sagittal Plane. The initial scan should be made slightly to the right of midline with the patient in full inspiration. The dilated inferior vena cava is seen as the posterior border (Figure 8-17). The main portal vein or right branch of the portal vein is the next landmark seen anterior to the cava. The pancreas lies just inferior to the portal vein and anterior to the inferior vena cava. As the pancreas enlarges, a slight indentation is apparent on the anterior border of the cava. This view is also good for visualizing the common bile duct because it lies anterior to the portal vein before dropping posterior to enter the head of the pancreas (Figure 8-18). The hepatic artery is sometimes visible as a circular tube when the common duct is seen (Figure 8-19). The use of color Doppler may help the sonographer separate the hepatic artery from the common duct.

Subsequent scans are made slightly to the left of the midline to image the aorta and superior mesenteric artery and vein because they form the posterior border of the body of the pan-

creas. The superior mesenteric vein flows cephalad to join the portal vein and may be seen as a long, tubular structure posterior to the neck of the pancreas and anterior to the uncinate process (Figure 8-20). The tail of the pancreas is more difficult to see, but may be imaged as the sonographer angles slightly to the left of the aorta. The patient may be rolled into a steep right decubitus position to image the tail of the gland as it lies in the hilum of the spleen near the left kidney.

The antrum of the stomach appears as a collapsed bull's-eye and may be identified anterior and slightly caudal to the body of the pancreas (Figure 8-21). The splenic vein is a circular sonolucent structure posterior to the cephalic portion of the gland (Figure 8-22). The left renal vein is a slitlike sonolucency between the aorta and the superior mesenteric artery.

Figure 8-18   The common bile duct *(markers)* is seen along the posterior border of the pancreas with the patient in a decubitus position.

Figure 8-19   Sagittal scan of the pancreas and its surrounding vascular landmarks. *GDA,* Gastroduodenal artery; *IVC,* inferior vena cava.

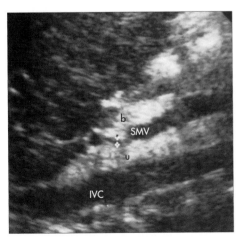

Figure 8-20   Sagittal scan of the right upper quadrant shows the superior mesenteric vein *(SMV)* as it flows anterior to the uncinate process *(u)* and posterior to the body *(b)* of the pancreas. *IVC,* Inferior vena cava.

Figure 8-21   The collapsed antrum of the stomach *(ST)* is seen as a target lesion anterior to the body of the pancreas.

Figure 8-22   The splenic vein is seen as a circle on the sagittal plane as it flows along the posteromedial border of the pancreas *(arrow).*

Figure 8-23   The pancreatic duct is seen as two parallel lines *(arrows)* within the center of the pancreas *(P). A,* Aorta.

Pancreatic Duct. The main pancreatic duct may be visualized best on the transverse image as it courses through the body of the gland (Figure 8-23). The sonographer should be sure to identify pancreatic tissue on both sides of the duct so as not to confuse it with vascular structures that may lie near it. The splenic vein is usually too posterior and the hepatic artery too anterior to be confused with the duct. Color Doppler may be used to help distinguish a dilated duct from vascular structures. The duct appears as an echo-free area sharply marginated by two parallel echogenic lines. A thin strip of retroperitoneal fat may underlie the anterior aspect of the pancreas. This sonolucent linear pattern should not be mistaken for duct. On transverse scans, the posterior wall of the antrum can be seen overlying the pancreas. Care should be taken to distinguish the antrum of the collapsed stomach from the small pancreatic duct.

PATHOLOGY OF THE PANCREAS

PANCREATITIS

Pancreatitis is inflammation of the pancreas. It may be chronic or acute. Pancreatitis occurs when the pancreas becomes damaged and malfunctions as a result of increased secretion and blockage of ducts. When this occurs, the pancreatic tissue may be digested by its own enzymes. Pancreatitis may be classified as acute or chronic with a further subdescription of mild

to severe. In patients with acute pancreatitis, ultrasound may not always be the first imaging performed because often ileus is associated with this condition. Therefore the optimal imaging procedure is the dynamic intravenous and oral contrast-enhanced computed tomography. See Table 8-4 for clinical findings, sonographic findings, and differential considerations for pancreatitis.

Acute Pancreatitis. Acute pancreatitis is an inflammation of the pancreas caused by the inflamed acini releasing pancreatic enzymes into the surrounding pancreatic tissue. Normally these enzymes do not become active until they reach the duodenum where they enable the breakdown of food in the system. The acute process of pancreatitis usually does not last more

TABLE 8-4 PANCREATITIS FINDINGS

Clinical Findings	Sonographic Findings	Differential Considerations
Acute Pancreatitis		
• Sudden onset of moderate to severe abdominal pain with radiation to back • Nausea and vomiting • History of gallstones (localized) or alcoholism (generalized) • Mild fever • ↑ Pancreatic enzymes in blood (amylase, lipase) • Leukocytosis (↑white blood cells) • Abdominal distention	• Ranges from normal size to focal/diffuse enlargement • Hypoechoic texture (edema) • Borders distinct but irregular • Enlargement of head causes depression on inferior vena cava • 40% to 60% have gallstones • Pancreatic duct may be enlarged • Parapancreatic fluid collections	• Hemorrhagic pancreatitis • Pancreatic neoplasm • Lymphoma • Retroperitoneal neoplasm
Hemorrhagic Pancreatitis		
• ↓ Hematocrit and serum calcium level • Intense, severe pain radiating to back, with subsequent shock and ileus • Hypotension despite volume replacement, with metabolic acidosis and adult respiratory distress syndrome	• Depends on age of hemorrhage • Well-defined homogeneous mass in area of pancreas	• Chronic hemorrhage
Phlegmonous Pancreatitis		
See Acute pancreatitis (above)	• Hypoechoic, ill-defined mass	• Chronic hemorrhage
Pancreatic Abscess		
• Fever, chills • ↑ Leukocytosis • Hypotension • Tender abdomen	• Hypoechoic mass with smooth borders • Thick walls • Echo free to echogenic	• Acute pancreatitis • Chronic pancreatitis
Chronic Pancreatitis		
• Severe abdominal pain radiating to back • Malabsorption • Fatty stools • Signs of diabetes • Weight loss • Jaundice • ↑ Amylase and lipase	• Gland is small and fibrotic • Irregular borders • Mixed echogenicity • Dilated pancreatic duct (string of pearls sign with dilated duct) • Look for calculi within duct	• Acute pancreatitis • Thrombosis of portal system • Pancreatic pseudocyst • Dilated common bile duct
Pancreatic Pseudocyst		
• Asymptomatic unless large enough to put pressure on other organs • ↑ Amylase and lipase • ↑ Alkaline phosphatase if obstruction develops	• Well-defined mass, usually in area of pancreas • ↑ Through-transmission • Variable size (round or oval) • May have debris at bottom	• True cyst • Fluid-filled cystadenoma

Figure 8-24 Gross pathology of acute hemorrhagic pancreatitis. The pancreas has been completely obliterated by blood. (From Damjanov I, Linder J: *Pathology: a color atlas,* St. Louis, 2000, Mosby.)

Figure 8-25 Gross pathology of acute pancreatitis. The foci of fat necrosis appear as white opaque patches. (From Damjanov I, Linder J: *Pathology: a color atlas,* St. Louis, 2000, Mosby.)

than several days. The patient may be at risk for abscess and hemorrhage secondary to the pancreatitis (Figure 8-24).

An acute attack of pancreatitis is commonly related to biliary tract disease and alcoholism. The most common cause of pancreatitis in the United States is biliary tract disease. Gallstones are present in 40% to 60% of patients, and 5% of patients with gallstones have acute pancreatitis. Gallstone pancreatitis causes a relatively sudden onset of constant biliary pain. As the pancreatic parenchyma is further damaged, the pain becomes more severe and the abdomen becomes rigid and tender.

Alcohol abuse is the second most common cause of pancreatitis. Other less common causes include trauma, inflammation from adjacent peptic ulcer or abdominal infection, pregnancy, mumps, tumors, vascular thrombosis or embolism, and drugs.

The laboratory analysis of pancreatic enzymes (protease, lipase, and elastase) is the key to pancreatic destruction (see Table 8-4).

Acute pancreatitis may be severe. Damage to the acinar tissue and ductal system results in exudation of pancreatic juice into the interstitium of the gland, leakage of secretions into the peripancreatic tissues, or both (Figure 8-25). After the acini or duct disrupts, the secretions migrate to the surface of the gland. The common course is for fluid to break through the pancreatic connective tissue layer and thin posterior layer of the peritoneum and enter the lesser sac.

The pancreatic juice enters the anterior pararenal space by breaking through the thin layer of the fibrous connective tissue, or the fluid may migrate to the surface of the gland and remain within the confines of the fibrous connective tissue layer.

Collections of fluid in the peripancreatic area generally retain communication with the pancreas. A dynamic equilibrium is established so that fluid is continuously absorbed from the collection and replaced by additional pancreatic secretions. The drainage of juices may cease as the pancreatic inflammatory response subsides and the rate of pancreatic secretions returns to normal. The collections of extrapancreatic fluid

should be reabsorbed or, if drained, should not recur with recovery of proper drainage through the duct.

The symptoms begin with severe pain that usually occurs after a large meal or alcohol binge. The serum amylase value increases within 24 hours, whereas the serum lipase value increases within 72 to 94 hours and remains elevated for a period of time. (Note: the serum lipase takes a longer time to elevate, but remains elevated longer than the serum amylase value.) The disease may be mild and respond to medical therapy or it may progress to multisystem failure. Patients with acute pancreatitis may go on to develop other complications, such as pseudocyst formation (10%), phlegmon (18%), abscess (1% to 9%), hemorrhage (5%), or duodenal obstruction.

Sonographic Findings. In the early stages of acute pancreatitis the gland may not show swelling (Figure 8-26). When swelling does occur, the gland is hypoechoic to anechoic and is less echogenic than the liver because of the increased prominence of lobulations and congested vessels (Figure 8-27). The borders may be somewhat indistinct but smooth. On a longitudinal scan, the anterior compression of the inferior vena cava by the swollen head of the pancreas may be apparent. Thus pancreatic enlargement and decreased pancreatic echogenicity are sonographic landmarks for acute pancreatitis.

If localized enlargement is present, it may be difficult to separate from neoplastic involvement of the gland (Figure 8-28). Analysis of patient history and laboratory values should enable the clinician to make the distinction.

The pancreatic duct may be obstructed in acute pancreatitis as a result of inflammation, spasm, edema, swelling of the papilla, or pseudocyst formation. The detection of biliary obstruction is important as so many of the patients have coexisting liver disease. Obstruction of the biliary system may be due to stricture in the distal common duct or to compression of the common bile duct by a pseudocyst or inflammation of the head of the pancreas.

The alteration in the size and echogenic texture of the pancreas may be subtle; therefore, the diagnosis of pancreatitis may

Figure 8-26 A 45-year-old male presented with midepigastric pain, elevated amylase and lipase levels, and tenderness. The pancreas is diffusely enlarged representing acute pancreatitis. **A** and **B,** Transverse scans over the upper abdomen show the inflamed pancreatic tissue. *A,* Aorta; *IVC,* inferior vena cava; *P,* pancreas; *SV,* splenic vein.

Figure 8-27 A 29-year-old female presented with back pain, nausea, and vomiting for 1 week, and elevated lipase. The pancreas was found to be diffusely enlarged with decreased echogenicity representing pancreatitis. **A** and **B,** Transverse image. *A,* Aorta; *IVC,* inferior vena cava; *P,* pancreas; *SV,* splenic vein. **C** and **D,** Sagittal image. *IVC,* Inferior vena cava; *P,* pancreas; *SMV,* superior mesenteric vein; *SV,* splenic vein.

Figure 8-28 **A,** Gross specimen of an inflamed pancreas. **B,** A 37-year-old male patient with AIDS presented with pancreatitis, hepatosplenomegaly, and peripancreatic adenopathy. The pancreas is enlarged and slightly hypoechoic. *A,* Aorta; *IVC,* inferior vena cava; *P,* pancreas; *SV,* splenic vein. **C,** Sagittal scan of the enlarged pancreas *(P)* with adenopathy *(arrows).*

be based on the visualization of peripancreatic fluid collections in a patient with abnormal pancreatic enzymes and clinical history suggestive of pancreatitis. Fluid collections around the pancreatic bed, along the pararenal spaces, within Morison's pouch, and around the duodenum may be present in a patient with acute pancreatitis.

Acute pancreatitis in children. The pediatric pancreas is more easily seen because there is less body fat to interfere with visualization (Figure 8-29). Often the left lobe of the liver is more prominent and the gland is more isotonic than hyperechoic. In acute pancreatitis, the gland is increased in size with a hypoechoic pattern and an indistinct outline. Acute pancreatitis may result from trauma, drugs, infection, or congenital anomalies, or it may be familial or idiopathic.

Hemorrhagic Pancreatitis. Hemorrhagic pancreatitis is a rapid progression of acute pancreatitis with rupture of pancreatic vessels and subsequent hemorrhage (see Table 8-4). In hemorrhagic pancreatitis, there is diffuse enzymatic destruction of the pancreatic substance caused by a sudden escape of

active pancreatic enzymes into the glandular parenchyma (Figure 8-30). These enzymes cause focal areas of fat necrosis in and around the pancreas, which leads to rupture of pancreatic vessels and hemorrhage. Nearly half of these patients have sudden necrotizing destruction of the pancreas after an alcoholic binge or an excessively large meal.

Sonographic Findings. Specific sonographic findings depend on the age of the hemorrhage. A well-defined homogeneous mass in the area of the pancreas may be seen with areas of fresh necrosis (Figure 8-31). Foci of extravasated blood and fat necrosis are also seen. Further necrosis of the blood vessels results in the development of hemorrhagic areas referred to as Grey Turner's sign (discoloration of the flanks). At 1 week the mass may appear cystic with solid elements or septation. After several weeks the hemorrhage may appear cystic.

Phlegmonous Pancreatitis. A phlegmon is an inflammatory process that spreads along fascial pathways, causing localized areas of diffuse inflammatory edema of soft tissue that may proceed to necrosis and suppuration. Extension outside

Figure 8-29   A 9-year-old female presented with pancreatitis and a dilated common bile duct. **A,** Transverse scan of the pancreas *(P),* liver *(L),* and aorta *(Ao).* **B,** Sagittal scan of the dilated common bile duct *(calipers)* as it enters the pancreas *(P). L,* Liver.

Figure 8-30   Gross pathology of acute hemorrhagic pancreatitis. Hemorrhagic fat necrosis and a pseudocyst filled with blood are seen on cross section. (From Damjanov I, Linder J: *Pathology: a color atlas,* St. Louis, 2000, Mosby.)

Figure 8-31   Pancreatitis with hemorrhage. The gland is enlarged and echogenic secondary to freshly clotted blood. *L,* Liver; *P,* pancreas; *SMV,* superior mesenteric vein.

the gland occurs in 18% to 20% of patients with acute pancreatitis.

Sonographic Findings. The phlegmonous tissue appears hypoechoic with good through-transmission (Figure 8-32). The phlegmon usually involves the lesser sac, left anterior pararenal space, and transverse mesocolon. Less commonly, it involves the small bowel mesentery, lower retroperitoneum, and pelvis. See Table 8-4 for sonographic findings and differential considerations for phlegmonous pancreatitis.

Pancreatic Abscess.   Pancreatic abscess has a low incidence, although it is a serious complication of pancreatitis; the condition is related to the degree of tissue necrosis (see Table 8-4). The majority of patients develop abscess secondary to pancreatitis that develops from postoperative procedures. A

very high mortality rate is associated with this condition if left untreated. An abscess may rise from a neighboring infection, such as a perforated peptic ulcer, acute appendicitis, or acute cholecystitis. A pancreatic abscess may be unilocular or multilocular and can spread superiorly into the mediastinum, inferiorly into the transverse mesocolon, or down the retroperitoneum into the pelvis.

Sonographic Findings. A pancreatic abscess is imaged on ultrasound as a poorly defined hypoechoic mass with smooth or irregular thick walls, causing few internal echoes; it may be echo-free to echodense (Figure 8-33). The sonographic appearance depends on the amount of debris present. If air bubbles are present, an echogenic region with a shadow posterior is imaged.

Figure 8-32   Hemorrhagic phlegmon is a complication of pancreatitis. The phlegmon is ill-defined as it lies anterior to the kidney.

Figure 8-34   Gross pathology of chronic pancreatitis. The main pancreatic duct is dilated and contains calculi. The pancreatic acini have been replaced by fibrous tissue. (From Damjanov I, Linder J: *Pathology: a color atlas,* St. Louis, 2000, Mosby.)

Figure 8-33   Gross pathology of peritonitis complicating acute pancreatitis. The mesentery shows foci of fat necrosis and hemorrhage. Bloody ascites has already been removed. (From Damjanov I, Linder J: *Pathology: a color atlas,* St. Louis, 2000, Mosby.)

Chronic Pancreatitis. Chronic pancreatitis results from recurrent attacks of acute pancreatitis and causes continuing destruction of the pancreatic parenchyma (see Table 8-4). It generally is associated with chronic alcoholism or biliary disease, although patients with **hypercalcemia** (elevated calcium levels) and **hyperlipidemia** (elevated fat levels) are more predisposed to chronic pancreatitis. The chronic destructive process is progressive, resulting in fibrous scarring and loss of acinar cells. The pancreatic ducts become obstructed with a build-up of protein plugs with resultant calcifications along the duct.

Patients with chronic pancreatitis may have pseudocysts (20%), a dilated common bile duct, or thrombosis of the splenic vein with extension into the portal vein develop. Patients with chronic pancreatitis have an increased risk of developing pancreatic cancer.

On pathologic examination, the pancreas shows an increase in the interlobular fibrous tissue and chronic inflammatory infiltration changes. Stones of calcium carbonate may be found inside the ductal system, and pseudocysts are common (Figure 8-34). There is calcification of the gland in 20% to 40% of the patients.

Sonographic Findings. Chronic pancreatitis on ultrasound appears as a mixed pattern. The tissue may appear as a diffuse or localized involvement of the gland (Figure 8-35). Echogenicity of the pancreas is increased beyond normal because of fibrotic and fatty changes. The size of the gland is reduced and the borders are irregular, and the pancreatic duct may be dilated secondary to stricture or as the result of an extrinsic stone moving from a smaller pancreatic duct into a major duct. The classic sonographic finding is calcifications. With pancreatic ductal lithiasis, shadowing may be present. The most common site of obstruction is at the papilla. The incidence of carcinoma with pancreatic calcification is 25%.

INFLAMMATORY AND INFECTIOUS PANCREATIC LESIONS

Pancreatic Pseudocysts. Pancreatic and parapancreatic fluid collections are most often complications of pancreatitis. These fluid collections may resolve spontaneously, but those that do not are recognized as pseudocysts on imaging studies when the well-defined wall becomes visible. Pseudocysts are always acquired; they result from trauma to the gland or acute or chronic pancreatitis (see Table 8-4). In approximately 11% to 18% of patients with acute pancreatitis, a pseudocyst develops. A **pseudocyst** may be defined as a collection of fluid that arises from the loculation of inflammatory processes, necrosis, or hemorrhage (Figure 8-36). The pancreatic enzymes that escape the ductal system cause enzymatic digestion of the surrounding tissue and pseudocyst development. The walls of the pseudocyst form in the various potential spaces in which the escaped pancreatic enzymes are found. The pseudocyst usually creates few symptoms until it becomes large enough to cause pressure on the surrounding organs. Pseudocysts usually develop through the lesser omentum, displacing the stomach or widening the duodenal loop.

Locations of a pseudocyst. The most common location of a pseudocyst is in the lesser sac anterior to the pancreas and posterior to the stomach. The second most common location

Figure 8-35 Ultrasound patterns in chronic pancreatitis. **A,** Calcifications are seen along the body of the pancreas *(P)*. *L,* Liver; *SV,* splenic vein. **B,** The pancreas is shrunken in size. **C,** The pancreatic duct is enlarged.

Figure 8-36 Gross pathology of pancreatic pseudocyst filled with hemorrhagic fluid in the tail with extension into the hilum of the spleen. (From Damjanov I, Linder J: *Pathology: a color atlas,* St. Louis, 2000, Mosby.)

is in the anterior pararenal space (posterior to the lesser sac, bounded by Gerota's fascia). The spleen is the lateral border of the anterior pararenal space on the left. Fluid occurs more commonly in left pararenal space than the right. Sometimes the posterior pararenal space is fluid-filled; fluid spreads from the anterior pararenal space to the posterior pararenal space on the same side. Fluid may enter the peritoneal cavity via the foramen of Winslow or by disrupting the peritoneum in the anterior surface of the lesser sac. It may extend into the mediastinum by extending through the esophageal or aortic hiatus, or it may extend into small bowel mesentery or down into the retroperitoneum into the pelvis and groin.

A **pancreatic pseudocyst** develops when pancreatic enzymes escape from the gland and break down tissue to form a sterile abscess somewhere in the abdomen. Its walls are not true cyst walls; hence the name *pseudo-,* or false, cyst. Pseudocysts generally take on the contour of the available space around them and therefore are not always spherical, as are normal cysts. There may be more than one pseudocyst, so the sonographer should search for daughter collections.

Sonographic Findings. Sonographically, pseudocysts usually appear as well-defined masses with essentially sonolucent, echo-free interiors. Because of debris, scattered echoes may be seen at the bottom of the cysts, and increased through-transmission is present (Figure 8-37). The borders are very echogenic, and the cysts usually are thicker than other simple cysts. When a suspected pseudocyst is located near the stomach, the stomach should be drained so the cyst is not mistaken for a fluid-filled stomach. If the patient has been on continual drainage before the ultrasound examination, this problem is eliminated.

Figure 8-37 **A** through **C**, Ultrasound patterns of a typical pancreatic pseudocyst. *A,* Aorta; *F,* fluid; *L,* liver; *P,* pancreas; *PS,* pseudocyst.

Unusual sonographic patterns. A series of pseudocysts have been found to contain unusual internal echoes (Figure 8-38). There were three classifications: (1) septated, which presents with multiple internal septations; (2) excessive internal echoes, caused by an associated inflammatory mass, hemorrhage, or clot formation; and (3) pseudocyst, with absence of posterior enhancement caused by the rim of calcification.

Spontaneous rupture of a pseudocyst. Spontaneous rupture is the most common complication of a pancreatic pseudocyst, occurring in 5% of patients. In half of this 5%, drainage is directly into the peritoneal cavity. Clinical symptoms are sudden shock and peritonitis. The mortality rate is 50%. **Pancreatic ascites** occurs when the pancreatic pseudocyst ruptures into the abdomen. Pancreatic ascites that develops as a consequence of spontaneous rupture may be differentiated from pancreatic ascites associated with cirrhosis in patients who have known rupture of a pseudocyst by analysis of the fluid for elevated amylase and protein content (Figure 8-39).

In the other half of the 5% of patients, the rupture is into the gastrointestinal tract. Such patients may present a confusing picture sonographically. The initial scan shows a typical pattern for a pseudocyst formation, but the patient may have intense pain develop secondary to the rupture, and consequent examination shows the disappearance of the mass.

CYSTIC LESIONS OF THE PANCREAS

A wide variety of cystic lesions of the pancreas may be seen on imaging studies of the abdomen, but pseudocysts are the most common. Cystic neoplasms may be misdiagnosed as pseudocysts if careful analysis of the clinical history is not obtained. Ultrasound, CT, MRI, and ERCP are imaging modalities that are used to help narrow the differential diagnosis to aid the clinician in arriving at a diagnosis when correlated with clinical, pathologic, and laboratory findings. See Table 8-5 for clinical findings, sonographic findings, and differential considerations for pancreatic cysts.

Congenital Cystic Lesions of the Pancreas. Most congenital pancreatic cysts are multiple, and nearly all are associated with underlying congenital diseases that primarily affect other organ systems. Solitary congenital cysts are very rare.

Multiple Pancreatic Cysts

Autosomal dominant polycystic disease. Extrarenal cysts are most commonly found in the liver, but they may also be

Figure 8-38 Atypical ultrasound patterns of a pancreatic pseudocyst. **A,** Septations with low-level internal echoes. **B,** Excessive internal echoes. **C,** Calcification around the rim.

TABLE 8-5 CONGENITAL PANCREATIC LESIONS		
Clinical Findings	Sonographic Findings	Differential Considerations
Autosomal Dominant Polycystic Kidney Diseases		
• Asymptomatic, often found in patients with polycystic renal disease	• Well-defined mass with serous fluid • Size varies from microscopic to several centimeters	• Pseudocyst • Other cystic lesions of the pancreas
Von Hippel-Lindau Disease		
• Asymptomatic • Patients may have central nervous system and retinal hemangioblastomas, visceral cysts, pheochromocytomas, and renal cell carcinoma	• Well-defined mass with thick fluid; calcifications • Single or multiple • Size varies from microscopic to several centimeters	• Pseudocyst • Other cystic lesions of the pancreas
Cystic Fibrosis		
• Asymptomatic	• Well-defined mass with serous fluid • Size varies from microscopic to several centimeters	• Pseudocyst • Other cystic lesions of the pancreas
True Pancreatic Cysts		
• Asymptomatic, often found in infants	• Well-defined mass with serous fluid • Unilocular or multilocular	• Pseudocyst • Other cystic lesions of the pancreas

Figure 8-39 Gross pathology of a pancreatic pseudocyst rupture. (From Damjanov I, Linder J: *Pathology: a color atlas*, St. Louis, 2000, Mosby.)

Figure 8-40 Gross pathology of acute hemorrhagic pancreatitis. Hemorrhagic fat necrosis and a pseudocyst filled with blood are seen on cross-section. (From Damjanov I, Linder J: *Pathology: a color atlas*, St. Louis, 2000, Mosby.)

found in the pancreas, spleen, endometrium, ovaries, seminal vesicles, epididymis, and thyroid gland. The incidence of cysts increases with age. These cysts vary from microscopic to several centimeters in diameter and have an epithelial lining.

Von Hippel-Lindau disease. Von Hippel-Lindau disease is an autosomal dominant condition characterized by central nervous system and retinal hemangioblastomas, visceral cysts, pheochromocytomas, and renal cell carcinoma. Pancreatic cysts are found in 75% of cases at autopsy. Cysts vary in size from millimeters to centimeters. Other pancreatic lesions include microcystic adenomas, islet cell tumors, angiomas, and vascular neoplasms.

Cystic fibrosis. Cystic fibrosis is a hereditary disease that causes excessive production of thick mucus by the endocrine glands. The most common pancreatic abnormality found is fatty replacement of the pancreas, sometimes with calcifications. The cysts develop from inspissated mucin that obstructs the pancreatic ducts. The cysts are either single or multiple. Most are microscopic, but they can also be several centimeters in diameter.

Solitary pancreatic cysts. This category includes true cysts and lymphoepithelial cysts.

True cysts. True cysts are microscopic sacs that may be congenital or acquired. Congenital cysts are the result of anomalous development of the pancreatic duct and may be single, but are usually multiple and without septation. True pancreatic cysts rise from within the gland, more commonly in the head first, then in the body and tail. They have a lining epithelium, which may be lost with inflammation. The cysts contain pancreatic enzymes or may be found to be continuous with the pancreatic duct.

Both true cysts and pseudocysts may protrude anteriorly in any direction, although the true cyst is generally associated directly with the pancreatic area.

Lymphoepithelial cysts. These are very rare, usually found in middle-aged to elderly males. Lesions vary from 1 to 17 cm, have a squamous lining, and contain keratinous material.

EXOCRINE PANCREATIC LESIONS

See Table 8-6 for clinical findings, sonographic findings, and differential considerations for pancreatic tumors.

Adenocarcinoma. The most common primary neoplasm of the pancreas is adenocarcinoma. This fatal tumor involves the exocrine portion of the gland (ductal epithelium) and accounts for greater than 90% of all malignant pancreatic tumors (Figure 8-40). Pancreatic carcinoma accounts for approximately 5% of all cancer deaths and is the fourth most common cause of cancer-related mortality, after lung, breast, and colon cancer. It usually occurs in elderly males and less often in patients under 40.

The most frequent site of occurrence is in the head of the gland (60% to 70%), with 20% to 30% in the body and 5% to 10% in the tail (Figure 8-41). One fifth of the tumors are diffuse. Tumors in the pancreatic head present early, causing obstruction of the common bile duct with subsequent jaundice and subsequent hydrops of the gallbladder.

Sonographic Findings. The sonographic appearance of adenocarcinoma is the loss of the normal pancreatic parenchymal pattern (Figures 8-42 to 8-43). The lesions represent localized change in the echogenicity of the pancreas texture. The echo pattern is hypoechoic or less dense than the pancreas or liver. The borders become irregular and the pancreas may be enlarged. There may be secondary enlargement of the common duct resulting from edema or tumor invasion of the pancreatic head. Usually there is dilation of the pancreatic duct. The sonographer should look for metastatic spread into the liver, para-aortic nodes (abnormal displacement of the superior mesenteric artery), or portal venous system. The superior mesenteric vessels may be displaced posteriorly by the pancreatic mass; anterior displacement is present when the carcinoma is in the uncinate process, and posterior displacement is present when the tumor is in the head or body. A soft tissue thickening caused by neoplastic infiltration of perivascular lymphatics may be seen surrounding the celiac axis or superior mesenteric artery; this occurs more with carcinoma of the body and tail.

TABLE 8-6 PANCREATIC TUMOR FINDINGS

Clinical Findings	Sonographic Findings	Differential Considerations
Adenocarcinoma		
• Depends on size and location of tumor (Symptoms occur late if located in body or tail) • Weight loss • Decreased appetite • Nausea, vomiting • Stool changes • Pain radiating to back • Painless jaundice if tumor is located in the head (hydrops of GB—Courvoisier's sign) • Metastasizes to lymph nodes, liver, lungs, bone, duodenum, peritoneum, and adrenal glands	• Loss of normal pancreatic parenchyma • Hypoechoic poorly defined mass • Focal mass with irregular borders • Enlargement of pancreas • If mass is located in head of pancreas, look for hydrops, compression of IVC, and dilated ducts	• Pseudocyst • Cystadenoma • Lymphoma
Cystadenoma		
• ↑Amylase	• Anechoic mass with posterior enhancement • May have internal septa • Thick walls • Small size of tumor makes it difficult to image • Single or multiple • Occur in body and tail • Hypoechoic	• Pseudocyst • Metastases
Cystadenocarcinoma	**Differential Considerations**	
• Epigastric pain or palpable mass • Abdominal pain	• Irregular lobulated cystic tumor • Thick walls • Hypoechoic mass	• Pseudocyst • Cystadenoma • Adenocarcinoma • Islet cell tumor

Most patients have **obstructive jaundice** and anterior wall compression of the inferior vena cava when the tumor involves the head of the pancreas. A tumor in the tail can compress the splenic vein, producing secondary splenic enlargement. A tumor may displace or invade the splenic or portal vein or produce thrombosis.

CYSTIC PANCREATIC NEOPLASMS

The cystic neoplasms of the pancreas account for less than 5% of the pancreatic tumors. There are two types: microcystic adenoma and macrocystic adenoma. Microcystic adenoma (serous cystadenoma) is a rare, benign disease found more often in middle-aged and elderly females. The tumor is well circumscribed and usually consists of a large mass with multiple tiny cysts (Figure 8-44). Macrocystic adenoma (mucinous cystadenoma/cystadenocarcinoma) may be either malignant or benign with a malignant potential. It occurs predominantly in middle-aged females, usually in the body or tail. It typically comprises well-defined cysts containing thick mucinous fluid, internal septations, or mural nodules.

Mucinous Adenocarcinoma (Colloid Carcinoma). Adenocarcinoma is by far the most common pancreatic neoplasm. Mucinous adenocarcinoma is an uncommon variant of adenocarcinoma. This neoplasm produces a large volume of mucin that results in a cystic appearance on imaging studies.

Other findings include tumor calcification and inspissated mucin or tumor obstructing bile ducts. The prognosis is poor.

Microcystic Adenoma (Cystadenoma, Serous Adenoma, Glycogen-Rich Adenoma). Microcystic adenoma is a rare benign lesion of the pancreas that is found most frequently in women in the seventh decade. The microcystic adenoma is one of the pancreatic lesions found in von Hippel-Lindau disease. The cysts can be either single or multiple and can involve any part of the pancreas. Most of the cysts are smaller than 2 cm in diameter. On ultrasound examination, the lesions may appear cystic, solid, or even echogenic if the cysts are very small. A minority of the cysts have an echogenic central stellate scar that may have calcification. It is difficult to differentiate a benign microcystic adenoma from a malignant mucinous cystic tumor without pathologic confirmation.

Sonographic Findings. The coarsely lobulated cystic tumors sometimes present sonographically with cyst walls thicker than the membranes between multilocular cysts (Figures 8-45 and 8-46). These cystic neoplasms look similar to pseudocysts and may have one of the following four ultrasound patterns:

1. Anechoic mass with posterior enhancement and irregular margins
2. Anechoic mass with internal homogeneous echoes

A   B

C

Figure 8-41   Fifty-two-year-old female with mucinous adenoma of the appendix with increased alkaline phosphatase. **A** and **B,** Transverse images of the pancreas demonstrate a rounded hypoechoic lesion within the body of the gland. This lesion may represent a metastatic focus to the gland. Color Doppler shows no sign of flow to the lesion. **C,** The gallbladder is markedly heterogeneous with a thickened wall. This may represent metastatic tumor.

3. Anechoic mass with irregular internal vegetations protruding into the lumen and showing no movement
4. Completely echogenic mass with inhomogeneous pattern

Mucinous Cystic Tumor (Cystadenoma, Cystadenocarcinoma, Macrocystic Adenoma). This lesion is more common in women in the fifth and sixth decades. Lesions may be premalignant to malignant. The overall survival if the lesion is intact is better than with adenocarcinoma. This is an uncommon, slow-growing tumor that rises from the ducts as a cystic neoplasm. It consists of a large cyst with or without septations and has a significant malignant potential. Patients present with epigastric pain or a palpable mass. Many patients have concurrent diseases: diabetes, calculous disease of biliary tract, or arterial hypertension. It occurs more commonly in the tail and body, with 60% in the tail, 35% in the body, and 5% in the head of the pancreas. Frequently, foci of calcification may be seen within the pancreas.

Cystadenocarcinoma may be difficult to separate from carcinoma arising from a true cyst or cystic degeneration of a solid carcinoma. It is an irregular, lobulated cystic tumor with thick cellular walls. Metastases rise most commonly in the lymph nodes and liver (see Figure 8-47). The course of this tumor may be slowly progressive with a tendency for the recurrent disease to remain localized.

Intraductal Papillary Mucinous Tumor (Ductectatic Cystadenoma, Cystadenocarcinoma, Ductectatic Mucinous Tumor). This slow-growing lesion affects both men and women in the sixth and seventh decades. Clinical symptoms of abdominal pain are accompanied by an elevated serum amylase level, so pancreatitis is a differential. The main pancreatic duct may include chronic pancreatitis as a differential. On ultrasound, a dilated pancreatic duct may be seen with dilatation so great that it resembles tiny cysts.

ENDOCRINE PANCREATIC NEOPLASMS

These endocrine tumors rise from the islet cells of the pancreas. There are several types of islet cell tumors; they may be functional or nonfunctional. The tumors may be classified as benign

Figure 8-42 Adenocarcinoma of the pancreas. **A,** Transverse image; arrow points to the hypoechoic abnormal tissue in the head of the pancreas. **B,** Sagittal image of the dilated pancreatic duct *(crossbars)*. **C,** Transverse image of a dilated pancreatic duct *(arrows)* measuring more than 3 mm in a patient with a large mass *(M)* in the head of the gland.

adenomas or malignant tumors. Nonfunctioning islet cell tumors comprise one third of all islet cell tumors, with 92% being malignant. The growth rate is very slow and they usually do not spread beyond the regional lymph nodes and the liver.

The most common functioning islet cell tumor is insulinoma (60%) followed by gastrinoma (18%). The tumor size is small (1 to 2 cm), and they are well encapsulated with a good vascular supply (Figure 8-47). A large percentage of insulinoma tumors occur in patients with hyperinsulinism and hypoglycemia. Most gastrinomas are malignant, with up to 40% appearing with metastatic disease at the time of diagnosis.

These endocrine tumors may be isolated or associated with the multiple endocrine neoplasia syndrome type 1 (MEN 1), which is characterized by the triad of parathyroid, pituitary, and pancreatic lesions. The lesions may be solitary, multiple, or diffuse.

Insulinoma. Insulinoma is the most common functioning islet cell tumor. The clinical triad is fasting hypoglycemia, symptoms of hypoglycemia, and immediate relief of symptoms

after the administration of IV glucose. Clinical symptoms include palpitations, headache, confusion, pallor, sweating, slurred speech, and coma. A small percent of insulinomas are multiple, 10% are malignant, and 10% of patients have hyperplasia rather than neoplasia. Most of the insulinomas are small and hypervascular. Some of the lesions contain calcification.

Gastrinoma. Gastrinoma is the second most common functioning islet cell tumor. These lesions usually affect young adults who have peptic ulcer disease (when ulcers are recurrent, intractable, multiple, or in unusual locations). Diarrhea is common due to the increased gastrin on the small bowel. Gastrinomas are frequently multiple, extrapancreatic, difficult to locate, and malignant.

Sonographic Findings. Sonographically, islet cell tumors are difficult to image because of their small size. The greatest success is when they are located in the head of the pancreas. The tumors may be multiple and occur mostly in the body and tail, where there is the greatest concentration of Langerhans islets (Figure 8-48).

Figure 8-43   Adenocarcinoma of the pancreas. **A,** Transverse image of the pancreas with a hypoechoic mass in the head (*A* marks first caliper measurement; *B* marks second caliper measurement). **B,** The pancreatic duct is prominent; the mass is still present in the head of the pancreas. The common bile duct is dilated, measuring 13 mm. **C,** Sagittal image of the dilated common duct as it flows posterior to the head of the pancreas. *A,* Aorta. **D,** Dilated gallbladder with sludge. **E,** Magnified transverse image of the head of the pancreas and the dilated common bile duct. *A,* Aorta.

Figure 8-44   Gross pathology of serous cystadenoma. **A,** Well-circumscribed tumor. **B,** Tumor appears microcystic. (From Damjanov I, Linder J: *Pathology: a color atlas,* St. Louis, 2000, Mosby.)

Figure 8-45   A 65-year-old patient with cystadenoma in the head of the pancreas that is not causing obstruction of the pancreatic duct. **A,** Transverse image of the pancreas *(P),* pancreatic duct *(arrows),* splenic vein *(SV),* superior mesenteric artery *(a),* left renal vein *(LRV),* and aorta *(A).* **B,** Large mass *(M)* in the head of the pancreas seen compressing the inferior vena cava *(IVC).*

Figure 8-46   Pancreatic cystadenoma was found in the body of the pancreas in this 53-year-old female.

Figure 8-47   Gross specimen of a pancreatic mass *(M)* in the tail of the gland. *P,* Pancreas; *SP,* spleen.

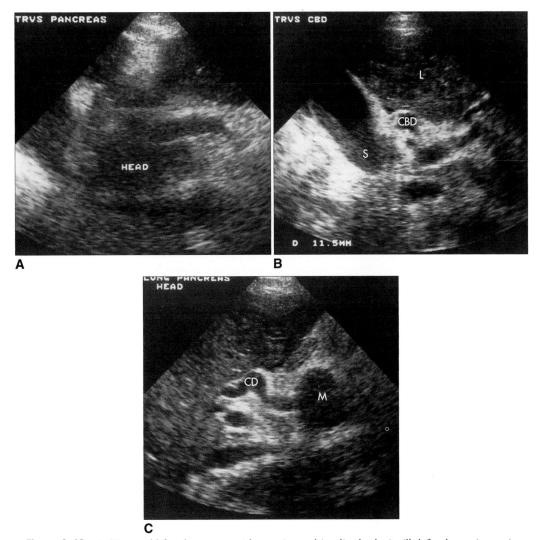

Figure 8-48 A 46-year-old female presents with sweating and insulin shock. An ill-defined mass is seen in the head of the pancreas, compressing the common bile duct. This was an islet cell tumor of the pancreas. **A,** Transverse scan of the head of the pancreas shows the irregularly margined mass. **B,** The dilated common bile duct *(CBD)* measures 11.5 mm. The distended gallbladder is half filled with sludge *(S). L,* Liver. **C,** Sagittal scan of the distended common duct *(CD)* and mass *(M)* in the head of the pancreas.

METASTATIC DISEASE TO THE PANCREAS

Generally speaking, metastasis to the pancreas is uncommon, but has been reported to be found in 10% of patients with cancer. Primaries that can metastasize to the pancreas include melanomas, breast, gastrointestinal, and lung tumors.

PARAPANCREATIC NEOPLASMS

Lymphomas are malignant neoplasms that rise from the lymphoid tissues. They are the most frequent parapancreatic neoplasm. It may be difficult to separate a parapancreatic lymphadenopathy from a primary lesion in the pancreas. An intraabdominal lymphoma may appear as a hypoechoic mass or with necrosis, a cystic mass in the pancreas (Figure 8-49). The superior mesenteric vessels may be displaced anterior instead of posterior as seen with a primary pancreatic mass.

Multiple nodes are seen along the pancreas, duodenum, porta hepatis, and superior mesenteric vessels; they may be difficult to distinguish from a pancreatic mass. The enlarged nodes appear hypoechoic and well defined.

Other types of retroperitoneal neoplasms that may appear as a cystic lesion near the area of the pancreas include lymphangiomas, paragangliomas, cystic teratomas, and metastases. The lymphangiomas are most often thin-walled, homogeneous, small cysts, but they have also been seen to have septa, thick walls, calcification, and internal debris. The paragangliomas are usually found near the inferior mesenteric artery or near the kidney. The cystic teratomas are found more frequently in children and young adults. Their appearance is a mixed sonographic pattern of cystic, solid, fat, and calcifications.

Figure 8-49 Patient with lymphoma who presented with epigastric pain. Multiple nodes *(calipers)* were seen in the peripancreatic area. *AO,* Aorta; *IVC,* inferior vena cava.

SELECTED BIBLIOGRAPHY

Carpenter SL, Scheiman JM: Pancreatic imaging, *Curr Opin Gastroenterol* 12:442, 1996.

Demos TC, Posniak HV, Harmath C and others: Cystic lesions of the pancreas, *AJR* 179:1375-1388, 2002.

DingH and others: Sonographic diagnosis of pancreatic islet cell tumor: value of intermittent harmonic imaging, *J Clin Ultrasound* 29:411-416, 2001.

Filly RA, Freimanis AK: Echographic diagnosis of pancreatic lesions, *Radiology* 96:575, 1970.

Filly RA, London SS: The normal pancreas: acoustic characteristics and frequency of imaging, *J Clin Ultrasound* 7:121, 1979.

Grogan JR, SaeianK, Taylor AJ and others: Marking sense of mucin-producing pancreatic tumors, *AJR* 176:921-929, 2001.

Grube J: *"Epigastric pain" in clinical guide to ultrasonography by Charlotte Henningsen,* St Louis, 2004, Mosby.

Gumaste VV, Pitchumoni CS: Pancreatic pseudocyst, *Gastroenterologist* 4:33, 1996.

Hadidi A: Pancreatic duct diameter: sonographic measurement in normal subjects, *J Clin Ultrasound* 11:17, 1983.

Kim YH, Auh YH, Kim KW and others: Lymphoepithelial cyst of the pancreas: CT and sonographic findings, *Abdom Imaging* 23:185-187, 1998.

Laing FC and others: Atypical pseudocysts of the pancreas: an ultrasonographic evaluation, *J Clin Ultrasound* 7:27, 1979.

Leopold GR, Berk RN, Reinke RT: Echographic-radiological documentation of spontaneous rupture of a pancreatic pseudocyst into the duodenum, *Radiology* 120:699, 1972.

Lim JH, Lee G, Oh YL: Radiologic spectrum of intraductal papillary mucinous tumor of the pancreas, *RadioGraphics* 21:323-337, 2001.

Lundstedt C, Dawiskiba S: Serous and mucinous cystadenomas/cystadenocarcinomas of the pancreas, *Abdomn Imaging* 25:201-206, 2000.

Marks WM, Filly RA, Callen PW: Ultrasonic evaluation of normal pancreatic echogenicity and its relationship to fat deposition, *Radiology* 137:475, 1980.

Megibow AJ, Lavelle MT, Rofsky NM: Cystic tumors of the pancreas: the radiologist, *Surg Clin North Am* 81:489-495, 2001.

Middleton WD and Kurtz AB: *Ultrasound, the requisites,* St Louis, 2004, Mosby.

Morgan DE, Baron TH: Practical imaging in acute pancreatitis, *Semin Gastrointest Dis* 9:41, 1998.

Neumyer MM: Ultrasonographic assessment of renal and pancreatic transplants, *J Vasc Technol* 19:321, 1995.

Nicolau C, Torra R, Bianchi L and others: Abdominal sonographic study of autosomal dominant polycystic disease, *J Clin Ultrasound* 28:277-282, 2000.

Patti MG, Pellegrini CA: Gallstone pancreatitis, *Surg Clin North Am* 70:1277, 1990.

Ralls PW and others: Color flow sonography in evaluating the resectability of periampullary and pancreatic tumors, *J Ultrasound Med* 16:131, 1997.

Riker A, Libutti SK, Bartlett DL: Advances in the early detection, diagnosis, and staging of pancreatic cancer, *Surg Oncol* 6:157, 1997.

Scott J and others: Mucinous cystic neoplasm of the pancreas: imaging features and diagnostic difficulties, *Clin Radiolo* 55:187-192, 2000.

Stott MA and others: Ultrasound of the common bile duct in patients undergoing cholecystectomy, *J Clin Ultrasound* 19:73, 1991.

Swobodnik W and others: Ultrasound characteristics of the pancreas in children with cystic fibrosis, *J Clin Ultrasound* 13:469, 1985.

Todd KE, Reber HA: Pancreatic neoplasms, *Curr Opin Gastroenterol* 12:436, 1996.

Ueno N and others: Contrast enhanced color Doppler ultrasonography in diagnosis of pancreatic tumor, *J Ultra Med* 15:527, 1996.

Weighall SL, Wolfman NT, Watson N: The fluid-filled stomach: a new sonic window, *J Clin Ultrasound* 7:353, 1979.

Yassa NA and others: Gray-scale and color flow sonography of pancreatic ductal adenocarcinoma, *J Clin Ultrasound* 25:473, 1997.

CHAPTER 9

The Gastrointestinal Tract

Sandra L. Hagen-Ansert

OBJECTIVES

- Describe the anatomy and relational landmarks of the gastrointestinal system
- Discuss the size of wall thickness and diameters of the gastrointestinal tract
- Describe the sonographic technique used to image the gastrointestinal tract
- Differentiate the sonographic appearances of the following conditions or diseases: duplication cyst, bezoar, benign tumor, malignant tumor, obstruction, appendicitis, mucocele, Meckel's diverticulitis, and Crohn's disease
- Describe the sonographic technique used to image the appendix

KEY TERMS

abscess – localized collection of pus surrounded by inflamed tissue

absorption – process of nutrient molecules passing through wall of intestine into blood or lymph system

alimentary tract – also known as the digestive tract; includes the mouth, pharynx, esophagus, stomach, duodenum, and small and large intestine

appendicolith – a fecalith or calcification located in the appendix

ascites – free fluid in the abdomen

cardiac orifice – entrance of the esophagus into the stomach

cholecystokinin – hormone released by the presence of fat in the intestine; regulates gallbladder contraction and gastric emptying

Crohn's disease – inflammation of the bowel, accompanied by abscess and bowel wall thickening

diverticulum – a pouch-like herniation through the muscular wall of a tubular organ that occurs in the stomach, the small intestine, or most commonly, the colon

duodenal bulb – first part of the duodenum

fecalith – calculus that may form around fecal material associated with appendicitis

gastrin – endocrine hormone released from the stomach (stimulates secretion of gastric acid)

gastrohepatic ligament – helps support the lesser curvature of the stomach

gastrophrenic ligament – helps support the greater curvature of the stomach

gastrosplenic ligament – helps support the greater curvature of the stomach

greater omentum – known as the "fatty apron" double fold of the peritoneum attached to the duodenum, stomach, and large intestine; helps support the greater curve of the stomach

haustra – normal segmentation of the wall of the colon

hemorrhage – collection of blood

hepatic flexure – ascending colon rises from the right lower quadrant to bend at this point to form the transverse colon

lesser omentum – suspends the stomach and duodenum from the liver; helps to support the lesser curvature of the stomach

lienorenal ligament – helps support the greater curvature of the stomach

lymphoma – malignancy of the lymph nodes, spleen, or liver

McBurney's point – located by drawing a line from the right anterosuperior iliac spine to the umbilicus; at approximately the midpoint of this line lies the root of the appendix

McBurney's sign – site of maximal tenderness in the right lower quadrant; usually with appendicitis

Meckel's diverticulum – congenital sac or blind pouch found in the lower portion of the ileum

mesentery – projects from the parietal peritoneum and attaches to the small intestine, anchoring it to the posterior abdominal wall

mesothelium – fifth layer of bowel

mucosa – first layer of bowel

muscularis – third layer of bowel

paralytic ileus – dilated fluid-filled bowel loops without peristalsis

peristalsis – rhythmic dilatation and contraction of the gastrointestinal tract as food is propelled through it

polyp – a small tumorlike growth that projects from a mucous membrane surface

pyloric canal – muscle that connects the stomach to the proximal duodenum

rugae – inner folds of the stomach wall

secretin – released from small bowel as antacid; stimulates secretion of bicarbonate

serosa – fourth layer of bowel; thin, loose layer of connective tissue, surrounded by mesothelium covering the intraperitoneal bowel loops

splenic flexure – the transverse colon travels horizontally across the abdomen and bends at this point to form the descending colon

submucosa – one of the layers of the bowel, under the mucosal layer; contains blood vessels and lymph channels

target sign – characteristic of gastrointestinal wall thickening consisting of an echogenic center and a hypoechoic rim

valvulae conniventes – normal segmentation of the small bowel

villi – inner folds of the small intestine

The gastrointestinal tract may be difficult to image with ultrasound in most patients unless they ingest fluids or some other acoustic transmittable contrast agent. Many laboratories have begun to investigate various contrast agents in pursuit of the ideal medium for imaging the stomach, duodenum, small bowel, and colon.

ANATOMY OF THE GASTROINTESTINAL TRACT

NORMAL ANATOMY

The digestive tract, also known as the **alimentary tract,** is a long tube (about 8 m long) extending from the mouth to the anus (Figure 9-1). The gastrointestinal tract is that part of the digestive system below the diaphragm. The sequential parts of the digestive system include the mouth, pharynx, esophagus, stomach, small intestine (duodenum, jejunum, and ileum), and large intestine (cecum, ascending colon, transverse colon, descending colon, and rectum). Three types of accessory digestive glands—the salivary glands, liver, and pancreas—secrete digestive juices into the digestive system.

Esophagus. The esophagus extends from the pharynx through the thoracic cavity, then passes through the diaphragm and empties into the stomach (see Figure 9-1). The lower end of the esophagus is a circular muscle that acts as a sphincter, constricting the tube so that the entrance to the stomach, at the **cardiac orifice,** is generally closed. This helps to prevent gastric acid from moving up into the esophagus.

Stomach. The stomach is a large, smooth, muscular organ that has two surfaces: the lesser curvature and greater curvature (Figure 9-2). The stomach is divided into three parts: the fundus is found in the superior aspect, the body comprises the major central axis, and the pylorus is the lower aspect. The pylorus is further subdivided into the antrum, the pyloric canal, and the pyloric sphincter. The **pyloric canal** is a muscle that connects the stomach to the proximal duodenum.

Supporting ligaments of the greater curvature of the stomach include: the **greater omentum,** the **gastrophrenic ligament,** the **gastrosplenic ligament,** and the **lienorenal ligament.** The ligaments that support the lesser curvature of the stomach include the **gastrohepatic ligament** of the **lesser omentum.** Folds of the **mucosa** and **submucosa** are called **rugae.**

Small Intestine. The small intestine is a long coiled tube about 5 m long by 4 cm in diameter (see Figure 9-1). The first 22 cm is the duodenum, which is curved like the letter C. The duodenum is subdivided into four segments: (1) superior, (2) descending, (3) transverse, and (4) ascending (Figure 9-3). The first part of the duodenum is not attached to the mesentery; the remainder of the small intestine, including the rest of the duodenum, is attached to the mesentery. The **mesentery** projects from the parietal peritoneum and attaches to the small intestine to anchor it to the posterior abdominal wall.

The first part of the duodenum begins at the pylorus and terminates at the neck of the gallbladder, posterior to the left lobe of the liver and medial to the gallbladder. The **duodenal bulb** is peritoneal, supported by the hepatoduodenal ligament, and passes anterior to the common bile duct, gastroduodenal artery, common hepatic artery, hepatic portal vein, and head of the pancreas.

The second part (descending) of the duodenum is retroperitoneal and runs parallel, posterior, and to the right of the spine. The transverse colon crosses anterior to the middle third of the descending duodenum. The pancreatic head is medial to the duodenum at this point. The common bile duct joins the pancreatic duct to enter the ampulla of Vater.

The third part (transverse) of the duodenum begins at the right of the fourth lumbar vertebra and passes anterior to the aorta, inferior vena cava, and crura of the diaphragm. The superior mesenteric vessels course anterior to the duodenum.

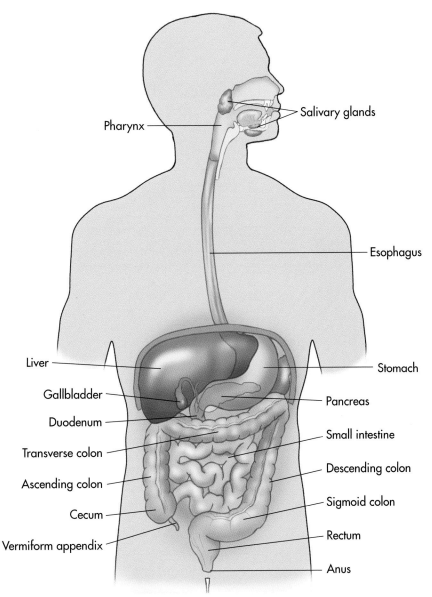

Figure 9-1 The digestive system includes the mouth, pharynx, esophagus, stomach, small intestine, large intestine, rectum, and anus.

The fourth part (ascending) of the duodenum ascends superiorly to the left of the spine and aorta to the second lumbar vertebra, where it joins the proximal jejunum (duodenojejunal flexure). This portion lies on the left crus of the diaphragm. It is held in place by the ligament of Treitz (which courses from the left toward the right crus of the diaphragm).

As the tube turns downward, it is called the jejunum; the jejunum extends for about 2 m before becoming the ileum. The inner wall of the small intestine is marked by circular folds of the mucous membrane, **villi.** The **valvulae conniventes** are large folds of mucous membrane that project into the lumen of the bowel and help retard the passage of food to provide greater absorption. The lower part of the small intestine is the ileum. The ileocecal orifice marks the entry into the large intestine and prevents food from reentering the small intestine.

Large Intestine. The large intestine is larger in diameter and shorter in length than the small intestine. The vermiform appendix; cecum; ascending, transverse, and descending colon; rectum; and anus all comprise the large intestine (see Figure 9-1). The colon is divided into segments called **haustra.** The ascending colon extends from the cecum vertically to the lower part of the liver. It turns horizontally at the **hepatic flexure** and moves to become the transverse colon. On the left side of the abdomen, at the **splenic flexure,** it then descends vertically to become the descending colon and eventually the sigmoid colon, which empties into the rectum. The rectum is 12 cm long, terminating at the anus.

The mucosa of the large intestine lacks villi and produces no digestive enzymes. The surface epithelium consists of cells specialized for absorption and goblet cells that secrete mucus.

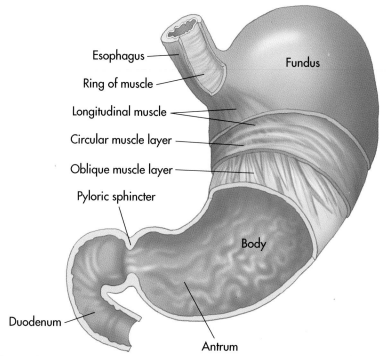

Figure 9-2   Food enters the stomach after leaving the esophagus through the gastroesophageal junction at the level of the diaphragm. The three parts of the stomach (fundus, body, and antrum) are shown. Food leaves the stomach through the pylorus and pyloric sphincter to enter the duodenum.

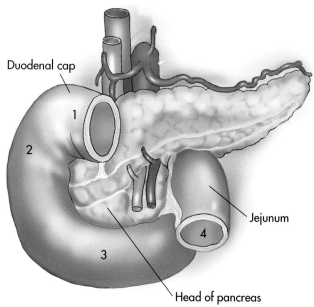

Figure 9-3   The duodenal cap is an excellent landmark for the head of the pancreas. The duodenum is divided into four sections. See text for explanation. (The fourth part of the duodenum is posterior to the jejunum).

VASCULAR ANATOMY

Esophagus. The arteries that supply the esophagus rise from the high, mid, and lower sections of this muscular tube. The inferior thyroid branch of the subclavian artery supplies the upper esophagus, the descending thoracic aorta supplies the midesophagus, and the gastric branch of the celiac axis and the left inferior phrenic artery of the abdominal aorta supply the lower end of the esophagus. Varices may be seen to rise from the gastroesophageal arteries (Figure 9-4).

Stomach. Vascular supply to the stomach is supplied by the right gastric arterial branch, pyloric and right gastroepiploic branches of the hepatic artery, left gastroepiploic branch and vasa brevia of the splenic artery, and left gastric artery (see Figure 9-4). The venous system of the stomach is parallel to the arterial vessels, which drain into the portal venous system.

Small Intestine. The **mesentery** outlines the small intestine and contains the superior mesenteric vessels, nerves, lymphatic glands, and fat between its two layers. The celiac axis supplies the duodenum through its right gastric, gastroduodenal, and superior pancreaticoduodenal branches (Figure 9-5). The superior mesenteric artery has multiple branches to the small bowel, which include the inferior pancreaticoduodenal, jejunal, and ileal arteries. The venous system parallels the arterial system and empties into the portal venous system.

Large Intestine. The celiac, superior mesenteric, and inferior mesenteric arteries supply both the small and large intestine. The superior mesenteric arterial branches include the ileocolic, the right colic, and the middle colic arteries (see Figure 9-5). The inferior mesenteric artery supplies the intestine from the left border of the transverse colon to the rectum, rising from the anterior surface of the abdominal aorta at the level of the third lumbar vertebra and descending

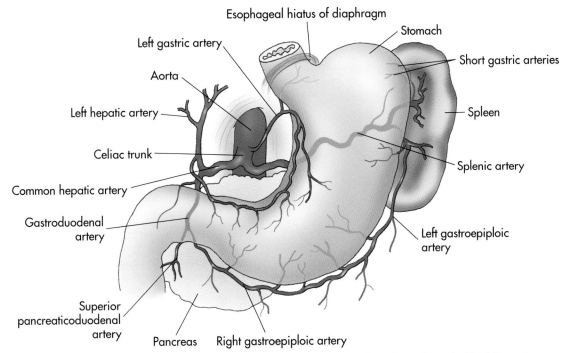

Figure 9-4 Vascular supply to the stomach is received from the branches of the celiac axis. The left gastric artery supplies the lower third of the esophagus and upper right part of the stomach. The right gastric artery supplies the lower right part of the stomach. The short gastric arteries supply the fundus. The left gastroepiploic artery supplies the upper part of the greater curvature of the stomach, and the right gastroepiploic artery supplies the lower part of the greater curvature of the stomach.

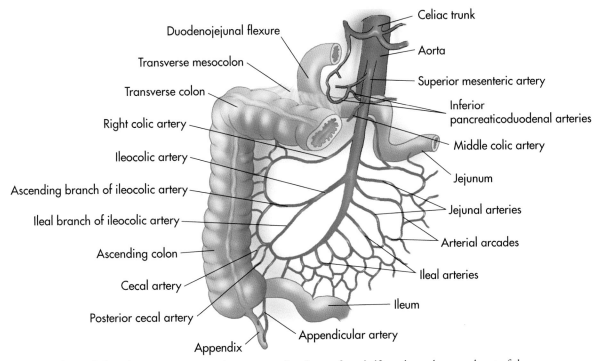

Figure 9-5 The superior mesenteric artery supplies the gut from halfway down the second part of the duodenum to the distal third of the transverse colon.

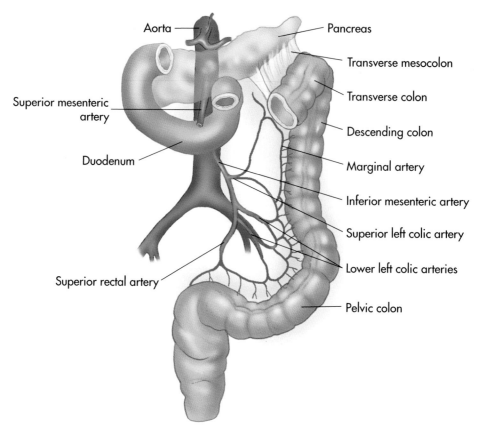

Aorta

Pancreas

Transverse mesocolon

Superior mesenteric
artery

Transverse colon

Descending colon

Duodenum

Marginal artery

Inferior mesenteric artery

Superior left colic artery

Lower left colic arteries

Superior rectal artery

Pelvic colon

Figure 9-6   The inferior mesenteric artery supplies the large bowel from the distal third of the transverse colon to halfway down the anal canal. It forms an anastomosis with the middle colic branch of the superior mesenteric artery.

retroperitoneally (Figure 9-6). Branches of the inferior mesenteric artery include the left colic, sigmoid, and superior rectal arteries. The venous system parallels the arterial system and empties into the portal venous system.

PHYSIOLOGY AND LABORATORY DATA OF THE GASTROINTESTINAL TRACT

Digestion and absorption are the primary functions of the gastrointestinal tract. In fact, the gastrointestinal tract is the largest endocrine organ in the body.

Food is ingested through the mouth, chewed, and swallowed. The molecules of food must be further digested, or mechanically broken down, and chemically split into small molecules. The chemical digestion of food breaks down long-chain organic molecules (i.e., polysaccharides or proteins). Each reaction is carried on with the help of a specific enzyme produced by cells of the digestive tract or its accessory glands. When these particles are small enough, the nutrient molecules pass through the wall of the intestine into the blood or lymph system by **absorption.**

The nutrients are transported to the liver after being absorbed by the blood; the liver processes and stores the nutrients. The remaining nutrients in the blood are transported to cells throughout the body. The undigested and unabsorbed food is eliminated from the digestive tract by the process of defecation.

When food enters the stomach, the rugae gradually smooth out, causing the stomach to stretch and increase its capacity for food intake. Contractions of the stomach help to mix the food. The three layers of smooth muscle in the wall enable the stomach to mash and churn food and move it along with **peristalsis.** Large amounts of mucus are secreted in the stomach. Gastric glands secrete gastric juice containing hydrochloric acid and enzymes.

Over a 3- to 4-hour period, food is converted into chyme. This soupy mixture is moved toward the pylorus and into the small intestine. Small amounts of water, salts, and lipid-soluble substances, such as alcohol, are absorbed through the stomach mucosa, with little absorption taking place in the stomach. The pyloric sphincter is a strong band of muscle that relaxes at the time necessary to release the food.

The villi within the small intestine increase its surface area for digestion and absorption of nutrients; otherwise food would move quickly through the intestine without time for absorption. The intestinal glands are found between the villi and secrete large amounts of fluid that serve as a medium for digestion and absorption of nutrients. The hormone **gastrin,** which is released by the stomach mucosa, stimulates the gastric glands to secrete. Most of the digestion occurs within the duodenum. Bile and enzymes from the liver and pancreas are secreted into the duodenum to act on the chyme and break down the food particles for absorption. The intestinal glands are stimulated to release their fluid mainly by local reflexes initiated when the small intestine is distended by chyme.

Other gastrointestinal hormones include **cholecystokinin** and **secretin.** Cholecystokinin is released by the presence of fat in the intestine and regulates gallbladder contraction and gastric emptying. Secretin is released from the small bowel to stimulate the secretion of bicarbonate to decrease the acid content of the intestine.

A period of 1 to 3 days or longer may be required for the journey through the large intestine. Bacteria within the large intestine devour the chyme and in turn produce vitamins that can be absorbed and used by the body. Most of the absorption process of sodium and water occurs in the cecum. Sodium is absorbed by active transport and water follows by osmosis.

The most common laboratory data the sonographer may come across in a patient with gastrointestinal disease relate to the presence of blood in the stool. Anemia may be present as a result of chronic blood loss. Blood in the stool indicates the presence of a bleed somewhere in the gastrointestinal system. Infection would show elevation of the white blood count. An increase in the carcinoembryonic antigen is found in patients with inflammatory bowel disease.

Clinical signs and symptoms of nausea, vomiting, and diarrhea are common with gastrointestinal problems. Abdominal pain and fever may also be present with gastrointestinal conditions, such as colitis, bowel **abscess,** acute diverticulitis, and appendicitis.

SONOGRAPHIC EVALUATION OF THE GASTROINTESTINAL TRACT

Visualization of the gastrointestinal tract with ultrasound may be difficult because intraluminal air is echogenic. The scattering and reflection effect of gas in the gastrointestinal tract often produces an incomplete or mottled distal acoustic shadow. The rim of lucency represents the wall (i.e., intima, media, and serosa), and its periserosal fat produces the outer echogenic border of the tract wall.

There are five layers of the bowel wall (Box 9-1). The odd-numbered walls (first, third, and fifth) are echogenic, and the even-numbered walls (second and fourth) are hypoechoic, with an average total thickness of 3 mm if distended and 5 mm if undistended.

The technique used to observe the upper gastrointestinal tract is for the patient to drink 10 to 40 oz of water through a straw after a baseline ultrasound study of the upper abdomen. The straw helps prevent ingestion of excess air when the water is consumed. The patient should be in an upright position for the examination; this causes air in the stomach to rise to the fundus of the stomach and not interfere with the ultrasound beam (Figure 9-7). The lower gastrointestinal tract requires no preparation. To image the lower colon, it may be useful to give the patient a water enema in order to help better delineate the colon.

BOX 9-1   LAYERS OF BOWEL

1. **Mucosa:** Directly contacts the intraluminal contents; lined with epithelial folds; echogenic
2. **Submucosa:** Contains blood vessels and lymph channels
3. **Muscularis:** Contains circular and longitudinal bands of fiber
4. **Serosa:** Thin, loose layer of connective tissue
5. **Mesothelium:** Covers intraperitoneal bowel loops

STOMACH

The gastroesophageal junction is seen on the sagittal scan to the left of the midline as a bulls-eye or target-shaped structure anterior to the aorta, posterior to the left lobe of the liver, and inferior to the hemidiaphragm (Figure 9-8). The left lobe of the patient's liver must be large enough to be able to image the gastroesophageal junction.

The gastric antrum can be seen as a target shape in the midline (Figure 9-9). The remainder of the stomach usually is not visualized unless dilated with fluid (Figure 9-10).

When pathology is present, the serosal layer of the normal gastric wall is seen running toward the serous side of a tumor, which allows differentiation of intramural from extraserosal tumors. If a serosal bridging layer (three layers are seen on the mucosal side of the tumor, and at least two of them are continuous with the first and second layers of normal gastric wall) is present, the tumor lies within the gastric wall. If mucosal bridging is continuous with the mucosal layers of the normal gastric wall, intramucosal or deeply infiltrated carcinoma can be excluded. The sonographer should orient the transducer vertical to the area of transition between the lesion and stomach wall to show their relationship.

Cystic Mass in the Left Upper Quadrant. If a patient has a cystic mass in the left upper quadrant, several measurements can be taken to determine if the mass is the fluid-filled stomach or another mass arising from adjacent organs. The sonographer may give the patient a carbonated drink to see bubbles in the stomach, ask the clinician to place a nasogastric tube for drainage, watch for a change in the shape or size of the "stomach" mass with the ingestion of fluids, alter the patient's position by scanning in an upright or left or right lateral decubitus position, watch for peristalsis, or ask the patient to drink water to see the swirling effect.

DUODENUM

Usually only the gas-filled duodenal cap is seen to the right of the pancreas. The duodenum is divided into the following four portions (see Figure 9-3):

1. A superior portion that courses anteroposteriorly from the pylorus to the level of the neck of the gallbladder
2. A sharp bend in the duodenum into the descending portion that runs along the inferior vena cava at the level of L4

Figure 9-7   A, Gross specimen of the stomach showing the internal rugae of the wall. **B,** Sagittal image of the fluid-filled stomach. The rugae may be seen along the peripheral margins of the wall. **C,** Transverse image of the prominent stomach and rugae. **D,** Contracted stomach after fluid has passed through the pylorus.

Figure 9-8 Sagittal image of the gastroesophageal *(Ge)* junction, which is shown as a small bull's-eye shape anterior to the aorta *(Ao)* and posterior to the left lobe of the liver, inferior to the hemidiaphragm.

Figure 9-9 Transverse view of the left lobe of the liver *(L)*. The antrum of the stomach *(St)* is seen posterior to the liver and anterior to the splenic vein *(SV)*.

Figure 9-10 Transverse view of the fluid-filled stomach. Real-time imaging shows movement throughout the stomach *(ST)*.

Figure 9-11 The duodenum, when filled with a small amount of fluid *(arrows)*, serves as an excellent landmark for the head of the pancreas *(P)*. *A,* Aorta; *IVC,* inferior vena cava.

3. A transverse portion that passes right to left with a slight inclination upward in front of the great vessels and crura
4. An ascending portion that rises to the right of the aorta and reaches the upper border at L2, where at the duodenojejunal flexure it turns forward to become the jejunum (usually not seen with ultrasound)

The duodenum can be outlined easily with water ingestion or a change in position (Figure 9-11). Generally the right lateral decubitus position allows the fluid to drain from the antrum of the stomach into the duodenum. Observation of peristalsis is useful to delineate the duodenum.

SMALL BOWEL

The sonographer usually cannot see the small bowel with ultrasound; the valvulae conniventes may be seen as linear echo densities spaced 3 to 5 mm apart (Figure 9-12). This is called the "keyboard sign" and can be seen in the duodenum and

jejunum. The ileum is smooth walled, and the small bowel wall is under 3 mm thick.

The small bowel is more difficult to image with ultrasound unless contrast or fluid is present. When there is fluid in the bowel loops, the sonographer may be able to look for peristalsis, air movement, or movement of intraluminal fluid contents to rule out obstruction.

APPENDIX

The vermiform appendix is a remnant of what was originally the apex of the cecum. It is a long, tubular structure extending from the cecum in one of several directions; it may lie superiorly behind the cecum, medially behind the ileum and mesentery, or downward and medial into the true pelvis (see Figure 9-1). The appendix is located on the abdominal wall under **McBurney's point.** McBurney's point is located by drawing a line from the right anterosuperior iliac spine to the umbilicus. At approximately the midpoint of this line lies the root of the appendix.

The appendix varies from 1 to 9 inches in length, averaging 3 inches. It is retained in position by a fold of the peritoneum that forms a mesentery for it, which is derived from the left leaf of the mesentery. This triangular structure covers two thirds of the appendix, leaving the distal one third completely uncovered by peritoneum. A branch of the ileocolic artery, the artery of the appendix, lies between the layers of this mesentery (see Figure 9-5). This artery runs the entire length of the appendix.

The small canal of the appendix communicates with the cecum by an orifice that is below and behind the ileocecal opening. The cellular layers that make up the appendix are the serosa or adventitia, muscularis propria, submucosal, and mucosal, the same layers as in the intestine. An abundant amount of retiform tissue is found in the mucosa layer, especially in younger ages.

The appendix has no known physiologic significance.

COLON

A prominent fluid-filled colon may present as a mass (Figures 9-13 and 9-14). The water-enema technique should be used to help delineate if the mass is within the colon, separate from the colon, or just the colon itself. The patient should have a full bladder when scanned to help push the small bowel out of the pelvis. The water in the enema should be lukewarm and the patient rolled into the left lateral decubitus position. Only a small amount of water needs to be given as the sonographer follows the rectum and rectosigmoid colon. The normal wall thickness measures 4 mm. There are five layers in the colon: from innermost to outermost, the first two layers are mucosa, the third is submucosa, the fourth is muscularis propria, and the fifth is subserosal fatty tissue.

If the colon is dilated, the sonographer should measure from the fluid to the outside of the wall. Distention is considered adequate if the stomach diameter is greater than 8 cm, the small bowel is greater than 3 cm, and the lower bowel is greater than 5 cm; the entire halo should measure less than 2 cm (target sign).

Figure 9-12 **A,** Gross specimen showing the valvulae conniventes within the small bowel lumen. **B** and **C,** Ultrasound images of prominent small bowel with valvulae conniventes.

Figure 9-13 Gross specimens of the colon.

Figure 9-14 Target or bull's eye sign. Ultrasound images of the prominent colon.

PATHOLOGY OF THE GASTROINTESTINAL TRACT

UPPER GASTROINTESTINAL TRACT

See Table 9-1 for clinical findings, sonographic findings, and differential considerations for upper gastrointestinal tract diseases and conditions.

Duplication Cyst. Duplication cysts are embryologic mistakes. They may cause symptoms, depending on their size, location, and histology (see Table 9-1). The criteria for a duplication cyst are as follows: (1) the cyst is lined with alimentary tract epithelium, (2) the cyst has a well-developed muscular wall, and (3) the cyst is contiguous with the stomach. These cysts may come from the pancreas or duodenum and occur more often in females than in males. They usually are found on the greater curvature of the stomach. Clinical symptoms are high intestinal obstruction-distention, vomiting, and abdominal pain; **hemorrhage** and fistula formation may also occur. Differential considerations include mesenteric or omental cyst, pancreatic cyst or pseudocyst, enteric cyst, renal cyst, splenic cyst, congenital cyst of the left lobe of the liver, and gastric distention.

Sonographic Findings. On ultrasound examination, duplication cysts appear anechoic with a thin inner echogenic rim (mucosa) and wider outer hypoechoic rim (muscle layer).

Gastric Bezoar. Bezoars are divided into the following three categories: (1) trichobezoars—hair balls in young women, (2) phytobezoars—vegetable matter (e.g., unripe persimmons), and (3) concretions—inorganic materials (e.g., sand, asphalt, and shellac).

Gastric bezoars are movable intraluminal masses of congealed ingested materials that are seen on upper gastrointestinal radiographs. Clinically, patients present with nausea, vomiting, and pain (see Table 9-1). Their symptoms may simulate those of a tumor.

Sonographic Findings. On ultrasound examination, a complex mass is seen, with internal mobile echogenic components. In the fasting patient the sonographer would see a broad band of high-amplitude echoes or a hyperechoic curvilinear dense strip at the anterior margin.

Benign Tumors

Polyp. A **polyp** is a small, tumorlike growth that projects from a mucous membrane surface. A gastric polyp is an outgrowth of tissue from the gastric wall. Patients are asymptomatic when the polyp is small. As the polyp grows, abdominal pain may be present. See Table 9-1 for clinical findings, sonographic findings, and differential considerations for upper gastrointestinal tract polyps.

Sonographic Findings. Polyps are seen with fluid distention of the stomach and appear as solid masses that adhere to the gastric wall. The polyp has variable echogenicity. A large polyp may be inhomogeneous; its contours may be sharply defined, depending on the nature of the surface; the detection of a pedicle may be possible.

Leiomyomas. Leiomyoma is the most common tumor of the stomach. Leiomyoma is seen as a mass similar to carcinoma; it is usually small and asymptomatic for the patient (see Table 9-1). It is often associated with other gastrointestinal abnormalities, such as cholelithiasis, peptic ulcer disease, adenocarcinoma, and leiomyosarcoma.

Sonographic Findings. On ultrasound examination, the mass is seen as hypoechoic and continuous with the muscular layer of the stomach. It may also be seen as a circular or oval space-occupying lesion with a homogeneous echo pattern and hemispheric bulging into the lumen, frequently separated from the lumen by two or three layers continuous with those of normal wall. The mass may appear as a solid with cystic areas that represent necrosis.

Malignant Tumors

Gastric carcinoma. At least 90% to 95% of malignant tumors of the stomach are carcinomas. Gastric carcinoma is the sixth leading cause of death; it occurs more in older males. One half of the tumors occur in the pylorus, with one fourth occurring in the body and fundus of the stomach. The lesions may be ulcerated, diffuse, polypoid, superficial, or some combination of these (see Table 9-1) (Figure 9-15).

Sonographic Findings. On ultrasound examination, the sonographer should look for the target or pseudokidney sign; the patient may have gastric wall thickening.

Lymphoma. **Lymphoma** can occur as a primary tumor of the gastrointestinal tract (3% of stomach tumors). In patients with

TABLE 9-1 UPPER GASTROINTESTINAL TRACT FINDINGS

Clinical Findings	Sonographic Findings	Differential Considerations
Duplication Cysts		
↓ Hematocrit with hemorrhage	Anechoic mass with thin inner echogenic rim Wide outer hypoechoic rim	Mesenteric or omental cyst Pancreatic cyst Enteric cyst Renal cyst Splenic cysts Hepatic cyst in LLL
Gastric Bezoar		
Nausea Vomiting Pain	Complex mass with internal mobile components Hyperechoic curvilinear dense strip at anterior margin	Tumor Cyst
Polyps		
Abdominal pain	Echogenic Heterogeneous	Leiomyoma
Leiomyomas		
N/A	Hypoechoic and contiguous with muscular layer of stomach Solid with cystic areas (necrosis)	Carcinoma Polyp
Gastric Carcinoma		
↑ LFTs Abdominal pain	Target or pseudokidney sign Gastric wall thickening	Leiomyoma Lymphoma Metastatic disease
Lymphoma		
Nausea, vomiting Weight loss	Large, hypoechoic mass Thickened gastric walls Spoke-wheel pattern	Gastric carcinoma Leiomyosarcoma Metastatic disease
Leiomyosarcoma		
N/A	Target lesion with variable pattern Irregular echoes Cystic cavity	Lymphoma Gastric carcinoma Metastatic disease
Metastatic Disease		
Secondary to other cancers	Target pattern Circumscribed thickening Uniform widening of wall without layering	Lymphoma Gastric carcinoma Leiomyosarcoma

LLL, Left lobe of the liver; *N/A,* not applicable.

disseminated lymphoma, a primary tumor occurs as a multifocal lesion in the gastrointestinal tract. The stomach has enlarged and thickened mucosal folds, multiple submucosal nodules, ulceration, and a large extraluminal mass. Clinical symptoms include nausea and vomiting with weight loss (see Table 9-1).

Sonographic Findings. On ultrasound examination, the sonographer will see a large and poorly echogenic (hypoechoic) mass, thickening of gastric walls, and a spoke-wheel pattern within the mass.

Leiomyosarcoma. The second most common malignant tumor is the leiomyosarcoma gastric sarcoma (1% to 5% of tumors). It occurs in the fifth to sixth decades of life. The mass is generally globular or irregular; it may become huge, out-

stripping its blood supply, with central necrosis leading to cystic degeneration and cavitation (see Table 9-1).

Sonographic Findings. On ultrasound examination, a target-shaped lesion is visible. Although the pattern is variable, hemorrhage and necrosis may occur, causing irregular echoes or a cystic cavity.

Metastatic disease. Metastatic disease to the stomach is rare; it may come from a melanoma or lung or breast cancer. The tumor is found in the submucosal layer, forming circumscribed nodules or plaques (see Table 9-1).

Sonographic Findings. On ultrasound examination, a target pattern, circumscribed thickening, or uniform widening of the stomach wall without layering is visible.

Figure 9-15   Gross specimen of adenocarcinoma of the stomach.

Figure 9-16   **A,** Gross specimen example of small bowel obstruction. **B,** Small bowel obstruction secondary to gallstones. **C** and **D,** Small bowel adenocarcinoma. The tumor may cause obstruction of the small bowel.

LOWER GASTROINTESTINAL TRACT

See Table 9-2 for clinical findings, sonographic findings, and differential diagnoses for lower gastrointestinal tract diseases and conditions.

Obstruction and Dilation. A small bowel obstruction is associated with dilation of the bowel loops proximal to the site of the obstruction (Figure 9-16). In 6% of cases the dilated loops are fluid-filled and can be mistaken for a soft tissue mass on x-ray examination (see Table 9-2).

Sonographic Findings. The dilated loops have a tubular or round echo-free appearance. In adynamic ileus, the dilated bowel has normal to somewhat increased peristaltic activity and less distention than with dynamic ileus. In dynamic ileus the loops are round, with minimal deformity at the interfaces with adjacent loops of distended bowel; valvulae conniventes

TABLE 9-2 LOWER GASTROINTESTINAL FINDINGS

Clinical Findings	Sonographic Findings	Differential Considerations
Obstruction and/or Dilation		
Epigastric pain	Tubular, round, echo-free lesion Compressibility of bowel	Appendicitis
Acute Appendicitis		
Pain rebound tenderness over McBurney's point Diarrhea Fever Nausea, vomiting	Thickened muscular wall and ↑ appendiceal diameter (6 mm) Lack of peristalsis Not compressible ↑ Blood flow (Doppler)	Ruptured ectopic pregnancy Fluid-filled colon Inflammation of Meckel's diverticulum
Mucocele		
↑ Leukocytes RLQ pain Asymptomatic	Variable: anechoic, hypoechoic, complex	Appendicitis
Meckel's Diverticulitis		
Rectal bleeding Tenderness	Loop-pattern	Acute appendicitis
Crohn's Disease		
Diarrhea Fever RLQ pain	Symmetrically swollen bowel Target pattern with preserved parietal layers around stenotic and hyperdense lumen ↑ Wall thickening Rigidity to pressure Peristalsis absent or sluggish	Appendicitis Meckel's diverticulum Diverticulitis
Lymphoma		
Abdominal pain Palpable mass Weight loss Blood loss	Large, discrete mass Exoenteric pattern	Pseudokidney Leiomyosarcoma
Leiomyosarcoma		
Abdominal pain Palpable mass	Large, solid mass Contained in necrotic areas	Lymphoma

RLQ, Right lower quadrant.

and peristalsis are seen. The fluid loops are not always associated with obstruction; they can occur with gastroenteritis and **paralytic ileus,** or in dilated, fluid-filled bowel loops without peristalsis. The sonographer should demonstrate pliability and compressibility of bowel wall.

With volvulus (closed-loop obstruction), the involved loop is doubled back on itself abruptly, so that a U-shaped appearance is seen on sagittal scan and a C-shaped anechoic area with a dense center is seen on a transverse scan. The dense center represents medial bowel wall and mesentery.

Abnormalities of the Appendix

Acute appendicitis. Acute appendicitis is the result of luminal obstruction and inflammation, leading to ischemia of the vermiform appendix (Figure 9-17). This may produce necrosis, perforation, and subsequent abscess formation and peritonitis.

The appendix lumen may be obstructed by fecal material, a foreign body, carcinoma of the cecum, stenosis, inflammation, kinking of the organ, or even lymphatic hypertrophy resulting from systemic infection. Obstruction results in edema, which can compromise the vascular supply to the appendix. Subsequently the permeability of the mucosa increases, and bacterial invasion of the wall of the appendix results in infection and inflammation. The increased intraluminal pressure may cause occlusion of the appendicular end artery. If the condition persists, the appendix may necrose, leading to gangrene, rupture, and subsequent local or generalized peritonitis. Periappendiceal abscess or peritonitis does not necessarily mean perforation; the organism may permeate the wall in the absence of perforation to cause these extraappendiceal complications.

The symptoms of acute appendicitis are pain and rebound tenderness, which is usually localized over the right lower quadrant **(McBurney's sign).** Typically the pain is followed by

Figure 9-17 Gross specimens of appendicitis.

nausea and vomiting, diarrhea, and systemic signs of inflammation, such as leukocytosis and fever (see Table 9-2). Acute appendicitis can occur at any age, but it is more prevalent at younger ages.

Diagnosis of even the classic case of appendicitis is complicated by the fact that many disorders present with a similar clinical picture of an acute condition in the abdomen. Differential diagnosis may include the following: (1) acute gastroenteritis, (2) mesenteric lymphadenitis in children, (3) ruptured ectopic pregnancy, (4) mittelschmerz, (5) inflammation of Meckel's diverticulum, (6) regional enteritis, and (7) right ovarian torsion.

Progression of acute appendicitis to frank perforation is more rapid in the younger child, sometimes occurring within 6 to 12 hours. The rate of perforation in the preschool child can be as high as 70% compared with the overall figure of 30% for children and 21% to 22% for adults. Women ages 20 to 40 years are at high risk of the condition being misdiagnosed on initial physical examination.

Acute appendicitis is one of the most frequent causes of abdominal surgery in nearly all age groups. Abdominal ultrasound has proven to be useful in diagnosing acute appendicitis and its complications. Before high-resolution sonography, no noninvasive imaging technique was available to enable direct visualization of the inflamed vermiform appendix. Barium enema examination traditionally has been used to aid diagnosis, but the appendix does not fill with barium in 15% of patients.

Sonographic Findings. The normal appendix can occasionally be visualized with gradual compression sonography. The maximal outer diameters of the normal appendix can measure up to 6 mm. The wall of the inflamed appendix is greater than 2 mm thick, and perforation may be present when asymmetric wall thickening is seen. In inflamed specimens, both the integrity and stratification of wall layers are altered. The distinction of layers is impaired, and each layer sonographically inhomogeneous. Only the sum of the two opposite wall measurements shows a statistical increase in thickness. The sum of the wall thickness in vitro may be similar to measurements of the overall appendix thickness when gentle external compression is applied.

Wall appearance should not be the only criterion for confirmation of appendicitis. The ultrasound pattern of acute appendicitis is characterized by a target-shaped appearance of the appendix in transverse view. Views of the appendix in the transverse plane should demonstrate a thickened muscular wall and increased appendiceal diameter (Figure 9-18). The typical target-shaped lesion consists of a hypoechoic, fluid-distended lumen, a hyperechoic inner ring representing mainly the mucosa and submucosa, and an outer hypoechoic ring representing the **muscularis** externa. The inflamed appendix is further characterized by a lack of peristalsis and compressibility and demonstration of its blind end tip. It is important to carefully survey the entire length of the appendix to prevent a false-negative examination.

Retrocecal appendicitis represents approximately 28% of pediatric appendicitis patients and is easy to diagnose by ultrasound. There are no bowel loops interposed between the appendix and the lateral wall of the abdomen. The inflamed appendix is identified on cross-sections as a **target sign** underneath the abdominis muscle. The incidence of complex masses is greater in retrocecal appendicitis, reflecting a higher incidence of perforation. The sonographic appearance of an appendiceal abscess is a complex mass. Sometimes you can recognize the appendix inside the mass. The omentum wrapping the appendix is in the form of an echogenic band and some bowel loops.

The initial inflammatory changes in appendicitis are more pronounced in the distal half of the appendix and may be focally confined to the appendiceal tip. Ulcerations and necrosis may cause loss of the echogenic submucosal layer in the tip of the appendix. The appendix should be compressed to the tip and visualized longitudinally and transversely to its blind termination. **Appendicoliths** are fecaliths or calculi in the appendix. They are seen as intraluminal foci of high-amplitude echoes with acoustic shadowing.

In infancy and childhood the appendix frequently becomes decompressed after perforation, and the inflammatory process may not wall off or form a well-defined abscess, as is typically seen in adults. With perforation and decompression and an abnormally thickened wall, a collapsed appendix may still be identified. In some patients, however, no appendix may be found and only questionable remnants remain. Supplemental findings, such as free abdominal fluid with debris or thickening of the adjacent abdominal wall, may suggest the diagnosis. However, the possibility of appendicitis cannot be ruled out even in a patient

Figure 9-18   Appendicitis. Transverse **(A)** and sagittal **(B)** images of the inflamed appendix that was not compressed with the linear array transducer.

who lacks an abnormal appendix or a well-defined abscess. Radiographic contrast studies may help diagnosis.

Gas collections within the appendix may be a pitfall in ultrasound evaluation. Gas within the appendix is diagnosed on the basis of sonographic findings of high-amplitude echogenic foci, causing distal reverberation artifacts (i.e., "comet-tails" or "dirty" acoustic shadowing). Although this is a relatively rare finding, its importance lies in the fact that it may be misconstrued as either a normal bowel loop or a gas-forming appendiceal abscess. Gas collections from within the bowel loops should be distinguished from an inflamed appendix. The inflamed appendix is noncompressible and demonstrates other specific anatomic features.

Graded compression ultrasound is an alternative technique for diagnosing appendicitis; it has a sensitivity of 88% and a specificity of 96%. Color Doppler ultrasound imaging can be used to detect increased flow, demonstrating hyperperfusion associated with inflammation. Vessels can be seen coursing through the periphery of the dilated appendix. Addition of color Doppler alone does not increase the sensitivity for detecting appendicitis compared with ultrasound alone. Color Doppler is a simple means of confirming gray scale sonographic findings.

Mucocele. Mucocele of the appendix is a rare pathologic entity. This term designates gross enlargement of the appendix from accumulation of mucoid substance within the lumen. It was recognized in 0.2% to 0.3% of 45,000 appendectomies. Scarring or **fecalith** after an appendectomy is the most common cause of mucocele, although proximal obstruction of the lumen by inflammatory fibrosis, cecal carcinoma, carcinoid polyp, and even endometriosis has been reported. Mucoceles have been classified into three distinct entities: mucosal hyperplasia (an innocuous hyperplastic process), mucinous cystadenoma (a benign neoplasm), and mucinous cystadenocarcinoma (a malignant tumor).

There are several classifications of mucoceles. If the tumor remains encapsulated and there are no malignant cells, this lesion is called a mucocele. If the mucus spreads through the abdominal cavity without evidence of malignant cells, this condition is called pseudomyxoma peritonei. The pseudomyxoma assumes a malignant potential only when epithelial cells occur within the gelatinous peritoneal fluid in association with carcinoma.

Appendiceal mucoceles reportedly show a female-to-male predominance of 4:1, with an average age at presentation of 55 years. The most common clinical complaint is right lower quadrant pain (see Table 9-2). About 25% of cases are asymptomatic. Other symptoms are right iliac fossa mass, sepsis, and urinary symptoms. Bloating of the abdomen is specific to patients with pseudomyxoma peritonei. Laboratory values show an increased erythrocyte sedimentation rate and an elevated leukocyte count. Also, elevated levels of carcinoembryonic antigen have been reported. Pseudomyxoma peritonei significantly decreases survival of patients with appendiceal cystadenocarcinomas.

Preoperative diagnosis of mucocele is helpful. If a mucocele is suspected, needle aspiration is not advised. Careful mobilization surgically may reduce the possibility of rupture, peritoneal contamination, and development of pseudomyxoma peritonei. Radiographically, a mucocele is seen as a soft tissue mass, typically with a rimlike, curvilinear calcification of the mucocele wall. A barium enema examination classically describes nonfilling of the appendix and an extrinsic or submucosal mass at the cecal tip with intact overlying mucosa.

Sonographic Findings. On ultrasound, the examiner should locate the appendix in the right lower quadrant, referencing the psoas muscle and iliac vessels. The ultrasound image varies according to the content of the mucocele, which may be anechoic when mucoid material is more fluid. The following patterns have been defined: (1) a purely cystic lesion with anechoic fluid; (2) a hypoechoic mass containing fine internal echoes; and (3) a complex mass with high-level echoes (Figure 9-19). As it enlarges, inspissation of the mucoid material creates this internal echo pattern. This mass has an irregular inner wall

Figure 9-19   **A** and **B,** Ultrasound image of a mucocele. This patient shows a complex mass with high-level echoes. **C,** Computed tomographic image of the mucocele.

caused by mucinous debris with varying degrees of epithelial hyperplasia. Calcification of the rim can produce acoustic shadowing. Internal, thin septations have been seen along with variable degrees of mucosal atrophy and ulceration.

Pseudomyxoma peritonei is seen as septated **ascites** (fluid in the abdomen) with numerous suspended echoes that do not mobilize as the patient changes position. Combined with ultrasound, paracentesis may accurately establish the diagnosis of gelatinous ascites.

Meckel's Diverticulitis. A **diverticulum** is a pouchlike herniation through the muscular wall of a tubular organ that occurs in the stomach, the small intestine, or most commonly the colon. **Meckel's diverticulum** is located on the antimesenteric border of the ileum, approximately 2 ft from the ileocecal valve. It is present in 2% of the population. In Meckel's diverticulitis, adults may present with intestinal obstruction, rectal bleeding, or diverticular inflammation (see Table 9-2). Acute appendicitis and acute Meckel's diverticulitis may not be distinguished clinically.

Sonographic Findings. The wall of Meckel's diverticulum consists of mucosal, muscular, and serosal layers. Noncompressibility of the obstructed, inflamed diverticulum indicates

Figure 9-20   Gross specimen of ulcerative colitis.

that intraluminal fluid is trapped. The area of maximal tenderness is evaluated along with its distance from the cecum.

Crohn's Disease. Crohn's disease is regional enteritis, a recurrent granulomatous inflammatory disease that affects the terminal ileum, colon, or both at any level (Figures 9-20 through 9-22). The reaction involves the entire thickness of the bowel wall. Clinical symptoms include diarrhea, fever, and right lower quadrant pain (see Table 9-2).

Figure 9-21   Gross specimens show complications of colitis. **A,** Hematoma in the colon. **B,** Gangrenous colon.

Figure 9-22   Ulcerative colitis. **A,** Small bowel colitis. **B** and **C,** Dilated colon with colitis. **D,** Prominent colon with increased vascularity.

Sonographic Findings. On ultrasound examination, a symmetrically swollen bowel target pattern with preserved parietal layers around the stenotic and echogenic lumen is seen. The findings are most prominent in ileocolonic disease, with uniformly increased wall thickness involving all layers, especially the mucosa and submucosa. A matted-loop pattern is found in the late stages. Patients with Crohn's disease show rigidity to pressure exerted with the transducer. Peristalsis is absent or sluggish.

Tumors

Lymphoma. Lymphoma is a tumor that usually occurs late in life, near the sixth decade; it is also the most common tumor of the gastrointestinal tract in children under 10 years of age. The intraperitoneal masses frequently involve the mesenteric vessels that encase them. Clinical signs include intestinal blood loss, weight loss, anorexia, and abdominal pain (see Table 9-2). The patient may have an intestinal obstruction or palpable mass.

Sonographic Findings. On ultrasound examination, the sonographer may see a large, discrete mass with a target pattern, an exoenteric pattern with a large mass on the mesenteric surface of bowel, and a small anechoic mass representing subserosal nodes or mesenteric nodal involvement.

Lymphomatous involvement of the intestinal wall may lead to pseudokidney or hydronephrotic pseudokidney. The lumen may be dilated with fluid and demonstrate a lack of peristalsis. The bowel wall is uniformly thickened, with homogeneous low echogenicity between the well-defined mucosal and serosal surfaces that contain a persistent, echo-free, wide, and long lumen.

Leiomyosarcoma. Leiomyosarcoma represents 10% of primary small bowel tumors. Approximately 10% to 30% of these occur in the duodenum, 30% to 45% in the jejunum, and 35% to 55% in the ileum. The patients are in their fifth to sixth decades of life.

Sonographic Findings. On ultrasound examination, a large solid mass containing necrotic areas anterior to solid viscus may be found.

SELECTED BIBLIOGRAPHY

Birnbaum BA, Jeffrey RB Jr: CT and sonographic evaluation of acute right lower quadrant abdominal pain, *Am J Roentgenol* 170:361-371, 1998.

Curry R, Tempkin B, editors: *Abdominal sonography*, Philadelphia, 2004, WB Saunders.

Eisen K: *"Gastrointestinal imaging" in clinical guide to ultrasonography by Charlotte Hennignsen*, St Louis, 2004, Mosby.

Gray HFRS: *Anatomy: descriptive and surgical*, London, 1989, Crown.

Landen S and others: Appendiceal mucoceles and pseudomyxoma peritonei, *Surg Gynecol Obstet* 175:401, 1992.

Limberg B: Sonographic features of colonic Crohn's disease: comparison of in vivo and in vitro studies, *J Clin Ultrasound* 18:161, 1990.

Mittelstaedt CA: *General ultrasound*, New York, 1992, Churchill Livingstone.

Quillin SP, Siegel MJ: Appendicitis: efficacy of color Doppler sonography, *Radiology* 191:557, 1994.

Rapp CL, Stavros AT, Meyers PR: Ultrasound of the normal appendix: the how and why. *J Diag Med Sonogr* 14:195, 1998.

Rumack C: *Diagnostic ultrasound*, ed 3, St Louis, 2005, Mosby.

Stavros AT, Rapp CL, Thickman D: Sonography of inflammatory conditions, *Ultrasound Q* 13:1, 1995.

Wilson SR, Toi A: The value of sonography in the diagnosis of acute diverticulitis of the colon, *Am J Roentgenol* 154:1199, 1990.

Worlicek H, Dunz H, Engelhard K: Ultrasonic examination of the wall of the fluid-filled stomach, *J Clin Ultrasound* 17:5, 1989.

Worrell JA et al: Graded compression ultrasound in the diagnosis of appendicitis: a comparison of diagnostic criteria, *J Ultrasound Med* 9:145, 1990.

Wright LL, Baker KR, Meny RG: Ultrasound demonstration of gastroesophageal reflux, *J Ultrasound Med* 7:471, 1988.

Yacoe ME, Jeffrey RB Jr: Sonography of appendicitis and diverticulitis, *Radiol Clin North Am* 32:899-912, 1994.

CHAPTER *10*

The Urinary System

Kerry Weinberg

OBJECTIVES

- List the organs in the urinary system and describe their basic functions
- Identify the internal anatomy of the kidney including the renal pelvis, calyces, renal sinus, medulla pyramids, cortex, and hilum and describe the sonographic appearance of each
- Describe the sonographic scanning technique to image the urinary system
- Identify the common locations of ectopic kidneys, their sonographic appearance, and their relationship to genital anomalies
- Identify and describe renal variants and anomalies, their sonographic appearance, and other secondary findings associated with renal anomalies
- Describe the clinical signs and symptoms, and list the laboratory tests (urinalysis, urine pH, specific gravity, blood, creatinine, and blood urea nitrogen) that are used to evaluate urinary tract problems
- Describe the different types of congenital renal cystic diseases: von Hippel-Lindau, tuberous sclerosis, polycystic, multicystic dysplastic, and medullary cystic disease, including sonographic appearance and involvement of other organs
- Identify and define sonographic appearance of benign and malignant urinary system neoplasms
- Describe the process of hydronephrosis, including the causes, stages, clinical symptoms, laboratory findings, sonographic appearance, and Doppler findings
- Describe prerenal, renal, and postrenal causes of renal failure, including the sonographic appearance of each
- Identify the sonographic appearance of the kidneys with acquired immune deficiency syndrome (AIDS), sickle cell anemia, and uncontrolled hypertension
- Define the following renal infections: pyonephrosis, emphysematous pyelonephritis, xanthogranulomatous pyelonephritis, and nephrocalcinosis
- Discuss the role of ultrasound in postrenal transplant patients, including parenchymal pattern, color flow and Doppler findings, and medical complications associated with rejection
- Describe the extraperitoneal fluid collections that may occur after transplant: lymphocele, lymph fistula, urinary fistula, urinoma, perinephric abscess, and hematoma
- List the factors that must be considered when an increased resistive index is found in a native and transplanted kidney and describe the uses and limitations of power, color, and Doppler to evaluate the intrarenal vascularity
- Identify lower urinary tract abnormalities and describe the sonographic appearance of each and scanning technique used for evaluation of the urinary bladder
- Describe the sonographic appearance of benign and malignant urinary bladder neoplasms
- Identify causes that prohibit the complete emptying of the urinary bladder

ANATOMY OF THE URINARY SYSTEM
NORMAL ANATOMY
VASCULAR SUPPLY

PHYSIOLOGY AND LABORATORY DATA OF THE URINARY SYSTEM
EXCRETION
LABORATORY TESTS FOR RENAL DISEASE

SONOGRAPHIC EVALUATION OF THE URINARY SYSTEM

Kidneys
Lower Urinary Tract
Bladder

PATHOLOGY OF THE URINARY SYSTEM

Renal Cystic Disease
Renal Neoplasms
Renal Disease
Renal Failure, Hydronephrosis, Renal Infections,
    Renal Artery Stenosis, and Renal Infarction
Renal Transplant
Kidney Stone (Urolithiasis)
Bladder Diverticulum
Bladder Inflammation (Cystitis)
Bladder Tumors

Key Terms

afferent arteriole – carry blood into the glomerulus of the nephron

arcuate arteries – small vessels found at the base of the renal pyramids

blood urea nitrogen (BUN) – measures amount of nitrogenous waste (along with creatinine); waste products accumulate in the blood when kidneys malfunction

Bowman's capsule – part of the filtration process; contains water, salts, glucose, urea, and amino acids

calyx – part of the collecting system adjacent to the pyramid that collects urine and is connected to the major calyx

columns of Bertin – bands of cortical tissue that separate the renal pyramids; a prominent column of Bertin may mimic a renal mass on sonography

cortex – refers to the outer parenchyma of the kidney that contains the renal corpuscle and proximal and distal convoluted tubules of the nephron

creatinine (Cr) – one of the laboratory tests used to measure the ability of the kidney to get rid of waste; waste products accumulate in the blood when the kidneys are malfunctioning

dromedary hump – normal variant that occurs on the left kidney as a bulge on the lateral border

ectopic kidney – located outside of the normal position, most often in the pelvic cavity

efferent arteriole – blood from this structure supplies the peritubular capillaries, which also supply the convoluted tubules

Gerota's fascia – another term for the renal fascia; the kidney is covered by the renal capsule, perirenal fat, Gerota's fascia, and pararenal fat

glomerulus – part of the filtration process in the kidney

hilus – area of kidney where vessels, ureter, and lymphatics enter and exit

homeostasis – maintenance of normal body physiology

horseshoe kidney – congenital malformation in which both kidneys are joined together by an isthmus, most commonly at the lower poles

hydronephrosis – dilation of the renal collecting system

loop of Henle – portion of a renal tubule lying between the proximal and distal convoluted portions; reabsorption of fluid, sodium, and chloride occurs in the proximal convoluted tubule and the loop of Henle

major calyces (also known as the infundibulum) – receives urine from the minor calyces to convey to the renal pelvis

medulla (also known as the pyramid) – refers to the inner portion of the renal parenchyma that contains the loop of Henle

minor calyces – receive urine from the renal pyramids; form the border of the renal sinus

Morison's pouch – right posterior subhepatic space located anterior to the kidney and inferior to the liver where fluid may accumulate

nephron – functional unit of the kidney; includes a renal corpuscle and a renal tubule

pyramids – convey urine to the minor calyces

renal agenesis – interruption in the normal development of the kidney resulting in absence of the kidney; may be unilateral or bilateral

renal capsule – first layer adjacent to the kidney that forms a tough, fibrous covering

renal corpuscle – part of the nephron that consists of Bowman's capsule and the glomerulus

renal hilum – area in the midportion of the kidney where the renal vessels and ureter enter and exit

renal pelvis – area in the midportion of the kidney that collects urine before entering the ureter

renal sinus – central area of the kidney that includes the calyces, renal pelvis, renal vessels, fat, nerves, and lymphatics

retroperitoneum – space behind the peritoneal lining of the abdominal cavity

specific gravity – laboratory tests that measure how much dissolved material is present in the urine

splaying – widening

tadpole sign – seen as narrow bands of acoustic shadowing posterior to the margins of the cyst along the lateral borders of enhancement

ureters – retroperitoneal structures that exit the kidney to carry urine to the urinary bladder

urethra – small, membranous canal that excretes urine from the urinary bladder

urinary bladder – muscular retroperitoneal organ that serves as a reservoir for urine

urolithiasis – stone within the urinary system

The urinary system has two principal functions: excreting wastes and regulating the composition of blood. Blood composition must not be allowed to vary beyond tolerable limits, or the conditions in tissue necessary for cellular life will be lost. Regulating blood composition involves not only removing harmful wastes but also conserving water and metabolites in the body.

ANATOMY OF THE URINARY SYSTEM

NORMAL ANATOMY

Kidneys. The urinary system is located posterior to the peritoneum lining the abdominal cavity in an area called the **retroperitoneum**. The kidneys lie in the retroperitoneal cavity near the posterior body wall, just below the diaphragm (Figure 10-1). The lower ribs protect both kidneys. The right kidney lies slightly lower than the left kidney because the large right lobe of the liver pushes it inferiorly. The kidneys move readily with respiration; on deep inspiration, both kidneys move downward approximately 1 inch.

The kidneys are dark red, bean-shaped organs that measure 9 to 12 cm long, 5 cm wide, and 2.5 cm thick. The outer **cortex** of the kidney is darker than the inner **medulla** because of the increased perfusion of blood. The inner surface of the medulla is folded into projections called *pyramids*, which empty into the renal pelvis. The **arcuate arteries** are located at the base of the pyramids and separate the medulla from the cortex. Numerous collecting tubules bring the urine from its sites of formation in the cortex to the pyramids. The renal tubules, or **nephrons**, are the functional units of the kidney.

On the medial surface of each kidney is a vertical indentation called the **renal hilum**, where the renal vessels and ureter enter and exit. Within the **hilus** of the kidney are other vascular structures, a ureter, and the lymphatics. The renal artery is the most posterior and superior structure. The two branches of the renal vein are anterior to the renal artery (Figure 10-2). The ureter is located slightly inferior to the renal artery. When present, the third branch of the renal artery may be seen to arise from the hilus. The lymph vessels and sympathetic fibers also are found within the renal hilus.

A fibrous capsule called the true capsule surrounds the kidney. Outside of this fibrous capsule is a covering of perinephric fat. The perinephric fascia surrounds the perinephric fat and encloses the kidneys and adrenal glands. The perinephric fascia is a condensation of areolar tissue, which is continuous laterally with the fascia transversalis. The renal fascia, known as **Gerota's fascia,** surrounds the true capsule and perinephric fat.

Anterior to the right kidney are the right adrenal gland, liver, **Morison's pouch,** second part of the duodenum, and right colic flexure (Figure 10-3). Anterior to the left kidney are the left adrenal gland, spleen, stomach, pancreas, left colic flexure, and coils of jejunum.

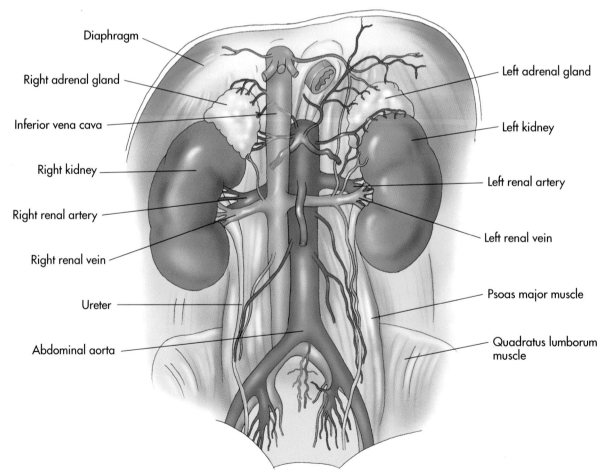

Figure 10-1   Relationship of the kidneys, suprarenal glands (adrenal), and vascular structures to one another.

Figure 10-2   The kidney cut longitudinally to show the internal structure.

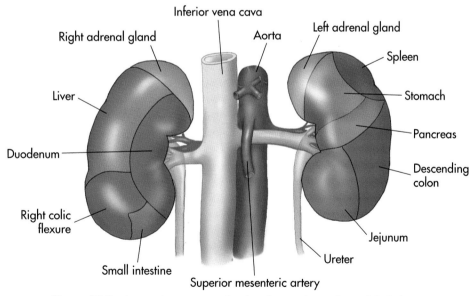

Figure 10-3   Anatomic structures related to the anterior surfaces of the kidneys.

Posterior to the right kidney are the diaphragm, costodiaphragmatic recess of the pleura, twelfth rib, psoas muscle, quadratus lumborum, and transversus abdominis muscles. The subcostal (T12), iliohypogastric, and ilioinguinal (L1) nerves run downward and laterally. Posterior to the left kidney are the diaphragm, costodiaphragmatic recess of the pleura, eleventh and twelve ribs, psoas muscle, quadratus lumborum, and transversus abdominis muscles. The same nerves are seen near the left kidney as in the right.

Within the kidney, the upper expanded end of the ureter, known as the **renal pelvis** of the ureter, divides into two or three **major calyces,** each of which divides further into two or three **minor calyces** (see Figure 10-2). The apex of a medullary pyramid, called the renal papilla, indents each minor **calyx.** The kidney consists of an internal medullary portion and an external cortical substance. The medullary substance consists of a series of striated conical masses, called the *renal pyramids.* The pyramids vary from 8 to 18 in number, and their bases are directed toward the outer circumference of the kidney. Their apices converge toward the **renal sinus,** where their prominent papillae project into the lumina of the minor calyces. Spirally arranged muscles surround the calyces and may exert a milking action on these tubes, aiding in the flow of urine into the renal pelvis. As the pelvis leaves the renal sinus, it rapidly becomes smaller and ultimately merges with the ureter.

Nephron. A nephron consists of two main structures—a renal corpuscle and a renal tubule. Nephrons filter the blood and produce urine. Blood is filtered in the renal corpuscle. The filtered fluid passes through the renal tubule. As the filtrate moves through the tubule, substances needed by the body are returned to the blood. Waste products, excess water, and other substances not needed by the body pass into the collecting ducts as urine.

The **renal corpuscle** consists of a network of capillaries called the **glomerulus,** which is surrounded by a cuplike structure known as **Bowman's capsule.** Blood flows into the glomerulus through a small **afferent arteriole** and leaves the glomerulus through an **efferent arteriole.** This arteriole conducts blood to a second set of capillaries, the peritubular capillaries, which surround the renal tubule.

There is an opening in the bottom of Bowman's capsule through which filtrate passes into the renal tubule. The first part of the renal tubule is the coiled proximal convoluted tubule. After passing through the proximal convoluted tubule, filtrate flows into the **loop of Henle** and then into the distal convoluted tubule. Urine from the distal convoluted tubules of several nephrons drains into a collecting duct. A portion of the distal convoluted tubule curves upward and contacts the afferent and efferent arterioles. Some cells of the distal convoluted tubule and some cells of the afferent arteriole are modified to form the juxtaglomerular apparatus, a structure that helps regulate blood pressure in the kidney.

The renal corpuscle, the proximal convoluted tubule, and the distal convoluted tubule of each nephron are located within the renal cortex. The loops of Henle dip down into the medulla.

Ureter. The **ureter** is a 25-cm tubular structure whose proximal end is expanded and continuous with the funnel shape of renal pelvis. The renal pelvis lies within the hilus of the kidney and receives major calyces. The ureter emerges from the hilus of the kidney and runs vertically downward behind the parietal peritoneum along the psoas muscle, which separates it from the tips of the transverse processes of the lumbar vertebrae. It enters the pelvis by crossing the bifurcation of the common iliac artery anterior to the sacroiliac joint. The ureter courses along the lateral wall of the pelvis to the region of the ischial spine and turns forward to enter the lateral angle of the bladder. The ureter from the ureteropelvic junction to the bladder is not routinely visualized with ultrasound. The superior and distal ends of the ureters are more readily visualized than the midsection. The ureters are located in the retroperitoneal cavity and are obscured by bowel gas.

There are three constrictions along the ureter's course: (1) where the ureter leaves the renal pelvis, (2) where it is kinked as it crosses the pelvic brim, and (3) where it pierces the bladder wall.

Urinary Bladder. The **urinary bladder** is a large muscular bag. It has a posterior and lateral opening for the ureters and one anterior opening for the urethra. The interior of the bladder is lined with highly elastic transitional epithelium. When the bladder is full, the lining is smooth and stretched; when it is empty, the lining is a series of folds. In the middle layer, a series of smooth muscle coats distend as urine collects and contract to expel urine through the urethra. Urine is produced almost continuously and accumulates in the bladder until the increased pressure stimulates the organ's nervous receptors to relax the urethra's sphincter and urine is released from the urinary bladder. The urinary bladder is visualized sonographically when it is distended with fluid.

Urethra. The **urethra** is a membranous tube that passes from the anterior part of the urinary bladder to the outside of the body. There are two sphincters: the internal sphincter and the external sphincter. The urethra is not routinely visualized sonographically.

VASCULAR SUPPLY

The arterial supply to the kidney is through the main renal artery. This vessel is a lateral branch of the aorta and rises just inferior to the superior mesenteric artery (Figure 10-4). Each artery divides into three branches to enter the hilus of the kidney—two anterior and one posterior to the pelvis of the ureter. The branches of the renal artery may vary in size and number. In most cases the renal artery divides into two primary branches: a larger anterior and a smaller posterior. These arteries break down into smaller segmental arteries, then into interlobar arteries, and finally into tiny arcuate arteries.

Five to six veins join to form the main renal vein. This vein emerges from the renal hilus anterior to the renal artery. The renal vein drains into the lateral walls of the inferior vena cava (see Figure 10-4).

The lymphatic vessels follow the renal artery to the lateral aortic lymph nodes near the origin of the renal artery. Nerves originate in the renal sympathetic plexus and are distributed along the branches of the renal vessels.

Blood supply to nephrons begins at the renal artery. The artery subdivides within the kidneys. A small vessel (afferent arteriole) enters Bowman's capsule, where it forms a tuft of capillaries, the glomerulus, which entirely fills the concavity of the capsule. Blood leaves the glomerulus via the efferent arteriole, which subdivides into a network of capillaries that surrounds the proximal and distal tubules and eventually unites as veins, which become the renal vein.

The renal vein returns the cleansed blood to the general circulation. Movements of substances between the nephron and the capillaries of the tubules change the composition of the blood filtrate moving along in the tubules. From the nephrons, the fluid moves to collecting tubules and into the ureter, leading to the bladder where urine is stored.

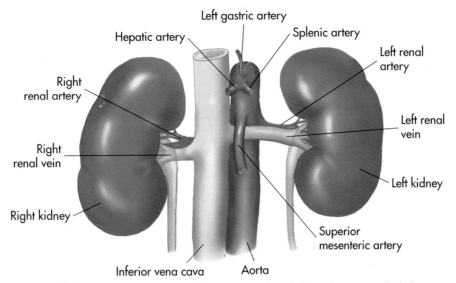

Figure 10-4   Vascular relationship of the great vessels and their tributaries to the kidneys.

The arterial supply to the ureter is from the following three sources: the renal artery, the testicular or ovarian artery, and the superior vesical artery.

PHYSIOLOGY AND LABORATORY DATA OF THE URINARY SYSTEM

The urinary system consists of two kidneys, which remove wastes from the blood and produce urine, and two ureters, which act as tubal ducts leading from the hilus of the kidneys and drain into the urinary bladder. The bladder collects and stores urine, which is eventually discharged through the urethra. The urinary system is located posterior to the peritoneum lining the abdominal cavity in an area called the retroperitoneum.

The function of the kidneys is to excrete urine. More than any other organ, the kidneys adjust the amounts of water and electrolytes leaving the body so that these equal the amounts of substances entering the body. The formation of urine involves the following three processes: glomerular filtration, tubular reabsorption, and tubular secretion.

EXCRETION

Cells in the body continually carry on metabolic activities that produce waste products. If permitted to accumulate, metabolic wastes eventually reach toxic concentrations and threaten **homeostasis.** To prevent this, metabolic wastes must be quickly excreted. The process of excretion entails separating and removing substances harmful to the body. The skin, lungs, liver, large intestine, and kidneys carry out excretion.

The principal metabolic waste products are water, carbon dioxide, and nitrogenous wastes (including urea, uric acid, and **creatinine**). Nitrogen is derived from amino acids and nucleic acids. Amino acids break down in the liver, and the nitrogen-containing amino group is removed. The amino group is then converted to ammonia, which is chemically converted to urea. Uric acid is formed from the breakdown of nucleic acids. Both

urea and uric acid are carried away from the liver into the kidneys by the vascular system. Creatinine is a nitrogenous waste produced from phosphocreatine in the muscles.

LABORATORY TESTS FOR RENAL DISEASE

The clinical symptoms of a patient with specific renal pathology may be nonspecific. A patient's history of infection, previous urinary tract problems (renal stones), or hypertension or family history of renal cystic disease is useful information. A patient with a renal infection or disease process may present with any of the following symptoms: flank pain, hematuria, polyuria, oliguria, fever, urgency, weight loss, or general edema.

A patient who presents with symptoms of renal infection, renal insufficiency, or disease may undergo a number of laboratory tests to help the clinician determine the cause of the problem.

Urinalysis. Urinalysis is essential to detect urinary tract disorders in patients whose renal function is impaired or absent. Most renal inflammatory processes introduce a characteristic exudate for a specific type of inflammation into the urine. The presence of an acute infection causes hematuria, red blood cells in the urine; pyuria causes pus in the urine.

Urine pH. Urine pH is very important in managing diseases such as bacteriuria and renal calculi. The pH refers to the strength of the urine as a partly acidic or alkaline solution. The abundance of hydrogen ions in a solution is called pH. If urine contains an increased concentration of hydrogen ions, the urine is acidic. The formation of renal calculi partly depends on the pH of urine. Other conditions, such as renal tubular acidosis and chronic renal failure, are associated with alkaline urine.

Specific Gravity. The **specific gravity** is the measurement of the kidney's ability to concentrate urine. The concentration factor depends on the amount of dissolved waste products. An excessive intake of fluids or a decrease in perspiration may cause a large output of urine and a decrease in the specific gravity. A low fluid intake, excessive perspiration, or diarrhea can cause the output of urine to be low and the specific gravity to increase. The specific gravity is especially low in cases of renal failure, glomerular nephritis, and pyelonephritis. These diseases cause renal tubular damage, which affects the ability of the kidneys to concentrate urine.

Blood. Hematuria is the appearance of blood cells in the urine; it can be associated with early renal disease. An abundance of red blood cells in the urine may suggest renal trauma, neoplasm, calculi, pyelonephritis, or glomerular or vascular inflammatory processes, such as acute glomerulonephritis and renal infarction.

Leukocytes may be present whenever there is inflammation, infection, or tissue necrosis originating from anywhere in the urinary tract.

Hematocrit. The hematocrit is the relative ratio of plasma to packed-cell volume in the blood. A decreased hematocrit occurs with acute hemorrhagic processes secondary to disease or blunt trauma.

Hemoglobin. The presence of hemoglobin in urine occurs whenever there is extensive damage or destruction of the functioning erythrocytes. This condition injures the kidney and can cause acute renal failure.

Protein. When glomerular damage is evident, albumin and other plasma proteins may be filtered in excess, allowing the overflow to enter the urine, which lowers the blood serum albumin concentration. Albuminuria is commonly found with benign and malignant neoplasms, calculi, chronic infection, and pyelonephritis.

Creatinine Clearance. Specific measurements of creatinine concentrations in urine and blood serum are considered an accurate index for determining the glomerular filtration rate. Creatinine is a by-product of muscle energy metabolism, which is normally produced at a constant rate as long as the body muscle mass remains relatively constant. Creatinine goes through complete glomerular filtration without normally being reabsorbed by the renal tubules. A decreased urinary creatinine clearance indicates renal dysfunction because creatinine blood levels are constant and only decreased renal function prevents the normal excretion of creatinine.

Blood Urea Nitrogen. The blood urea nitrogen (BUN) is the concentration of urea nitrogen in blood and is the end product of cellular metabolism. Urea is formed in the liver and carried to the kidneys through the blood to be excreted in urine. Impairment of renal function and increased protein catabolism result in BUN elevation that is relative to the degree of renal impairment and rate of urea nitrogen excreted by the kidneys.

Serum Creatinine. Renal dysfunction also results in serum creatinine elevation. Blood serum creatinine levels are said to be more specific and more sensitive in determining renal impairment than BUN.

SONOGRAPHIC EVALUATION OF THE URINARY SYSTEM

KIDNEYS

Ultrasound evaluation of the kidneys is a noninvasive, relatively inexpensive, reproducible diagnostic test to evaluate renal problems. Until recently, an intravenous pyelogram (IVP) was the initial diagnostic test performed on patients who presented with renal colic (flank pain). In patients who presented with renal colic without a history of renal stones, a noncontrast computerized tomography (NCCT) is typically performed. NCCT requires no patient preparation and is not operator or patient dependent. The main disadvantages of NCCT are cost and the use of ionizing radiation. Patients who present with a history of renal stones require a plain film x-ray, and a renal ultrasound with Doppler is usually the first diagnostic test performed. In many areas where computerized tomography (CT) is not readily available, an IVP is performed if the patient can tolerate the contrast agent used and not have an allergic reaction to it.

Magnetic resonance imaging (MRI) using magnetic resonance urography (MRU) is currently being investigated for diagnosing renal disease. MRU can also assess renal function, which is similar to an IVP, in addition to diagnosing obstructive uropathy. MRI can also assess other abdominal organs for disease.

A renal ultrasound is able to demonstrate the acoustic properties of a mass, delineate an abnormal lie of a kidney resulting from an extrarenal mass, or determine if hydronephrosis is secondary to renal stones. In addition, ultrasound can define perirenal fluid collections, such as a hematoma or abscess; determine renal size and parenchymal detail; detect dilated ureters and **hydronephrosis**; and image renal congenital anomalies.

Normal Texture and Patterns. The kidneys are imaged by ultrasound as organs with smooth outer contours surrounded by reflected echoes of perirenal fat. The renal parenchyma surrounds the fatty central renal sinus, which contains the calyces, infundibula, pelvis, vessels, and lymphatics (Figure 10-5). Because of the fat interface, the renal sinus is imaged as an area of intense echoes with variable contours. If two separate collections of renal sinus fat are identified, a double collecting system should be suspected.

Generally, patients are given nothing by mouth before ultrasound or other imaging examinations. This state of dehydration causes the infundibula and renal pelvis to be collapsed and thus indistinguishable from the echo-dense renal sinus fat. If on the other hand the bladder is distended from rehydration, the intrarenal collecting system also will become distended. An extrarenal pelvis may be seen as a fluid-filled structure medial to the kidney on transverse scans. Differentiation of the normal

Figure 10-5   Transverse section of the abdominal cavity through the epiploic foramen.

variant from obstruction is made by noting the absence of a distended intrasinus portion of the renal pelvis and infundibula. Dilation of the collecting system has also been noted in pregnant patients. (The right kidney is generally involved with a mild degree of hydronephrosis. This distention returns to normal shortly after delivery.)

Patient Position and Technique. The most efficient way to examine the kidneys is to use the liver as a window to image the right kidney (Figures 10-6 and 10-7) or through the spleen for the left kidney (Figure 10-8). The patient should be in a supine and/or decubitus position. There are several alternative scanning windows to image the kidney. These include the right posterior oblique, right lateral decubitus, and left lateral decubitus views. Having the patient take in a deep breath will move the liver and spleen distally, which may create a better window to increase visualization of the kidneys. A subcostal or intercostal transducer approach may also be used for visualization of the upper and lower poles of the kidneys.

A proper adjustment of time gain compensation (TGC) with adequate sensitivity settings allows a uniform acoustic pattern throughout the image. The renal cortical echo amplitude should be compared with the liver parenchymal echo amplitude at the same depth to effectively set the TGC and sensitivity.

If the patient has a substantial amount of perirenal fat, a high-frequency transducer may not provide the penetration necessary to optimally visualize the area. The deeper areas of the kidney may appear hypoechoic. Renal detail may also be obscured if the patient has hepatocellular disease, gallstones, rib interference (Figure 10-9), or other abnormal collections between the liver and kidney (Figure 10-10). The use of harmonic imaging or tissue contrast enhancement technology TCE (Figure 10-11) may aid in optimizing visualization of the kidneys.

Renal Parenchyma. The parenchyma is the area from the renal sinus to the outer renal surface (Figure 10-12). The arcuate arteries and interlobar vessels are found within and are best demonstrated as intense specular echoes in cross-section or oblique section at the corticomedullary junction.

The cortex generally is echo producing (Figure 10-13) (although its echoes are less intense than those from normal liver), whereas the medullary pyramids are hypoechoic (Figure 10-14). The two are separated from each other by bands of cortical tissue, called columns of Bertin, which extend inward to the renal sinus.

Diseases of the renal parenchyma are those that accentuate cortical echoes but preserve or exaggerate the corticomedullary junction (type I) and those that distort the normal anatomy, obliterating the corticomedullary differentiation in either a focal or diffuse manner (type II).

The criteria for type I changes include (1) the echo intensity in the cortex be equal to or greater than that in the adjacent liver or spleen and (2) the echo intensity in the cortex equal that in the adjacent renal sinus. Minor signs would include the loss of identifiable arcuate vessels or the accentuation of corticomedullary definition.

Type II changes can be seen in a focal disruption of normal anatomy with any mass lesion, including cysts, tumors, abscesses, and hematomas.

Renal Vessels. The arteries are best seen with the supine and left lateral decubitus views. The right renal artery extends from the lateral wall of the aorta to enter the central renal sinus (Figure 10-15). On the longitudinal scan, the right renal artery can be seen as a round anechoic structure posterior to the inferior vena cava (Figure 10-16). The right renal vein extends from the central renal sinus directly into the inferior vena cava (Figure 10-17). Both vessels appear as tubular structures in the transverse plane.

The renal arteries have an echo-free central lumen with highly echogenic borders that consist of a vessel wall and surrounding retroperitoneal fat and connective tissue. They lie posterior to the veins and can be demonstrated with certainty if their junction with the aorta is seen.

Figure 10-6   **A** and **B,** Transverse scan of the normal upper pole of the right kidney imaged through the homogeneous liver. Scans are made from the upper pole, mid pole to include the right renal vein *(RRV),* and inferior vena cava *(IVC)* to the lower pole. **C,** Normal blood flow through the right renal vein to the IVC. **D,** A slight decubitus position allows the liver *(L)* to roll anterior to the right kidney *(RK)* and gallbladder *(GB)* for better visualization. (**A** through **C,** Courtesy Shpetim Telegrafi, New York University.)

Figure 10-7   Longitudinal scans through the long axis of the right kidney *(RK)* and psoas muscle. Measurements are made along the maximum length of the right kidney from upper pole to lower pole. (Courtesy Shpetim Telegrafi, New York University.)

A   **B**

C   **D**

Figure 10-8   **A,** Longitudinal scan of the normal left kidney as imaged through the homogeneous spleen. The psoas muscle is the posterior medial border of the kidney. **B,** Measurements are made along the maximum length of the kidney from the upper pole to lower pole. **C,** The patient may be rolled into a right lateral decubitus position for better visualization of the renal medullary pyramids and parenchyma. **D,** Splenomegaly *(S)* aids in the visualization of the upper pole of the left kidney *(LK).* (Courtesy Shpetim Telegrafi, New York University.)

Figure 10-9   The ribs may interfere with uniform visualization of the kidney. Variations in respiration help the sonographer find the best window to image the renal parenchyma without rib interference.

Figure 10-10   Transverse view of right kidney with ascites in Morison's pouch. (Courtesy Siemens.)

Figure 10-11 Sagittal view of normal liver/kidney using TCE tissue contrast enhancement technology. (Courtesy Siemens Medical Solutions USA, Inc.)

Figure 10-13 Sagittal scan of the normal kidney. The cortex is the brightest of the echoes within the renal parenchyma. The medullary pyramids are echo free. The pyramids are separated from the cortex by bands of cortical tissue and the columns of Bertin that extend inward to the renal sinus. (Courtesy Joseph Yee, New York University.)

Figure 10-14 Longitudinal scan of the hypoechoic renal pyramids. (Courtesy Shpetim Telegrafi, New York University.)

Figure 10-12 Thickness of the renal substance. **A,** Maximal in the polar regions, medium in the middle zone. **B,** Medial plane showing the pelvis *(PV)* emerging through the hilum and minimal thickness anteriorly and posteriorly. **C,** Hypertrophy. **D,** Normal adult proportions of the renal substance. **E,** Senile atrophy. **F,** Normal appearance in a 2-year-old child.

Figure 10-15 Transverse scan of the right renal artery *(RRA)* as it extends from the posterior lateral wall of the aorta *(Ao)* to enter the central renal sinus.

Figure 10-16 On the longitudinal scan of IVC and aorta at renal bifurcation, the right renal artery *(RRA)* can be seen as a circular structure posterior to the inferior vena cava *(IVC)*. (Courtesy Siemens Medical Solutions USA, Inc.)

Figure 10-17 The right renal vein *(RRV)* extends from the central renal sinus directly into the inferior vena cava *(IVC)*. (Courtesy Shpetim Telegrafi, New York University.)

The left renal artery flows from the lateral wall of the aorta to the central renal sinus (Figure 10-18). The left renal vein flows from the central renal sinus, anterior to the aorta and posterior to the superior mesenteric artery, to join the inferior vena cava (Figure 10-19). It is seen as a tubular structure on the transverse scan.

The diaphragmatic crura run transversely in the para-aortic region. The crura lie posterior to the renal arteries and should be identified by their lack of pulsations and absence of Doppler flow (Figure 10-20). They vary in echogenicity, depending on the amount of surrounding retroperitoneal fat. They may appear hypoechoic, like lymph nodes.

Renal Medulla. The renal medulla consists of hypoechoic pyramids disbursed in a uniform distribution, separated by bands of intervening parenchyma that extend toward the renal sinus. The pyramids are uniform in size, shape (triangular), and distribution. The apex of the pyramid points toward the sinus, and the base lies adjacent to the renal cortex. The arcuate vessels lie at the base of the pyramids. The pyramids are located at the junction between the more peripheral renal cortex and the central sinus (see Figure 10-2).

Figure 10-18 The left renal artery *(arrows)* flows from the posterior lateral wall of the aorta *(A)* to the central renal sinus.

Figure 10-19 The left renal vein *(LRV)* flows from the central renal sinus, anterior to the aorta *(A)* and posterior to the superior mesenteric artery *(SMA)* to join the inferior vena cava.

Figure 10-20 The crura of the diaphragm lie posterior to the renal arteries and should be identified by their lack of pulsations and no Doppler flow *(arrows)*.

Renal Variants. Renal variants include slight alterations in anatomy that may lead the sonographer to suspect an abnormality is present when it really is a normal variation. See Table 10-1 for a description of renal variants and anomalies.

Columns of Bertin. The **columns of Bertin** are prominent invaginations of the cortex located at varying depths within the medullary substance of the kidneys. These areas are normal cortex. The columns may be the fusion of two septa into a single column of twice normal thickness. The columns are most exaggerated in patients with complete or partial duplication (Figure 10-21).

Sonographic features of a renal mass effect produced by a hypertrophied column of Bertin include the following: a lateral indentation of the renal sinus, a clear definition from the renal sinus, or a maximum dimension that does not exceed 3 cm. There is contiguity with the renal cortex, and the overall echogenicity is similar to that of the renal parenchyma.

Dromedary hump. The **dromedary hump** is a cortical bulge that occurs on the lateral border of the kidney, typically more on the left side (Figure 10-22). In some patients, it may be so prominent that it resembles a neoplasm. The dromedary hump probably results from pressure on the developing fetal kidney by the spleen. The echogenicity is identical to that of the rest of the renal cortex.

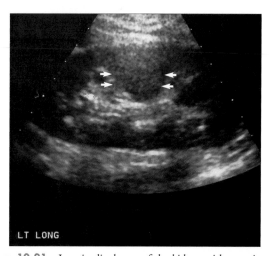

Figure 10-21   Longitudinal scan of the kidney with prominent column of Bertin *(arrows)*. (Courtesy Shpetim Telegrafi, New York University.)

Figure 10-22   Coronal view of the left kidney. The dromedary hump *(arrows)* is a cortical bulge that occurs on the lateral border of the kidney, typically on the left more than the right. (Courtesy Shpetim Telegrafi, New York University.)

TABLE 10-1   RENAL ANOMALIES AND VARIANTS

Type	Location	Sonographic Appearance	Differential Considerations	Distinguishing Characteristics
Column of Bertin	Medulla	Indentation of the renal sinus	Renal mass effect	Similar to renal parenchyma; contiguous with cortex
Dromedary hump	Lateral border of the kidney	Identical to the renal cortex	Mass effect	Usually seen on the left kidney
Junctional parenchymal defect	Upper pole of renal parenchyma	Echogenic triangular area	Mass effect	Best seen on sagittal scans
Fetal lobulation	Surface of the kidney	Indentations between the calyces	Mass effect	Best seen on sagittal scans
Lobar dysmorphism	Middle and upper calyces	Elongation of upper and middle calyces	Column of Bertin	Best seen on sagittal scans
Duplex collecting system	Central renal sinus	Two echogenic regions separated by moderately echogenic parenchymal tissue	Mass effect	"Faceless"; no echogenic renal pelvis seen on transverse view at the level of the mid pole
Extrarenal pelvis	Long renal pelvis that extends outside the renal border	Central cystic region that extends beyond the medial renal border	Renal aneurysm, dilated proximal ureter	Best seen on a transverse view at the level of the midpole
Horseshoe kidney	Kidneys seen more medial and anterior to the spine	Fusion of the polar region, usually the lower poles		Inferior poles lie more medial, associated with pyelocaliectasis, anomalous extrarenal pelvis, urinary calculi

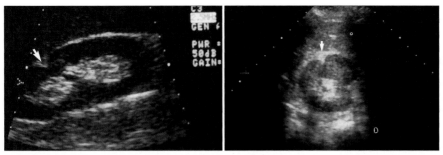

Figure 10-23 Junctional parenchymal defect *(arrow)* is a triangular area in the upper pole of the renal parenchyma. (Courtesy Shpetim Telegrafi, New York University.)

Figure 10-24 An 89-year-old male with renal lobulations (an irregularly shaped renal border). (Courtesy Shpetim Telegrafi, New York University.)

Junctional parenchymal defect. A junctional parenchymal defect is a triangular, echogenic area in the upper pole of the renal parenchyma that can be seen during normal scanning (Figure 10-23). The defect results from the normal extensions of the renal sinus in cases in which there is distinct division between the upper and lower poles of the kidney.

The kidneys develop from fusion of two embryonic parenchymatous masses referred to as ranunculi. In cases of partial fusion, parenchymal defects occur at the junction of the ranunculi and are best demonstrated on sagittal scans.

A lobar dysmorphism is a lobar fusion variant in which there is a malrotation of the renal lobe. The middle and upper calyces may be splayed. The dysmorphic lobe may resemble a mass or prominent column of Bertin on ultrasound.

Fetal lobulation. Fetal lobulation is developmental variation that is typically seen in children and may be seen in adults. The surfaces of the kidneys are generally indented in between the calyces, giving the kidneys a slightly lobulated appearance (Figure 10-24).

Duplex collecting system. The duplex collecting system is a common normal variant. It is difficult to tell if it is complete or incomplete because the ureters are not routinely visualized on sonograms. The way to confirm a complete collecting system is to demonstrate two ureteral jets entering the bladder on the same side. The duplex kidney is usually enlarged with smooth margins. The central renal sinus appears as two echogenic regions separated by a cleft of moderately echogenic tissue similar in appearance to the normal renal parenchyma (Figure 10-25). On a transverse view, the area separating the renal pelvis is called "faceless" because the tissue is homogeneous with no central echogenic renal pelvis. The pelvis of the lower pole is usually larger than the upper pole.

Sinus lipomatosis. Sinus lipomatosis is a condition characterized by deposition of a moderate amount of fat in the renal sinus (Figures 10-26 and 10-27). The degree of proliferation of fibrofatty tissue varies. The renal sinus consists of fibrous tissue, fat, lymphatic vessels, and renal vascular structures. In normal kidneys, this central zone appears as a bright area. In sinus lipomatosis, the abundant fibrous tissue may cause enlargement of the sinus region and increased echogenicity.

Extrarenal pelvis. The normal renal pelvis is a triangular structure. Its axis points inferiorly and medially. An intrarenal pelvis lies almost completely within the confines of the central renal sinus. This is usually small and foreshortened. The extrarenal pelvis tends to be larger with long major calyces. Using sonography, the pelvis appears as a central cystic area that is either partially or entirely beyond the confines of the bulk of the renal substance. Transverse views are the best to view continuity with the renal sinus. The dilated extrarenal pelvis will usually decompress when the patient is placed in the prone position (Figure 10-28).

Renal Anomalies. Renal anomalies comprise abnormalities in number, size, position, structure, or form (Figures 10-29 and 10-30) (see Table 10-1). Anomalies in number include agenesis or dysgenesis and supernumerary kidneys. Agenesis of the kidney is the absence or failure of formation of the organ. Dysgenesis is the defective embryonic development of the kidney. A pseudotumor is an overgrowth of cortical tissue that indents the echogenic renal sinus. This overgrowth may be mistaken for a renal tumor (Figure 10-31). A supernumerary kidney is a complete duplication of the renal system.

Solitary kidney. A solitary kidney results from unilateral **renal agenesis.** It is very rare. The sonographer must look for a small, nonfunctioning kidney. Renal compensatory hyper-

A   **B**   **C**

Figure 10-25   **A,** Duplex collecting system. The central sinus appears as two echogenic regions separated by a cleft of moderate echogenic tissue similar to the normal renal parenchyma. **B,** Transverse view of the echogenic tissue separates the renal sinus "faceless." **C,** Double right ureteral jets confirming complete duplex collecting system. (Courtesy Shpetim Telegrafi, New York University.)

Figure 10-26   Longitudinal scan of the right kidney showing increased renal sinus fat consistent with the renal sinus lipomatosis.

trophy (enlargement) generally occurs with a solitary kidney (Figure 10-32).

Pelvic kidney. If the kidney is not seen in the normal position in the renal fossa, the retroperitoneum and pelvis should be scanned. Most true **ectopic kidneys** are located in the bony pelvis and may be malrotated. The pelvic kidney may simulate a solid adnexal mass. It may be associated with other abnormalities, such as vesicoureteral reflux and anomalous extrarenal pelvis. Three complications that are associated with ectopic kidneys are chronic pyelonephritis, hydronephrosis, and stones.

Horseshoe kidney. Fusion anomalies of the kidneys include crossed renal ectopia and horseshoe kidney (most common). In a patient with a **horseshoe kidney,** there is fusion of the polar regions of the kidneys during fetal development that almost invariably involves the lower poles. Commonly, it is associated with improper ascent and malrotation of the kidneys, usually in a lower retroperitoneal position. The renal pelvis and ureters are more ventrally located. These kidneys generally lie closer to the spine. The inferior poles lie more medially. The isthmus of the kidney lies anterior to the spine and may simulate a solid pelvic mass or enlarged lymph nodes (Figure 10-33). Associated pathology includes pyelocaliectasis, anomalous extrarenal pelvis, and urinary calculi.

Thoracic kidney. A thoracic kidney migrates through the diaphragm into the thoracic cavity. It is a rare finding and not easily diagnosed with ultrasound.

Crossed-fused kidney. Both kidneys are located on the same side of the body. In the majority of the cases, the upper pole of the ectopic kidney will be fused to the lower pole of

Figure 10-27   Transverse **(A)** and longitudinal **(B)** scans of a patient with renal sinus lipomatosis.

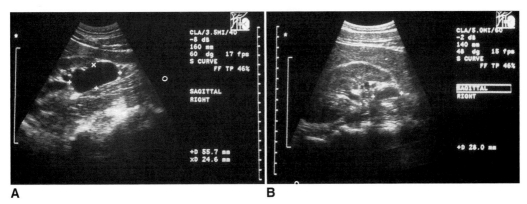

Figure 10-28   Extrarenal pelvis. **A,** Scan of the right kidney with an extrarenal pelvis appearing as a cystic area that extends beyond the confines of the renal borders. **B,** Patient lying in a prone position shows the collapsed extrarenal pelvis. (Courtesy Shpetim Telegrafi, New York University.)

the other kidney. It is a rare finding and is difficult to determine with ultrasound (Figure 10-34).

Evaluation of a Renal Mass.   Before the ultrasound examination for the evaluation of a renal mass, the sonographer should review the patient's chart, including the laboratory findings and previous diagnostic examinations, which may include a plain radiograph of the abdomen, IVP, CT, or MRI study. Whenever possible, these films should be obtained before the ultrasound study to tailor the examination to address the clinical problem. The sonographer should evaluate the ultrasound images to determine the shape and size of the kidney and the location of the mass lesion, to look for distortion of the renal or ureter structure, and to look for calcium stones or gas within the kidney.

Renal masses are categorized as cystic, solid, or complex by ultrasound evaluation. A cystic mass sonographically displays several characteristic features: (1) a smooth, thin, well-defined border; (2) round or oval shape; (3) sharp interface between the cyst and renal parenchyma; (4) no internal echoes (anechoic); and (5) increased posterior acoustic enhancement.

A solid lesion projects as a nongeometric shape with irregular borders, a poorly defined interface between the mass and the kidney, low-level internal echoes, a weak posterior border

because of the increased attenuation of the mass, and poor through-transmission.

Areas of necrosis, hemorrhage, abscess, or calcification within the mass may alter the classification and cause the lesion to fall into the complex category. This means the mass shows characteristics associated with both the cystic and solid lesions.

Real-time ultrasound allows the sonographer to carefully evaluate the renal parenchyma in many stages of respiration. If the mass is very small, respiratory motion may cause it to move in and out of the field of view. Careful evaluation of the best respiratory phase combined with use of the cine-loop feature will allow the sonographer to adequately image most renal masses to determine their characteristic composition.

Ultrasonic aspiration techniques.   Most renal masses that have met the criteria for a simple cystic mass do not require a needle aspiration. The Bosniak classification of cysts is used to determine the appropriate work-up for a cystic mass (Table 10-2). A needle aspiration may be recommended to obtain fluid from the lesion to evaluate its internal composition.

The patient should be placed in a prone position with sandbags or rolled sheets under the abdomen to help push the kidneys toward the posterior abdominal wall and provide a flat scanning surface. The renal mass should be located in the

A Horsehoe kidney

B Cake kidney

C Pelvic kidney

D Extrarenal pelvis

E Double collecting system

F Polycystic kidney

Figure 10-29   Variations of renal anatomy, position within the retroperitoneal cavity, and pathology. **A,** Horseshoe kidney shown as two kidneys connected by an isthmus anterior to the great vessels and inferior to the inferior mesenteric artery. **B,** Cake kidney with a double collecting system. **C,** Pelvic kidney with one kidney in the normal retroperitoneal position. **D,** Extrarenal pelvis. **E,** Double collecting system in a single kidney. **F,** Polycystic kidney.

Figure 10-30   Oblique view of a malrotated right kidney, unable to image the normal bean shape of the kidney. (Courtesy Shpetim Telegrafi, New York University.)

Figure 10-31   Pseudotumor. A longitudinal scan showing an overgrowth of cortical tissue indenting the renal pelvis. (Courtesy Shpetim Telegrafi, New York University.)

transverse and longitudinal planes, with scans performed at midinspiration. Hold the transducer lightly over the scanning surface so as not to compress the subcutaneous tissue. The depth of the mass should be noted from its posterior to anterior borders so the exact depth can be given to aid in placement of the needle. Compression of the subcutaneous tissue results in an inaccurate depth measurement.

A beveled needle causes multiple echoes within the walls of the lesion. If the needle is slightly bent, many echoes appear until the bent needle is completely out of the transducer's path. The larger the needle gauge, the stronger the reflection.

Sterile technique is used for aspiration and biopsy procedures. The transducer must be gas sterilized. Sterile lubricant is used to couple the transducer to the patient's skin.

Figure 10-32 Enlarged solitary kidney with unilateral renal agenesis. (Courtesy Joseph Yee, New York University.)

When the area of aspiration is outlined on the patient's back, the distance is measured from the posterior surface to the middle of the lesion.

The volume of the cyst may be determined by measuring the radius of the mass and using the following formula:

$$V = 4/3\pi r^3$$

The diameter of the mass can be applied to this formula:

$$V = d^3/2$$

The patient's skin is painted with tincture of benzalkonium (Zephiran), and sterile drapes are applied. A local anesthetic agent is administered over the area of interest, and the sterile transducer is used to relocate the lesion. The needle is inserted into the central core of the cyst. The needle stop helps ensure

Figure 10-33 **A** and **B**, Longitudinal scans of the right and left kidney in a pediatric patient. It was very difficult to record the lower poles of both kidneys. *LK*, Left kidney; *RK*, right kidney. **C**, Transverse scan of the renal area shows a hypoechoic tissue mass connected to both kidneys. This represents the isthmus of the horseshoe kidney. *A*, Aorta.

TABLE 10-2   BOSNIAK CYST CATEGORIES, CRITERIA, AND WORK-UP

Category	Criteria	Work-up
Simple cyst (I)	Thin smooth wall, anechoic, round or oval in shape; increased through-transmission	None
Mildy complex cyst (II)	Thin septation or calcified wall	2-3 month follow-up with CT or ultrasound
Indeterminate lesion (III)	Multiple septa, thickened septa, internal echoes	Biopsy or partial nephrectomy—increased risk for malignancy
Malignant lesion (IV)	Solid component, irregular walls	Nephrectomy

that the needle does not go through the cyst. The fluid is then withdrawn according to the volume calculations.

LOWER URINARY TRACT

Congenital Anomalies

Duplication of ureters. Duplication of the ureters can be complete, with separate ureters draining the upper and lower collecting systems of the kidneys and entering the bladder separately. The ureter draining the upper pole enters the bladder more caudad than the ureter draining the lower pole. Duplications can be either unilateral or bilateral. Duplication of the ureters is more common in females than males. Incomplete duplication occurs when the ureters join together and enter the bladder as one.

Ureterocele. Ureterocele is a cystlike enlargement of the lower end of the ureter (Figure 10-35). Ureteroceles are caused by either a congenital or an acquired stenosis of the distal end of the ureter. They usually are small and asymptomatic. Ureteroceles may cause obstruction and infection of the upper urinary system; if large, they may cause bladder outlet obstruction. They are found more often in adults than in children.

A large ureterocele may fill the urinary bladder and have the same sonographic appearance as diverticula. Having the patient partially empty the bladder will help make a better diagnostic-quality image because the ureterocele will be empty.

Figure 10-34 Crossed fused kidney measuring 16.9 cm. (Courtesy Shpetim Telegrafi, New York University.)

The alternate filling and emptying of the ureterocele because of peristalsis may be demonstrated with real-time ultrasound imaging. Calculi may also be present.

Ectopic ureterocele. Ectopic ureteroceles are rare and found more commonly in children and young adults, especially in females. They usually are associated with complete ureteral duplication. The ureter, which empties the upper pole, inserts low in the bladder by the bladder neck, urethra, or lower genital tract. The ectopic ureter may become stenotic and cause ureteral obstruction, which is associated with hydroureter and hydronephrosis. The ureterocele sac may obstruct the bladder outlet or prolapse through the urethra.

The sonographic appearance is a round, thin-walled cystic structure that may contain debris protruding into the bladder. The sonographic appearance is similar to a Foley catheter.

BLADDER

Ultrasound is not the imaging modality of choice to examine the bladder. Cystoscopy is usually used to examine the bladder because of its ability to diagnose early neoplasms. Transabdominal ultrasound will allow visualization of most lesions greater than 5 mm. A transurethral intravesicular sonographic approach has been used to evaluate bladder tumors.

The examination of the urinary bladder should be performed at the same time as the examination of the upper urinary tract. A complete review of the patient's chart, including previous diagnostic imaging procedures, should be obtained before beginning the ultrasound study of the bladder.

Ultrasound of the bladder is performed with a distended bladder. The patient lies in a supine position. A right or left decubitus position may be used to demonstrate calculi movement. Proper adjustment of the TGC allows for minimization of the anterior wall reverberations, anechoic bladder, with posterior acoustic enhancement. The depth of the image should be set to visualize any structure that may lie posterior or caudal to the bladder. A 3.5-MHz transducer is usually used. In very thin patients a 5-MHz transducer may be used. If evaluation of the anterior bladder wall is indicated, a high-frequency, curved linear array transducer will give a larger field of view than a sector transducer.

A   **B**

Figure 10-35 **A,** Longitudinal scan of a left ureterocele with ureteral jet known as the "candle sign." **B,** Transverse view of a ureterocele *(arrow).*

CONDITIONS THAT CAUSE INCOMPLETE EMPTYING OF BLADDER

Bladder calculi
Diabetes mellitus
Foley catheter
Inflammation
Neogenic bladder
Neoplasms—benign or malignant
Postsurgical intervention
Pregnancy
Radiation therapy
Rectal or vaginal fistulas
Renal disease
Sexual intercourse
Trauma (blood clot)
Tuberculosis (lower ureteric stricture)
Urethral stricture

SYMPTOMS IN DISEASES OF THE KIDNEY

RENAL CYSTIC DISEASE
Inflammatory or Necrotic Cysts
Clinical symptoms include the following:

- Flank pain
- Hematuria
- Proteinuria
- White blood cells in urine
- ↑ Protein

RENAL SUBCAPSULAR HEMATOMA
- Hematuria
- ↓ Hematocrit

RENAL INFLAMMATORY PROCESSES
Abscess
- Acute onset of symptoms
- Fever
- May have palpable mass
- ↑ White blood cell count
- Pyuria

Acute Focal Bacterial Nephritis
- Symptoms
  Fever
  Flank pain
  Pyuria
- ↑ Blood urea nitrogen
- ↑ Albumin
- ↑ Total plasma proteins

Acute Tubular Necrosis
- Symptoms (caused by renal calculi):
  Moderate to severe intermittent flank pain
  Vomiting
- Hematuria
- Infection
- Leukocytosis with infection

Chronic Renal Failure
- ↑ Concentration of urea in blood
- High urine protein excretion
- ↑ Creatinine
- Presence of granulocytes

RENAL CELL CARCINOMA
- Erythrocytosis may occur
- Leukocytosis
- Red blood cells in urine
- Pyuria
- ↑ Lactic acid dehydrogenase

The transducer should be placed in the middle of the filled urinary bladder and angled laterally, inferiorly, and superiorly. The bladder walls should be smooth and thin (3 to 6 mm). The bladder should be midline and not deviated to either side or have any irregular or asymmetric indentations.

Ultrasound is used to evaluate residual bladder volume in patients with outflow obstruction. The postvoid bladder is scanned in two planes: anteroposterior and transverse. Measurements are obtained in three planes: anterior-posterior, transverse, and longitudinal. Images and measurements are obtained at the largest dimensions. Since the bladder shape varies, any volume measurement can be used to approximate volume. A residue of less than 20 cc of urine is considered normal in an adult.

Ureteral jets should be identified as flashes of Doppler color entering the bladder from the lateral posterior border of the bladder and coursing superior and medial.

An enlarged prostate, enlarged uterus, pelvic mass, or filled loop of bowel may indent the urinary bladder (Box 10-1).

The urethra is not routinely visualized sonographically. A transvaginal approach has been used in females; a transrectal or transperineal approach can also successfully image the urethra in both females and males. Doppler has been used in sonourethrography to image the penile urethra in cases of erectile dysfunction. The use of drugs for erectile dysfunction has decreased the number of sonourethrograms performed.

PATHOLOGY OF THE URINARY SYSTEM

See Table 10-3 for clinical findings, sonographic findings, and differential considerations for various renal diseases and conditions. See Box 10-2 for symptoms of renal diseases.

RENAL CYSTIC DISEASE
Simple renal cystic disease encompasses a wide range of disease processes, which may be typical, complicated, or atypical. The disease may be acquired or inherited (e.g., von Hippel-Lindau disease or tuberous sclerosis). More complex cystic disease includes adult polycystic, infantile polycystic, or multicystic disease. There may be cystic disease in the renal medulla or sinus (see Table 10-3).

Simple Renal Cyst. The exact pathogenesis of a simple renal cyst is not known. Generally the cyst is believed to

Text continues on p. 314

Table 10-3 Renal Findings

Clinical Findings	Sonographic Findings	Differential Considerations
Simple Cysts		
Usually asymptomatic Usually normal laboratory findings	Found anywhere in the kidney, but usually in cortex Round or ovoid in shape, anechoic Thin, well-defined walls Tadpole sign No color flow or Doppler in mass	Hemorrhagic cyst, infected cyst, necrotic cyst, malignant cyst, obstruction of upper pole, calyceal diverticula, pseudoaneurysm, arteriovenous malformation
Parapelvic Cysts		
Usually asymptomatic May present with hypertension or obstruction (hilum cyst) Pain Usually normal laboratory findings	Found in the renal hilum or renal sinus Well-defined sonolucent mass with regular or irregular borders Good through-transmission Not connected to the renal collecting system	Hydronephrosis
von Hippel-Lindau Cysts		
Flank pain General discomfort Involves many body systems Usually presents in third to fifth decade Initial clinical symptoms caused by cerebellar or spinal cord hemangioblastomas, not abdominal If renal involvement occurs, there is an ↑ chance of renal carcinoma No hypertension or renal failure	Bilateral cysts and masses Other organs are affected Masses may develop within the cysts Hyperplastic linings of cysts Pancreatic cysts	Multiple cysts Renal adenoma
Tuberous Sclerosis		
Involves several body systems Patient usually presents with mental retardation, seizures, and cutaneous lesions	Multiple cysts or angiomyolipomas Multiple organs involved Multiple angiomyolipomas that may become large	Angiomyolipomas
Acquired Cystic Disease of Dialysis		
Usually occurs in patients on renal dialysis for ≥3 yr Flank pain	Found in cortex Simple cysts Atypical because of hemorrhage Normal or small echogenic kidneys with ↓ in corticomedullary distinction with simple or atypical cysts	Renal cyst Adenoma Renal cell carcinoma
Adult Polycystic Kidney Disease		
Hypertension Renal failure Abdominal, flank pain Fever, chills (infection) Uremia Palpable mass Polycythemia Hematuria	Bilateral enlarged kidneys with multiple cysts of varied size Kidneys lose their reniform shape; in the late stages, no normal renal parenchyma may be identified Cysts may be atypical because of infection or hemorrhage Cysts may be found in liver, spleen, testes, pancreas	Cortical cysts Localized hydronephrosis Renal tuberculosis Multilocular cyst
Infantile Polycystic Kidney Disease		

May be seen in utero
Renal insufficiency
Lung hypoplasia, usually fatal depending on the amount of renal function
In juvenile form:
  Portal hypertension
  Hepatic fibrosis
  GI hemorrhage
	Bilateral enlarged echogenic kidneys
	Cysts too small to be seen
	No distinction between the corticomedullary region
		In utero—ADPKD, dysplasia, glomerulocystic kidney disease

TABLE 10-3   RENAL FINDINGS—cont'd

Clinical Findings	Sonographic Findings	Differential Considerations
Multicystic Dysplastic Kidney		
Most common palpable mass in neonates Restricted growth in children Polyuria Hypertension Infection Usually unilateral; bilateral is incompatible with life	Multiple cysts of varying size No renal parenchyma surrounding the cyst Enlarged kidneys in children Small kidneys in adults	Hydronephrosis
Medullary Sponge Kidney		
Usually asymptomatic unless calculus is present, then hematuria and infections Pain Hydronephrosis Infection	Normal or small kidneys with echogenic parenchyma (cysts too small to be resolved on ultrasound) Or Small cysts in medulla and corticomedullary region with ↑ echogenicity	Papillary necrosis Nephrocalcinosis Renal cystic disease Pyelonephritic cysts
Medullary Cystic Disease		
Normal renal function Anemia Salt loss Progressive azotemia Polyuria Pain Infection	Normal or small echogenic kidneys with small cysts under 2 cm Widening of the renal sinus *after 2* cm in the medulla or corticomedullary junction	Medullary sponge kidney
Renal Cell Carcinoma		
Hematuria Weight loss Fatigue Fever Flank pain Palpable mass Hypertension	Cystic or complex mass that may have areas of calcifications May displace renal pyramids and invade renal architecture Irregular margins Hypervascular Renal vein or IVC thrombosis	Angiomyolipoma Transitional cell carcinoma Lymphoma Oncocytoma Column of Bertin Renal vein or IVC thrombus
Transitional Cell Carcinoma		
Hematuria Weight loss Fatigue Fever Flank pain	Solid hypoechoic mass Not well defined within the renal sinus May be multiple	Squamous cell tumor Renal cell carcinoma Adenoma Blood clot Fungus ball
Squamous Cell Carcinoma		
Gross hematuria History of chronic irritation Palpable kidney if severe hydronephrosis is present	Large bulky mass Invasion of the renal vein and IVC	Transitional cell carcinoma
Renal Lymphoma		
Not a primary site; usually caused by adjacent lymph involvement More common in patients with non-Hodgkin's lymphoma Usually no renal symptoms Asymptomatic Pain Hematuria	Hypoechoic mass may be bilateral Enlarged kidney	Renal cell carcinoma Cyst

Continued

TABLE 10-3	RENAL FINDINGS—cont'd	
Clinical Findings	Sonographic Findings	Differential Considerations
Wilms' Tumor		
Palpable abdominal mass in children Abdominal pain Nausea and vomiting Hematuria	Usually unilateral, may be bilateral Heterogeneous Look for extension into renal vein and inferior vena cava	Nephroblastoma Renal cell carcinoma Mesoblastoma Multicystic kidney Retroperitoneal sarcoma
Benign Renal Tumor		
Usually asymptomatic May cause painless hematuria	Well-defined mass—hyperechoic to hypoechic	Angiomyolipoma Transitional cell carcinoma Oncocytoma Lymphoma Column of Bertin
Adenoma		
Asymptomatic	Well-defined mass with calcifications	Renal cell carcinoma
Angiolipoma		
Usually asymptomatic Possible flank pain Normal laboratory values Hematuria if tumor hemorrhages	Usually echogenic homogeneous mass with well-defined borders Hemorrhagic neoplasm	Oncocytoma Renal cell carcinoma
Lipoma		
Usually asymptomatic Normal laboratory values	Well-defined echogenic mass	Fibromas Adenoma
Oncocytoma		
Asymptomatic	Well-defined mass with spoke-wheel patterns of enhancement and central scar	Renal abscess
Acute Glomerulonephritis		
Nephrotic syndrome Hypertension Anemia Peripheral edema	↑ Cortical echoes	Chronic glomerulonephritis Acute tubular nephrosis AIDS Lupus nephritis Acute interstitial nephritis
Acute Interstitial Nephritis		
Uremia Hematuria Rash Fever Eosinophilia	Enlarged kidneys with ↑ cortical echoes	Acute glomerulonephritis Chronic glomerulonephritis Acute tubular necrosis AIDS Lupus nephritis
Lupus Nephritis		
Hematuria Proteinuria Renal vein thrombus Renal insufficiency	↑ Cortical echoes and renal atrophy	Acute glomerulonephritis Chronic glomerulonephritis Acute tubular necrosis AIDS Acute interstitial nephritis
Acquired Immunodeficiency Syndrome (AIDS)		
Renal dysfunction	Kidneys are either normal or enlarged Echogenic parenchyma ↑ Cortical echoes	Acute glomerulonephritis Chronic glomerulonephritis Acute tubular necrosis Lupus nephritis Acute interstitial nephritis

TABLE 10-3 RENAL FINDINGS—cont'd

Clinical Findings	Sonographic Findings	Differential Considerations
Sickle Cell Nephropathy		

Hematuria
Renal vein thrombosis
	Varies—*patients with acute renal vein thrombosis*:
	  Enlarged kidneys with ↓ echogenicity
	Subacute:
	  Enlarged kidneys with ↑ cortical echogenicity
		Lupus nephritis

Hypertensive Nephropathy		
Uncontrolled hypertension	Small kidneys with smooth borders may have distortion of intrarenal anatomy	Hypoplasia
Papillary Necrosis		
Hematuria Flank pain Hypertension Dysuria Acute renal failure	Fluid-filled spaces at the corticomedullary junction Round or triangular Mimics calculi	Congenital megacalyces Hydronephrosis Postobstruction atrophy
Renal Atrophy		
Renal failure	Small echogenic kidneys	Renal hypoplasia Chronic renal failure
Renal Sinus Lipomatosis		
Asymptomatic	Enlarged kidneys with ↑ echogenicity of renal sinus Hyperechoic areas ↓ Renal parenchyma	Infection Atrophy Hydronephrosis
Acute Renal Failure		
Renal insufficiency ↓ Urine output	Hydronephrosis Enlarged hypoechoic kidneys Renal artery stenosis	Prerenal, renal, or postrenal causes
Obstructive Hydronephrosis		
Renal insufficiency ↓ Urine output Hypertension	Fluid-filled renal collecting system Thin parenchyma Hydroureter ↓ or absent ureteral jets	Extrarenal collecting system Parapelvic cyst Reflux Renal artery aneurysm Transient diuresis Congenital megacalyces Papillary necrosis Arteriovenous malformation
Renal Infarction		
Asymptomatic	Irregular triangle masses in the renal parenchyma Lobulated renal contour	Renal lobulations Dromedary hump
Acute Tubular Necrosis		
Renal insufficiency Hematuria	Bilaterally enlarged kidneys with hyperechoic pyramids	Nephrocalcinosis
Chronic Renal Failure		
Renal failure Hypertension	Bilateral small echogenic kidneys	Multiple causes AIDS Chronic parenchymal infections

Continued

TABLE 10-3   RENAL FINDINGS—cont'd

Clinical Findings	Sonographic Findings	Differential Considerations
Pyonephrosis		
Renal insufficiency Hematuria	Dilated collecting system with low-level echoes or ↓ through-transmission	Hydronephrosis Hemorrhage Blood clot Uroepithelial tumors
Xanthogranulomatous Pyelonephritis		
Multiple infections Nonfunctioning kidneys	"Staghorn appearance" Destruction of renal parenchyma ↑ Echogenicity ↑ Renal size Dilated calyces	Hydronephrosis Renal calculi

↑, Increase; ↓, decrease; *GI,* gastrointestinal; *IVC,* inferior vena cava.

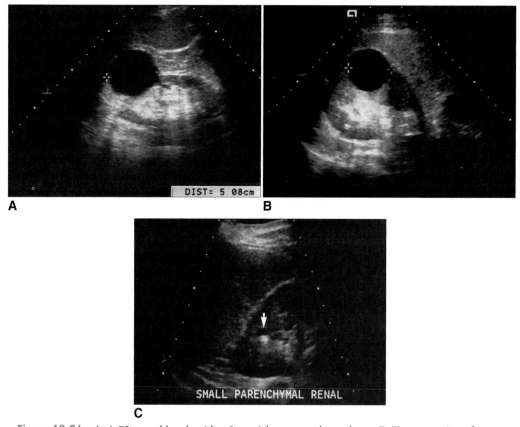

Figure 10-36   **A,** A 75-year-old male with a 5-cm right upper pole renal cyst. **B,** Transverse view of a right upper pole cyst. The borders are smooth and well defined. No internal echoes are seen. **C,** Small parenchymal renal cyst with increased posterior enhancement. (Courtesy Shpetim Telegrafi, New York University.)

represent retention cysts that occur secondary to tubular obstruction, vascular occlusion, or focal inflammation. Simple renal cysts are common, occurring in half of adults over 50 years of age. Renal cysts may be located anywhere in the kidney and are not clinically significant unless they distort the adjacent calyces or produce hydronephrosis or pain (see Table 10-3).

Sonographic Findings. Sonographic features of a simple renal cyst include a well-defined anechoic mass lesion with smooth walls with good through-transmission and no color flow within the cyst (Figures 10-36 to 10-37). The **tadpole sign** may be seen as narrow bands of acoustic shadowing posterior to the margins of the cyst along the lateral borders of

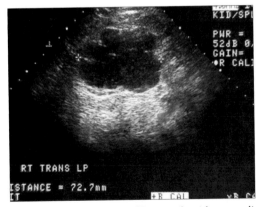

Figure 10-37 **A,** Upper pole renal cyst with no blood flow to the cyst. **B,** CT scan of the lower pole complicated cyst. **C,** Sagittal view of the left kidney with a cystic mass. (**A** courtesy Shpetim Telegrafi, New York University; **B** and **C** courtesy Joseph Yee, New York University.)

enhancement. A septum is occasionally seen within the cyst as a well-defined linear line. This indicates that the cyst is not a simple cyst, but a cyst with septations (Figure 10-38). Sonographically, it is difficult to differentiate between a septated cyst and small, adjacent cortical cysts known as "kissing" cysts (Figure 10-39). A cyst may also have a cyst or mass within it (Figure 10-40). Sometimes small sacculations or infoldings of the cystic wall produce wall irregularity; a cyst puncture or aspiration may be recommended to ascertain the pathology of the fluid within the mass.

Low-level echoes within a renal cyst may be artifacts (sensitivity too high or transducer frequency too low) or result from infection, hemorrhage (Figure 10-41), or a necrotic cystic tumor and in rare cases malignancy.

Parapelvic Cyst. The parapelvic cyst (renal sinus cyst) is found in the renal hilum, but does not communicate with the renal collecting system (Figure 10-42). Clinical symptoms are infrequent; the cyst can cause pain, hypertension, or obstruction (see Table 10-3).

Sonographic Findings. Ultrasound shows a well-defined mass with no internal septations. It can have irregular borders because it may compress the adjacent renal sinus structures. The parapelvic cyst may obstruct the kidney; the peripelvic cyst does not. The sonographer should be able to differentiate

Figure 10-38 Transverse view of lower pole with a complicated cyst.

the parapelvic cyst from hydronephrosis by trying to connect the dilated renal pelvis centrally. The dilated renal pelvis may present as a cauliflower appearance, whereas the parapelvic cyst is more spherical in appearance.

Cysts Associated With Multiple Renal Neoplasms
von Hippel-Lindau. von Hippel-Lindau disease is an autosomal-dominant genetic disorder. Several areas of the body

Figure 10-39   A, A single upper-pole cortical cyst with a thin septation. **B,** Two small adjacent renal cysts; "kissing" cysts. (Courtesy Shpetim Telegrafi, New York University.)

Figure 10-40 A 70-year-old man with a mass within a cyst. The calipers are measuring the mass. (Courtesy Shpetim Telegrafi, New York University.)

may be affected (see Table 10-3). Disease investigation has found retinal angiomas, cerebellar hemangioblastomas, and a variety of abdominal cysts and tumors, including renal and pancreatic cysts, renal adenomas, and frequent multiple and bilateral renal adenocarcinoma tumors.

Tuberous sclerosis. Tuberous sclerosis is an autosomal-dominant genetic disorder that may cause multiple renal cysts or angiomyolipomas or cutaneous, retinal, and cerebral hamartomas (see Table 10-3).

Acquired cystic disease of dialysis. Patients on renal dialysis have been shown to have an increased incidence of renal cysts, adenomas, and renal carcinoma. The incidence increases with time, particularly after the first 3 years of dialysis. Renal cysts can show spontaneous bleeding and hemorrhage, causing pain and flank discomfort (see Table 10-3).

Congenital Cystic Disease. Polycystic renal disease may present in one of two forms: the infantile autosomal-recessive form and the adult autosomal-dominant form.

Autosomal-recessive polycystic kidney disease. Autosomal-recessive polycystic kidney disease (ARPKD) is a fairly rare genetic disorder. The gene that causes this disorder has been located on chromosome 6. There is dilatation of the renal collecting tubules, which cause renal failure, and in the later forms there is also liver involvement. There are four forms of ARPKD: perinatal, neonatal, infantile, and juvenile. The earlier the clinical symptoms manifest themselves, the less the kidneys are functioning. The earliest form is found in utero (perinatal), which usually progresses to renal failure causing pulmonary hypoplasia and intrauterine demise. There is less renal function in the neonatal form than in the infantile form, but it can also progress to renal failure. In addition, there is usually some liver involvement. The juvenile form may present with hypertension, renal insufficiency, nephromegaly, hepatic cysts, bile duct proliferation, Caroli's disease of the liver, and periportal fibrosis, which causes portal hypertension. The decrease in renal function is usually secondary to the hepatic problems the later in life ARPKD appears.

Sonographic Findings. In the perinatal form, the fetus may have oligohydramnios, which are enlarged echogenic kidneys. In the later forms of ARPKD, the kidneys are enlarged with echogenic cortex and medulla and lack of corticomedullary differentiation. There may also be macroscopic or small cysts (1 to 2 mm) located in the medulla. In children there may also be hepatic fibrosis and splenomegaly.

Autosomal-dominant polycystic kidney disease. Autosomal-dominant polycystic kidney disease (ADPKD) is a common genetic disease that is found in both men and women. The severity of the disease varies depending upon the genotype. The most common type is PKD1 (located on the short arm of the 16th chromosome), which affects the kidneys more severely than PKD2 (located on the long arm of the 4th chromosome). There are a number of people who have no known genetic disposition to ADPKD; it may result by spontaneous mutations. It is a bilateral disease that is characterized by multiple cysts located in the renal cortex and medulla. The cysts vary in size and may be asymmetrical. The disease is progressive, which does not usually clinically manifest itself until the fourth or fifth decade. By the age of 60, approximately 50% of the patients will have end-stage renal disease (ESRD).

Figure 10-41   **A,** Transverse scan of a hemorrhagic cyst with no increase in blood flow. **B,** CT scan of hemorrhagic cyst. (Courtesy Joseph Yee, New York University.)

Figure 10-42   Transverse **(A)** and longitudinal **(B)** scans of a renal sinus cyst. Good through-transmission is noted beyond the renal parenchyma.

Clinical symptoms include pain (common complaint), hypertension, palpable mass, hematuria, headache, urinary tract infection, and renal insufficiency (Table 10-3).

Associated complications include infection, hemorrhage, stone formation, rupture of cyst, and renal obstruction.

Associated abnormalities include cysts in the liver, spleen, pancreas, thyroid, ovary, testes, breast, cerebral berry aneurysm, and abdominal aortic aneurysm. Patients who are on renal dialysis have an increased incidence of renal cell carcinoma.

Sonographic Findings. The sonographic appearance of ADPKD in the fetus has been described as moderately enlarged hyperechogenic kidneys with increased corticomedullary differentiation (CMD). This appearance is not unique to ADPKD, but further screening is warranted when noted on prenatal sonographic examination.

In the adult patient there is bilateral renal enlargement with multiple cysts in both the cortex and medulla. In the most advanced cases the normal renal parenchyma is replaced bilaterally with multiple cysts (Figures 10-43 to 10-48) and the kidneys lose their reniform shape. The cysts may grow large enough to obliterate the renal sinus. The cysts may become infected or hemorrhagic, which is characterized sonographically by internal debris within the cysts or thickened walls. The walls of the cysts maybe calcified or stones may form within the cysts. A complicated cyst may result in spontaneous bleeding, causing flank pain for the patient (see Table 10-3).

Multicystic Dysplastic Kidney. Multicystic dysplastic kidney disease is nonhereditary renal dysplasia that usually occurs unilaterally (see Table 10-3). Bilateral disease is incompatible with life. This disease is the most common form of cystic disease in neonates. There is a slight increased risk of malignant transformation that can occur if the kidney is not removed. There is research occurring that tries to identify specific tumor markers for multicystic dysplastic kidney disease to identify the patients who are at risk for malignant degeneration. Complications of multicystic dysplastic kidneys that are not removed include hypertension, hematuria, infection, and flank pain.

Sonographic Findings. In neonates and children the kidneys are enlarged; in adults, they may be small and calcified. The typical pattern is multiple cysts of varying size with no normal renal parenchyma. Other findings may also be present, including ureteral atresia (failure of the ureter to develop from the calyceal system), contralateral ureteropelvic

Figure 10-43   A 54-year-old male with polycystic renal disease. Longitudinal scans of both kidneys show multiple small cystic structures replacing the renal parenchyma.

Figure 10-44   Longitudinal and transverse scans of a patient with bilateral polycystic renal disease.

obstruction in 30% of patients (development of the ureter from the bladder with retrograde filling), nonfunctioning kidney, or an atretic renal artery.

Medullary Cystic Disease

Medullary sponge kidney. Medullary sponge kidney is a rare, nonhereditary, benign renal disease found in children (see Table 10-3).

Sonographic Findings. Common findings include tubular ectasia and calcium stones in 40% to 80% (nephrocalcinosis) (Figures 10-49 and 10-50). It is also associated with Caroli's disease of the liver.

Medullary cystic disease (nephronophthisis). Medullary cystic disease is autosomal-recessive. It is characterized by salt-wasting nephropathy in young adults.

Sonographic Findings. The patient presents with small echo-dense kidneys, tubular atrophy, and glomerular sclerosis. There are multiple small cysts under 2 cm.

RENAL NEOPLASMS

The sonographic appearance of most renal masses is nonspecific. Usually an abnormal renal contour is the first finding that

a mass may be present and require further investigation. Very often the sonographic characteristic patterns between a benign and malignant tumor cannot be differentiated from one another. In most clinical settings, ultrasound is usually the next step after the discovery of a renal mass on an IVP. If a solid mass is detected, renal cell carcinoma, oncocytomas, angiomyolipoma, transitional cell carcinoma, or secondary neoplasms (e.g., metastasis and lymphoma) must be considered.

Renal Cell Carcinoma. Renal cell carcinoma is the most common of all renal tumors (85% of all kidney tumors). It is twice as common in males as in females, usually in the sixth to seventh decade of life. The classic clinical presentation is nonspecific; however, the patient may report hematuria, flank pain, and palpable mass. The tumor appears bilaterally in 0.1% to 1.5% of patients. The incidence is increased in patients with von Hippel-Lindau disease and patients on long-term dialysis. The incidence of adenomas has also been reported.

Staging of renal cell carcinoma may be performed initially with ultrasound, although CT (with and without contrast) and

Figure 10-45   Patients with polycystic disease show enlargement of both kidneys with multiple small cystic areas throughout. **A** to **C,** Right kidney. **D** to **F,** Left kidney.

MRI are superior in tumor staging. Staging of renal cell carcinoma using the Robson system is as follows:

   I. Confined to kidney
  II. Spread to perinephric fat but within Gerota's fascia (Figure 10-51)
IIIa. Perinephric involvement with spread to renal vein and/or inferior vena cava (Figure 10-52)
IIIb. Perinephric involvement with regional lymph node enlargement
IIIc. Perinephric involvement with venous and lymph node involvement
  IV. Invasion of adjacent structures; distant metastases

Sonographic Findings. The increase in technical improvements in harmonic imaging has increased the detection of

Figure 10-46   A 45-year-old female with polycystic disease presented with huge cystic masses throughout the renal parenchyma. All of the cysts are distinct lesions and do not connect with the central renal sinus to indicate hydronephrosis.

Figure 10-47   About one third of patients with polycystic renal disease also have polycystic liver disease. This severe case shows multiple cysts throughout the liver parenchyma. Often the cysts are so complex that it becomes difficult to distinguish the renal parenchyma from the liver.

Figure 10-48   A 30-year-old male with a solitary left polycystic kidney and hematuria was sent to rule out obstruction. It is very difficult to rule out obstruction with so many small cysts.

small renal cell carcinomas. When found, renal cell carcinoma usually presents as a solid parenchymal mass, frequently with areas of hemorrhage and necrosis (see Table 10-2). Renal cell carcinoma is not usually echogenic unless the mass is very small or calcification is present. Characteristically the mass is isoechoic to hypoechoic or complex on ultrasound (Figure 10-53). Occasionally, renal cell carcinoma appears predominately as an echogenic mass. Irregular tumor calcification can be seen in a small number of patients. Any calcified mass within the kidney indicates the possibility of tumor. When a mass is found, the sonographer should define the extent of involvement in the renal veins, inferior vena cava, and right atrium of the heart. Color flow Doppler is useful to image the renal vein to observe flow rate; a low velocity may be seen if tumor obstruction is severe.

Transitional Cell Carcinoma. Transitional cell carcinoma is the most common tumor of the renal collecting system. The tumor is often multiple. The incidence is three to four times higher in males and increases with age. The differential

Figure 10-49   Longitudinal scans of a young patient with medullary sponge kidney show nephrocalcinosis and an echogenic medullary renal parenchyma.

Figure 10-50   A 6-year-old male with medullary sponge kidneys. **A** and **B**, Transverse scans. **C**, Longitudinal scan of the right kidney.

Figure 10-51 Transverse view of renal cellular carcinoma extending through the renal border. (Courtesy Shpetim Telegrafi, New York University.)

diagnosis includes other tumors of the renal pelvis, such as squamous cell tumor or adenoma, a blood clot, or a fungus ball (see Table 10-2).

Sonographic Findings. On ultrasound examination, the mass in the renal pelvis shows low-level echoes, widening of the central sinus echoes, and a hypoechoic central area (Figure 10-54). Clinically the patient may present with a history of blood in the urine.

Squamous cell carcinoma. Squamous cell carcinoma is a rare, highly invasive tumor with a poor prognosis. Clinically the patient usually presents with a history of chronic irritation and gross hematuria, with a palpable kidney secondary to severe hydronephrosis.

Sonographic Findings. The sonographic finding is usually a large mass in the renal pelvis. Obstruction from kidney stones may also be present (Figure 10-55).

Renal Lymphoma. The lymphomatous involvement of the kidneys is usually a secondary process, via either hematogenous spread or contiguous spread from the retroperitoneum (see Table 10-2). Non-Hodgkin's lymphoma is more common than Hodgkin's. Lymphoma is more common as a bilateral invasion with multiple nodules.

Sonographic Findings. The sonographic findings are not specific in patients with lymphoma involving the kidneys. The kidneys are enlarged and hypoechoic and usually no definite mass is identified (Figure 10-56).

Metastases. Metastases to the kidneys are a relatively common finding at autopsy, but metastases may also present when the patient is alive. The most common primaries are from malignant melanoma, lymphoma, and carcinoma of the lungs, breast, stomach, cervix, colon, or pancreas.

Wilms' Tumor. Nephroblastoma or Wilms' tumor is the most common solid renal mass of childhood. It is rare in the newborn; the incidence peaks in the second year of life. Half of the tumors occur before the child's third birthday. The tumor may recur, so careful follow-up of the patient is important.

Wilms' tumor is associated with Beckwith-Widemann syndrome, sporadic aniridia (no color in the eye), omphalocele, and hemihypertrophy (one side of body is larger than other).

Most patients present with a palpable abdominal mass. Other clinical findings include abdominal pain, anorexia, nausea and vomiting, fever, and gross hematuria. Venous obstruction may result with findings of leg edema, varicocele, or Budd-Chiari syndrome.

Sonographic Findings. The tumor may spread beyond the **renal capsule** and invade the venous channel, with tumor cells extending into the inferior vena cava and right atrium and with eventual metastasis into the lungs (Figures 10-57 to 10-59). The tumor may be multifocal in a small percentage of patients.

Benign Renal Tumors. Benign renal tumors are rare. All renal tumors are treated as malignant until proven otherwise. The patient usually is asymptomatic and only presents with flank pain if the mass is large or if there is hemorrhage from the mass. Adenomas and oncocytomas are two common benign renal tumors.

Adenoma. Adenoma is one of the most common benign renal tumors. The tumors consist of tubular epithelial cells. Patients are usually asymptomatic and there are usually incidental findings; in some cases they may cause hematuria.

Sonographic Findings. Adenomas are well-defined hyperechoic masses with calcifications located in the renal cortex (see Table 10-3).

Angiomyolipoma. Angiomyolipoma (AML) is an uncommon benign renal tumor composed mainly of fat cells and commonly found in the renal cortex. It is intermixed with smooth muscle cells and aggregates of thick-walled blood vessels. There may be hemorrhage in the tumor itself or in the subcapsular or perinephric space.

Sonographic Findings. On ultrasound, a focal, solid hyperechoic mass located in the cortex, which may have posterior acoustic enhancement, is typical of an angiomyolipoma (see Table 10-3). There are two primary patterns of occurrence; the most common is the tumor that is solitary, nonhereditary, and found in young to middle-aged women (Figures 10-60 and 10-61). The other multiple tumors with bilateral renal involvement are found in patients with tuberous sclerosis.

Lipomas. A lipoma consists of fat cells and is the most common of the mesenchymal type of tumors. The tumor is found more often in females than males. The patient is typically asymptomatic, but the tumor has been reported to cause hematuria.

Sonographic Findings. Lipomas appear as a well-defined echogenic mass (Figure 10-62) (see Table 10-3).

Oncocytomas. Oncocytomas consist of large epithelial cells. They are found more often in older men than women and can also occur in the parathyroid glands, thyroid gland, and adrenal glands. They range in size from small to large. The patient is typically asymptomatic, but the tumor may also cause pain and hematuria.

Sonographic Findings. Oncocytomas resemble "spokewheel" patterns of enhancement with a central scar (see

Text continued on p. 327

Figure 10-52 Stage III renal cell carcinoma with invasion into the inferior vena cava. **A,** Longitudinal scan shows lower pole mass with no normal renal parenchyma. **B,** Measurement of the lower pole mass. **C,** Longitudinal scan demonstrating the thrombus-filled inferior vena cava (IVC). **D,** Longitudinal scan of IVC with color flow showing obstruction. **E,** Transverse view of the dome of the liver with patent hepatic veins and nonvisualization of the IVC. (Courtesy Joseph Yee, New York University.)

Figure 10-53   Renal cell carcinoma seen in a 62-year-old male who presented with hematuria. **A,** Longitudinal scan shows the mass forming an irregular border at the lower pole of kidney. **B,** Another patient with renal cell carcinoma seen to displace the central renal sinus on this transverse image.

Figure 10-54   Longitudinal **(A)** and transverse **(B)** scans of a transitional cell carcinoma. The mass *(M)* is hypoechoic and is located near the renal sinus. *LK,* Left kidney.

Figure 10-55   Sixty-year-old patient with metastatic disease. **A,** Sagittal image of right kidney shows irregular-shaped mass filling the renal sinus. **B,** Transverse image of the squamous cell carcinoma. (From Henningsen C: *Clinical guide to ultrasonography,* St. Louis, 2004, Mosby.)

Figure 10-56   Sixty-year-old patient with bilateral renal lymphomas. **A,** Sagittal image of right kidney with hypoechoic upper pole mass. **B,** Transverse image of upper pole of right kidney with hypoechoic lymphoma. (From Henningsen C: *Clinical guide to ultrasonography,* St. Louis, 2004, Mosby.)

Figure 10-57   This 2-year-old presented with a large palpable abdominal mass *(M)* and nausea and vomiting. The tumor arises from the right kidney *(RK)* and compresses the renal sinus. It is clearly separate from the liver *(L).* This is a Wilms' tumor of the kidney.

Figure 10-58 **A** and **B,** One of the complications of a Wilms' tumor *(M)* is spread beyond the renal capsule into the renal vein and inferior vena cava *(IVC).* This 18-month-old child had a large, complex tumor with extension into the inferior vena cava *(IVC, arrows). RK,* Right kidney. **C** and **D,** Longitudinal scan, showing the dilated inferior vena cava with tumor echoes along the posterior border. The tumor may extend into the right atrium of the heart. *L,* Liver; *RK,* right kidney.

Figure 10-59 **A** through **D,** A 14-month-old child with a large Wilms' tumor *(M)* extending from the right kidney *(KID)* into the inferior vena cava *(IVC).* On the coronal scan **(D),** the tumor mass is seen within the IVC. The patient is rolled into a slight decubitus position to better image the IVC and aorta *(Ao). LIV,* Liver.

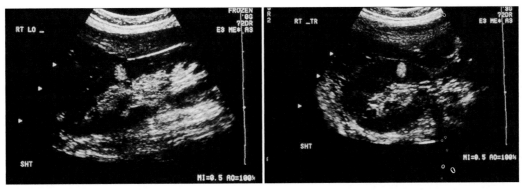

Figure 10-60   Angiomyolipoma appears as an echogenic focal mass in the renal parenchyma. (Courtesy Shpetim Telegrafi, New York University.)

Figure 10-61   Angiolipomas are uncommon benign tumors that usually appear as unilateral echogenic masses in middle-aged women. A common location is adjacent to the collecting system. Renal function is normal. (Courtesy Shpetim Telegrafi, New York University.)

Figure 10-62   Sagittal view of left kidney with lipoma. (Courtesy Siemens Medical Solutions USA, Inc.)

Table 10-3). To differentiate malignant from benign tumors, the sonographer should look at the vascular flow patterns, the presence of nodes, or metastasis surrounding the structure or adjacent to the kidney. Ultrasound may distinguish the composition of a tumor, but it cannot indicate the histologic nature of the mass (Figure 10-63).

RENAL DISEASE

Intrinsic renal disease can be demonstrated by examining the renal parenchyma with ultrasound. Two classifications of disease processes have been described. One group produces a generalized increase in cortical echoes, believed to result from deposition of collagen and fibrous tissue. This group includes interstitial nephritis, acute tubular necrosis, amyloidosis, diabetic nephropathy, systemic lupus erythematosus, and myeloma.

The second group of diseases causes loss of normal anatomic detail, resulting in the inability to distinguish the cortex and medullary regions of the kidneys. This group of diseases includes chronic pyelonephritis, renal tubular ectasia, and acute bacterial nephritis.

Lack of specificity and the overlapping appearances of different disease entities prevented this schematic from gaining wide acceptance. The end stage of many of these disease processes is renal atrophy, which can be seen on ultrasound by measuring renal length and cortical thickness. Some acute renal disorders can produce exactly the opposite findings— decreased parenchymal echogenicity and renal enlargement. Examples include renal vein thrombosis, pyelonephritis, and renal-transplant rejection. Interstitial edema is thought to be the most likely cause of these findings.

Acute Glomerulonephritis. In acute glomerulonephritis, necrosis or proliferation of cellular elements (or both) occurs in the glomeruli (see Table 9-2). The vascular elements, tubules, and interstitium become secondarily affected; the end result is enlarged, poorly functioning kidneys.

Sonographic Findings. Different forms of glomerulonephritis, including membranous, idiopathic, membranoproliferative, rapidly progressive, and poststreptococcal, can be associated with abnormal echo patterns from the renal parenchyma on ultrasound (Figure 10-64). The increased cortical echoes probably result from changes within the glomerular, interstitial, tubular, and vascular structures. Patients have many symptoms, including nephrotic syndrome, hypertension, anemia, and peripheral edema.

Acute Interstitial Nephritis. Acute interstitial nephritis has been associated with the infectious processes scarlet fever

A

B

C

Figure 10-63 **A,** Longitudinal view of right kidney shows large oncocytoma mass. **B,** Transverse image of oncocytoma with compression of right kidney. **C,** Computer tomography of transverse cross-section of the abdomen at the level of right renal oncocytoma shows central scar, which is characteristically used in diagnosis of oncocytoma. (From Henningsen C: *Clinical guide to ultrasonography,* St. Louis, 2004, Mosby.)

and diphtheria. It may be a manifestation of an allergic reaction to certain drugs. Patient signs and symptoms include uremia, proteinuria, hematuria, rash, fever, and eosinophilia.
Sonographic Findings. The kidneys are enlarged and mottled. On ultrasound, the renal cortical echogenicity is

Figure 10-64 Acute glomerulonephritis may be suspected when the echogenicity of the renal parenchyma exceeds that of the liver.

Figure 10-65 Patients with lupus nephritis demonstrate a very echogenic renal parenchymal pattern compared with the liver. Renal atrophy is usually present.

increased. The increase in echogenicity is greatest in cases of diffuse active disease. There is less increase in diffuse scarring.

Lupus Nephritis. Systemic lupus erythematosus is a connective tissue disorder believed to result from an abnormal immune system. Females are affected more, and the incidence peaks between 20 and 40 years of age. The kidneys are involved in more than 50% of patients. The renal manifestations are hematuria, proteinuria, hypertension, renal vein thrombosis, and renal insufficiency.
Sonographic Findings. Sonography shows increased cortical echogenicity and renal atrophy (Figure 10-65).

Acquired Immunodeficiency Syndrome. Acquired immunodeficiency syndrome (AIDS) is a highly contagious disease, mainly spread by unprotected sexual activity or infected needles. The virus destroys T cells and then replicates rapidly within the body. It affects many organs. Patients have various symptoms (see Table 19-2). Unexplained uremia or azotemia may indicate renal dysfunction resulting from AIDS; it is usually a late finding. Causes of renal dysfunction in AIDS patients include acute tubular necrosis, nephrocalcinosis, interstitial nephritis, and focal segmental glomerulosclerosis.

Sonographic Findings. An echogenic parenchymal pattern is present on ultrasound. Cortical echogenicity is increased. Kidneys are normal in size or enlarged (Figures 10-66 to 10-68). If there is AIDS-related lymphoma or Kaposi sarcoma, the kidneys will appear enlarged and hypoechoic on a sonogram.

Sickle Cell Nephropathy. Renal involvement is common in patients with sickle cell disease. Abnormalities include glomerulonephritis, renal vein thrombosis, and papillary necrosis; hematuria is common.

Sonographic Findings. The sonographic appearance depends on the type of disorder. In acute renal vein thrombosis, the kidneys are enlarged with decreased echogenicity secondary to edema. In patients with subacute cases, renal enlargement is present with increased cortical echoes.

A   **B**

Figure 10-66   Longitudinal (**A**) and transverse (**B**) scans in a patient with acquired immunodeficiency syndrome (AIDS) show cortical echogenicity with normal to slightly increased renal size.

Figure 10-67   Transverse scans of a young male with acquired immunodeficiency syndrome (AIDS) show a mildly echogenic renal parenchyma.

Figure 10-68 Longitudinal scans of a 26-year-old male with acquired immunodeficiency syndrome (AIDS).

Figure 10-69 A 73-year-old man with chronic renal disease. Small echogenic kidney with inability to distinguish the medulla from the cortex region of the kidney. (Courtesy Shpetim Telegrafi, New York University.)

Figure 10-70 Renal sinus lipomatosis appears as enlarged kidneys with echogenic, enlarged renal sinus and a thin cortical rim. Renal sinus fat is easily seen on ultrasound as very echogenic reflections.

Hypertensive Nephropathy. Uncontrolled hypertension can lead to progressive renal damage and azotemia.

Sonographic Findings. Sonographically the kidneys are small with smooth borders. Superimposed scars of pyelonephritis or lobar infarction may distort the intrarenal anatomy. Bilateral small kidneys occur secondary to end-stage disease as a result of hypertension, inflammation, or ischemia (Figure 10-69).

Papillary Necrosis. Papillary necrosis occurs when the cells at the apex of the renal pyramids are destroyed. Many conditions may lead to papillary necrosis (e.g., analgesic abuse, sickle cell disease, diabetes, obstruction, pyelonephritis, and renal transplant). Necrosis may develop within weeks or months after transplantation. Patients previously treated for rejection and those with cadaveric kidney are at greatest risk. Ischemia is thought to have an important role in necrosis.

Symptoms suggest calculus or an inflammatory process. Complaints include hematuria, flank pain, dysuria, hyperten-

sion, and acute renal failure (see Table 10-2). Differential considerations include congenital megacalyces, hydronephrosis, and postobstructive atrophy.

Sonographic Findings. Sonographic findings include one or more fluid spaces at the corticomedullary junction that correspond to the distribution of the renal pyramids. The cystic spaces may be round or triangular. Sometimes the arcuate vessels are seen.

Renal Atrophy. Renal atrophy results from numerous disease processes. Intrarenal anatomy is preserved with uniform loss of renal tissue. Renal sinus lipomatosis occurs secondary to renal atrophy. More severe lipomatosis results from a tremendous increase in renal sinus fat content in cases of marked renal atrophy because of hydronephrosis and chronic calculus disease.

Sonographic Findings. The kidneys appear enlarged with a highly echogenic, enlarged renal sinus and thin cortical rim. Renal sinus fat is easily seen on ultrasound as very echogenic reflections (Figure 10-70).

RENAL FAILURE, HYDRONEPHROSIS, RENAL INFECTIONS, RENAL ARTERY STENOSIS, AND RENAL INFARCTION

The excretory and regulatory functions of the kidneys are decreased in both acute and chronic renal failure. Acute renal failure (ARF) is a common medical condition that can be caused by a number of medical diseases or pathophysiological mechanisms. ARF is typically an abrupt transient decrease in renal function often heralded by oliguria. The pathophysiologic states that cause varying degrees of renal malfunction have been categorized as prerenal, renal, and postrenal (Box 10-3). Decreased perfusion of the kidneys can cause prerenal failure (e.g., renal vein thrombus, CHF, and renal artery occlusion) and can be diagnosed by clinical, laboratory data and also by color Doppler. The renal causes of acute azotemia include parenchymal disease (e.g., acute glomerulonephritis, acute interstitial nephritis, and acute tubular necrosis) and hydronephrosis. Major postrenal causes of acute renal failure include bladder, pelvic, or retroperitoneal tumors and calculi. Prompt diagnosis and treatment are crucial for postrenal failure, which is potentially reversible.

The etiologic basis of chronic renal failure includes obstructive nephropathies, parenchymal diseases, renovascular disorders, and any process that progressively destroys nephrons. See Table 10-2 for clinical findings, sonographic findings, and differential considerations for malfunctioning kidney conditions.

Numerous studies have previously documented that ultrasound is extremely sensitive in diagnosing hydronephrosis. Patients in whom laboratory test results indicate compromised renal function should receive rule-out obstruction studies (Box 10-4). Most agree that sonography is the initial procedure of choice in evaluating all patients with known or suspected renal failure.

Acute Renal Failure. Acute renal failure may occur in prerenal, renal, or postrenal failure stages. The prerenal stage is secondary to the hypoperfusion of the kidney. The renal stages may be caused by parenchymal diseases (i.e., acute glomerulonephritis, acute interstitial nephritis, or acute tubular necrosis). It may also be caused by renal vein thrombosis or renal artery occlusion. In postrenal failure, radiologic imaging plays a major role. This condition is usually the result of outflow obstruction and is potentially reversible. Postrenal failure is usually increased in patients with a malignancy of the bladder, prostate, uterus, ovaries, or rectum. Less frequent causes include retroperitoneal fibrosis and renal calculi. See Table 10-3 for clinical findings, sonographic findings, and differential considerations for renal failure.

Sonographic Findings. The cause of the acute renal disease urinary outflow obstruction can be differentiated from parenchymal disease. The kidneys may appear normal in size or enlarged and hypoechoic with parenchymal disease. Obstruction is responsible for approximately 5% of acute renal failure. The most important issue is the presence or absence of urinary tract dilation. The degree of dilation does not necessarily reflect either the presence or severity of an obstruction. A sonographer should try to determine the level of obstruction. A normal ultrasound does not totally exclude urinary obstruction. In the clinical setting of acute obstruction secondary to calculi, a nondistended collecting system can be present.

Acute Tubular Necrosis. Acute tubular necrosis (ATN) is the most common medical renal disease to produce acute renal failure, although it can be reversible.

Sonographic Findings. Ultrasound shows bilaterally enlarged kidneys with hyperechoic pyramids (see Table 10-2); this can revert to a normal appearance. The differential considerations include nephrocalcinosis. In pediatric patients, the

---

BOX 10-3   CAUSES OF RENAL FAILURE

PRERENAL
Hypoperfusion
Hypotension
Congestive heart failure (CHF)

RENAL
Infection
Nephrotoxicity
Renal artery occlusion
Renal mass or cysts

POSTRENAL
Lower urinary tract obstruction (ureter, bladder)
Retroperitoneal fibrosis

BOX 10-4   CAUSES OF HYDRONEPHROSIS

ACQUIRED
Bladder tumors
Carcinoma of the cervix
Calculi
Neurogenic bladder
Normal pregnancy
Pelvic mass
Prostatic enlargement
Retroperitoneal fibrosis

INTRINSIC
Calculus
Stricture
Inflammation
Pyelonephritis
Congenital
Bladder neck obstruction
Posterior urethral valves
Ureterocele
Ureteropelvic junction (UPJ) obstruction

Figure 10-71   Transverse **(A)** and longitudinal **(B)** scans of the pediatric patient with acute tubular necrosis and nephrocalcinosis. The echogenic renal pyramids are well seen.

Figure 10-72   Hydronephrosis of the kidney. The dilated pyelocaliceal system appears as separation of the renal sinus echoes by fluid-filled areas that conform anatomically to the infundibula, calyces, and pelvis. (Courtesy Shpetim Telegrafi, New York University.)

Figure 10-73   Slight dilation of the collecting system seen. A longitudinal left kidney scan with dilation of the proximal ureter caused by a stone *(arrows)*. (Courtesy Shpetim Telegrafi, New York University.)

renal pyramids are very echogenic without shadowing. The calculi may be too small to cause dilation and shadowing of the pyramids (Figure 10-71). As renal function improves, the echogenicity decreases. This can occur in the medulla or cortex. If it reverses, it is probably acute tubular necrosis.

Chronic Renal Disease. Chronic renal disease is the loss of renal function as a result of disease, most commonly parenchymal diseases. There are three primary types of chronic renal failure: nephron, vascular, and interstitial abnormalities. Glomerulonephritis, chronic pyelonephritis, renal vascular disease, and diabetes are a few of the diseases that lead to renal failure.

Sonographic Findings. Chronic renal disease is a diffusely echogenic kidney with loss of normal anatomy. It is a nonspecific ultrasound finding; chronic renal disease can have multiple causes (AIDS can produce echogenic kidneys). If chronic

renal disease is bilateral, small kidneys are identified. This may result from hypertension, chronic inflammation, or chronic ischemia.

Hydronephrosis. Hydronephrosis is the separation of renal sinus echoes by interconnected fluid-filled areas. The dilated pyelocalyceal system appears as separation of the renal sinus echoes by fluid-filled areas that conform anatomically to the infundibula, calyces, and renal pelvis (Figure 10-72). In patients with progressive obstruction, the pyelocalyceal system continues to dilate, compressing the parenchyma. In cases of end-stage hydronephrosis, multiple cystic areas are seen with little or no renal parenchyma identified.

Whenever the renal collecting system is dilated, the ureters and bladder are scanned to locate the level of obstruction. It is possible to identify the site of obstruction using ultrasound (Figure 10-73). A congenital obstruction of the ureteropelvic junction can be seen in utero and in infants. The collecting system will be dilated and only the proximal portion of where the ureter enters into the renal pelvis is imaged. A localized hydronephrosis occurs as a result of strictures, calculi, focal masses, or a duplex collecting system. Hydronephrosis with a dilated ureter and bladder indicate obstruction of the ureterovesical junction or of the urethra.

A mildly distended collecting system can be caused by overhydration, a normal variant of extrarenal pelvis, or a previous urinary diversion procedure (Figure 10-74). Postvoid scanning techniques are helpful to prevent these errors.

Sonographic Findings. If hydronephrosis is suspected, the sonographer should examine the bladder. If it is full, a postvoid longitudinal scan of each kidney should be done to show that hydronephrosis has disappeared or remained the same. At the level of the obstruction, the sonographer should sweep the transducer back and forth in two planes to see if a mass or stone can be distinguished.

There are three grades of hydronephrosis. *Grade I* entails a small separation of the calyceal pattern, also known as **splay-**ing (Figure 10-75). The sonographer must be able to rule out a parapelvic cyst (the septations may be numerous) or renal vessels in the peripelvic area (color flow Doppler is extremely useful). An extrarenal pelvis would protrude outside of the renal area, and the sonographer probably would not confuse this pattern with hydronephrosis (Figure 10-76). *Grade II* shows the bear-claw effect, with fluid extending into the major and minor calyceal systems and thinning of the renal parenchyma (Figures 10-77 and 10-78). *Grade III* represents massive dilation of the renal pelvis with loss of renal parenchyma (Figure 10-79).

In evaluating the patient for hydronephrosis, a sonographer must be sure to look for a dilated ureter (Figure 10-80), an enlarged prostate (which may cause the ureter to become obstructed), or an enlarged bladder (may be secondary to an enlarged prostate). Bladder carcinoma may obstruct the pathway of the urethra, causing urine to back into the ureter and renal pelvis. A ureterocele may also block urine output. This condition occurs where the ureter inserts into the bladder wall. The ureter can turn inside out and obstruct the orifice.

Figure 10-74 **A** and **B,** A distended urinary bladder may cause pseudohydronephrosis of both kidneys and ureters. The patient should be scanned after the bladder has been emptied. **C** and **D,** Distended ureters in transverse and longitudinal sections.

Obstructive Hydronephrosis. Dilation of the renal pelvis is just one factor present in patients with obstructive hydronephrosis. (See Table 10-3 for clinical findings, sonographic findings, and differential considerations for obstructive hydronephrosis.)

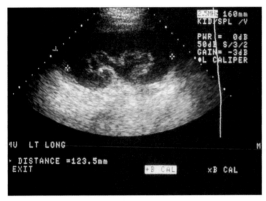

Figure 10-75　Sagittal scan of the kidney with mild hydronephrosis. Slight widening of the renal collecting system. (Courtesy Shpetim Telegrafi, New York University.)

Figure 10-76　An extrarenal pelvis should not be confused with hydronephrosis.

Sonographic Findings. In cases of acute obstruction, the RI (resistive index) of the intrarenal vessels may be greater than 0.70 for 48 to 72 hours after obstruction (Figure 10-81). The RI returns to normal. There will be no ureteral jet on the affected side, or there will be decreased flow if the obstruction is partial.

Nonobstructive hydronephrosis. Dilation of the renal pelvis does not always mean that obstruction is present. Several other factors may cause the renal pelvis to be dilated, such as reflux, infection, large extrarenal pelvis, high flow states (polyuria), distended renal bladder, atrophy after obstruction *(once obstruction is relieved the obstruction can remain),* or pregnancy dilation (the enlarged uterus can compress the ureter; usually occurs more on the right).

Sonographic Findings. Ureteral jets are present when there is nonobstructive hydronephrosis. Ureteral jets are best visualized by color Doppler imaging (Figure 10-82). The Doppler shift is caused by the difference between the higher specific gravity of the urine in the bladder and the lower specific gravity level of urine entering the bladder. Urine fills the bladder at a rate up to 2 ml/min. Patients who have voided before the renal examination and are rehydrated may have a false-positive

Figure 10-77　Grade II hydronephrosis shows moderate splaying of the renal pelvis. (Courtesy Shpetim Telegrafi, New York University.)

A　　　　　　　　**B**

Figure 10-78　Conventional **(A)** and harmonic **(B)** imaging of the kidney with moderate hydronephrosis. The use of harmonics allows more contrast between the parenchyma and dilated renal pelvis.

absence of ureteral jets. This results from the concentration of the urine in the recently distended bladder being of similar density as the urine entering the bladder. A comparison of both ureteral jets is necessary to confirm that nonvisualization of the symptomatic side is not due to the density of urine in the ureter and bladder being similar. A partial obstruction of the ureter may cause absence of ureteral jets or decreased flow (Figure 10-83).

False-positive hydronephrosis. Many conditions may mimic hydronephrosis (Box 10-5), such as extrarenal pelvis, parapelvic cysts, reflux, multicystic kidney, central renal cyst, transient diuresis, congenital megacalyces, papillary necrosis, renal artery aneurysm (color can help distinguish that this enlargement is vascular, not the renal pelvis), or an arteriovenous malformation (color can distinguish this abnormality).

Localized hydronephrosis may be secondary to strictures, calculi, or focal masses (transitional). It can also occur in a duplex system when one of the systems can be obstructed because of an ectopic insertion of the ureter. In females it can insert below the external urinary sphincter and cause dribbling.

False-negative hydronephrosis. A dilated renal pelvis may be distinguished from other conditions by the use of other techniques. In patients with retroperitoneal fibrosis or necrosis, give liquids to see if the renal pelvis dilates. In patients with a distal calculi, no obstruction can be seen unless the calculi has been there for several days. A staghorn calculus can mask an associated dilation.

The condition of adult polycystic disease and multicystic renal disease with severe hydronephrosis may be confused. In patients with severe hydronephrosis, the image shows dilated calyces as they radiate from a larger central fluid collection in the renal pelvis. The kidney usually retains a normal shape. The sonographer sees fluid-filled sacs in a radiating pattern or cauliflower configuration. In patients with adult polycystic renal disease and multicystic renal disease, the renal cysts are randomly distributed, the contour is disturbed, and the cysts are variable in size.

Once obstruction has been ruled out, consider renal medical disease, which is the leading cause of acute renal failure.

Renal Infections. There is a spectrum of severity in renal infections. The disease can progress from pyelonephritis to focal bacterial nephritis to an abscess. An abscess can be transmitted through the parenchyma into the blood. Most renal infections stay in the kidney and are resolved with antibiotics

Figure 10-79　Grade II to grade III hydronephrosis caused by a ureteropelvic junction *(UPJ)* obstruction. (Courtesy Shpetim Telegrafi, New York University.)

BOX 10-5	CONDITIONS THAT MIMIC HYDRONEPHROSIS

- Extrarenal pelvis
- Parapelvic cysts
- Reflux
- Persistent diuresis
- Congenital megacalyces
- Papillary necrosis
- Renal artery aneurysm
- Arteriovenous malformation

A   B

Figure 10-80　**A,** Mild hydronephrosis is seen. **B,** The longitudinal scan of the bladder shows a distended distal ureter with a large stone *(arrow).* (Courtesy Shpetim Telegrafi, New York University.)

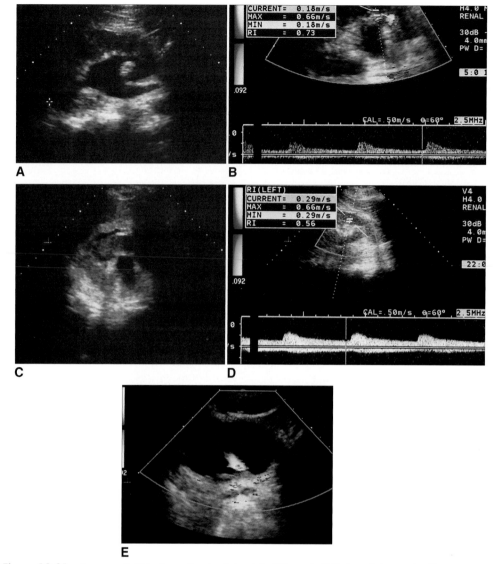

Figure 10-81   Acute grade II hydronephrosis of the right kidney. **A,** Dilation of the renal collecting system and proximal ureter. **B,** Increased intrarenal vascularity with an RI of 0.73. **C,** A small amount of perinephric fluid is seen surrounding the kidney. **D,** Normal contralateral kidney with an RI of 0.56. **E,** Normal ureteral jet seen on the left side. No ureteral jet seen on the obstructed side. (Courtesy Shpetim Telegrafi, New York University.)

Figure 10-82   Normal right **(A)** and left **(B)** ureteral jets seen in the fluid-filled bladder. (Courtesy Shpetim Telegrafi, New York University.)

Figure 10-83   **A,** Transverse scan of a fluid-filled bladder with a normal right ureteral jet. A partially obstructed left ureter with decreased flow. **B,** Transverse scan of a partial obstructed distal left ureter. *Arrows* indicate the stone with shadowing posterior to the stone. **C,** Transvaginal scan of the dilated distal ureter with a ureteral stone. **D,** Normal RI of 0.59 for left kidney. (Courtesy Shpetim Telegrafi, New York University.)

Figure 10-84   This patient presented with an elevated white blood count and spiking fever. **A,** The supine sagittal scan reveals a homogeneous, slightly irregular mass arising from the upper pole of the right kidney. **B,** Transverse scan of the renal abscess. Note the decreased through-transmission posterior to the abscess wall.

(Figure 10-84). A perirenal abscess occurs from a direct extension.

Pyonephrosis. Pyonephrosis occurs when pus is found within the obstructed renal system. It is often associated with severe urosepsis and represents a true urologic emergency that requires urgent percutaneous drainage. It usually occurs secondary to long-standing ureteral obstruction from calculus disease, stricture, or a congenital anomaly (Figure 10-85).

(See Table 10-3 for clinical findings, sonographic findings, and differential considerations for pyonephrosis.)

Figure 10-85 Longitudinal (**A**) and transverse (**B**) scans of the left kidney showing an irregular mass lesion in the lower pole. This patient was found to have pyonephrosis of the kidney secondary to ureteral obstruction.

Figure 10-86 Other findings in a patient with pyonephrosis include a fluid and/or debris level within a well-defined mass lesion.

Sonographic Findings. The sonographic findings include the presence of low-level echoes with a fluid-debris level (Figure 10-86). The sonographer should be aware that an anechoic dilated system can occur. (Ultrasound-guided aspiration or CT may be necessary.)

Emphysematous Pyelonephritis. Emphysematous pyelonephritis occurs when there is air in the parenchyma (diffuse gas-forming parenchymal infection). It may be caused by *Escherichia coli* bacteria. When this occurs in diabetic patients, they become very sick. It generally is found unilaterally and may be cause for an emergency nephrectomy.

Sonographic Findings. On ultrasound examination, the enlarged kidneys appear hypoechoic and inflamed.

Xanthogranulomatous Pyelonephritis. Xanthogranulomatous pyelonephritis is an uncommon renal disease associated with chronic obstruction and infection. It involves destruction of renal parenchyma and infiltration of lipid-laden histiocytes. Clinically the patient presents with a large, non-

functioning kidney, staghorn calculus, and multiple infections (Figure 10-87) (see Table 10-3). The disease is more common in females and is poorly understood. It is thought to be an impaired host response to an infection in a chronically obstructed and infected kidney.

Sonographic Findings. The ultrasound appearance may show the bright echogenicity from the staghorn calculus. (Peripelvic fibrosis can prevent the staghorn from shadowing.) The renal parenchyma is replaced by cystic spaces. The overall renal size is increased. The disease process may be diffuse or segmental.

Nephrocalcinosis. Nephrocalcinosis is diffuse foci calcium deposits, which are usually located in the medulla and infrequently can also be seen in the renal cortex. Both kidneys are affected. The patient may present with fever; this may indicate infection with hydronephrosis.

Sonographic Findings. The nephrocalcinosis disease process shows very echogenic pyramids with or without associated shadowing (see Figure 10-71).

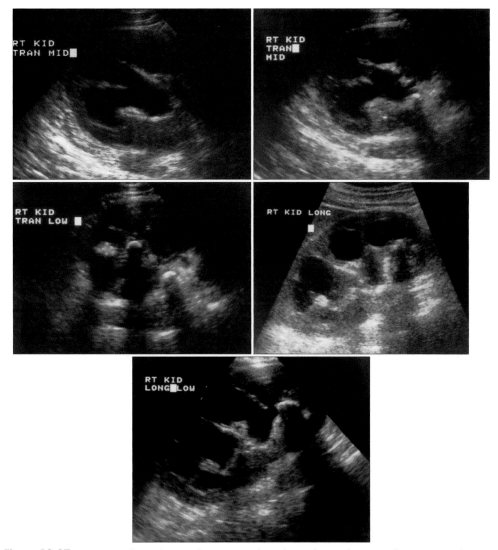

Figure 10-87 Patient with xanthogranulomatous pyelonephritis shows a large, nonfunctioning right kidney secondary to a stone. Multiple areas of shadowing are seen within the renal parenchyma from the renal stones.

Renal Artery Stenosis. The major cause of renal artery stenosis in an adult is arteriosclerosis. Fibromuscular hyperplasia of the distal segment of the renal artery is seen in young adults, especially women. Two Doppler methods are used to evaluate for renal artery stenosis (RAS): direct evaluation of the main renal artery and indirectly by evaluating the arcuate and intralobar renal arteries. Both methods are difficult to perform, and the accuracy rates vary because of technical problems and the experience of the person performing the examination.

The most reliable signs for diagnosing renal artery stenosis (RAS) using the main renal artery are increased velocity through the stenotic area greater than 150 to 190 cm/sec and turbulence distal to the narrowing. The use of peak systolic velocity (PSV) has not proven to be accurate because of overestimating caused by suboptimal angles of incidence. The use of frequency ranges has also been shown to be of little value because of the tortuosity of the renal artery, which causes varied frequencies throughout the vessel.

One of the problems that occur when using the main renal artery to evaluate renal blood flow is that there may be more than one renal artery. The main renal artery may have normal blood flow and a stenotic accessory renal artery causing hypertension. Evaluating the entire course of the main renal arteries is a long and tedious study and one that sonographers and sonologists try to avoid. There are several technical factors (body habitus, tortuosity of the vessel, overlying bowel gas, respiratory motion, and underlying arteriosclerotic disease) that prohibit the visualization of the entire length of the renal artery. The proximal portion of the renal arteries may be difficult to evaluate because of cardiac or aortic pulse frequencies.

A resistive index (RI) of 0.70 has generally been accepted as the upper limit of normal. In two exceptions, patients under the age of 6 and older patients, an RI greater than 0.70 may not be indicative of renal dysfunction (Figure 10-88). Proper sonographic technique is essential for diagnosing RAS. A 3.5- to 2.5-MHz transducer is used because of the depth of the kidney and to prevent aliasing of a stenotic renal artery. The lowest pulse repetitive frequency (PRF) and a low wall filter setting are also used. The mean of at least 3 to 5 distinct waveforms is used to calculate the RI.

Evaluating the segmental and intralobar renal vessels is an indirect method for evaluating for RAS. They are easier to demonstrate than the main renal artery with the use of convergent color or power color (Figure 10-89). It is very difficult to obtain a 60-degree angle of the renal vessels. Convergent color and power color are not angle dependent.

Patients with RAS have a decrease of the intravascular blood flow; therefore, it is more difficult to demonstrate blood flow in the arcuate and intralobar vessels. Comparison of the ipsilateral kidney to the contralateral kidney is necessary to determine that the decrease of blood flow is not caused by technical factors, but is real.

Studies have been performed using various Doppler parameters to assist in the evaluation of RAS. The normal intrarenal Doppler signal has a rapid systolic upstroke and early systolic peak (ESP) (Figures 10-90 and 10-91). The absence of early systolic peak and a prolonged systolic upstroke or acceleration time (AT) together with decreased peak systole and a dampening of the distal waveform are indications of RAS. The term tardus-parvus is used to describe the decreased acceleration time and the decreased peak.

Renal arteriography is still the gold standard for the evaluation of RAS and occlusion. Doppler analysis of the main renal artery and the intrarenal arteries has limitations because of technical factors and skill of the person performing the examination. Clinical studies with the use of contrast agents are continuing to improve the uses of ultrasound and Doppler for the evaluation of renal vascularity. The use of 3-D imaging for demonstrating renal vasculature is also being investigated (Figure 10-92).

Renal Infarction. A renal infarction occurs when part of the tissue undergoes necrosis after the cessation of the blood supply, usually as a result of artery occlusion. Renal function is usually normal. This may result from a thrombus, tumor infiltration, or obstruction. (See Table 10-3 for clinical findings, sonographic findings, and differential considerations for renal infarction.)

Sonographic Findings. Infarcts within the renal parenchyma appear as irregular masses, somewhat triangular in shape, along the periphery of the renal border. The renal contour may be somewhat "lumpy-bumpy." Remember that lobulations in the pediatric patient may be normal, except for the dromedary hump variant. In the adult patient the renal contour should be smooth. In a patient with a renal infarct, the irregular area may be slightly more echogenic than the renal parenchyma.

RENAL TRANSPLANT

Renal transplantation and dialysis are currently used to treat chronic renal failure or end-stage renal disease. Ultrasound has emerged as an excellent tool in monitoring such transplant patients and may complement nuclear medicine and laboratory values in distinguishing the course of rejection. Because the sonogram does not rely on the function of the kidney, serial studies can be readily incorporated in determining the diagnosis and the treatment to be administered.

Complications may arise after transplantation, including rejection, acute tubular necrosis (ATN), obstructive nephropathy, extraperitoneal fluid collections, hemorrhage or infarction,

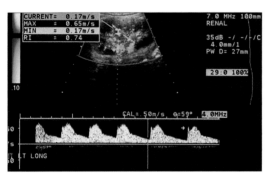

Figure 10-88 Normal RI of 0.74 in a 4-year-old female. The *arrow* indicates an early systolic peak. (Courtesy Shpetim Telegrafi, New York University.)

A   B

Figure 10-89 Longitudinal **(A)** and transverse **(B)** color Doppler of normal intrarenal vessels with vascular flow throughout the renal cortex. (Courtesy Shpetim Telegrafi, New York University.)

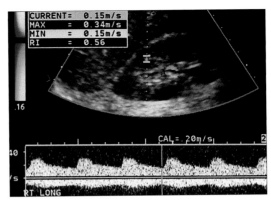

Figure 10-90   Normal arcuate vessel Doppler spectral signal. A rapid systolic rise with an RI of 0.56. A gradual decrease into diastole. (Courtesy Shpetim Telegrafi, New York University.)

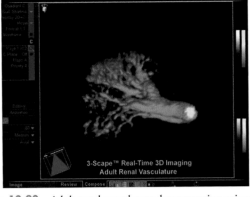

Figure 10-92   Adult renal vasculature demonstration using 3-Scape™ real-time 3-D imaging. (Courtesy Siemens Medical Solutions USA, Inc.)

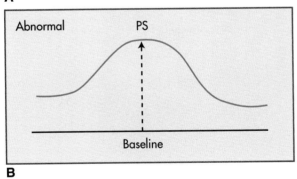

Figure 10-91   **A,** Diagram of a normal renal artery spectral waveform with early systolic peak *(ESP)* and a rapid systolic upstroke followed by peak systole *(PS)* and a gradual decrease into diastole. **B,** Diagram of an abnormal renal artery spectral waveform with absence of early systolic peak and a long systolic upstroke.

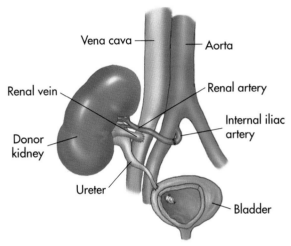

Figure 10-93   Surgical placement of the renal transplant into the iliac fossa.

recurrent glomerulonephritis, graft rupture, and renal emphysema. Decreased renal function is commonly the main indication for ultrasonic evaluation.

The Procedure. Most renal transplant patients have had long-standing renal failure without obstructive nephropathy. Before the procedure, patient risk factors to be considered are age, primary diagnosis, secondary medical complications, and

transplant source. It is found that recipients between 16 and 45 years of age with primary renal disease have the lowest risk for morbidity and mortality.

The major problem encountered with transplantation is graft rejection. The success of the transplant is directly related to the source of the donated kidney. Living relatives and cadavers are the two donor types.

The surgical procedure begins with removal of the donor's left kidney, which is then rotated and placed in the recipient's right iliac fossa or groin region. The renal artery is attached by an end-to-end anastomosis, with either the common or the external iliac artery (Figure 10-93).

The ureter is inserted into the bladder above the normal ureteral orifice through a submucosal tunnel in the bladder wall. The tunnel creates a valve in the terminal ureter to prevent reflux of urine into the transplanted kidney.

Although the kidney is more vulnerable to trauma when it is placed in the iliopelvic region, this has rarely been a problem. The advantage of such a location is its observation accessibility. Complications may arise after transplantation, however, so a variety of examinations may be incorporated to detect and follow the transplant. Useful information may be accumulated through laboratory tests, nuclear medicine, sonography, intravenous pyelography, and renal arteriography.

Sonographic Evaluation. As early as 48 hours after surgery, a baseline sonographic examination is performed to determine renal size, calyceal pattern, and extrarenal fluid collections. Hydronephrosis can be easily recognized sonographically with calyceal dilation. Perirenal fluid collections (hematoma, abscess, lymphocele, or urinoma) can be diagnosed reliably and differentiated from acute rejection. Serial

scans at 3- to 6-month intervals may be made to detect fluid collections at an early, asymptomatic stage. The patient should be examined at the first sign of tenderness in the graft area or mass development.

Technique for sonographic examination. To locate the kidney precisely by ultrasound, transverse supine scans are made from the pubic symphysis to above the level of the graft. Longitudinal and transverse scans are made parallel with and perpendicular to the long axis of the kidney. From these scans, accurate measurements of the renal length, width, and anteroposterior dimensions can be determined (Figures 10-94 and 10-95).

Figure 10-94 **A** to **C,** Multiple transverse scans of the renal transplant taken in the transverse planes at the upper, middle, and lower segments. **D** to **F,** Longitudinal scans should be made along the longest axis of the kidney in the midline, medial, and lateral planes.

Figure 10-95   Normal evaluation of the renal transplant includes evaluation of the size, evaluation of the renal parenchyma, evaluation for the presence of abnormal fluid collections, and Doppler assessment of the renal vessels. **A,** Main renal vein flow. **B,** Main renal artery flow. **C,** Interlobar arterial flow. **D,** Arcuate artery flow.

Figure 10-96   A 41-year-old female with a kidney transplant. The medullary pyramids are discrete sonolucent structures surrounded by homogeneous grainy texture of the cortex. (Courtesy Shpetim Telegrafi, New York University.)

Figure 10-97   The psoas muscle *(PS)* is posterior to the renal transplant *(RT)* and appears as parallel linear echoes along the posterior border.

Sonographic Findings. The normal transplant should appear as a smooth structure surrounding the homogeneous parenchymal pattern. A dense band of echoes in the midportion of the transplant represents the renal pelvis, calyces, blood vessels, and fatty fibrous tissues. The medullary pyramids are discrete sonolucent structures surrounded by the homogeneous grainy texture of the cortex (Figure 10-96). The psoas appears as parallel linear echoes posterior to the kidney transplant (Figure 10-97). The Doppler flow pattern for a healthy transplant kidney is the same as a normally functioning native kidney (Figure 10-98).

A sonolucent appearance of the anterior portion of the kidney and, at times, an increased echogenic band across the anterior kidney occur on some scans because of inaccurate set-

Figure 10-98 Normal flow patterns in a recent renal transplant patient. **A,** Main renal vein. **B,** Main segmental renal artery. **C,** Interlobar artery. **D,** Arcuate artery.

tings in the near field. Decreased amplification of the near gain in the first few centimeters of the slope obliterates the decreased echoes of the near field and allows for better fill-in of the anterior portion of the kidney. This difference in anterior structure delineation is probably because of the attenuation of sound by subcutaneous fat, muscle thickness, skin texture, and scarring or the fact that some patients transmit the sound frequency more readily than others.

The opposite is true for the problem of increased echoes in the near field. By decrease in the near gain, suppression of the echoes in the near field yields an image with uniform texture. Thus it is important to maintain proper penetration and delineation of internal structures with a good outline of adjacent musculature.

To record echoes from the parenchyma and distinguish the cortex from the medulla, the sonographer should scan the patient with low-gain and high-gain settings. The scans include both kidneys and the pararenal area (i.e., iliac wing and iliopsoas).

Medical Complications

Renal transplant rejection. Rejection has been the most difficult of the medical complications to accurately diagnose without percutaneous needle biopsy. No single imaging method permits accurate diagnosis with sufficient specificity and sensitivity to totally obviate renal biopsy.

There are four types of rejection: hyperacute, acute, immunologic, and chronic. Hyperacute rejection occurs within hours of transplantation and is caused by vasculitis

leading to thrombosis and usually loss of the graft. Acute rejection occurs within days to months after transplant. Immunologic rejection causes include preformed antibodies, immune complexes, and cell-mediated responses. Pathologically, acute rejection is separated into vascular and interstitial forms. Without aggressive therapy the graft can be lost. Lastly, chronic rejection can occur months after transplantation with gradual onset. It tends to be secondary to mononuclear infiltration and fibrosis. Steroid therapy and antilymphocyte serum are of little benefit in improving renal function and can lead to opportunistic infections.

Sonographic Findings. Sonography can be useful in the diagnosis of rejection. Care must be taken to observe the size and shape; the appearance of the pyramids, cortex, and parenchyma; and the presence of any surrounding fluid collections. The following five changes in the renal parenchymal echo pattern have been observed during the process of rejection:

1. Enlargement and decreased echogenicity of the pyramids. This appearance is not at all uniform, and only a few pyramids may appear as such (Figure 10-99).
2. Hyperechogenic cortex. The swollen, sonolucent pyramids stand out against the background of increased echogenicity of the outer and interpyramidal cortex (Figure 10-100).
3. A localized area of renal parenchyma, including both the cortex and the medulla presenting an anechoic appearance,

Figure 10-99 Transverse view of a chronic renal transplant rejection. Enlargement and decreased echogenicity of the pyramids caused by edema and congestion with hemorrhage of the interstitial tissue. Ischemia and cellular infiltration (fibrosis) result in hyperechogenicity of the cortex. (Courtesy Shpetim Telegrafi, New York University.)

is very difficult to fill in even when using high sensitivity and TGC settings. This is usually seen in polar regions.

4. Distortion of the renal outline because of localized areas of swelling involving both the cortex and the pyramids. The renal sinus echoes may appear compressed and displaced (Figure 10-101).
5. Patchy sonolucent areas involving both cortex and medulla with coalescence on follow-up studies. These areas can become quite extensive, affecting a large portion of the renal parenchyma.

In long-standing rejection, two patterns have been observed:

1. A normal-size renal transplant with very little differentiation between the parenchymal and renal sinus echoes.
2. A small kidney with irregular margins and an irregular parenchymal echo pattern.

These sonographic appearances correlate with the pathologic occurrences. When swelling is present with increased

Figure 10-100 The hyperechogenic cortex appears as swollen sonolucent pyramids against the background of increased echogenicity of the outer and interpyramidal cortex. In addition, this patient had obstruction near the distal ureter, causing mild dilation of the renal pelvis and ureter.

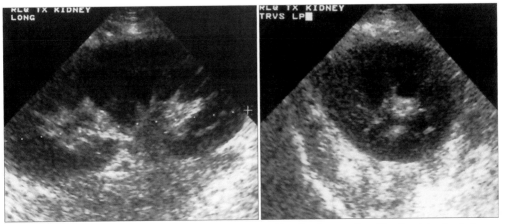

Figure 10-101 Distortion of the renal outline because of localized areas of swelling involving both the cortex and the pyramids. The renal sinus echoes may appear compressed and displaced.

internal echoes within the cortex, rejection can be diagnosed. Edema, congestion, and hemorrhage of the interstitium produce swelling of the pyramids, which appears as decreased echogenicity. Ischemia and cellular infiltration produce the increased echogenicity of the cortex. Increased areas of sonolucency may also occur in the cortex as a result of necrosis and infarction. These areas are usually seen in the polar regions of the transplant. If actual necrosis begins, the affected part appears as an area of decreased echogenicity, which suggests partial liquefaction. Irregular parenchymal echo patterns may result from parenchymal atrophy with fibrosis and shrinkage resulting from long-standing renal rejection.

Acute tubular necrosis. Acute tubular necrosis (ATN) is a common cause of acute posttransplant failure. Some degree occurs in almost every transplant patient, and it has been suggested that as many as 50% of the recipients of cadaver kidneys experience ATN after transplantation. The incidence of ATN is usually higher in cadaveric transplants than in donor-relative transplants or in kidneys that undergo warm ischemia or prolonged preservation, kidneys with multiple renal arteries, or kidneys obtained from elderly donors. ATN usually occurs as a medical complication after a loss of blood supply to the transplant tissue. This can occur in the donor before harvesting the kidney; during the process of harvesting, preserving, and transportation; during surgery; or as a result of poor circulation after the transplant. ATN is associated with prolonged severe ischemia; therefore, the likelihood of it occurring after any incidence of cardiac arrest cannot be ruled out. This pertains to the donor and the recipient.

ATN usually resolves early in the postoperative period. Uncomplicated ATN is often reversible and can be treated by immediate use of diuretics and satisfactory hydration. It is important to recognize uncomplicated ATN and distinguish it from acute rejection because the therapy for the two conditions is very different.

Clinically, ATN may present a variety of different patterns. Urine volumes may be good initially, followed by oliguria or anuria, or there may be low urine output from the time of transplantation. The serum creatinine level is always elevated. If urine output remains low and BUN and creatinine remain elevated, ATN may be difficult to distinguish from rejection. Other indications of rejection (e.g., hematuria, elevated eosinophil counts, or pain over the transplant) are helpful but may be late signs.

Sonographic Findings. Sonographically, there are usually no changes seen within the renal parenchyma. In the initial postoperative period the kidney may enlarge slightly as a result of secondary hypertrophy. This is believed to be a normal physiologic response of the newly transplanted kidney or is caused by swelling that often regresses within a week. However, if the swelling persists, either ATN or rejection should be considered. With ATN the renal parenchymal pattern remains unchanged, in contrast to the earlier description of the parenchymal changes during rejection. If these changes are lacking and the transplant fails to function, the cause is most likely ATN, provided the radionuclide evaluation has confirmed the patency of the vascular supply to the transplant.

Cyclosporine toxicity. Cyclosporine A toxicity (drug toxicity) is a reaction to the antirejection drug cyclosporine A with azathioprine and steroids. Over time, this drug can prove to be toxic to the transplant. At present, a biopsy best documents this diagnosis.

Malignancy. Malignancy is a newly discovered delayed complication now becoming prevalent as the life of transplants has improved. A total of 55% of renal transplant recipients in a long-term (17-year) study developed at least one malignancy. The two major types of neoplasms found in transplant patients are non-Hodgkin's lymphoma and skin cancer. Research on the incidence of occurrence of these malignancies has shown a strong correlation to the immunosuppressive drug used to maintain the transplant. A cyclosporine regimen has shown an increased incidence of non-Hodgkin's lymphoma (38% over azathioprine). Azathioprine produces an increased incidence of skin and lip tumors (40% over cyclosporine A). Cases have been documented of a neoplasm from a transplant primary, but this is uncommon. Even so, prescreening donor kidneys may reduce this occurrence.

Extraperitoneal fluid collections. Numerous extraperitoneal fluid collections may occur after transplantation, including lymphocele and lymph fistula, urinary fistula and urinoma, perinephric abscess, and hematoma (Box 10-6). These collections consist of lymph, blood, urine, pus, or a combination of these substances. A sign common to several of the complications is a decrease in renal function manifested by increased creatinine values.

Sonographic Findings. Sonographically the fluid collections may appear as round or oval structures with irregular and slightly thickened walls. Usually clinical or laboratory correlation suggests the cause of the fluid. Because the transplant is superficial, scans can easily be made and, if necessary, sonographic guidance can be rendered for aspiration of the contents for further analysis (Figure 10-102).

Hematoma. A hematoma may develop shortly after surgery. One of the major indications for an ultrasound scan may be a drop in the hematocrit value. Other clinical findings pertinent to hematomas include signs of bleeding, perinephric hemorrhage, a palpable mass, hypertension, and impaired renal function. The hematoma may also be an incidental finding during scanning.

Sonographic Findings. Hematomas appear as walled-off, well-defined areas whose sonolucent echo production depends on the age or stage of the hematoma. It may appear sonolu-

---

BOX 10-6　FLUID COLLECTIONS ASSOCIATED WITH RENAL TRANSPLANT

Haul (ORDER OF POSTOPERATIVE OCCURRENCE)
Hematoma
Abscess
Urinoma
Lymphocele

Figure 10-102 A 29-year-old male with a right lower quadrant renal transplant. Two fluid collections *(F)* were noted, one adjacent to the lower pole of the renal transplant and another within the anterior abdominal wall at the incision site. *UB,* Urinary bladder.

cent while the blood is fresh and be difficult to distinguish from a lymphocele or urinoma. As the clot becomes organized, the hematoma may tend to fragment and have low-level internal echoes develop. The mass then appears complex and eventually solid. After a time it may revert to a sonolucent mass and form a seroma.

Perinephric abscess. Perinephric infections can be very hazardous to the transplant patient undergoing immunosuppressive therapy. It is an uncommon complication reported as early as 12 days or many months after transplantation. If the patient has a fever of unknown origin, care must be taken to rule out abscess formation.

Sonographic Findings. Sonographically an abscess may appear with septa in it. Edema and inflammation may be present around the mass, making the borders appear less distinct compared with those found with lymphoceles and hematomas.

Lymphocele. Lymphoceles are a common complication of transplantation, occurring in approximately 12% of all transplant patients. The source of the lymph collection is probably vessels severed during the preparation of recipient vessels, or it may be the kidney itself in the form of leakage from injured capsular and hilar lymphatics. The lymph drains into the peritoneal cavity, provoking a fibrous reaction and eventually walling itself off. Primary clinical signs are deterioration of renal function (usually within 2 weeks to 6 months of transplantation), development of painless fluctuant swelling over

the transplant, ipsilateral leg edema, or wound drainage of lymph cells. If an IVP was performed, a mass indenting the bladder, ureteral deviation, ureteral obstruction, or kidney deviation will be seen.

Sonographic Findings. Sonographically the lymphocele is a well-defined anechoic area, occasionally with numerous septations (Figure 10-103). Urinomas may appear similar to lymphoceles, although usually they appear early, whereas lymphoceles are more common chronically. If the mass is complex with solid components, hematoma or abscess must be considered. Percutaneous aspiration and drainage with ultrasound or CT guidance has a success rate of 80%, with little risk of urinoma or abscess. Lymphoceles often recur after catheter drainage, and further surgery may be required.

Obstructive nephropathy. Early signs of obstruction are anuria or severe oliguria in a patient with satisfactory renal volumes. Numerous conditions may cause obstruction, such as ureteral necrosis, abscess, lymphocele, fungus ball, retroperitoneal fibrosis, stricture at the ureterovesical junction, ureteral calculus, and hemorrhage into the collecting system with obstruction from clots.

Sonographic Findings. Obstruction can be identified sonographically as hydronephrosis. There are many causes of obstruction after renal transplantation. In the early postoperative period, edema at the ureteric implantation site can cause temporary mild obstruction (Figure 10-104), or extrinsic mass effect from perinephric fluid collections can impinge on and

Figure 10-103 A 30-year-old female with a renal transplant 14 years previously presented with right upper quadrant and midabdominal pain. She had rigors and chills, but was afebrile. A tender cystic collection of fluid located above and to the right of the umbilicus and anterior to the inferior vena cava represented an infected lymphocele. She also had mild to moderate hydronephrosis.

Figure 10-104 **A,** Renal transplant with mild hydronephrosis and thrombus after a biopsy procedure. **B,** Normal color flow image in a renal transplant patient. (Courtesy Shpetim Telegrafi, New York University.)

impair ureteral drainage (Figure 10-105). In the later postoperative period, rejection or vascular insufficiency may predispose to distal ureteric stricture. Ureteric blood clots or calculi can also cause the obstruction. A very common benign form of pelvic dilation of the collecting system, pyelocaliectasis, can mimic obstruction. Analysis of laboratory values and an increased RI help rule this out. Finally, the sonographer should be wary of functional obstruction caused simply by an over-distended urinary bladder. Have the patient void and rescan to confirm.

Vascular insufficiency in the form of arterial stenosis or venous thrombus can best be diagnosed with color and duplex Doppler imaging. When trying to rule out renal artery stenosis, look for a high-velocity jet with distal turbulence.

Graft Rupture. Graft ruptures can occur in the first 2 weeks after surgery, presenting with an abrupt onset of pain and swelling over the graft, oliguria, and shock.

Sonographic Findings. Sonographically, a graft rupture appears as a gross distortion of the graft contour and a perinephric or paranephric hematoma.

Improvement of RI specificity. Perhaps the most confusing and frustrating problem presently is determining the use of the RI to accurately determine and specify transplant disease. Because many transplant complications exhibit increased RI, is there a way to help limit the differentials with time since a transplant? Knowing that many transplant complications tend to surface at particular times after surgery, a more holistic approach to interpretation of increased RIs may be the answer at present.

Sonographic Findings. If there is high renovascular impedance immediately after surgery, patency of the renal vein must be tested. With the use of color and pulsed Doppler imaging, renal thrombosis displays a distinctive spectral pattern with a plateaulike reversal of diastolic flow (accentuated at end diastole) (Figure 10-106). Renal artery stenosis exhibits a high-

Figure 10-105 In the early postoperative stages, the ureter may be compressed by extrarenal fluid collections, mass effect, or kinks within the ureter. The result is mild obstruction, extending into the renal ureter.

Figure 10-106 Observation of renal vein patency is very important after renal transplantation. This patient showed a normal renal vein flow pattern.

velocity jet with distal turbulence. After venous patency has been established, the sonographer must question if the RI increase is caused by extrarenal compression (e.g., an adult allograft in a child is a common initial cause of extrarenal compression; for evaluation, the child's position should be changed to alleviate vascular compromise).

Although ATN does not commonly become abnormal until 24 hours after reperfusion of the graft, this is still a possible cause of increased RI immediately after surgery (Figures 10-107 to 10-108). Percutaneous biopsy will confirm ATN or rejection (hyperacute or acute). If there is an abnormally high renovascular impedance within the first few days after surgery (after a previous normal sonogram), obstructive uropathy should be suspected. The renal transplant should be evaluated with color (lack of color confirms hydronephrosis). Pyelocaliectasis is common, and its appearance of hydronephrosis can lead to a false-positive diagnosis of ureteral obstruction.

Clinically the patient should next be examined for pyelonephritis, pyuria, and extrarenal compression. At this later period, fluid collections can be the cause of extrarenal compression. The patient should be examined for periallograft fluid collections.

When there is increased renovascular impedance in the second week after surgery, rejection is by far the most common cause, especially if rejection has a vascular component. Biopsy is necessary to confirm rejection and determine whether rejection is from a vascular or interstitial pathologic cause.

Finally, if the creatinine levels increase in the first weeks after transplant, if RIs reveal increased renovascular impedance, and if no evidence of obstruction, compression, or infection can be found, the most common cause by far is acute rejection, which biopsy can confirm.

Color and Doppler Imaging. Arteriovenous malformations after biopsy, such as pseudoaneurysms and arteriovenous fistulas, can be readily seen using color Doppler imaging (Figure 10-109).

The color shows turbulent flow in the affected area. Duplex Doppler has not proved to be as sensitive for these arteriovenous malformations. Although color Doppler can identify them, it cannot distinguish one from the other. Power Doppler used in conjunction with color Doppler improves the evaluation of vessels. Power Doppler is not angle dependent and has a greater sensitivity to detect blood flow. It has the potential to increase the detection rate for intrarenal arteriovenous fistulas. Convergent color, which is not angle dependent and can detect direction of blood flow, may be the color imaging modality of the future.

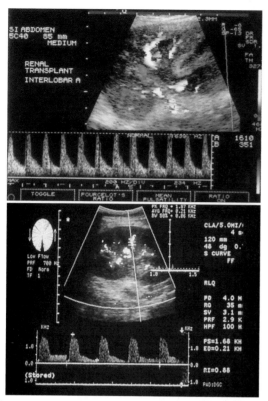

Figure 10-107 Color flow and Doppler of a normal flow pattern with good perfusion versus an abnormal flow pattern with high RI, as seen in a patient with chronic rejection. (*Bottom*, Courtesy Shpetim Telegrafi, New York University.)

Heart rate has a statistically significant effect on the RI in renal arteries. Increasing the heart rate of patients and taking measurements at paced rate intervals (70, 80, 90, 100, and 120 beats per minute), researchers have found that the RI decreased with increasing heart rate in six of eight patients. This suggests that in interpreting RI renal arteries, the actual heart rate must always be considered.

In conclusion, many factors must be considered when interpreting the meaning of increased RI in the transplanted kidney. Knowledge of the different complications and their relation to postoperative time, patient history, donor history, and clinical findings plays an integral part in helping to understand and find the cause of an increased RI.

Contrast Agents. The use of contrast agents for visualization of renal arteries has not been FDA approved. There have been some research studies performed using contrast agents to visualize the main renal arteries. The results have been encouraging: there has been an increase in visualization of normal renal arteries with the use of contrast agents and a decrease in scanning time.

KIDNEY STONE (UROLITHIASIS)

A stone located in the urinary system is called **urolithiasis**. The majority of urinary tract stones are formed in the kidney and course down the urinary tract. Stones consist of a combination of chemicals that precipitate out of urine. The most common chemical found in stones is calcium along with either oxalate or phosphate. Uric acid, cystine, and xanthine can also be found in kidney stones. Kidney stones are one of the most common kidney problems that can occur; they may cause obstruction, and this obstruction can be extremely painful. Most kidney stones are small and can travel through the urinary system without treatment or with increased hydration. Stones that are large and fill the renal collecting system are called staghorn calculi. Some kidney stones that travel down the urinary system may obstruct the ureter in the constricted areas.

There has been an increase in the number of people with kidney stones in the United States in the past 20 years. Kidney stones are more common in men. Some people tend to form kidney stones more than others, and once a kidney stone has formed, the person is at an increased risk of getting stones in the future. Kidney stones are associated with renal acidosis (a rare hereditary disorder), and people taking the protease inhibitor Indinavir are at an increased risk of developing kidney stones. The initial clinical sign of a kidney stone is extreme pain typically followed by cramping on the side that the stone is located on; nausea and vomiting may also occur. The pain may subside while the stone is traveling down the ureter.

Treatment for stones that cause obstruction varies depending upon the size and location of the stone. Treatment can include extracorporeal shockwave lithotripsy (ESWL), percutaneous nephrolithotomy, and ureteroscopic stone removal. Extracorporeal shockwave lithotripsy uses ultrasound or x-ray to locate the stone, and shock waves are used to break up the stone to smaller particles, which can readily pass through the urinary system. Percutaneous nephrolithotomy is a surgical procedure where an opening is made in the kidney and a nephroscope is used to remove the stone from the kidney. For mid and lower urinary tract stones, a ureteroscope (which has a basket-like end) can be placed through the urethra and bladder and guided up to the level of the stone to capture and remove the stone. Early treatment of stones that cause obstruction is important to reverse any renal damage that the obstruction may cause.

Sonographic Findings. Renal stones are very echogenic foci with posterior acoustic shadowing. When searching for renal stones, sonographer should scan along the lines of the renal fat; usually stones less than 3 mm may not shadow by using traditional B-mode (Figures 10-110 and 10-111). Prominent renal sinus fat, mesenteric fat, and bowel have high attenuation and may appear as an indistinct echogenic focus with questionable posterior acoustic shadowing, making it difficult to differentiate from stones. The use of tissue harmonics can demonstrate the shadowing of small stones measuring millimeters in size (Figure 10-112). Color and power Doppler have increased the sensitivity of confirming the presence of stones. Color and power Doppler cause a twinkling artifact posterior to the stone. The artifact is also referred to as the *twinkling sign* and is imaged as a rapidly changing mixture of red and blue colors posterior to the stone (Figure 10-113). Color and power Doppler are more sensitive when an "all-digital"

Figure 10-108   Abnormal flow patterns in a patient with rejection. **A,** Large, hypoechoic area along the anterior border of the kidney with compression of the calyceal system. **B,** Abnormal flow pattern in the segmental artery with decreased diastolic flow and increased RI to 0.9. **C,** Abnormal flow in the interlobar artery. **D,** Abnormal flow in the arcuate artery. **E** and **F,** The patient had a renal biopsy; status after biopsy shows fine, stippled echoes throughout the bladder indicating hematoma within the bladder. Before and after biopsy, scans should routinely be made to search for hematoma collections around the kidney or within the bladder.

processing technology is used because of its increased color sensitivity and acoustic power.

If the stone causes obstruction, there will be hydronephrosis, and, depending upon the location of the stone, the ureter may be dilated superior to the level of obstruction (Figure 10-114). The ureter—from the ureteropelvic junction to the bladder—is not routinely visualized on ultrasound unless they are dilated. The superior and distal ends of the ureters are more readily visualized than the midsection. The ureters lie in the retroperitoneal cavity and are obscured by bowel gas. Stones can also be imaged when the urinary bladder is distended with fluid (Figure 10-115).

BLADDER DIVERTICULUM

Bladder diverticulum is the herniation of the bladder wall. These outpouchings may be singular or multiple and are thinner than the normal bladder wall (Figure 10-116).

Diverticula can be either congenital or acquired. Congenital diverticulum entails herniation of all layers of the bladder wall and is located in the posterior angle of the trigone. Acquired diverticula are herniations of only the two inner layers through the muscle layer. Acquired bladder diverticula have higher prevalence in patients with chronic bladder outlet obstruction or neurogenic bladders.

Sonographic Findings. The sonographic finding is a neck of varying size connecting the adjacent fluid-filled structure to the bladder. The diverticula may still be filled with fluid after the patient empties the bladder. The urine stasis leads to recurring infections and stone formation (Figure 10-117).

BLADDER INFLAMMATION (CYSTITIS)

There are several infectious and noninfectious causes for inflammation of the bladder. Cystitis is usually secondary to another condition that causes stasis of urine in the bladder. Conditions that cause incomplete emptying of the bladder are urethral stricture, benign and malignant neoplasms, bladder calculi, trauma (blood clot), tuberculosis (lower ureteric strictures), pregnancy, neurogenic bladder, and radiation therapy. Other causes of cystitis include Foley catheter,

Figure 10-109 Longitudinal view of the left kidney with renal arteriovenous fistula.

Figure 10-110 Arrow indicating a small stone in the renal sinus. (Courtesy Shpetim Telegrafi, New York University.)

Figure 10-111 A 69-year-old male presented with right flank pain. A midpole echogenic structure, with *arrows* indicating posterior shadowing, representative of a renal stone. (Courtesy Shpetim Telegrafi, New York University.)

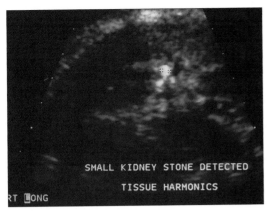

Figure 10-112   A small (31 mm) right renal stone detected using tissue harmonics. (Courtesy Shpetim Telegrafi, New York University.)

A

B

Figure 10-113   **A,** Sagittal image of the right kidney with large calculi. Posterior shadowing is seen with no renal obstruction. **B,** Sagittal image of right kidney with large calculi. Multiple colors are seen posterior to the stone *twinkle sign.* (From Henningsen C: *Clinical guide to ultrasonography,* St. Louis, 2004, Mosby.)

common rectal or vaginal fistulas, renal disease, sexual intercourse, poor hygiene, diabetes mellitus, and inflammation following surgical intervention.

Sonographic Findings. Sonographically the bladder wall may appear normal in the early stages of inflammatory disease. As the inflammation duration increases, the smooth bladder wall will become diffuse or nondiffuse with hypoechoic thickening. As the inflammatory process progresses, the bladder wall will become fibrotic and scarred. The bladder wall will appear more echogenic on ultrasound.

BLADDER TUMORS

The majority (95%) of bladder tumors in adults are transitional cell carcinoma (TCC). Bladder tumors are usually not detected until they have become advanced. Patients usually present with gross hematuria and may also present with dysuria, urinary frequency, or urinary urgency. Ultrasound cannot distinguish between benign and malignant masses. Either a cystoscopy or biopsy may obtain differentiation between a benign or malignant neoplasm. The bladder may also be the secondary site of malignancy. The most common site is the prostate. Invasion of the bladder may also be from colon, uterine, or ovarian carcinoma or endometriosis.

Sonographic Findings. The sonographic appearance of bladder masses varies and commonly appears as a focal bladder wall thickness. Ultrasound, CT, or MRI may be used to perform staging of bladder carcinoma. A transabdominal ultrasound approach can detect intravesical lesions as small as 3 to 4 mm. Ultrasound is limited and is unable to detect a perivesi-

cal extension and pelvic wall involvement. A transrectal approach can be used to detect intravesicular involvement.

Benign tumors are typically hypoechoic when compared with malignant bladder tumors, but they may also have the same echogenicity. All primary bladder tumors, which includes squamous cell carcinoma, adenocarcinoma, and rhabdomyosarcoma in children, have the same sonographic appearance: an irregular echogenic mass that projects into the lumen of the bladder. Color Doppler can be used to determine increased vascularity (Figure 10-118). Any bladder mass may cause outflow obstruction, and the kidneys should be evaluated for hydronephrosis.

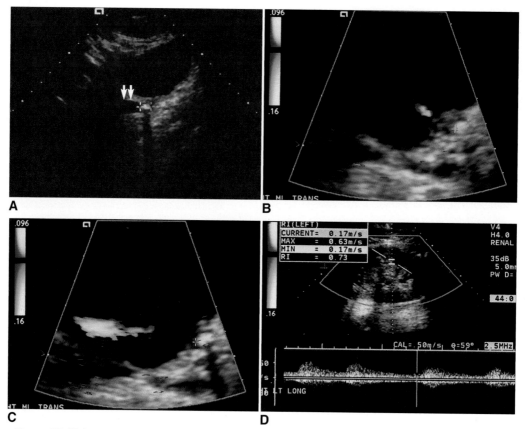

Figure 10-114 **A,** Longitudinal scan of a 65-year-old man with a stone in the distal left ureter *(arrows).* **B,** Partial obstruction of left ureter with decreased ureteral jet. **C,** Transverse scan of bladder with left ureteral stone measuring 8 mm and normal right ureteral jet. **D,** Increased left intrarenal RI of 0.73. (Courtesy Shpetim Telegrafi, New York University.)

Figure 10-116 Transverse scan of two bladder diverticula, one on either side. (Courtesy Shpetim Telegrafi, New York University.)

Figure 10-115 Transverse scan of the bladder stone with shadowing measuring 1.21 cm. (Courtesy Shpetim Telegrafi, New York University.)

Figure 10-117 Transverse scan of the urinary bladder with a stone in the diverticulum. (Courtesy Shpetim Telegrafi, New York University.)

Figure 10-118 Carcinoma of the urinary bladder with blood flow seen within the mass. (Courtesy Shpetim Telegrafi, New York University.)

SELECTED BIBLIOGRAPHY

Aytac SK, Özcan H: Effect of color Doppler system on the twinkling sign associated with urinary tract calculi, *Jour of Clin Med* vol 27, No 8, 1999.

Bajwa ZH and others: Pain management in polycystic kidney disease, *Int Soc of Nephrol* 60(5):1631-1644, 2001.

Brun M, Maugey-Laulom B and others: Prenatal sonographic patterns in autosomal dominant polycystic kidney disease: a multicenter study, *Ultrad in Obsts & Gyny* 24(1):55-61, 2004.

Buturovic-Ponikvar J, Visnar-Perovic A: Ultrasonography in chronic renal failure, *Eur Jour of Rad* 46(2):115-122, 2003.

Coyne SC and others: Surgically correctable renal transplant complications: an integrated clinical and radiologic approach, *Am J Roentgenol* 136:1113, 1981.

Don S and others: Detection of rejection in renal allografts, *J Ultrasound Med* 9:503, 1990.

Fischbach F: *A manual of laboratory diagnostic tests,* Philadelphia, 1980, JB Lippincott.

Genkins SM, Sanfilippo FP, Carroll BA: Duplex Doppler sonography of renal transplants: lack of sensitivity and specificity in establishing pathological diagnosis, *Am J Roentgenol* 152:535, 1989.

Ghosh AK, Ghosh K: *Medullary sponge kidney,* http://www.emedicine.com/med/topic1413.htm, retrieved February 24, 2004.

Gordon D: Imaging in cystic renal disease, *Archives of Disease in Childhood* 83(5):533, 2000.

Grant EG, Perrella RR: Wishing won't make it so: duplex Doppler sonography in the evaluation of renal transplant dysfunction, *Am J Roentgenol* 155:538, 1990.

Helenon O, Correas JM and others: Ultrasound renal tumors, *Euro Radio* 11(10):1890-1901, 2001.

Hennerici M, Neuerbrug-Hensler D: *Vascular diagnosis with ultrasound,* New York, 1998, Thieme.

Henningsen C: *Clinical guide to ultrasonography,* St. Louis, 2004, Mosby.

Jeffrey RB Jr, Ralls PW: *Sonography of the abdomen,* New York, 1995, Raven.

Kamaya A, Tuthill T, Rubin J: Twinkling artifact on color doppler sonography: depending on machine parameters and underlying cause, *AJR* January 2003.

Kaveggia LP and others: Duplex Doppler sonography in renal allografts: the significance of reversed flow in diastole, *Am J Roentgenol* 155:295, 1990.

King BF, Matsumoto JS: Diagnostic imaging of renal cystic diseases (Chap 8). In Watson ML, Torres VE, editors. *Polycystic kidney disease,* Oxford, 1996, Oxford University Press.

Kumar R, Wilson DD, Santa-Cruz FR: Postoperative urological complications of renal transplantation, *Radiographics* 4:531, 1984.

Lee HI, Grant: Sonography in renovascular hypertension, *J Ultrasound Med* 21:431-441, 2002.

Lee JY, Kim AH and others: Color and power Doppler twinkling artifacts from urinary stones, *AJR* 176:1441-1445, 2001.

Letourneau JG, Day DD, Ascher NL: Imaging of renal transplants, *Am J Roentgenol* 150:833, 1988.

Maklad NF, Wright CH, Rosenthal SJ: Gray scale ultrasonic appearances of renal transplant rejection, *Radiology* 131:711, 1979.

Mallek R and others: Distinction between obstructive and nonobstructive hydronephrosis: value of diuresis duplex Doppler sonography, *Am J Roentgenol* 166(1):133, 1996.

McGahan J, Goldberg B: *Diagnostic ultrasound: a logical approach,* Philadelphia, 1998, Lippincott-Raven.

Mostbeck GH, Gossinger HD, Mallek R: Effect of heart rate on Doppler measurements of RI in renal arteries, *Radiology* 175:511, 1990.

National Kidney and Urologic Diseases Information and Clearinghouse: Kidney stones in adults, http://niddk.nih.gov/health/kidney/pubs/stonadul/stonadul.htm, retrieved February 2000.

Nicolau C and others: Abdominal sonographic study of autosomal dominant polycystic kidney disease, *J Clin Ultrasound* 22:277-282, 2000.

Olcott ER, Goldstein RB, Salvatierra O: Lymphoma presenting as allograft hematoma in a renal transplant recipient, *J Ultrasound Med* 9:239, 1990.

Pepe P, Motta L and others: Functional evaluation of the urinary tract by color-Doppler ultrasonography (CDU) in 100 patients with renal colic, *Eur Rad* 53(1):131-135, 2005.

Platt JF, Ellis JM, Rubin JM: Examination of the native kidneys with duplex Doppler ultrasound, *Semin Ultrasound CT MR* 12:308, 1991.

Platt JF, Ellis JH, Rubin JM: Renal transplant pyelocaliectasis: role of duplex Doppler US in evaluation, *Radiology* 179:425, 1991.

Platt JF, Ellis JM, Rubin JM: Assessment of internal ureteral stent patency with pyelocaliectasis: value of renal duplex sonography, *Am J Roentgenol* 161:87, 1993.

Redmond A, McDevitt M, Barnes S: Acute renal failure: recognition and treatment in ward patients, *Nur Stan* vol 18(22):46-55, 2004.

Reuther GR, Wanjukra D, Bauer H: Acute renal vein thrombosis in renal allografts: detection with duplex Doppler US, *Radiology* 170:557, 1989.

Shokeir AA: Renal colic: new concepts related to pathophysiology, diagnosis and treatment, *Current Opinion in Urology* 12(4):263-269, 2002.

Silver TM: Peritransplant fluid collections, *Radiology* 138:145, 1981.

Snider JF and others: Transplant renal artery stenosis: evaluation with duplex sonography, *Radiology* 172:1027, 1989.

Stavros T, Harshfield D: Renal artery stenosis and renovascular hypertension: the clinical problem, *Ultrasound Q* 12(21):263-266, 1994.

Taylor JW, Marks WH: Use of Doppler imaging for evaluation of dysfunction in renal allografts, *Am J Roentgenol* 155:536, 1990.

Taylor KJ and others: Vascular complications in renal allografts: detection with duplex Doppler US, *Radiology* 162:31, 1987.

Tempkin B: *Ultrasound scanning: principles and protocols,* ed 2, Philadelphia, 1998, WB Saunders.

Tublin M, Murphy M, Tessler F: Duplex Doppler examination of native and transplant kidney dysfunction: technique applications and controversies, *Ultrasound Q* 15:2, 1999.

Wolf SJ Jr: State of the art article evaluation and management of solid and cystic renal masses, *J Urology* 159:1120, 1998.

The Spleen

Sandra L. Hagen-Ansert

KEY TERMS

accessory spleen – results from the failure of fusion of separate splenic masses forming on the dorsal mesogastrium; most commonly found in the splenic hilum or along the splenic vessels or associated ligaments

amyloidosis – a metabolic disorder marked by amyloid deposits in organs and tissue

autoimmune hemolytic anemia – anemia caused by antibodies produced by the patient's own immune system

culling – process by which the spleen removes abnormal red blood cells as they pass through

erythrocyte – red blood cell

gastrosplenic ligament – one of the ligaments between the stomach and spleen that helps to hold the spleen in place

Gaucher's disease – one of the storage diseases in which fat and proteins are deposited abnormally in the body

hematopoiesis – blood cell production

hemoglobin – oxygen-binding protein found in red blood cells

hemolytic anemia – anemia resulting from hemolysis of red blood cells

hemosiderin – pigment released from the hemoglobin process

Hodgkin's disease – a malignant disease that involves lymphoid tissue

infarction – an interruption in the blood supply to an area that may lead to necrosis of the area

intraperitoneal – within the peritoneal cavity

left hypochondrium – left upper quadrant of the abdomen that contains the left lobe of the liver, the spleen, and the stomach

leukopenia – abnormal decrease of white blood corpuscles; may be drug induced

lienorenal ligament – one of the ligaments that helps to hold the spleen in its place (attachment of spleen to kidney)

lymph – an alkaline fluid found in the lymphatic vessels

malpighian corpuscles – small masses found in the white pulp; lymph node in the spleen

mononucleosis – an acute infection caused by the Epstein-Barr virus that most commonly affects teenagers and young adults; symptoms include fever, sore throat, enlarged lymph nodes, abnormal lymphocysts, and hepatosplenomegaly

non-Hodgkin's lymphoma – a malignant disease of lymphoid tissue seen in increased frequency in individuals over 50 years of age

phagocytosis – process by which the red pulp destroys the degenerating red blood cells

phrenocolic ligament – the ligament between the spleen and the colon

pitting – process by which the spleen removes nuclei from blood cells without destroying the erythrocytes

polycythemia – an excess of red blood cells

polycythemia vera – chronic, life-shortening condition of unknown cause involving bone marrow elements; characterized by an increase in red blood cell mass and hemoglobin concentration

polysplenia – condition in which there is more than one spleen

red pulp – consists of reticular cells and fibers (cords of Billroth); surrounds the splenic sinuses

reticuloendothelial – certain phagocytic cells (found in the liver and spleen) make up the reticuloendothelial system (RES); plays a role in the synthesis of blood proteins and hemopoiesis

sickle cell anemia – inherited disorder transmitted as an autosomal recessive trait that causes an abnormality of the globin genes in hemoglobin

sickle cell crisis – condition in sickle cell anemia in which the sickled cells interfere with oxygen transport, obstruct capillary blood flow, and cause fever and severe pain in the joints and abdomen

spherocytosis – condition in which erythrocytes assume a spheroid shape; hereditary

splenic agenesis – complete absence of the spleen

splenic artery – branch of the celiac axis; tortuous course toward the spleen; serves as the superior border of the pancreas

splenic hilum – located in the middle of the spleen; site where vessels and lymph nodes enter and exit the spleen

splenic sinuses – long irregular channels lined by endothelial cells or flattened reticular cells

splenic vein – leaves the splenic hilum, travels transversely through the upper abdomen to join with the superior mesenteric vein to form the main portal vein; serves as the posterior medial border of the pancreas

splenomegaly – enlargement of the spleen

thalassemia – group of hereditary anemias occurring in Asian and Mediterranean populations

wandering spleen – spleen that has migrated from its normal location in the left upper quadrant

white blood cells – cells that defend the body by destroying invading microorganisms and their toxins

white pulp – consists of lymphatic tissue and lymphatic follicles

---

The spleen is part of the **reticuloendothelial** system that plays a part in the synthesis of blood proteins and is the largest single mass of lymphoid tissue in the body. The spleen is active in blood formation (**hematopoiesis**) during the initial part of fetal life. This function decreases gradually by the fifth or sixth month when the spleen assumes its adult characteristics and discontinues its hematopoietic (blood-producing) activities. The spleen plays an important role in the defense of the body. Although it is often affected by systemic disease processes, the spleen is rarely the primary site of disease.

ANATOMY OF THE SPLEEN

NORMAL ANATOMY

The spleen lies in the **left hypochondrium**, with its axis along the shaft of the tenth rib (Figure 11-1). Its lower pole extends forward as far as the midaxillary line. The spleen is an **intraperitoneal** organ covered with peritoneum over its entire extent except for a small area at its hilum, where the vascular structures and lymph nodes are located (Figure 11-2). The peritoneal ligaments attach the spleen to the stomach and the kidney. A protective capsule covers the spleen with peritoneum.

SIZE

The spleen is of variable size and shape (e.g., "orange segment," tetrahedral, or triangular), but generally is considered to be ovoid with smooth, even borders and a convex superior and concave inferior surface (Figure 11-3). The spleen is normally measured with ultrasound on a longitudinal image from the upper margin (near the diaphragm) to the inferior margin at the long axis. Normal measurements should be 8-13 cm in an adult.

VASCULAR SUPPLY

Blood is supplied to the spleen by the **splenic artery,** which is a tortuous vessel that travels horizontally along the superior border of the pancreas (see Figure 11-2). Upon entering the **splenic hilum,** this artery immediately branches into six smaller arteries to supply the organ with oxygenated blood to profuse the splenic parenchyma. Color Doppler imaging allows the sonographer to image the vascularity of the spleen; gray scale imaging will show small echogenic lines throughout the spleen that represent the arterial system. The splenic arteries are subject to **infarction** because there are not adequate anastomoses between the vessels.

The **splenic vein** is formed by multiple branches within the spleen and leaves the hilum in a horizontal direction to join the superior mesenteric vein, which is returning unoxygenated blood from the bowel to form the main portal vein (Figure 11-4). The splenic vein travels along the posteromedial border of the pancreas.

The **lymph** vessels emerge from the splenic hilum, pass through other lymph nodes along the course of the splenic artery, and drain into the celiac nodes. The nerves to the spleen accompany the splenic artery and are derived from the celiac plexus.

RELATIONAL ANATOMY

The spleen lies between the left hemidiaphragm and the stomach. The diaphragm may be seen as a bright, curvilinear, echogenic structure close to the proximal superolateral surface of the spleen. Posteriorly the diaphragm, left pleura, left lung, and ribs (eighth to eleventh) are in contact with the spleen.

The medial surface is related to the stomach, tail of the pancreas, left kidney, and splenic flexure of the colon (see Figure 11-2).

DISPLACEMENT OF THE SPLEEN

The spleen is held in place by the **lienorenal, gastrosplenic, and phrenocolic ligaments** (see Figure 11-2). These ligaments are derived from the layers of peritoneum that form the greater and lesser sacs. A mass in the left upper quadrant may displace the spleen inferiorly. Caudal displacement may be secondary to a subclavian abscess, splenic cyst, or left pleural effusion. Cephalic displacement may result from volume loss in the left

lung, left lobe pneumonia, paralysis of the left hemidiaphragm, or a large intraabdominal mass. A normal spleen with medial lobulation between the pancreatic tail and left kidney may be confused with a cystic mass in the tail of the pancreas.

WANDERING SPLEEN

The term **wandering spleen** describes a spleen that has migrated from its normal location in the left upper quadrant. It is the result of an embryologic anomaly of the supporting ligaments of the spleen. The patient presents with an abdominal or pelvic mass, intermittent pain, and volvulus (splenic torsion). The sonographer should use color Doppler to map

A

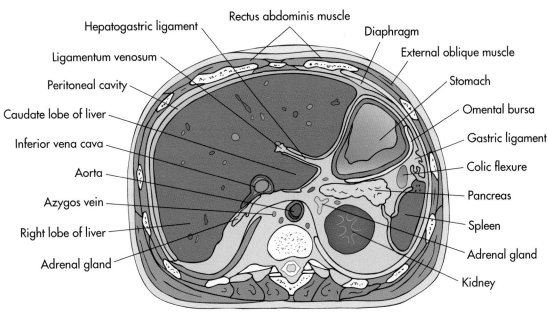

B

Figure 11-1   **A,** Transverse plane of the upper abdomen shows the posterior position of the spleen in the left upper quadrant. **B,** Transverse plane of the spleen.   *Continued*

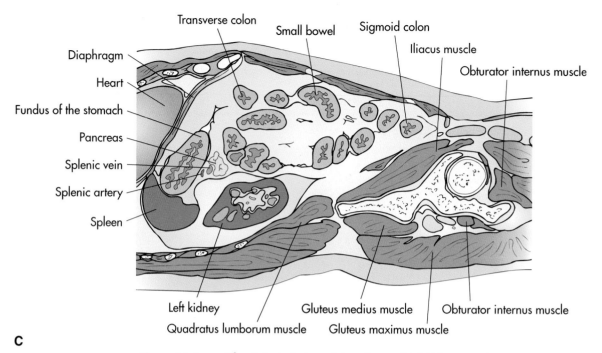

C

Figure 11-1, cont'd   C, Sagittal plane of the spleen and left kidney.

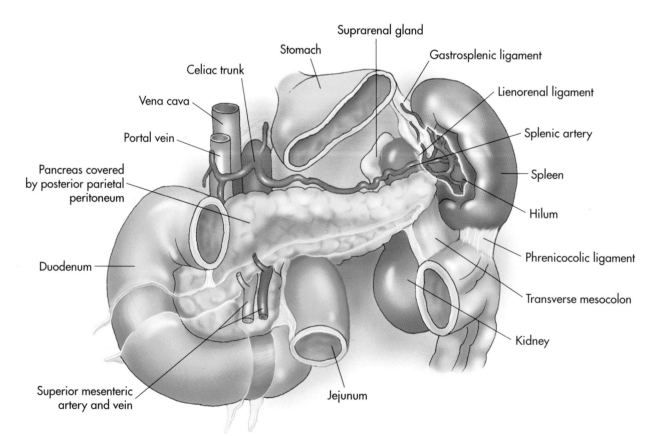

Figure 11-2   Anterior view of the spleen as it lies in the left hypochondrium. Note the relational anatomy, ligament attachments, and vascular landmarks.

the vascularity within the spleen. When torsion is complete, the vascular pattern shows decreased velocity.

CONGENITAL ANOMALIES

Splenic Agenesis. Complete absence of the spleen (asplenia), or **splenic agenesis,** is rare and by itself causes no difficulties. However, it may occur as part of asplenic or **polysplenia** syndromes in association with complex cardiac malformations, bronchopulmonary abnormalities, or visceral heterotaxis (anomalous placement of organs or major blood vessels, including a horizontal liver, malrotation of the gut, and interruption of the inferior vena cava with azygos continuation).

Splenic agenesis may be ruled out by demonstrating a spleen on ultrasound. The sonographer should be careful not to confuse the spleen with the bowel, which may lie in the area normally occupied by the spleen. Color Doppler helps determine the splenic vascular pattern and thus separate it from the colon.

Accessory Spleen. An **accessory spleen** is a more common congenital anomaly (Figure 11-5). The accessory spleen may be difficult to demonstrate by sonography if it is very small. However, when it is seen, it appears as a homogeneous pattern like that of the spleen. It is usually found near the hilum or inferior border of the spleen, but has been reported elsewhere in the abdominal cavity. Lesions affecting the normal spleen would also affect the accessory spleen.

An accessory spleen occasionally is found near the hilum of the spleen. An accessory spleen results from the failure of fusion of separate splenic masses forming on the dorsal mesogastrium; it is most commonly located in the splenic hilum or along the splenic vessels or associated ligaments. The location of the accessory spleen has been reported anywhere from the diaphragm to the scrotum and is usually solitary in number. It usually remains small and does not present as a clinical problem. The accessory spleen may simulate a pancreatic, suprarenal, or retroperitoneal tumor.

PHYSIOLOGY AND LABORATORY DATA OF THE SPLEEN

Although the spleen is the largest organ in the reticuloendothelial system, it is rarely the site of primary disease. More commonly it is involved in metabolic, hematopoietic, and infectious disorders. Blunt abdominal trauma to the spleen may result in splenic lacerations and rupture. The spleen is active in the body's defense against disease; its major function is to filter the peripheral blood.

The spleen is a soft organ with elastic properties that allow it to distend as blood fills the venous sinuses. These characteristics are related to the spleen's function as a blood reservoir. Within the lobules of the spleen are tissues called *pulp*. Two components are composed within the spleen: the red pulp and the white pulp.

Figure 11-3 Gross specimen of the spleen demonstrates its homogeneous texture and shape.

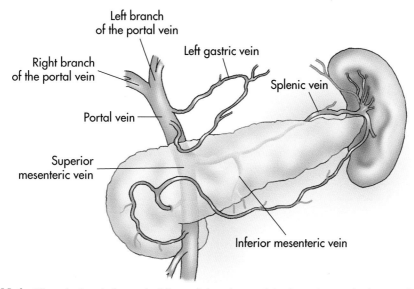

Figure 11-4 The splenic vein leaves the hilum of the spleen to join the main portal vein posterior to the head of the pancreas.

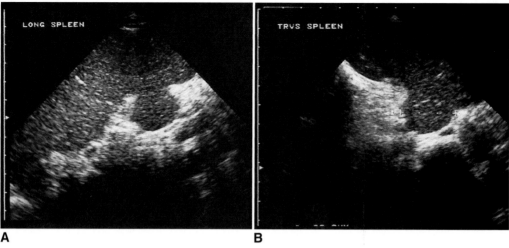

Figure 11-5 Accessory spleen. Long **(A)** and transverse **(B)** images of the small accessory spleen as it projects from the hilum of the spleen.

White pulp is distributed throughout the spleen in tiny islands. This tissue consists of splenic nodules, which are similar to those found in lymph nodes and contain large numbers of lymphocytes. Red pulp fills the remaining spaces of the lobules and surrounds the venous sinuses. The pulp contains relatively large numbers of red blood cells, which are responsible for its color, along with many lymphocytes and macrophages.

The **red pulp** of the spleen consists of **splenic sinuses** alternating with splenic cords. The blood capillaries within the red pulp are quite permeable. Red blood cells can squeeze through the pores in these capillary walls and enter the venous sinuses. The older, more fragile red blood cells may rupture as they make this passage, and the resulting cellular debris is removed by phagocytic macrophages located within the splenic sinuses. The macrophages engulf and destroy foreign particles, such as bacteria, that may be carried in the blood as it flows through the sinuses. The lymphocytes of the spleen help defend the body against infections.

The blood that leaves the splenic sinuses to enter the reticular cords passes through a complex filter. The venous drainage of the sinuses and cords is not well defined, but it is assumed that tributaries of the splenic vein connect with the sinuses of the red pulp.

The **white pulp** of the spleen consists of the **malpighian corpuscles,** small nodular masses of lymphoid tissue attached to the smaller arterial branches. Extending from the splenic capsule inward are the trabeculae, which contain blood vessels and lymphatics. The lymphoid tissue, or malpighian corpuscles, has the same structure as the follicles in the lymph nodes; however, it differs in that the splenic follicles surround arteries, so that on cross-section each contains a central artery. These follicles are scattered throughout the organ and are not confined to the peripheral layer or cortex, as are lymph nodes.

As part of the reticuloendothelial system, the spleen plays an important role in the defense mechanisms of the body and is also implicated in pigment and lipid metabolism. It is not essential to life and can be removed with no ill effects. The functions of the spleen may be classified under two general

---

BOX 11-1   FUNCTIONS OF THE SPLEEN

FUNCTIONS OF THE SPLEEN AS AN ORGAN OF THE RETICULOENDOTHELIAL SYSTEM
• Production of lymphocytes and plasma cells
• Production of antibodies
• Storage of iron
• Storage of other metabolites

FUNCTIONS CHARACTERISTIC OF THE SPLEEN
• Maturation of the surface of erythrocytes
• Reservoir
• Culling
• Pitting function
• Disposal of senescent or abnormal erythrocytes
• Functions related to platelet and leukocyte lifespan

---

headings: those that reflect the functions of the reticuloendothelial system and those that are characteristic of the organ itself (Box 11-1).

The role of the spleen as an immunologic organ concerns the production of cells capable of making antibodies (lymphocytes and plasma cells); however, antibodies are also produced at other sites.

Phagocytosis of **erythrocytes** and the breakdown of **hemoglobin** occur throughout the entire reticuloendothelial system, but roughly half the catabolic activity is localized in the normal spleen. In splenomegaly the major portion of hemoglobin breakdown occurs in the spleen. The iron that is liberated is stored in the splenic phagocytes. In anomalies such as the hemolytic anemias, the splenic phagocytes become engorged with **hemosiderin** when erythrocyte destruction is accelerated.

In addition to storing iron, the spleen is subject to the storage diseases, such as Gaucher's disease and Niemann-Pick disease. Abnormal lipid metabolites accumulate in all phagocytic reticuloendothelial cells, but may also involve the phagocytes in the spleen, producing gross splenomegaly.

The functions of the spleen that are characteristic of the organ relate primarily to the circulation of erythrocytes through it. In a normal individual, the spleen contains only about 20 to 30 ml of erythrocytes. In splenomegaly the reservoir function is greatly increased, and the abnormally enlarged spleen contains many times this volume of red blood cells. The transit time is lengthened, and the erythrocytes are subject to destructive effects for a long time. In part, ptosis causes consumption of glucose, on which the erythrocyte depends to maintain normal metabolism, and the erythrocyte is destroyed. Selective destruction of abnormal erythrocytes is also accelerated by the splenic pooling.

As erythrocytes pass through the spleen, the organ inspects them for imperfections and destroys those it recognizes as abnormal or senescent. **Pitting** is the process of removing the nuclei from the red blood cells. **Culling** is the process by which the spleen removes abnormal red blood cells. The normal function of the spleen keeps the number of circulating erythrocytes with inclusions at a minimum.

The spleen also pools platelets in large numbers. The entry of platelets into the splenic pool and their return to the circulation is extensive. In splenomegaly the splenic pool may be so large that it produces thrombocytopenia. Sequestration of leukocytes in the enlarged spleen may produce **leukopenia.**

Laboratory data include the following:

- *Hematocrit.* The hematocrit indicates the percentage of red blood cells per volume of blood. Abnormally low readings indicate hemorrhage or internal bleeding within the body.
- *Bacteremia.* The test for bacteremia indicates the presence of bacteria within the body. The term *sepsis* indicates bacteria in the bloodstream. Typical symptoms of fever and chills, along with other medical conditions, may indicate the presence of an infection.
- *Leukocytosis.* The increase in the number of white cells present in the blood is usually a typical finding in infection. This finding may also occur after surgery, in malignancies, or in the presence of leukemia.

- *Leukopenia.* Abnormal decrease in white blood corpuscles may be secondary to certain medications or bone marrow disorder.
- *Thrombocytopenia.* Thrombocytopenia is an abnormal decrease in platelets, which may be due to internal hemorrhage.

SONOGRAPHIC EVALUATION OF THE SPLEEN

NORMAL TEXTURE AND PATTERNS

Sonographically the splenic parenchyma should have a fine homogeneous low-level echo pattern, as is seen within the liver parenchyma (Figure 11-6). The spleen has two components joined at the hilum. On transverse scans it has a crescent appearance, usually with a large medial component. Moving inferiorly, only the lateral component is imaged. On longitudinal scans the superior component extends more medially than the inferior component. The irregularity of these components makes it difficult to assess mild splenomegaly accurately.

SIZE

The spleen is normally measured along its long axis (Figure 11-7). The normal spleen measures 8 to 13 cm in length, 7 to 8 cm in anteroposterior diameter, and less than 6 cm in thickness. In children, the formula for splenic length is 5.7 + 0.31 × age (in years). The length of the spleen usually measures greater than the length of the kidney. Splenomegaly is diagnosed when the spleen measures more than 13 cm in the adult patient or more than the normal length in the respective child.

PATIENT POSITION AND TECHNIQUE

The left upper quadrant may be imaged as the sonographer carefully manipulates the transducer between costal margins to image the left kidney, spleen, and diaphragm. The patient should be rolled into a steep right lateral decubitus position and instructed to raise his or her left arm over his or her head to further open up the intercostal spaces to allow the transducer better access to the spleen. The sector transducer may fit between the intercostal margins better than the larger curved array transducer.

Figure 11-6 Normal spleen. Long **(A)** and transverse **(B)** images of the normal spleen. The parenchyma is homogeneous throughout except for the area of the hilum where the vascular structures enter and leave the spleen.

Figure 11-7   Splenic size. The spleen is measured in the long axis and should be 8 to 13 cm in length.

Figure 11-8   Color Doppler shows the splenic arterial system within the spleen.

Figure 11-9   The splenic venous system is well demarcated with color Doppler.

When the patient is lying supine, the problem of overlying air-filled stomach or bowel anterior to the spleen may interfere with adequate visualization; thus the patient should be rotated into a slight right decubitus position to permit better transducer contact between the ribs without as much bowel interference. The right lateral decubitus, or axillary, position enables the sonographer to scan in an oblique fashion between the ribs. If the ultrasound laboratory has a cardiac bed with a drop-leaf component, the patient should be rolled onto his or her left side and the transducer directed along the left intercostal margin to image the spleen. Excellent visualization is made because the spleen will lie flush against the patient's abdominal wall.

Variations in patient respiration may also help to image the spleen; deep inspiration causes the diaphragm to move, with resultant displacement of the spleen from under the ribs.

In a routine abdominal examination, the spleen should be surveyed to make sure the parenchyma is uniform and the splenic hilum shows normal vascular patterns. At least two images of the spleen should be recorded in the longitudinal and transverse planes (see Figure 11-6). The longitudinal plane should demonstrate the left hemidiaphragm, the superior and inferior margins of the spleen, and the upper pole of the left kidney. The sonographer should look at the left pleural space superior to the diaphragm to see if fluid is present in the lower costal margin. The long axis of the spleen is measured from its superior-to-inferior border.

After the longitudinal scan is completed, the transducer is rotated 90 degrees to survey the spleen in a transverse plane. The sonographer should obtain at least one transverse image at the hilum of the spleen. The sonographer should observe the flow of the splenic artery and vein with color Doppler. Forward (positive to the baseline) arterial flow should be seen entering the main splenic artery as it bifurcates into multiple branches to supply the splenic parenchyma (Figure 11-8). Conversely, returning (negative to the baseline) flow from the multiple splenic venous branches enters into the splenic vein. The splenic vein leaves the hilum of the spleen to transverse horizontally across the abdomen to join the superior

mesenteric vein that leads into the main portal vein anterior to the inferior vena cava (Figure 11-9).

Increased hypoechoic structures in the area of the splenic hilum may indicate either portal hypertension with collateral vessels or enlarged lymph nodes. A correlation has been noted between the caliber of splenic arteries and the size of the spleen in cirrhotic patients with esophageal varices.[5] The splenic artery is larger in patients with splenomegaly (patients with cirrhosis with esophageal varices and patients with hematologic malignancies). The use of color Doppler imaging will help the sonographer determine if the structures are vascular or nonvascular in composition (Figure 11-10).

NONVISUALIZATION OF THE SPLEEN

The inability to image the spleen in its normal location may be a result of one of several conditions (e.g., asplenia syndrome, polysplenia syndrome, traumatic fragmentation of the spleen, or the wandering spleen).

Atrophy.   Atrophy of the spleen may be found in normal individuals. It may also occur in wasting diseases. In chronic hemolytic anemias, particularly sickle cell anemia, there is excessive loss of pulp, increasing fibrosis, scarring from multiple infarcts, and incrustation with iron and calcium deposits. In the final stages of atrophy, the spleen may be so small

Figure 11-10   Color Doppler shows the dilated splenic vessels that may be seen with portal hypertension and varices.

TABLE 11-1 SPLENIC FINDINGS		
Clinical Findings	Sonographic Findings	Differential Considerations
Splenomegaly		
Depends on cause	Long axis ≥13 cm Look for liver anomalies (e.g., cirrhosis, diffuse disease)	
Splenic Abscess		
Fever Leukocytosis	Splenomegaly Irregular, ill-defined borders May have internal septa	Hematoma Necrotic neoplasm Lymphoma Leukemia
Splenic Infarction		
Related to primary diagnosis	Acute: wedge-shaped, hypoechoic area Chronic: wedge-shaped, echogenic area (base points to periphery) Look for splenic atrophy	Infection Hemorrhage Neoplasm Lymphoma
Splenic Trauma		
↓ Hematocrit	Spleen may appear enlarged Hematoma may form later along subcapsular area or internally	
Splenic Cysts		
Asymptomatic	Solitary Anechoic ↑ Transmission Well-defined walls Look for tissue compression	Hematoma Lymphangioma Echinococcal cyst
Primary Tumors		
Depends on primary	Splenomegaly May be diffuse, single, or multiple Hypoechoic to hyperechoic	Infection

that it is hardly recognizable. Advanced atrophy is sometimes referred to as autosplenectomy.

PATHOLOGY OF THE SPLEEN

See Table 11-1 for clinical findings, sonographic findings, and differential considerations for selected splenic diseases and conditions.

SPLENOMEGALY

As the largest unit of the reticuloendothelial system, the spleen is involved in all systemic inflammations and generalized hematopoietic disorders and many metabolic disturbances (Table 11-2 and Boxes 11-2 and 11-3). It is rarely the primary site of disease. Whenever the spleen is involved in systemic disease, splenic enlargement usually develops; therefore,

TABLE 11-2 SONOGRAPHIC-PATHOLOGIC CLASSIFICATION OF SPLENIC DISORDERS

| Uniform Splenic Sonodensity | | | Focal Defects | |
Normal Sonodensity	Low Sonodensity	Sonodense	Sonolucent	Perisplenic Defects
Erythropoiesis (including myeloproliferative disorders) Reticuloendothelial Congestion Hyperactivity	Granulocytopoiesis (excluding myelo disorders) Lymphopoiesis Other (multiple myeloma) Congestion	Nonspecific (metastasis)	Nonspecific (benign primary neoplasm, cyst, abscess, malignant neoplasm [lymphopoietic])	Nonspecific (hematoma)

From Mittelstaedt CA, Partain CL: *Radiology* 134:697, 1980.

BOX 11-2 PATHOLOGIC CLASSIFICATION OF SPLENIC DISORDERS

HEMATOPOIETIC
Granulocytopoiesis
  Reactive hyperplasia to acute and chronic infection (low sonodensity)
Noncaseous granulomatous inflammation
Myeloproliferative syndromes (normal)
Chronic myelogenous leukemia
Acute myelogenous leukemia
Lymphopoiesis (low sonodensity or focal sonolucent)
Chronic lymphocytic leukemia
  Lymphoma
  Hodgkin's disease
Erythropoiesis (normal)
Sickle cell disease
  Hereditary spherocytosis
  Hemolytic anemia
  Chronic anemia
  Myeloproliferative syndrome
Other
  Multiple myeloma (low sonodensity)

RETICULOENDOTHELIAL HYPERACTIVITY (NORMAL)
Still's disease
Wilson's disease
Felty's syndrome
Reticulum cell sarcoma

Congestion (Normal or Low Sonodensity)
Hepatocellular disease

Nonspecific
Neoplasm-metastasis (focal sonodense)
Cyst (focal sonolucent)
Abscess (focal sonolucent)
Malignant neoplasm (focal sonolucent)
  Hodgkin's disease
  Lymphoma
Benign neoplasm (focal sonolucent)
  Lymphangiomatosis
Hematoma (perisplenic)

BOX 11-3 CAUSES OF SPLENOMEGALY

- Congestion
- Neoplasm
- Storage disease
- Infection
- Hemolytic anemia
- Extramedullary hematopoiesis
- Collagen-vascular disease
- Trauma

splenomegaly (Figure 11-11) is a major manifestation of disorders of this organ.

Although splenomegaly is the most common disease process the sonographer may encounter when evaluating this organ, careful evaluation of the splenic contour and homogeneity should be undertaken to determine if a disease process involves the spleen. Evaluation of the splenic parenchyma and vascular patterns may demonstrate changes in the size, texture, and vascularity of the organ, which could be helpful in the patient's clinical evaluation to rule out the presence of a diffuse disease process or focal lesion.

Clinical signs of splenomegaly may include left upper quadrant pain (secondary to stretching of the splenic capsule or ligaments) or fullness. Enlargement of the spleen may encroach upon surrounding organs, such as the left kidney, pancreas, stomach, and intestines.

CONGESTION OF THE SPLEEN

There are two types of splenic congestion: acute and chronic. In acute congestion, active hyperemia accompanies the reaction in the moderately enlarged spleen. In chronic venous congestion, there is diffuse enlargement of the spleen.

The venous congestion may be of systemic origin, caused by intrahepatic obstruction to portal venous drainage or by obstructive venous disorders in the portal or splenic veins. Systemic venous congestion is found in cardiac decompensation

Figure 11-11   Patterns of splenomegaly. **A** and **B,** The tip of the spleen covers the lower pole of the kidney in patients with splenomegaly. **C,** The dilated splenic hilum is secondary to portal hypertension. Both the liver and spleen are enlarged.

> **BOX 11-4** **CAUSES OF CONGESTIVE SPLENOMEGALY**
>
> - Heart failure
> - Portal hypertension
> - Cirrhosis
> - Cystic fibrosis
> - Portal or splenic vein thrombosis
> - Acute splenic sequestration crisis of sickle cell disease

involving the right side of the heart. It is particularly severe in tricuspid or pulmonary valvular disease and in chronic cor pulmonale.

The most common causes of striking congestive splenomegaly are the various forms of cirrhosis of the liver. It is also caused by obstruction to the extrahepatic portal or splenic vein (e.g., spontaneous portal vein thrombosis) (Box 11-4).

STORAGE DISEASE

Amyloidosis. In systemic diseases leading to **amyloidosis,** the spleen is the most frequently involved organ.

Sonographic Findings. The spleen may be of normal size or decidedly enlarged, depending on the amount and distribution of amyloid. Two types of involvement are seen—nodular and diffuse. In the nodular type, amyloid is found in the walls of the sheathed arteries and within the follicles but not in the red pulp (see Figure 11-11). In the diffuse type, the follicles are not involved, the red pulp is prominently involved, and the spleen is usually greatly enlarged and firm.

Gaucher's Disease. All age groups can be affected by **Gaucher's disease.** About 50% of patients are under 8 years of age, and 17% are under 1 year of age. Clinical features follow a chronic course, with bone pain and changes in skin pigmentation.

Sonographic Findings. On ultrasound examination, there is splenomegaly, diffuse inhomogeneity, and multiple splenic nodules (well-defined hypoechoic lesions). These nodules may be irregular, hyperechoic, or mixed. They represent focal areas of Gaucher's cells associated with fibrosis and infarction.

Niemann-Pick Disease. Niemann-Pick disease is a rapidly fatal disease that predominantly affects female infants. The clinical features consist of hepatomegaly, digestive disturbances, and lymphadenopathy.

DIFFUSE DISEASE

Erythropoietic abnormalities include the following: sickle cell, hereditary spherocytosis, hemolytic anemia, chronic anemia,

Figure 11-12 Sickle cell crisis. Patient with sickle cell anemia demonstrated a small spleen with the progressive infarction and fibrosis as seen in autosplenectomy.

Figure 11-13 A patient with thalassemia major shows a huge spleen extending into the lower abdominal cavity.

polycythemia vera, thalassemia, and myeloproliferative disorders. On ultrasound, they tend to produce an isoechoic pattern.

Sickle Cell Anemia. In the earlier stage of **sickle cell anemia,** as seen in infants and children, the spleen is enlarged with marked congestion of the red pulp. Later the spleen undergoes progressive infarction and fibrosis and decreases in size until, in adults, only a small mass of fibrous tissue may be found (autosplenectomy). It is generally believed that these changes result when sickle cells plug the vasculature of the splenic substance, effectively producing ischemic destruction of the spleen.

Sonographic Findings. On ultrasound examination, sickle cell disease has different sonographic appearances depending upon its disease state (Figure 11-12). An acute **sickle cell crisis** commonly occurs in children with homozygous sickle cell disease with splenomegaly and a sudden decrease in hematocrit. In addition, these patients may develop a subacute hemorrhage that appears as a hypoechoic area in the periphery of the spleen.

Congenital Spherocytosis. In congenital or hereditary **spherocytosis** an intrinsic abnormality of the red cells gives rise to erythrocytes that are small and spheroid rather than the normal, flattened, biconcave disks. The two results of this disease are the production by the bone marrow of spherocytic erythrocytes and the increased destruction of these cells in the spleen. The spleen destroys spherocytes selectively.

Sonographic Findings. The spleen may be enlarged.

Hemolytic Anemia. Hemolytic anemia is the general term applied to anemia referable to decreased life of the erythrocytes. When the rate of destruction is greater than the bone marrow can compensate for, then anemia results.

Autoimmune Hemolytic Anemia. Autoimmune hemolytic anemia can occur in its primary form without underlying disease, or it may be seen as a secondary disorder in patients already suffering from some disorder of the reticuloendothelial or hematopoietic systems, such as lymphoma, leukemia, or infectious **mononucleosis**.

Sonographic Findings. In the secondary form the splenic changes are dominated by the underlying disease; in the primary form the spleen is variably enlarged.

Polycythemia Vera. This is a chronic disease of unknown cause that involves all bone marrow elements. **Polycythemia vera** is characterized by an increase in red blood cell mass and hemoglobin concentration. Clinical symptoms include weakness, fatigue, vertigo, tinnitus, irritability, splenomegaly, flushing of the face, redness and pain in the extremities, and blue-and-black spots.

Sonographic Findings. In polycythemia vera the spleen is variably enlarged, rather firm, and blue-red. Infarcts and thromboses are common in polycythemia vera.

Thalassemia. The spleen is severely involved in **thalassemia.** This hemoglobinopathy differs from the others in that an abnormal molecular form of hemoglobin is not present. Instead, there is a suppression of synthesis of beta or alpha polypeptide chains, resulting in deficient synthesis of normal hemoglobin. The erythrocytes are not only deficient in normal hemoglobin but also abnormal in shape; many are target cells, whereas others vary considerably in size and shape. Their life span is short because they are destroyed by the spleen in large numbers. The disease ranges from mild to severe.

Sonographic Findings. The changes in the spleen are greatest in the severe form, called thalassemia major (Figure 11-13). The spleen is very large, often seeming to fill the entire abdominal cavity.

Myeloproliferative Disorders. Myeloproliferative disorders include acute and chronic myelogenous leukemias, polycythemia vera, myelofibrosis, megakaryocytic leukemia, and erythroleukemia (Figure 11-14).

Sonographic Findings. An isoechoic ultrasound pattern is seen because the parenchyma is hypoechoic compared with the liver (Figure 11-15).

Figure 11-14 Chronic myeloid leukemia shows infarcts in a gross specimen with splenomegaly. (From Damjanov I, Linder J: *Pathology: a color atlas,* St. Louis, 2000, Mosby.)

Figure 11-15 Patient with acute myelogenous leukemia shows a large mass within the splenic parenchyma and enlarged nodes in the hilum.

Granulocytopoietic Abnormalities. Granulocytopoietic abnormalities include cases of reactive hyperplasia resulting from acute or chronic infection (e.g., splenitis sarcoid and tuberculosis).

Sonographic Findings. On ultrasound examination, splenomegaly is seen with a diffusely hypoechoic pattern (less dense than the liver). Patients who have had a previous granulomatous infection have bright echogenic lesions on ultrasound, with or without shadowing. Histoplasmosis and tuberculosis are the most common causes; sarcoidosis is rare. The sonographer may also find calcium in the splenic artery.

Reticuloendotheliosis. Diseases characterized by reticuloendothelial hyperactivity and varying degrees of lipid storage in phagocytes are included in the category of reticuloendotheliosis.

Sonographic Findings. On ultrasound, the spleen appears isoechoic.

Letterer-Siwe Disease. In Letterer-Siwe disease, sometimes called *nonlipid reticuloendotheliosis,* there is proliferation of

Figure 11-16 Lymphoblastic lymphoma. Tumor cells form a discrete mass in the spleen. (From Damjanov I, Linder J: *Pathology: a color atlas,* St. Louis, 2000, Mosby.)

reticuloendothelial cells in all tissues but particularly in the splenic lymph nodes and bone marrow.

Sonographic Findings. This disease is generally found in children under the age of 2. Clinical features are hepatosplenomegaly, fever, and pulmonary involvement. It is rapidly fatal. Usually the spleen is only moderately enlarged, although the change may be more severe in affected older infants.

Hand-Schüller-Christian Disease. Hand-Schüller-Christian disease is benign and chronic, in spite of many features similar to those of Letterer-Siwe disease. It usually affects children over 2 years of age. The clinical features are a *chronic course,* diabetes, and moderate hepatosplenomegaly.

LYMPHOPOIETIC ABNORMALITIES

Lymphopoietic abnormalities include lymphocytic leukemias, lymphoma, and **Hodgkin's disease** (Figure 11-16).

Sonographic Findings. Ultrasound shows a diffusely hypoechoic splenic pattern with focal lesions. Patients with **non-Hodgkin's lymphoma** have been reported to have an isoechoic echo pattern.

Leukemia. Chronic myelogenous leukemia may be responsible for more extreme splenomegaly than any other disease. Chronic lymphocytic leukemia produces less severe splenomegaly.

FOCAL DISEASE

Focal disease of the spleen may be single or multiple and may be found in normal or enlarged spleens. The major nontraumatic causes of focal splenic defects include tumors (benign and malignant), infarction, abscesses, and cysts. Splenic defects may be discovered incidentally, as in another imaging study, or specifically, as in the case of a splenic infarct or abscess.

Splenic Abscess. Splenic abscesses are uncommon, probably because of the phagocytic activity of the spleen's efficient reticuloendothelial system and leukocytes. The system may be infected by the following: subacute bacterial endocarditis, septicemia, decreased immunologic states, or drug abuse. In the majority of patients the infection is spread from distant foci in the abdomen, or an inflammatory process extends directly from adjacent organs. Extrinsic processes (i.e., perinephric or subphrenic abscess, perforated gastric or colonic lesions, or pancreatic abscess) may invade the splenic parenchyma.

Clinical findings may be subtle and may include fever, left upper quadrant tenderness, abdominal pain, left shoulder and flank pain, and splenomegaly.

Sonographic Findings. Sonography shows a mixed echo pattern (Figure 11-17). The lesion may be hypoechoic, often with a hyperechoic foci that represents debris or gas. Other findings include the following: thick or shaggy walls, anechoic (without echoes within a mass) appearance, poor definition of the lesion, and increased to decreased transmission (depending on the presence of gas). An abscess may be difficult to distinguish from an infarct, neoplasm, or hematoma, and clinical correlation is necessary.

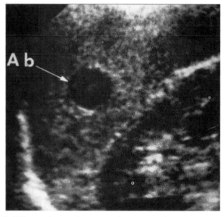

Figure 11-17 Splenic abscess (Ab). A small, well-defined hypoechoic lesion was seen within the spleen in a patient who had been febrile for 6 days.

Splenic Infection. Many infections can affect the spleen. The most prominent feature is splenomegaly. Many immunocompromised patients also have multiple nodules within the spleen.

Sonographic Findings. Patients with hepatosplenic candidiasis may show irregular masses within the spleen, the "wheels-within-wheels" pattern, with the outer wheel representing the ring of fibrosis surrounding the inner echogenic wheel of inflammatory cells and a central hypoechoic area (Figure 11-18). Other patterns found are bull's eye (hypoechoic rim with a echogenic central core), hypoechoic nodule, or hyperechoic nodule. On ultrasound examination, patients with mycobacterial infections show tiny, diffuse echogenic foci throughout the spleen. Active tuberculosis shows echo-poor or cystic masses representing small abscess lesions.

Acquired Immunodeficiency Syndrome. In patients with acquired immunodeficiency syndrome (AIDS), the most common finding is splenomegaly. These patients may have multiorgan involvement (i.e., liver, spleen, and kidneys). The focal lesions include candida, *Pneumocystis carinii* pneumonia, mycobacterium, disseminated pneumocystis, Kaposi's sarcoma, and lymphoma.

Sonographic Findings. In an AIDS study performed by Porcel and others,[4] the sonographic findings in such patients revealed focal splenic lesions displaying small round lesions that may be multiple, hypoechoic, and well defined. Many of these lesions were due to disseminated mycobacterium tuberculosis infection. All of the patients presented with splenomegaly. In addition, hepatomegaly with focal lesions, retroperitoneal lymphadenopathy, and ascites were also seen.

Splenic Infarction and Trauma. Splenic infarction is the most common cause of focal splenic lesions caused by occlusion of the major splenic artery or any of its branches (see Figure 11-11). They are almost always the result of emboli that arise in the heart, produced either from mural thrombi or from

Figure 11-18 Patient came to the emergency room with fever and upper abdominal pain after receiving dental work 2 days earlier. The spleen was enlarged, with areas of inhomogeneity representing a splenic infection.

vegetation on the valves of the left side of the heart. Other causes include septic emboli and local thrombosis in patients with pancreatitis, leukemia, lymphomatous disorders, sickle cell anemia, sarcoidosis, or polyarteritis nodosa.

Sonographic Findings. Ultrasound may show a localized hypoechoic area, depending on the time of onset (Figure 11-19). Fresh hemorrhage has a hypoechoic appearance; healed infarctions appear as echogenic, peripheral, wedge-shaped lesions with their base toward the subcapsular surface of the spleen. The infarction may become nodular or hyperechoic with time.

Splenic Trauma. The spleen is most commonly injured as a result of blunt abdominal trauma. If the patient has severe left upper quadrant pain secondary to trauma, a splenic hematoma or subcapsular hematoma should be considered. The tear may result in linear or stellate lacerations or capsular tears, puncture wounds from foreign bodies or rib fractures, or subcapsular hematomas.

Blunt trauma has two outcomes. If the capsule is intact, the outcome may be intraparenchymal or subcapsular hematoma; if the capsule ruptures, a focal or free intraperitoneal hematoma may form. In delayed ruptures, a subcapsular hematoma may develop with subsequent rupture. The quick assessment of free fluid that may surround the splenic capsule in a blunt abdominal trauma can be a life-saving diagnosis for the patient.

Sonographic Findings. Ultrasound is a sensitive and specific test to examine trauma patients for abdominal injury requiring surgery (Figure 11-20). Routine abdominal ultrasound examination can be performed at the bedside in the trauma center. The use of screening ultrasound can improve clinical decision making for the use of emergency laparotomy.

A study was conducted to evaluate the efficiency of emergency ultrasound scans for blunt abdominal trauma performed by surgeons and radiologists in a trauma center.[3] Two groups of medical personnel were compared; the first consisted of surgeons and residents with minimal training in emergency ultrasound, and the second group was radiologists attending in the emergency department. The overall results revealed an accuracy on ultrasound readings of 99% for the surgical team and 99% for the attending radiologists. The conclusion was that surgeons and surgical residents at different levels of training can accurately interpret emergency ultrasound examinations for blunt trauma from real-time images at a level comparable with attending radiologists.

The patient typically presents with left upper quadrant pain, left shoulder pain, left flank pain, or dizziness. On

Figure 11-19　Splenic infarct. **A,** Computed tomography demonstrates the area of infarct in the spleen. **B** and **C,** Ultrasound shows the hypoechoic area near the peripheral margin of the spleen.

Figure 11-20   Splenic hematoma. **A** to **C,** Separation of the splenic capsule from the spleen secondary to a large hematoma resulting from an automobile accident. **D,** Computed tomography demonstrates the splenic hematoma along the posterolateral wall of the abdomen.

clinical evaluation, the patient may have tenderness over the left upper quadrant, hypotension, and decreased hemoglobin, indicating a bleed. A timely response to this emergent situation may save the patient undergoing a peritoneal lavage or exploratory surgery. The sonographer should quickly examine the four abdominopelvic quadrants: the area surrounding the kidneys (Morison's pouch), the subdiaphragmatic areas, the liver and splenic capsule, and the bladder and anterior rectal area to determine if free fluid is present. The patient's bladder may be filled retrograde to help serve as a window in the pelvic cavity. The entire screening examination should take under 5 minutes and may be recorded on video tape.

If the spleen has been lacerated and blood is contained within the splenic capsule, the most prominent ultrasound finding is splenomegaly, with progressive enlargement as the

bleeding continues. In addition, an irregular splenic border, hematoma, contusion (splenic inhomogeneity), subcapsular and pericapsular fluid collections, free intraperitoneal blood, or left pleural effusion may be present.

Focal hematomas may have intrasplenic fluid collections. Perisplenic fluid is seen in patients with subcapsular hematomas. The sonographer should be aware that blood exhibits various echo patterns, depending on the time that has passed since the trauma. Fresh hemorrhage may appear hypoechoic and may be difficult to distinguish from normal splenic tissue. The sonographer should look for a double-contour sign depicting the hematoma as separate from the spleen. As the protein and cells resorb the hematoma, the fluid becomes organized, hyperechoic, and similar to splenic tissue. In focal areas, tiny splenic lacerations give rise to small collections of blood interspersed with disrupted splenic pulp (contusion). With time, the hematoma becomes more fluid or appears lucent.

The echo-free, intraperitoneal fluid is probably blood mixed with peritoneal transudate. Healing of the lesion takes time, often extending into months. The free fluid disappears quicker because the fluid is moved across the pleural and peritoneal membranes rapidly (2 to 4 weeks). Intrasplenic hematomas and contusions take longer because the fluid, protein, and necrotic debris must be resorbed from within a solid organ in which the blood supply has already been focally disrupted. When the spleen returns to normal, small irregular foci may remain, or the parenchyma may be normal.

Splenic Cysts. Splenic cysts may be classified as parasitic or nonparasitic in origin. Most cysts are considered secondary cysts caused by trauma, infection, or infarction.

Echinococcus is the only parasite that forms splenic cysts; it is uncommon in the United States. Parasitic cysts appear as anechoic lesions with possible daughter cysts and calcification, or as solid masses with fine internal echoes and poor distal enhancement. Nonparasitic cysts of the spleen have been categorized as either primary or true.

Primary, or epidermoid, cysts contain an epithelial lining and are considered to be of congenital origin. False or secondary cysts lack a cellular lining, probably developing as a result of prior trauma to the spleen, and account for 80% of nonparasitic splenic cysts. True cysts are usually solitary and unilocular and rarely contain calcification. The internal surface of the cyst may be smooth or trabeculated. The fluid may be clear or turbid, and may contain protein, iron, bilirubin, fat, and cholesterol crystals. Primary cysts occur more frequently in females; 50% occur in patients under 15 years of age. Clinically, they present with an asymptomatic left upper quadrant mass.

Sonographic Findings. Ultrasound examination shows a hypoechoic or anechoic foci with well-defined walls and increased through-transmission (Figure 11-21). Primary cysts can have internal echoes at increased gain. Hemorrhage within the cyst may produce a fluid level.

Benign Primary Neoplasms. Generally speaking, primary tumors of the spleen are rare. The tumors may be divided into two groups: benign or malignant. With the benign primary tumors, splenomegaly is the first indication of an abnormality. Most of these tumors appear isoechoic compared with the normal splenic parenchyma. Benign primary tumors include hamartoma, cavernous hemangioma, and cystic lymphangioma.

Hamartoma. The patient with hamartoma is asymptomatic. The tumor may be solitary or multiple and is considered well defined but not encapsulated. The hamartoma consists of lymphoid tissue or a combination of sinuses and structures equivalent to pulp cords of normal splenic tissue. Symptomatic splenic hamartomas are rare in the pediatric age group.

Sonographic Findings. Hamartoma has both solid and cystic components and is generally hyperechoic on an ultrasound (Figure 11-22).

Cavernous hemangioma. Cavernous hemangioma is a large inhomogeneous echogenic mass with multiple small hypoechoic areas (Figure 11-23). The patient displays no symptoms and only becomes symptomatic when the size of the spleen increases and compresses other organs. Complications occur when the tumor increases in size to cause a splenic rupture with peritoneal symptoms.

Sonographic Findings. The ultrasound appearance is a complex pattern; infarction with coagulated blood or fibrin in the cavities may be seen, but is unspecific. Hydatid cyst, abscess, dermoid cyst, and metastasis should be considered in the differential diagnosis.

Cystic lymphangioma. Cystic lymphangioma is a benign malformation of lymphatics, consisting of endothelium-lined cystic spaces. Lymphangiomatosis affects predominately the somatic soft tissue (found in the neck, axilla, mediastinum, retroperitoneum, and soft tissue of the extremities). It may involve multiple organ systems or be confined to solitary organs, such as the liver, spleen, kidney, or colon.

Sonographic Findings. Cystic lymphangioma appears as a mass with extensive cystic replacement of splenic parenchyma.

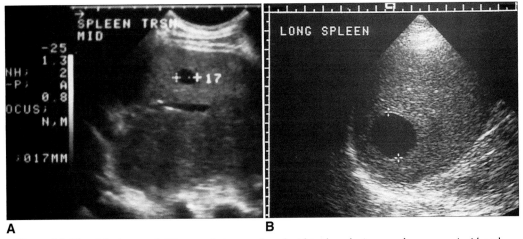

Figure 11-21 Splenic cyst. **A,** Tiny anechoic mass found within the splenic parenchyma as an incidental finding. **B,** Well-defined anechoic mass found within an asymptomatic young female.

Figure 11-22 Hamartoma of the spleen. Small solitary hyperechoic lesion within the spleen was seen in a young patient with ascites.

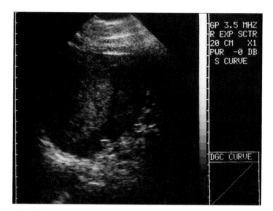

Figure 11-23 Cavernous hemangioma. A large inhomogeneous mass nearly fills the entire splenic parenchyma in this middle-aged male.

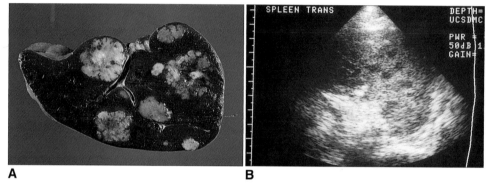

A   B

Figure 11-24 Metastases. **A,** Gross specimen of splenic metastases. **B,** Multiple diffuse hypoechoic lesions are seen throughout this spleen in a patient with primary breast cancer.

Splenic involvement is rare, but when it occurs a multicystic appearance is characteristic.

Malignant Primary Neoplasm

Hemangiosarcoma. Hemangiosarcoma is a rare malignant neoplasm arising from the vascular endothelium of the spleen. Malignant tumors of the spleen are also uncommon. Primary tumors found in the spleen may be lymphoma, Hodgkin's tumor, or hemangiosarcoma.

Sonographic Findings. The mixed cystic ultrasound pattern of hemangiosarcoma resembles that of a cavernous hemangioma, but it can also be hyperechoic.

Lymphoma. The spleen is commonly involved in lymphoma. *Sonographic Findings.* It may be difficult to detect splenic lymphoma by ultrasound. When it is seen, however, it appears to be typically hypoechoic; some focal areas are also seen. Four different sonographic patterns have been cited in patients with malignant lymphoma: (1) diffuse involvement, (2) focal small nodular lesions, (3) focal large nodular lesions, and (4) bulky disease. The diffuse or small nodular pattern was seen predominantly in low-grade lymphomas and in Hodgkin's disease.[1]

Metastases. Metastases are the result of a hematogenous spread from another primary site. The spleen is the tenth most common site of metastases, which may originate from the breast, lung, ovary, stomach, colon, kidney, or prostate or from melanoma (Figure 11-24). The metastatic tumors may be microscopic, causing no symptoms.

Sonographic Findings. The splenic parenchyma should be carefully examined by the sonographer to detect the abnormalities of the splenic parenchyma. Melanoma deposits appear hypoechoic, but are of higher echo amplitude than lymphoma; some are echodense.

Primary tumors and sonographic findings were evaluated in a small number of patients with isolated splenic metastasis to determine when these rare metastases should be suspected.[2] Four of the primary tumors were colonic cancer and one was renal cancer. Care should be taken to image the spleen carefully if focal lesions are identified elsewhere in the body.

REFERENCES

1. Gorg C, Weide R, Schwek W: Malignant splenic lymphoma: sonographic patterns, diagnosis and follow-up, *Clin Radiol* 52: 7-12, 1997.
2. Ishida H, Konno K, Ishida J and others: Isolated splenic metastases, *J Ultrasound Med* 16:11-15, 1997.
3. McKenney MG, McKenney KL, Compton RP and others: Can surgeons evaluate emergency ultrasound scans for blunt abdominal trauma? *J Trauma Infect Crit Care* 44:4-8, 1998.

4. Porcel MA, Rendon UP, Bascunana QA and others: Focal splenic lesions in patients with AIDS: sonographic findings, *Abdominal Imaging* 23:2-6, 1998.

5. Yang PM, Huang GT, Yang PJ and others: Caliber of splenic arteries in predicting the existence of esophageal varices, *J Med Ultrasound* 5:1-5, 1997.

SELECTED BIBLIOGRAPHY

Al-Salem AH, Qaisaruddin S, Al-Jam's A and others: Splenic abscess and sickle cell disease, *Am J Hematol* 58:2-8, 1998.

Aytac S and others: Multimodality demonstration of primary splenic angiosarcoma, *J Clin Ultrasound* 27:92-95, 1999.

Danaci M and others: Power Doppler sonographic diagnosis of torsion in a wandering spleen, *J Clin Ultrasound* 28:246-248, 2000.

Duddy MJ, Calder CJ: Cystic hemangioma of the spleen: findings on ultrasound and computed tomography, *Br J Radiol* 62:180, 1989.

Fitoz S and others: Post-traumatic intrasplenic pseudoaneurysms with delayed rupture: color Doppler sonographic and CT findings, *J Clin Ultrasound* 29:102-104, 2001.

Franquet T, Montes M, Lecumberri FJ and others: Hydatid disease of the spleen: imaging findings in nine patients, *Am J Roentgenol* 154:525, 1990.

Hicken P, Sauerbrei EE, Cooperberg PL: Ultrasonic coronal scanning of left upper quadrant, *J Can Assoc Radiol* 32:107, 1981.

Hill SC, Reinig JW, Barranger JA and others: Gaucher's disease: sonographic appearance of spleen, *Radiology* 160:631, 1986.

Kurtz AB, Middleton WB: *Ultrasound: the requisites,* ed 2, St Louis, 2004, Mosby.

Mostbeck G, Sommer G, Haller J and others: Accessory spleen: presentation as a large abdominal mass in an asymptomatic young woman, *Gastrointest Radiol* 12:337, 1987.

Pastakia B, Shawker TH, Thalar M and others: Hepatosplenic candidiasis: wheels within wheels, *Radiology* 166:417, 1988.

Perez Fontan FJ, Soler R, Santos M and others: Accessory spleen torsion: US, CT and MR findings, *Eur Radiol* 11:509-512, 2001.

Porter RS, Nester BA, Dalsy WC and others: Use of ultrasound to determine need for laparotomy in trauma patients, *Ann Emerg Med* 29:3-7, 1997.

Robertson F, Leander P, Ekberg O: Radiology of the spleen, *Eur Radiol* 11:80-95, 2001.

Solomon EP, Phillips GA: *Understanding human anatomy and physiology,* Philadelphia, 1987, WB Saunders.

Stevens PG, Kumari-Subaiya SS, Kahn LB: Splenic involvement in Gaucher's disease: sonographic findings, *J Clin Ultrasound* 15:397, 1987.

Tang S and others: Color Doppler sonographic findings in splenic hamartoma, *J Clin Ultrasound* 28:249-253, 2000.

Thibodeau GA, Patton KT: *The human body in health & disease,* ed 3, St Louis, 2002, Mosby.

Thompson SE, Walsh EA, Cramer BC and others: Radiological features of a symptomatic splenic hamartoma, *Pediatr Radiol* 26:9-12, 1996.

Vyborny CJ, Merrill TN, Reda J and others: Subacute subcapsular hematoma of the spleen complicating pancreatitis: successful percutaneous drainage, *Radiology* 169:161, 1989.

The Retroperitoneum

Kerry Weinberg

KEY TERMS

Addison's disease – condition caused by hyposecretion of hormones from the adrenal cortex

adenoma – smooth, round, homogeneous benign tumor of the adrenal cortex associated with Cushing's syndrome

adenopathy – multiple, enlarged lymph nodes

adrenocorticotropic hormone (ACTH) – a hormone secreted by the pituitary gland

cortex – outer parenchyma of the adrenal gland that secretes steroid hormones, commonly called corticoids

Cushing's syndrome – condition caused by hypersecretion of hormones from the adrenal cortex

false pelvis – portion of the pelvic cavity that is above the pelvic brim, bounded posteriorly by the lumbar vertebrae, laterally by the iliac fossae and iliacus muscles, and anteriorly by the lower anterior abdominal wall

hyperplasia – enlargement

lymphoma – malignancy that primarily affects the lymph nodes, spleen, or liver

medulla – central tissue of the adrenal gland that secrets epinephrine and norepinephrine

neuroblastoma – malignant adrenal mass that is seen in pediatric patients

neuroectodermal tissue – early embryonic tissue that will eventually develop into the brain and spinal cord

pheochromocytoma – benign adrenal tumor that secretes hormones that produce hypertension

ANATOMY OF THE RETROPERITONEUM

NORMAL ANATOMY

The retroperitoneal space is the area between the posterior portion of the parietal peritoneum and the posterior abdominal wall muscles (Figure 12-1). It extends from the diaphragm to the pelvis. Laterally the boundaries extend to the extraperitoneal fat planes within the confines of the transversalis fascia, and medially the space encloses the great vessels. It is subdivided into the following three categories: anterior pararenal space, perirenal space, and posterior pararenal space (Box 12-1).

The perirenal space surrounds the kidney, adrenal, and perirenal fat. The anterior pararenal space includes the duodenum, pancreas, and ascending and transverse colon. The posterior pararenal space includes the iliopsoas muscle, ureter, and branches of the inferior vena cava and aorta and their lymphatics.

The retroperitoneum is protected by the spine, ribs, pelvis, and musculature and has been a difficult area to assess clinically by ultrasound. Computerized tomography imaging is better to outline the retroperitoneal cavity. Occasionally, however, the sonographer is asked to rule out fluid collection, hematoma, urinoma, or ascitic fluid in the retroperitoneal space.

The retroperitoneum is delineated anteriorly by the posterior peritoneum, posteriorly by the transversalis fascia, and laterally by the lateral borders of the quadratus lumborum muscles and peritoneal leaves of the mesentery. Proceeding from a superior to inferior direction, the retroperitoneum extends from the diaphragm to the pelvic brim. Superior to the pelvic brim the retroperitoneum can be partitioned into the lumbar and iliac fossae. The pararenal and perirenal spaces are included in the lumbar fossa.

Pathologic processes can stretch from the anterior abdominal wall to the subdiaphragmatic space, mediastinum, and subcutaneous tissues of the back and flank. The retrofascial space, which includes the psoas, quadratus lumborum, and iliacus muscles (muscles posterior to the transversalis fascia), is often the site of extension of retroperitoneal pathologic processes.

Anterior Pararenal Space. The anterior pararenal space is bound anteriorly by the posterior parietal peritoneum and posteriorly by the anterior renal fascia. It is bound laterally by the lateroconal fascia formed by the fusion of the anterior and posterior leaves of the renal fascia. (This space merges with the bare area of the liver by the coronary ligament.) The pancreas, duodenum, and ascending and transverse colon are the structures included in the anterior pararenal space (Figure 12-2).

Perirenal Space. The perirenal space is surrounded by the anterior and posterior layers of the renal fascia (Gerota's fascia), attaching to the diaphragm superiorly. They are united loosely at their inferior margin at the iliac crest level or superior border of the **false pelvis**. Collections in the perinephric space can communicate within the iliac fossa of the retroperitoneum (Figure 12-3).

The lateroconal fascia (the lateral fusion of the renal fascia) proceeds anteriorly as the posterior peritoneum. The posterior renal fasciae fuse medially with the psoas or quadratus lumborum fascia (Figure 12-4). The anterior renal fascia fuses medially with connective tissue surrounding the great vessels. (This space contains the adrenal gland, kidney, and ureter; the great vessels, also within this space, are largely isolated within their connective tissue sheaths.) The perirenal space contains the adrenal gland and kidney (in a variable amount of echogenic

---

BOX 12-1 · ORGANS IN THE RETROPERITONEAL SPACES

ANTERIOR PARARENAL SPACE
- Pancreas
- Duodenal sweep
- Ascending and transverse colon

PERIRENAL SPACE
- Adrenal glands
- Kidneys
- Ureter
- Great vessel

POSTERIOR PARARENAL SPACE
- Blood
- Lymph nodes

ILIAC FOSSA
- Ureter
- Major branches of great vessels
- Lymphatics

RETROFASCIAL SPACE
Three Compartments
- Psoas
- Lumbar (quadratus lumborum)
- Iliacus

Retroperitoneal space

Figure 12-1 Schematic transverse section of the abdominal cavity at the level of the fourth lumbar vertebra. The retroperitoneal space is outlined in blue.

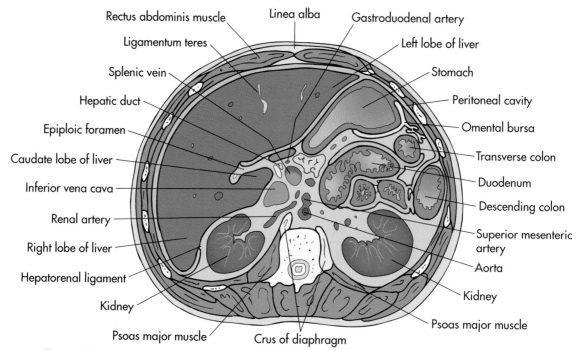

Rectus abdominis muscle
Ligamentum teres
Splenic vein
Hepatic duct
Epiploic foramen
Caudate lobe of liver
Inferior vena cava
Renal artery
Right lobe of liver
Hepatorenal ligament
Kidney
Psoas major muscle

Linea alba
Crus of diaphragm

Gastroduodenal artery
Left lobe of liver
Stomach
Peritoneal cavity
Omental bursa
Transverse colon
Duodenum
Descending colon
Superior mesenteric artery
Aorta
Kidney
Psoas major muscle

Figure 12-2 Transverse drawing of the anterior pararenal space. Cross-section of the abdomen at the first lumbar vertebra.

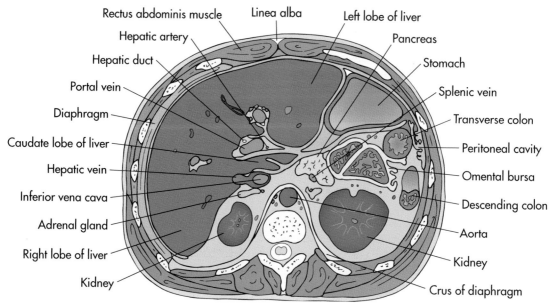

Rectus abdominis muscle
Hepatic artery
Hepatic duct
Portal vein
Diaphragm
Caudate lobe of liver
Hepatic vein
Inferior vena cava
Adrenal gland
Right lobe of liver
Kidney

Linea alba

Left lobe of liver
Pancreas
Stomach
Splenic vein
Transverse colon
Peritoneal cavity
Omental bursa
Descending colon
Aorta
Kidney
Crus of diaphragm

Figure 12-3 Transverse drawing of the perirenal space. Cross-section of the abdomen at the level of the twelfth thoracic vertebra.

perinephric fat, the thickest portion of which is posterior and lateral to the kidney's lower pole). The kidney is anterolateral to the psoas muscle, anterior to the quadratus lumborum muscle, and posteromedial to the ascending and descending colon.

The second portion of the duodenum is anterior to the renal hilum on the right. On the left, the kidney is bounded by the stomach anterosuperiorly, the pancreas anteriorly, and the spleen anterolaterally.

Adrenal Glands. In the adult patient the adrenal glands are anterior, medial, and superior to the kidneys (Figure 12-5). The right adrenal is more superior to the kidney, whereas the left adrenal is more medial to the kidney. The medial portion of the right adrenal gland is immediately posterior to the inferior vena cava (above the level of the portal vein and lateral to the crus). The lateral portion of the gland is posterior and medial to the right lobe of the liver and posterior to the duodenum.

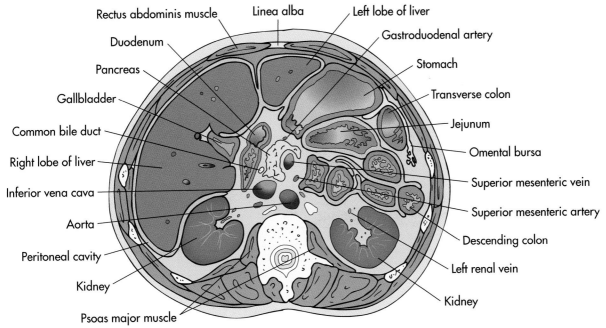

Rectus abdominis muscle

Duodenum

Pancreas

Gallbladder

Common bile duct

Right lobe of liver

Inferior vena cava

Aorta

Peritoneal cavity

Kidney

Psoas major muscle

Linea alba

Left lobe of liver

Gastroduodenal artery

Stomach

Transverse colon

Jejunum

Omental bursa

Superior mesenteric vein

Superior mesenteric artery

Descending colon

Left renal vein

Kidney

Figure 12-4   Transverse drawing of the posterior pararenal space. Cross-section of the abdomen at the level of the second lumbar vertebra. This space is located between the posterior renal fascia and the transversalis fascia. It communicates with the peritoneal fat. The space merges inferiorly with the anterior pararenal space and retroperitoneal tissue of the iliac fossa.

Inferior vena cava

Right inferior phrenic vein

Right superior suprarenal arteries

Right suprarenal vein

Right adrenal gland

Right middle suprarenal artery

Upper pole of the right kidney

Right inferior suprarenal artery and vein

Right renal artery and vein

Esophagus

Left inferior phrenic vein

Left inferior phrenic artery

Left adrenal gland

Left superior suprarenal arteries

Upper pole of the left kidney

Left middle suprarenal artery

Left inferior suprarenal artery and vein

Left renal artery and vein

Abdominal aorta

Figure 12-5   The adrenal glands are retroperitoneal organs that lie on the upper pole of each kidney. They are surrounded by perinephric fat. The right adrenal gland is triangular and caps the upper pole of the right kidney. It extends medially behind the inferior vena cava and rests posteriorly on the diaphragm. The left adrenal gland is semilunar and extends along the medial borders of the left kidney. It lies posterior to the pancreas, the lesser sac, and the stomach and rests posteriorly on the diaphragm.

The left adrenal gland is lateral or slightly posterolateral to the aorta and lateral to the crus of the diaphragm. The superior portion is posterior to the lesser omental space and posterior to the stomach. The inferior portion is posterior to the pancreas. The splenic vein and artery pass between the pancreas and the left adrenal gland.

The adrenal glands vary in size, shape, and configuration; the right adrenal is triangular and caps the upper pole of the right kidney. The left adrenal is semilunar in shape and extends along the medial border of the left kidney from the upper pole to the hilus. The internal texture is medium in consistency; the cortex and medulla are not distinguished.

The adrenal gland is a distinct hypoechoic structure; sometimes highly echogenic fat is seen surrounding the gland. The size is usually smaller than 3 cm (3 to 6 cm long, 3 to 6 mm thick, 2 to 4 cm wide).

Neonatal adrenal. The neonatal adrenal glands are characterized by a thin echogenic core surrounded by a thick transonic zone. This thick rim of transonicity represents the hypertrophied adrenal cortex, whereas the echogenic core is the adrenal medulla. An infant adrenal gland is proportionally larger than an adult adrenal gland (one third the size of the kidney; in adults it is one thirteenth the size)(Figure 12-6).

Diaphragmatic Crura. The diaphragmatic crura begins as tendinous fibers from the lumbar vertebral bodies, disks, and transverse processes of L3 on the right and L1 on the left (Figure 12-7). The right crus is longer, larger, and more lobular and is associated with the anterior aspect of the lumbar vertebral ligament. The right renal artery crosses anterior to the crus and posterior to the inferior vena cava at the level of the right kidney. The right crus is bounded by the inferior vena cava anterolaterally and the right adrenal and right lobe of liver posterolaterally.

The left crus courses along the anterior lumbar vertebral bodies in a superior direction and inserts into the central tendon of the diaphragm.

Para-aortic Lymph Nodes. There are two major lymph node bearing areas in the retroperitoneal cavity: the iliac and hypogastric nodes within the pelvis, and the para-aortic group in the upper retroperitoneum. The lymphatic chain follows the course of the thoracic aorta, abdominal aorta, and iliac arteries (Figure 12-8). Common sites are the para-aortic and para-caval areas near the great vessels, peripancreatic area, renal hilar area, and mesenteric region. Normal nodes are smaller than the tip of a finger, less than 1 cm, and are not imaged with ultrasound. However, if these nodes enlarge because of infection or tumor, they can be seen with ultrasound.

Posterior Pararenal Space. The posterior pararenal space is located between the posterior renal fascia and the transversalis fascia. It communicates with the peritoneal fat, lateral to the lateroconal fascia. The posterior pararenal space merges inferiorly with the anterior pararenal space and retroperitoneal tissues of the iliac fossa (see Figure 12-4).

The psoas muscle, the fascia of which merges with the posterior transversalis fascia, makes up the medial border of this posterior space. This space is open laterally and inferiorly. The blood and lymph nodes embedded in fat may be found in the posterior pararenal space.

Iliac Fossa. The iliac fossa is the region extending between the internal surface of the iliac wings, from the crest to the iliopectineal line. This area is known as the **false pelvis** and contains the ureter and major branches of the distal great vessels and their lymphatics. The transversalis fascia extends into the iliac fossa as the iliac fascia.

Retrofascial Space. The retrofascial space is made up of the posterior abdominal wall, muscles, nerves, lymphatics, and areolar tissue behind the transversalis fascia. It is divided into the following three compartments:

1. The psoas compartment: a muscle that spans from the mediastinum to the thigh (Figure 12-9). The fascia attaches to the pelvic brim.
2. The lumbar region consists of the quadratus lumborum, a muscle that originates from the iliolumbar ligament, the adjacent iliac crest, and the superior borders of the transverse process of L3 and L4, and inserts into the margin of the twelfth rib (Figure 12-10). It is adjoining and posterior to the colon, kidney, and psoas muscle.
3. The iliac area, which is made up of the iliacus and extends the length of the iliac fossa. The psoas passes through the iliac fossa medial to the iliacus and posterior to the iliac fascia (Figure 12-11). These two muscles merge together as they extend into the true pelvis. The iliopsoas takes on a more anterior location caudally to lie along the lateral pelvic side wall.

Pelvic Retroperitoneum. The pelvic retroperitoneum lies between the sacrum and pubis from back to front, between the pelvic peritoneal reflection above and pelvic diaphragm (coccygeus and levator ani muscles) below, and between the obturator internus and piriformis muscles. There are four subdivisions: (1) prevesical, (2) rectovesical, (3) presacral, and (4) bilateral pararectal (and paravesical) spaces.

Figure 12-6 Neonatal right kidney and adrenal gland. (Courtesy Siemens Medical Solutions USA, Inc.)

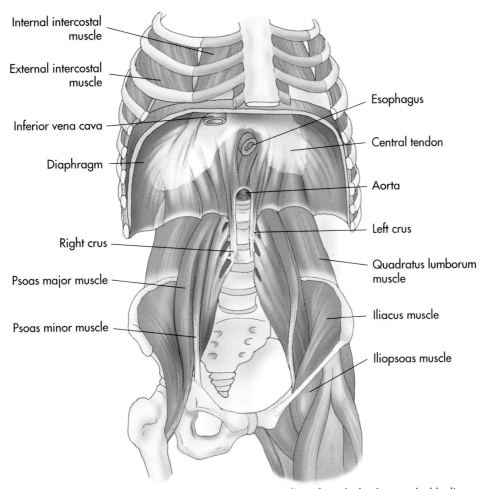

Figure 12-7 The crura of the diaphragm begin as tendinous fibers from the lumbar vertebral bodies, disks, and transverse processes of L3 on the right and L1 on the left.

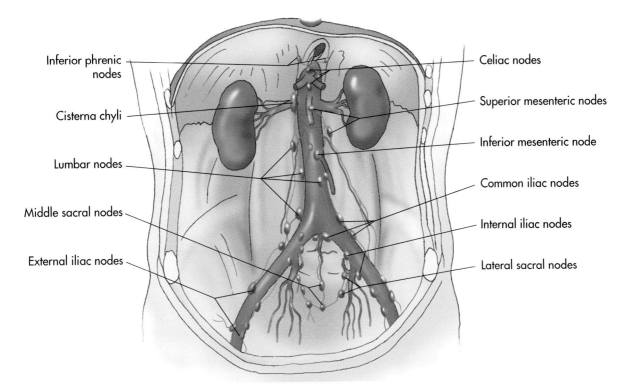

Figure 12-8 Lymphatic chain along the aorta and iliac artery.

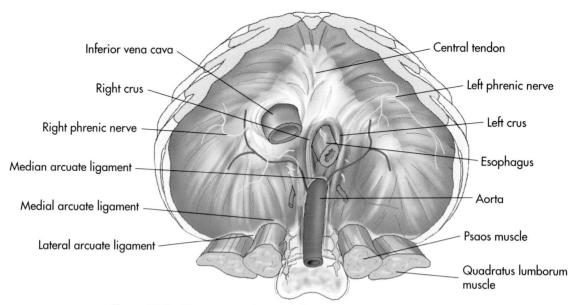

Figure 12-9   The psoas muscle extends from the mediastinum to the thigh.

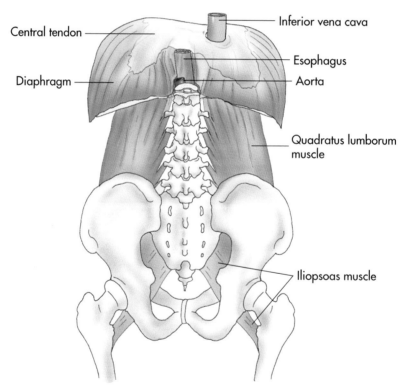

Figure 12-10   The quadratus lumborum muscle originates from the iliolumbar ligament, the adjacent iliac crest, and the superior borders of the transverse process of L3 and L4 and inserts into the margins of the twelfth rib.

Prevesical Space. The prevesical space spans from the pubis to the anterior margin of the bladder. It is bordered laterally by the obturator fascia. The connective tissue covering the bladder, seminal vesicles, and prostate is continuous with the fascial lamina within this space. The space is an extension of the retroperitoneal space of the anterior abdominal wall deep to the rectus sheath, which is con-

tinuous with the transversalis fascia. The space between the bladder and rectum is the rectovesicle space (Figure 12-12).

Presacral Space. The presacral space lies between the rectum and fascia covering the sacrum and posterior pelvic floor musculature.

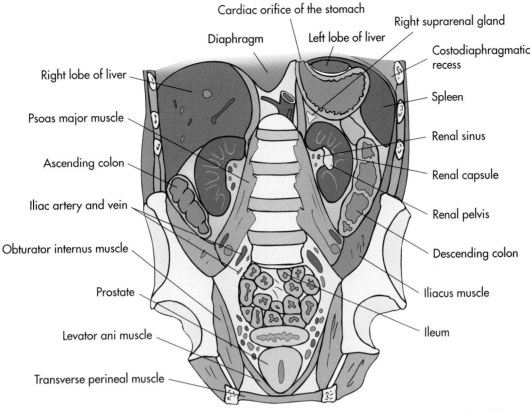

Cardiac orifice of the stomach

Diaphragm

Left lobe of liver

Right suprarenal gland

Costodiaphragmatic recess

Right lobe of liver

Psoas major muscle

Ascending colon

Iliac artery and vein

Obturator internus muscle

Prostate

Levator ani muscle

Transverse perineal muscle

Spleen

Renal sinus

Renal capsule

Renal pelvis

Descending colon

Iliacus muscle

Ileum

Figure 12-11 The iliacus muscle extends the length of the iliac fossa. The psoas muscle passes through the iliac fossa medial to the iliacus. The psoas and iliacus muscles merge as they extend into the true pelvis. The iliopsoas muscle takes on a more anterior location caudally to lie along the lateral pelvic side wall.

Bilateral Pararectal Space. The pararectal space is bounded laterally by the piriformis and levator ani fascia and medially by the rectum. It extends anteriorly from the bladder, medially to the obturator internus, and laterally to the external iliac vessels (Figures 12-13 and 12-14).

The paravesical and pararectal spaces are traversed by the two ureters. The pelvic wall muscles, iliac vessels, ureter, bladder, prostate, seminal vesicles, and cervix are retroperitoneal structures within the true pelvis. The obturator internus muscle lines the lateral aspect of the pelvis. Posteriorly the piriformis muscle is seen extending anterolaterally from the region of the sacrum.

VASCULAR SUPPLY

Aorta. The aorta enters the abdomen posterior to the diaphragm at the level of L1 and passes posterior to the left lobe of the liver. The aorta has a straight horizontal course to the level of L4, where it bifurcates into the common iliac arteries. A slight anterior curve of the aorta is the result of lumbar lordosis.

Inferior Vena Cava. The inferior vena cava extends from the junction of the two common iliac veins to the right of L5 and travels cephalad. Unlike the aorta, it curves anterior toward its termination into the right atrial cavity.

Adrenal Glands. Three arteries supply each adrenal gland: the suprarenal branch of the inferior phrenic, the suprarenal branch of the aorta, and the suprarenal branch of the renal artery (see Figure 11-5). A single vein from the hilum of each gland drains into the inferior vena cava on the right, and on the left, the vein drains into the left renal vein.

PHYSIOLOGY AND LABORATORY DATA OF THE RETROPERITONEUM

Each adrenal gland is made up of two endocrine glands. The **cortex**, or outer part, secretes a range of steroid hormones; the **medulla**, or core, secretes epinephrine and norepinephrine.

CORTEX

The steroids secreted by the adrenal cortex fall into the following three main categories: mineralocorticoids, glucocorticoids, and sex hormones.

Mineralocorticoids. Mineralocorticoids regulate electrolyte metabolism. Aldosterone is the principal mineralocorticoid. It has a regulatory effect on the relative concentrations of mineral ions in the body fluids and therefore on the water content of tissue. An insufficiency of this steroid leads to

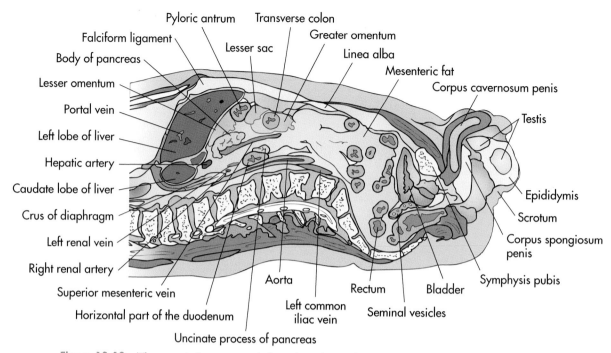

Figure 12-12 The prevesical space extends from the pubis to the anterior margin of the bladder. It is bordered by the obturator fascia on its lateral margins. The space between the bladder and rectum is the rectovesical space.

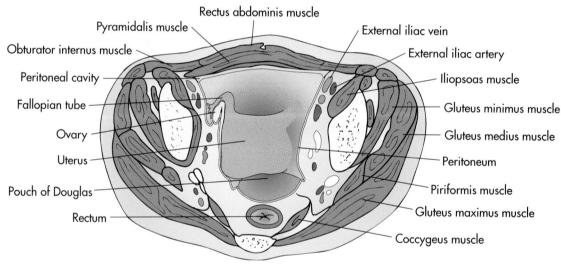

Figure 12-13 The pararectal space is bounded laterally by the piriformis and levator ani fascia and medially by the rectum.

increased excretion of sodium and chloride ions, and water into the urine. This is accompanied by a fall in sodium, chloride, and bicarbonate concentrations in the blood, resulting in a lowered pH or acidosis.

Glucocorticoids. Glucocorticoids play a principal role in carbohydrate metabolism. They promote deposition of liver glycogen from proteins and inhibit use of glucose by the cells, thus increasing blood sugar level. Cortisone and hydrocorti-

sone are the primary glucocorticoids. They diminish allergic response, especially the more serious inflammatory types (rheumatoid arthritis and rheumatic fever).

Sex Hormones. Androgens are the male sex hormones, and estrogens are the female sex hormones. The adrenal gland secretes both types of hormones regardless of the patient's gender. Normally these are secreted in minute quantities and have almost insignificant effects. With oversecretion, however,

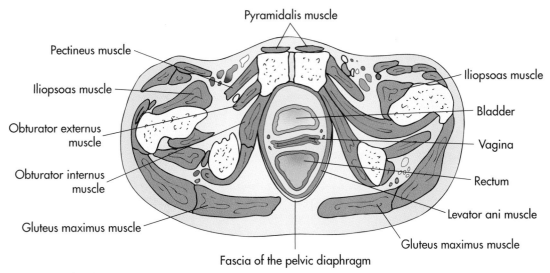

Pyramidalis muscle

Pectineus muscle

Iliopsoas muscle

Obturator externus
muscle

Obturator internus
muscle

Gluteus maximus muscle

Fascia of the pelvic diaphragm

Iliopsoas muscle

Bladder

Vagina

Rectum

Levator ani muscle

Gluteus maximus muscle

Figure 12-14   The pararectal space extends anteriorly from the bladder, medially to the obturator internus, and laterally to the external iliac vessels.

a marked effect is seen. Adrenal tumors in women can promote secondary masculine characteristics. Hypersecretion of the hormone in prepubertal boys accelerates adult masculine development and the growth of pubic hair. The adrenal cortex is controlled by **adrenocorticotropic hormone (ACTH)** from the pituitary. A diminished glucocorticoid blood concentration stimulates the secretion of ACTH. Consequent increase in adrenal cortex activity inhibits further ACTH secretion.

Hypofunction of the adrenal cortex in humans is called **Addison's disease.** Symptoms and signs include hypotension, general weakness, fatigue, loss of appetite and weight, and a characteristic bronzing of the skin (hyperpigmentation).

Oversecretion of the adrenal cortex may be caused by an overproduction of ACTH resulting from a pituitary tumor, **hyperplasia,** or a tumor in the cortex itself. Hypersecretion of the cortical hormones produces distinct syndromes. The features of the syndromes often overlap and can be either acquired or congenital. Adrenal hyperfunction can cause Cushing's syndrome, Conn's syndrome, or adrenogenital syndrome (see adrenal pathology).

MEDULLA

The adrenal medulla makes up the core of the gland in which groups of irregular cells are located amid veins that collect blood from the sinusoids. The adrenal medulla produces epinephrine and norepinephrine. Both of these hormones are amines, sometimes referred to as catecholamines. They elevate the blood pressure, the former working as an accelerator of the heart rate and the latter as a vasoconstrictor. The two hormones together promote glycogenolysis, the breakdown of liver glycogen to glucose, which causes an increase in blood sugar concentration.

The adrenal medulla is not essential for life and can be removed surgically without causing untreatable damage. An increase in the production of the medulla hormones may be caused by a **pheochromocytoma.**

SONOGRAPHIC EVALUATION OF THE RETROPERITONEUM

There is no specific patient preparation necessary to image the retroperitoneal cavity, although 6 to 8 hours of fasting may help to eliminate bowel gas. To image the retroperitoneum, scans should be made in the longitudinal and transverse planes from the diaphragm to the iliac crest, with the patient in a supine or prone position, and from the crest to the symphysis, with the patient in a supine position and having a full bladder. The upper abdomen may also be scanned with the patient in a decubitus position. All scans should include the kidneys and retroperitoneal muscles.

ADRENAL GLANDS

Although sonography has proven useful in evaluating soft tissue structures within the abdominal cavity, visualization of the adrenal glands has been difficult because of their small size, medial location, and surrounding perirenal fat. If the adrenal gland becomes enlarged secondary to disease, it is easier to image and separate from the upper pole of the kidney.

Visualization of the adrenal area depends on several factors: the size of the patient and the amount of perirenal fat surrounding the adrenal area, the presence of bowel gas, and the ability to move the patient into multiple positions.

With the patient in the decubitus position, the sonographer should attempt to align the kidney and ipsilateral paravertebral vessels (inferior vena cava or aorta). The right adrenal gland has a "comma" or triangular shape in the transaxial plane. The best visualization is obtained by a transverse scan with the patient in a left lateral decubitus position. As the patient assumes this position, the inferior vena cava moves forward and the aorta rolls over the crus of the diaphragm to offer a good window to image the upper pole of the right kidney and adrenal gland. If the patient is obese, it may be difficult to recognize the triangular- or crescent-shaped adrenal gland. The adrenal should not appear rounded; if it does, the finding suggests a pathologic process.

The longitudinal scan is made through the right lobe of the liver, perpendicular to the linear right crus of the diaphragm. The retroperitoneal fat must be recognized as separate from the liver, crus of the diaphragm, adrenal gland, and great vessel (Figure 12-15).

The left adrenal gland is closely related to the left crus of the diaphragm and the anterior-superior-medial aspect of the upper pole of the left kidney. It may be more difficult to image the left adrenal gland because of the stomach gas interference. The patient should be placed in a right lateral decubitus position and transverse scans made in an attempt to align the left kidney and the aorta. The left adrenal gland is seen by scanning along the posterior axillary line (Figure 12-16). The patient should be in deep inspiration in an effort to bring the adrenal and renal area into better view.

SONOGRAPHY PITFALLS
- Right crus of the diaphragm
- Second portion of the duodenum

Figure 12-15 Longitudinal scan of the right adrenal gland is made through the right lobe of the liver *(L)*, adrenal gland *(A)*, and upper pole of the right kidney *(RK)*. (Courtesy Shpetim Telegrafi, New York University.)

Figure 12-16 Longitudinal scan of the left adrenal gland *(LA)* and the anterior superior aspect of the upper pole of the left kidney *(LK)* and spleen *(S)*. (Courtesy Shpetim Telegrafi, New York University.)

- Gastroesophageal junction (cephalad to the left adrenal gland)
- Medial lobulations of the spleen
- Splenic vasculature
- Body-tail region of the pancreas
- Fourth portion of the duodenum

The normal right adrenal gland can be visualized in more than 90% of patients, whereas the left is seen in 80% of patients.

DIAPHRAMATIC CRURA
The crus of the diaphragm may be imaged in the transverse or longitudinal coronal plane. The right crus is seen in a plane that passes through the right lobe of the liver, kidney, and adrenal gland (Figure 12-17). The left crus is seen using the spleen and left kidney as a window, with the crus to the left of the aorta.

PARA-AORTIC LYMPH NODES
Ultrasound patterns associated with nodes include rounded, focal, echo-poor lesions (1 to 3 cm in size and larger), and confluent, echo-poor masses, which often displace the kidney laterally. The sonographer may also detect a "mantle" of nodes in the paraspinal location, a "floating" or anteriorly displaced aorta secondary to the enlarged nodes, or the mesenteric "sandwich" sign representing the anterior and posterior node masses surrounding mesenteric vessels (Figures 12-18 to 12-21).

The lymph nodes lie along the lateral and anterior margins of the aorta and inferior vena cava; thus the best scanning is done with the patient in the supine or decubitus position. A left coronal view using the left kidney as a window may be used to discover para-aortic nodes (Figure 12-22).

It is always important to examine the patient in two planes because in only one plane the enlarged nodes may mimic an aortic aneurysm or tumor.

Longitudinal scans may be made first to outline the aorta and to search for enlarged lymph nodes. The aorta provides an excellent background for the hypoechoic nodes. Scans should begin at the midline, and the transducer should be angled both to the left and right at small angles to image the anterior and lateral borders of the aorta and inferior vena cava.

Transverse scans are made from the level of the xiphoid to the symphysis. Careful identification of the great vessels, organ structures, and muscles is important (Figure 12-23). Patterns of a fluid-filled duodenum or bowel may make it difficult to outline the great vessels or may cause confusion in diagnosing **lymphadenopathy**.

Scans below the umbilicus are more difficult because of interference from the small bowel. Careful attention should be given to the psoas and iliacus muscles within the pelvis where the iliac arteries run along their medial border. Both muscles serve as a hypoechoic marker along the pelvic side wall. Enlarged lymph nodes can be identified anterior and medial to these margins. A smooth sharp border of the muscle indicates no nodal involvement. The bladder should be filled to help push the small bowel out of the pelvis and to serve as an

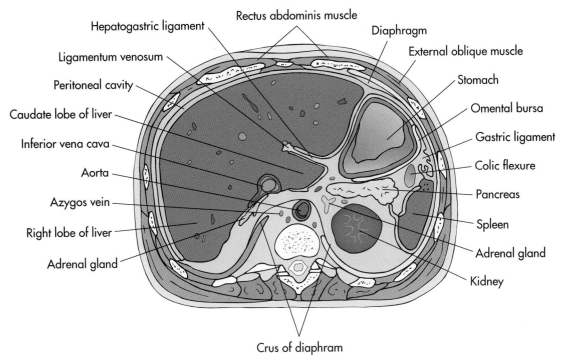

Rectus abdominis muscle

Hepatogastric ligament

Ligamentum venosum

Peritoneal cavity

Caudate lobe of liver

Inferior vena cava

Aorta

Azygos vein

Right lobe of liver

Adrenal gland

Diaphragm

External oblique muscle

Stomach

Omental bursa

Gastric ligament

Colic flexure

Pancreas

Spleen

Adrenal gland

Kidney

Crus of diaphram

Figure 12-17   The right crus of the diaphragm passes posterior to the inferior vena cava, and the left crus passes anterior to the aorta.

| 1 DIST= 6.87cm |
| 2 DIST= 2.05cm |
| 3 DIST= 3.11cm |

| 1 DIST= 7.40cm |
| 2 DIST= 2.74cm |

A   **B**

Figure 12-18   **A,** A 39-year-old female with lymphoma. Three nodes were seen peripancreatic *(crossbars):* *1,* anterior to the pancreas; *2,* lateral to the pancreas head; and *3,* paracaval. **B,** Two nodes paraportal *(crossbars):* *1,* anterior and compressing the main portal vein; and *2,* a smaller, sonolucent homogeneous node. (Courtesy Shpetim Telegrafi, New York University, NY.)

acoustic window to better image the vascular structures. Color Doppler may be used to help delineate the vascular structures.

Splenomegaly should also be evaluated in patients with lymphadenopathy. As the sonographer moves caudal from the xiphoid, attention should be on the splenic size and great vessel area to detect nodal involvement near the hilus of the spleen (Figures 12-24 and 12-25).

Lymph nodes remain as consistent patterns, whereas bowel and the duodenum display changing peristaltic patterns when imaged with ultrasound. As gentle pressure is applied with the transducer in an effort to displace the bowel, the lymph nodes remain constant in shape. The echo pattern posterior to each structure is different. Lymph nodes are homogeneous and thus transmit sound easily; the bowel presents a more complex pattern with dense central echoes from its mucosal pattern. Often the duodenum has air within its walls, causing a shadow posteriorly. Enlarged lymph nodes should be reproducible on ultrasound. After the abdomen is completely scanned, repeat sections over the enlarged nodes should demonstrate the same pattern as on the earlier scan.

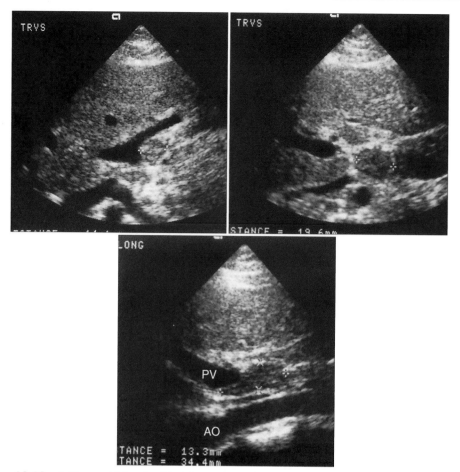

Figure 12-19   A 32-year-old female with right upper quadrant pain and fever. Two paracaval nodes were seen anterior to the aorta *(AO)* and inferior to the portal vein *(PV).*

Figure 12-20   Longitudinal view of the aorta *(Ao)* with the superior mesenteric artery *(sma).* If the angle of the SMA exceeds 15 degrees, lymphadenopathy should be considered. *N,* Node.

PATHOLOGY OF THE RETROPERITONEUM

ADRENAL CORTICAL SYNDROMES

The cortical syndromes that the sonographer may encounter while scanning for an adrenal mass are as follows:

- *Addison's disease (adrenocortical insufficiency):* It affects males and females equally and can be diagnosed in any age group. It is characterized by atrophy of the adrenal cortex with decreased production of cortisol and sometimes aldosterone. Usually the majority of the cortical tissue is destroyed before adrenal insufficiency is diagnosed. Primary causes of reduced adrenal cortical tissue include an autoimmune process, tuberculosis (TB), an inflammatory process, a primary neoplasm, or metastases. Secondary adrenal insufficiencies are caused by pituitary dysfunction and a decrease in production of the pituitary hormone ACTH (adrenocorticotropic hormone). The clinical signs and symptoms usually manifest during metabolic stress or trauma. Symptoms include increased sodium retention, which leads to tissue edema; increased plasma volume; increased potassium excretion; hyperpigmentation; and a mild alkalosis. Fatigue and muscle and bone weakness are common. Prognosis is good with steroid replacement therapy.

- *Adrenogenital syndrome (adrenal virilism):* Results from the excessive secretion of the sex hormones and adrenal androgens. It is caused either by an adrenal tumor or by hyperplasia. The symptoms and clinical signs vary depending upon the age and sex of the person. In a newborn there may be ambiguous genitalia with or without adrenal hyperplasia.

A

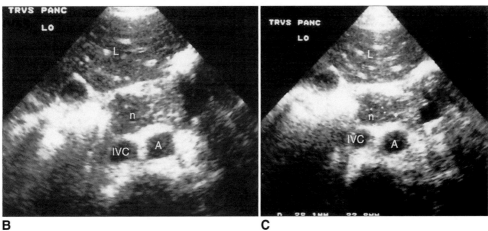

B   **C**

Figure 12-21 A 46-year-old male with a history of acquired immune deficiency syndrome (AIDS). Liver function tests were abnormal. Hepatosplenomegaly was present. Adjacent to the pancreas are numerous small nodal masses, the largest measuring 2 cm. **A,** Longitudinal view. *A,* aorta; *L,* liver; *n,* nodes; *v,* superior mesenteric vein. **B** and **C,** Transverse view. *A,* aorta; *IVC,* inferior vena cava; *L,* liver; *n,* nodes.

Figure 12-22 Decubitus scan using the left kidney as a window to see the aorta. (Courtesy Shpetim Telegrafi, New York University.)

Figure 12-23 Two homogeneous peripancreatic nodes. (Courtesy Thomas Hoffman and Jack D. Weiler, Albert Einstein Medical Center, Bronx, NY.)

(Ambiguous genitalia can also be caused by things other than adrenal hyperplasia.) Adrenal virilism has masculinizing effects on adult women. The clinical signs and symptoms in a female adult include hirsutism, baldness, and acne; deepening of the voice; atrophy of the uterus; decreased breast size; clitoral hypertrophy; and increased muscularity. Prepubescent males will have signs of masculine develop-

ment, deepening voice, and an increase in body hair. The imaging modality of choice to confirm the presence or absence of an adrenal tumor is CT and MRI scan.

• *Conn's syndrome (aldosteronism):* Caused by excessive secretion of aldosterone, usually because of a cortical **adenoma** of the glomerulosa cells or less frequent causes, including adrenal hyperplasia or adrenal carcinoma. Hyperplasia is

Figure 12-24   Splenomegaly should be evaluated in patients with lymphadenopathy. Enlarged nodes are seen in the area of the hilus of the spleen *(S)*. This patient also has a metastatic lesion near the periphery of the spleen. *L,* liver.

Figure 12-25   Axial and coronal scans of a patient with splenomegaly and enlarged nodes in the area of the splenic hilus. Color flow imaging should be used to document that the lesions are nodes and not dilated vascular structures. *Arrows,* nodes; *S,* spleen.

more common in males and adrenal adenomas are more common in females. Adenomas tend to be small, less than 2 cm in size. Clinical signs and symptoms include muscle weakness, hypertension, and abnormal electrocardiogram. If an adenoma is causing the hyperaldosteronism, removal of the adenoma is performed. In rare cases a bilateral adrenalectomy is necessary. In cases of secondary aldosteronism, the hypertension may be caused by renal artery disease.

- **Cushing's syndrome:** Produced by excessive secretion of cortisol resulting from adrenal hyperplasia, cortical adenoma, adrenal carcinoma, or elevated ACTH resulting from a pituitary adenoma. Cushing's syndrome symptoms include truncal obesity, pencil thin extremities, "buffalo hump," "moon face," hypertension, renal stones, irregular menses in females, and psychiatric disturbances. If an adrenal tumor is present, the secretion of androgens may increase and cause masculinizing effects in women. Cushing's syndrome can also be caused by an anterior pituitary tumor. Treatment to decrease the production of cortisol varies depending upon the cause of the hypersecretion. If an adrenalectomy is performed, the patient will require replacement steroids for life.

- *Waterhouse-Friderichsen syndrome:* This commonly results from bilateral hemorrhage into the adrenal glands, which is caused by severe meningococcal infection. It is characterized by acute adrenal gland insufficiency, which is fatal if not treated immediately (Table 12-1).

ADRENAL CYSTS

Adrenal cysts are uncommon lesions that produce no clinical symptoms when the lesion is small. The cysts affect females more often than males (3:1). Adrenal cysts are usually unilateral and tend to be found incidentally. They may vary in size and can be unilocular or multilocular.

Sonographic Findings. Sonographically, adrenal cysts present a typical cystic pattern, with a strong back wall, no internal echoes, and good through-transmission. Adrenal cysts have the tendency to become calcified, which gives them the ultrasound appearance of a somewhat solid mass with no internal echoes (a sharp posterior border with poor through-transmission) (Figures 12-26 and 12-27). The cyst may have hemorrhaged; then it appears as a complex mass with multiple internal echoes and good through-transmission.

ADRENAL HEMORRHAGE

Adrenal hemorrhage in adults is very rare and is usually caused by severe trauma or infection. Posttraumatic hemorrhage is usually unilateral and does not cause any major clinical problems. A bilateral hemorrhage may cause adrenal insufficiency. Adrenal hemorrhages are more common in neonates who experienced a traumatic delivery with stress, asphyxia, and septicemia. The adrenal glands in a neonate are very vascular and the glands are proportionally larger than in an adult. Clinical signs and symptoms include abdominal mass, anemia, and hyperbilirubinemia.

Sonographic Findings. The sonographic appearance of an adrenal hemorrhage will vary depending upon the age of the hemorrhage. The adrenal gland will appear as a solid mass initially and over time the mass will have a more cystic or complex appearance. As the hemorrhage resolves, the mass will decrease in size. The adrenal gland may go back to a normal size with focal areas of calcification (Figure 12-28).

ADRENAL TUMORS

Further pathology of the adrenal glands is related to the tumors arising within them and their hyposecretion or hypersecretion of hormones. Rare nonfunctional adrenal tumors include myelolipomas, hemangiomas, teratomas, lipomas, and fibromas. These tumors are typically not seen on a sonogram.

Adrenal Adenoma. Adrenal adenomas can account for hypersecretion of cortical hormones and may cause Cushing's syndrome, Conn's syndrome, or adrenogenital syndrome.

Sonographic Findings. Adrenal adenomas are usually solid, well-defined, and round.

TABLE 12-1 ADRENAL PATHOLOGY

Adrenal Diseases	Hormone Secreted	Distinguishing Characteristics
Addison's disease	Hypofunction	Increases when there is stress or trauma Hypotension, general weakness, loss of appetite, (hyperpigmentation) bronzing of skin, may have renal failure, low blood pressure
Adrenogenital syndrome	Excessive secretion of androgens (male) Excessive secretion of estrogen (female)	Prepubertal males accelerate adult masculine development and growth of pubic hair Female: masculine characteristics
Conn's syndrome	Excessive secretion of aldosterone	Cortical adenoma, carcinoma
Cushing's syndrome	Excessive secretion of glucocorticoids	Hyperplasia, benign tumor, carcinoma
Waterhouse-Friderichsen syndrome		Bilateral hemorrhage into adrenal glands
Medulla tumor Pheochromocytoma	Excessive secretion of epinephrine and norepinephrine	Intermittent hypertension; large tumor with varied sonographic pattern (cystic, solid, calcified components)

Figure 12-26   A through D, Small adrenal cyst is imaged on this longitudinal scan of the right kidney in two asymptomatic females. B, Different patient from A, C, and D. (B, Courtesy Shpetim Telegrafi, New York University.)

Figure 12-27   Adrenal cysts (a) may become calcified, which gives them the ultrasound appearance of a "solid" mass with decreased transmission. L, liver.

Adrenal Malignant Tumors. Primary adrenal carcinomas are rare and may be hyperfunctional or nonfunctional. Hyperfunctional malignant tumors are more common in females. Adrenal malignant tumors may be a cause of Cushing's syndrome, Conn's syndrome, or adrenogenital syndrome. The origin of the tumor should be clearly defined.

Figure 12-28   Adrenal hemorrhage in a 6-day-old neonate. The mass appears as a complex lesion with multiple echogenic internal echoes and general enlargement of the gland. (Courtesy Thomas Hoffman and Jack D. Weiler, Albert Einstein Medical Center, Bronx, NY.)

Sonographic Findings. Functional tumors tend to be smaller than nonfunctional tumors because they are typically diagnosed earlier. The tumors are homogeneous with the same echogenicity as the renal cortex. The larger neoplasms tend to be nonfunctional and heterogeneous, with a central area of necrosis and hemorrhage. The sonographic appearance of a mass cannot be used to differentiate between a benign or malignant tumor (Figure 12-29).

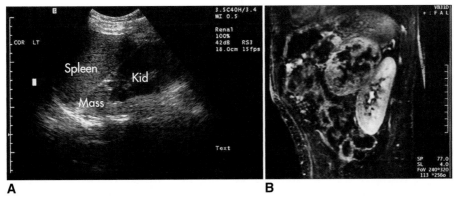

Figure 12-29   **A,** Coronal scan through the spleen of an 8-cm left adrenal carcinoma. **B,** Coronal view of a magnetic resonance image of the left adrenal mass. (Courtesy Heather Baum, New York University.)

Metastasis. Metastases to the adrenal glands are most commonly caused by a primary carcinoma of the lung, breast, stomach, colon, or kidney. Metastases to the adrenal gland typically cause adrenal insufficiency.

Sonographic Findings. Adrenal glands will vary in size and echogenicity (Figures 12-30 through 12-32). Often central necrosis causes sonolucent areas within the tumor.

ADRENAL MEDULLA TUMORS

Pheochromocytoma. The pheochromocytes of the adrenal medulla may produce a tumor called a **pheochromocytoma**, which secretes epinephrine and norepinephrine in excessive quantities. A small percentage of patients will have ectopic adrenal pheochromocytomas rising from the **neuroectodermal tissue**; these tumors tend to be malignant. The clinical symptoms include intermittent hypertension, severe headaches, heart palpitations, and excess perspiration. Treatment usually is removal of the tumor.

Sonographic Findings. The tumor has a homogeneous pattern that can be differentiated from a cyst by its weak posterior wall and poor through-transmission (Figure 12-33). Pheochromocytomas are usually unilateral and may be large, bulky tumors with a variety of sonographic patterns, including cystic, solid, and calcified components.

Adrenal Neuroblastoma. The adrenal **neuroblastoma** is the most common malignancy of the adrenal glands in childhood and the most common tumor of infancy. Generally, it develops within the adrenal medulla. Although children are usually asymptomatic, some do present with a palpable abdominal mass that must be differentiated from a neonatal hemorrhage and hydronephrosis.

Sonographic Findings. Sonographically the tumor appears as an echogenic mass. It may be large and evaluation of the surrounding retroperitoneum and liver should be made to rule out metastases.

RETROPERITONEAL FAT

The anatomic origin of the right upper quadrant mass may be difficult to determine. The reflection produced by the

Figure 12-30   Sagittal image of a 7.3 × 6.7 × 7.0 cm heterogeneous echogenic left adrenal mass. This mass represents either a metastatic mass or adrenal carcinoma. (Courtesy Elizabeth Polanno, Beth Israel Center North, NY.)

retroperitoneal fat is displaced in a characteristic manner by masses originating from this area. This pattern of displacement helps to localize the origin of the mass. Retroperitoneal lesions cause ventral and often cranial displacement of the lesion.

Sonographic Findings. The lesions in the liver or in Morison's pouch displace the echoes posterior and inferior, whereas renal and adrenal lesions cause anterior displacement of structures. An extrahepatic mass may shift the inferior vena cava anteromedially (anterior displacement of right kidney).

PRIMARY RETROPERITONEAL TUMORS

A primary retroperitoneal tumor is one that originates independently within the retroperitoneal space. The tumors can develop anywhere, and most are malignant. Like other tumors, they may exhibit a variety of sonographic patterns from homogeneous to solid to a mixture of complex tissue masses.

Neurogenic tumors are usually encountered in the paravertebral region, where they rise from nerve roots or sympathetic chain ganglia.

Sonographic Findings. Sonographically the pattern of neurogenic tumors is quite variable.

Figure 12-31 Ill-defined mass in the area of the adrenal gland in a patient with metastatic liver disease. *L*, liver; *RK*, right kidney; *S*, spleen.

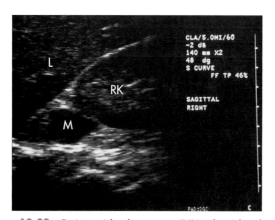

Figure 12-32 Patient with a large mass *(M)* in the right adrenal gland representing metastases from a melanoma. *L*, liver; *M*, mass; *RK*, right kidney. (Courtesy Shpetim Telegrafi, New York University.)

Leiomyosarcomas are prone to undergo necrosis and cystic degeneration. Their sonographic pattern is complex. Liposarcomas produce a highly reflective sonographic pattern because of their fat interface.

Fibrosarcomas and rhabdomyosarcomas may be quite invasive and may infiltrate widely into muscles and adjoining soft tissue. They often extend across the midline and appear very

similar to **lymphomas**. Sonographically, they are highly reflective tumors.

Teratomatous tumors may arise within the upper retroperitoneum and the pelvis. They may contain calcified echoes from bones, cartilage, teeth, and soft tissue elements.

Tumors of uniform cell type generally have a homogeneous appearance unless there is hemorrhage or necrosis. Often the presence of necrosis depends on the size and growth of the mass.

SECONDARY RETROPERITONEAL TUMORS
Secondary retroperitoneal tumors are primarily recurrences from previously resected tumors. Recurrent masses from previous renal carcinoma are common. Ascitic fluid along with a retroperitoneal tumor usually indicates seeding or invasion of the peritoneal surface. Evaluation of the para-aortic region should be made for extension to the lymph nodes. The liver should also be evaluated for metastatic involvement.

RETROPERITONEAL FLUID COLLECTIONS
Urinoma. A urinoma is a walled-off collection of extravasated urine that develops spontaneously after trauma, surgery, or a subacute or chronic urinary obstruction. Urinomas usually collect around the kidney or upper ureter in the perinephric space. Occasionally urinomas dissect into the pelvis and compress the bladder.

Figure 12-33 The pheochromocytoma is a homogeneous tumor that has a weak posterior wall and decreased through-transmission. This tumor can grow quite large. **A,** Longitudinal view. *L,* liver; *M,* mass. **B,** Transverse view. *IVC,* inferior vena cava; *M,* mass; *RK,* right kidney.

Figure 12-34 **A,** Longitudinal view of right kidney with a 9.4 × 2.0 × 6.8 cm perinephric hematoma inferior to liver, anterior to right kidney. **B,** Transverse view of right kidney with hematoma. (Courtesy Elizabeth Polanno, Beth Israel Center North, NY.)

Sonographic Findings. Generally the sonographic pattern of urinomas is sonolucent unless they become infected.

Hemorrhage. A retroperitoneal hemorrhage may occur in a variety of conditions, including trauma, vasculitis, bleeding diathesis, a leaking aortic aneurysm, or a bleeding neoplasm. *Sonographic Findings.* Sonographically the hemorrhage may be well localized and produce displacement of other organs, or it may present as a poorly defined infiltrative process (Figure 12-34). Fresh hematomas present as sonolucent areas, whereas an organized thrombus with clot formation shows echo densities within the mass. Calcification may be seen in long-standing hematomas.

Abscess. Abscess formation may result from surgery, trauma, or perforations of the bowel or duodenum. *Sonographic Findings.* Sonographically the abscess usually has a complex pattern with debris. Gas within the abscess is reflective and casts an acoustic shadow. The sonographer

should be careful not to mistake a gas-containing abscess for "bowel" patterns. The radiograph should be evaluated in this case. The abscess frequently extends along or within the muscle planes, is of an irregular shape, and lies in the most dependent portion of the retroperitoneal space.

RETROPERITONEAL FIBROSIS (ORMOND'S DISEASE)

Retroperitoneal fibrosis is a disease of unknown cause and in a small percentage of cases it is associated with a malignant process. The disease may occur in association with methysergide use, Crohn's disease, and abdominal aortic aneurysm surgery or leakage. It is characterized by thick sheets of fibrous tissue in the retroperitoneal cavity. The fibrosis may encase and obstruct the ureters and vena cava, with resultant hydronephrosis. The clinical signs and symptoms are flank pain, back pain, weight loss, and nausea and vomiting. *Sonographic Findings.* A discrete mass of abnormal tissue lies anterior and lateral to the great vessels; it may mimic lymphoma and further evaluation by computerized tomography

Figure 12-35 Transverse scan of retroperitoneal tumor anterior to the inferior vena cava *(C)*. *A,* aorta. (Courtesy Shpetim Telegrafi, New York University.)

(CT) may be necessary to establish whether there is a benign or malignant disease process. The kidneys should also be evaluated for obstruction (Figure 12-35).

SELECTED BIBLIOGRAPHY

Beer MH, Berkow R: *The Merck manual,* ed 17, Whitehouse Station, 1999, Merck Research Laboratories.

Choyke PL and others: Von Hippel-Lindau disease: genetic, clinical and imaging features, *Radiology* 194:629, 1996.

Dunnick NR, Korobkin M, Francis I: Adrenal radiology: distinguishing benign from malignant adrenal masses, *Am J Roentgenol* 167:861, 1996.

Gay S, Woodcock RJ: *Radiology recall,* Philadelphia, 2000, Lippincott Williams & Wilkins.

Henningsen C: *Clincial guide to ultrasonography,* St. Louis, 2004, Mosby.

Hsu CW and others: Adrenal insufficiency caused by primary aggressive non-Hodgkin's lymphoma of bilateral adrenal glands: report of a case and literature review, *Ann Hematol* 78:151, 1999.

Kawamura D: *Diagnostic medical sonography: a guide to clinical medicine: abdomen and superficial structures,* ed 2, Philadelphia, 1998, Lippincott-Raven.

Krebs C, Rawls K: Techniques for successful scanning: positioning strategy for optimal visualization of a left adrenal mass, *J Diag Med Sonogr* 5:286, 1990.

Little AF: Adrenal gland and renal sonography, *World J Surg* 24:171, 2000.

McGahan J, Goldberg B: *Diagnostic ultrasound: a logical approach,* Philadelphia, 1998, Lippincott-Raven.

Mittelstaedt CA: *General ultrasound,* New York, 1992, Churchill Livingstone.

Rumack CM, Wilson SR, Charboneau JW: *Diagnostic ultrasound,* ed 3, St Louis, 2005, Mosby.

Sample WF: Adrenal ultrasonography, *Radiology* 127:461, 1978.

Sample WF: Renal, adrenal, retroperitoneal, and scrotal ultrasonography. In Sarti DA, Sample WF, editors: *Diagnostic ultrasound: text and cases,* Boston, 1980, GK Hall.

Sample WF, Sarti DA: Computed tomography and gray scale ultrasonography of the adrenal gland: a comparative study, *Radiology* 128:377, 1978.

Sanders R: *Clinical sonography: a practical guide,* ed 3, Philadelphia, 2003, Lippincott.

Sivit CJ and others: Sonography in neonatal congenital adrenal hyperplasia, *Am J Roentgenol* 156:141, 1991.

Talmont CA: Adrenal glands. In Taylor KJW and others, editors: *Manual of ultrasonography,* New York, 1980, Churchill Livingstone.

Udelsman R, Fishman EK: Radiology of the adrenal, *Endocrinol Metab Clin North Am* 29(1):27-42, viii, 2000.

CHAPTER 13

The Peritoneal Cavity and Abdominal Wall

Sandra L. Hagen-Ansert

KEY TERMS

abscess – localized collection of pus

ascites – accumulation of serous fluid in the peritoneal cavity

gutters – most dependent areas in the flanks of the abdomen and pelvis where fluid collections may accumulate

hemorrhage – collection of blood

leukocytosis – increase in the number of leukocytes (white blood cells)

mesentery – the loops of the digestive tract are anchored to the posterior wall of the abdominal cavity by this large double fold of peritoneal tissue

Morison's pouch – space anterior to the right kidney and posterior to the inferior border of the liver where ascites or fluid may accumulate or an abscess may develop

omentum – pouchlike extension of the visceral peritoneum from the lower edge of the stomach, part of the duodenum, and the transverse colon. It hangs down over the intestines like an apron.

peritonitis – inflammation of the peritoneum

pyogenic – pus producing

sandwich sign – condition occurs when a vessel or organ is surrounded by a tumor on either side

sepsis – spread of an infection from its initial site to the bloodstream

septicemia – infection in the blood

subhepatic – inferior to the liver

subphrenic – below the diaphragm

urinoma – cyst containing urine

ANATOMY AND SONOGRAPHIC EVALUATION OF THE PERITONEAL CAVITY AND ABDOMINAL WALL

PERITONEAL CAVITY

The peritoneal cavity is made up of multiple peritoneal ligaments and folds that connect the viscera to each other and to the abdominopelvic walls. Within the cavity are found the lesser and greater **omentum**, the mesenteries, the ligaments, and multiple fluid spaces (lesser sac, perihepatic and **subphrenic** spaces). The peritoneum is a smooth membrane that lines the entire abdominal cavity and is reflected over the contained organs. The part that lines the walls of the cavity is the parietal peritoneum, whereas the part covering the abdominal organs to a greater or lesser extent is the visceral peritoneum. In the male, the peritoneum forms a closed cavity; in the female, there is a "communication" outside the peritoneum through the uterine tubes, uterus, and vagina. In reality, however, the complex linings of the uterus and fallopian tubes tend to close off any potential space and prohibit the entrance of air into the peritoneal cavity.

The relationship of the peritoneum to the abdominal structures may be understood with the visualization of an inflated balloon (the peritoneum) within an empty box (the abdominal cavity) (Figure 13-1). If one were to place objects within the box, yet outside the balloon, these objects might impinge on the balloon shape. This is the same condition that the kidneys and the ascending and descending colon have on the peritoneal cavity. Since these structures lie along the posterior surface of the peritoneal cavity, they are considered "retroperitoneal," and they are overlaid by visceral peritoneum. If an object bulges so far into the balloon that it loses contact with the box, the object would become surrounded by a fold of the balloon. This is the situation with the small intestine, transverse colon, and the sigmoid colon; they are suspended from the posterior abdominal wall by a double fold of peritoneum called the **mesentery**, transverse mesocolon, and sigmoid

mesocolon. Thus the peritoneal cavity is really empty of abdominal organs as they bulge into or are covered by the cavity, but are not located within the cavity.

The general peritoneal cavity is known as the greater sac of the peritoneum. With the development of the stomach and the spleen, a smaller sac, called the lesser sac (omental bursa), is the peritoneal recess posterior to the stomach (Figure 13-2). This sac communicates with the greater sac through a small vertical opening known as the epiploic foramen. The epiploic foramen is just inferior to the liver and superior to the first part of the duodenum; the inferior vena cava is posterior, and the portal vein is anterior.

The attachments of the peritoneum to the abdominal walls and organs help determine the way abnormal collections of fluid within the peritoneal cavity can collect or move. When the patient is lying supine, the lowest part of the body is the pelvis (Figure 13-3). On a transverse view, the flanks are lower than the midabdomen. Fluid will accumulate in the lowest parts of the body; therefore, the pelvis and lateral flanks (**gutters**) should be carefully examined for pathologic collections of fluid.

The lesser omentum is a double layer of peritoneum, extending from the liver to the lesser curvature of the stomach. This structure acts as a sling for the stomach, suspending it from the liver.

The greater omentum is an apronlike fold of peritoneum that hangs from the greater curvature of the stomach (Figure 13-4). The omentum lies freely over the intestine except for the upper part, which is fused with the transverse colon and

Figure 13-1 **A,** The "abdominal cavity" containing a "balloon" (peritoneum). **B,** An organ inside the abdomen and partly covered by peritoneum, such as the kidney, which is said to be in the retroperitoneal cavity. **C,** An organ suspended from the abdominal wall by a fold of peritoneum, such as the small intestine suspended by its mesentery. **D,** When supine, the backward tilt of the pelvis makes it the lowest part of the peritoneal cavity. *(Dotted line),* long axis of abdomen; *(solid line),* long axis of pelvis; *PC,* pelvic part of peritoneal cavity; *D,* diaphragm; *T,* thorax. (From McMinn: *Functional and clinical anatomy,* St. Louis, 1999, Mosby.)

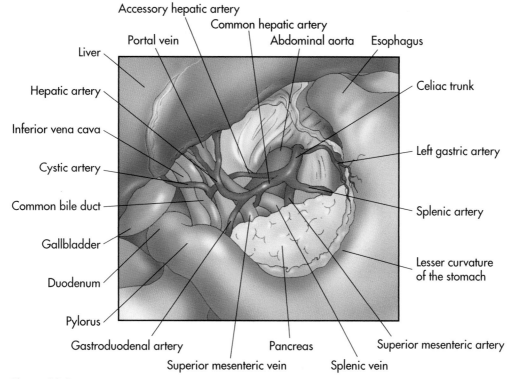

Figure 13-2 Upper abdominal dissection, with part of the left lobe of the liver and the lesser omentum removed to show the celiac trunk, portal vein, bile duct, and related structures.

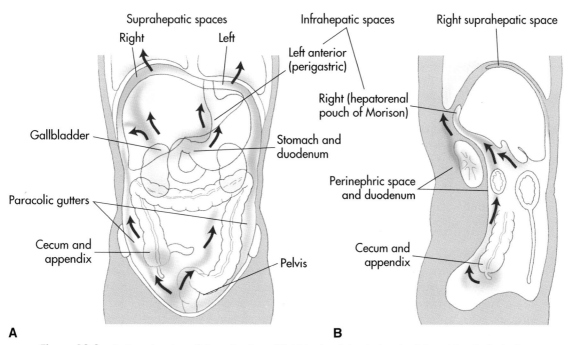

Figure 13-3 **A,** Anterior view of the collection of fluid in the abdominal and pelvic cavities. **B,** Sagittal view of the right abdomen shows how the fluid collects in the most dependent areas of the abdomen and pelvis.

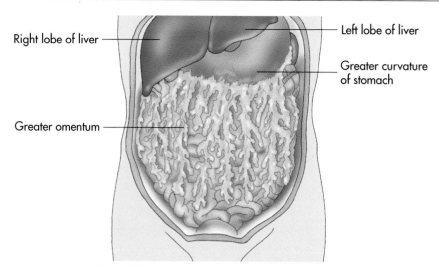

Figure 13-4   Anterior view of the greater omentum.

mesocolon. The greater omentum is able to adhere to diseased organs, which in turn helps prevent further spread of infected fluid by essentially "walling it off" from the rest of the body. The greater omentum is profusely supplied with blood vessels by the epiploic branches of the gastroepiploic vessels and thus can bring masses of blood phagocytes to the areas it adheres to, which helps combat infection.

Determination of Intraperitoneal Location. The determination of intraperitoneal fluid from pleural, subdiaphragmatic, subscapular, or retroperitoneal fluid is necessary to determine a differential diagnosis or to locate a fluid pocket for aspiration or a biopsy.

Pleural versus subdiaphragmatic. Because of the coronary ligament attachments, collections in the right posterior subphrenic space cannot extend between the bare area of the liver and the diaphragm. On the other hand, because the right pleural space extends medially to the attachment of the right superior coronary ligament, pleural collections may appear apposed to the bare area of the liver (Figure 13-5). Unless it is loculated, the pleural fluid tends to distribute posteromedially in the chest.

Subcapsular versus intraperitoneal. Subcapsular liver and splenic collections are seen when they are inferior to the diaphragm unilaterally, and they conform to the shape of an organ capsule (Figure 13-6). They may extend medially to the attachment of the superior coronary ligament.

Retroperitoneal versus intraperitoneal. A mass is confirmed to be within the retroperitoneal cavity when anterior renal displacement or anterior displacement of the dilated ureters can be documented (Figure 13-7). The mass interposed anteriorly or superiorly to kidneys can be located either intraperitoneally or retroperitoneally.

Fatty and collagenous connective tissues in the perirenal or anterior pararenal space produce echoes that are best demonstrated on sagittal scans. Retroperitoneal lesions displace echoes ventrally and cranially; hepatic and **subhepatic** lesions produce inferior and posterior displacement.

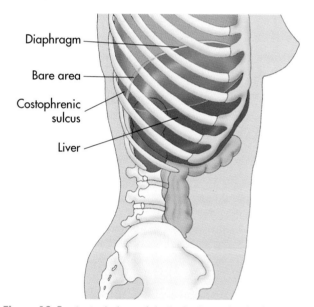

Figure 13-5   Sagittal plane of the body shows the diaphragm and liver with the highlighted "bare" area of the liver. The costophrenic sulcus forms the sharp border posterior to the liver and may be identified when fluid is present.

The anterior displacement of the superior mesenteric vessels, splenic vein, renal vein, and inferior vena cava excludes an intraperitoneal location. A large, right-sided retroperitoneal mass rotates the intrahepatic portal veins to the left. This causes the left portal vein to show reversed flow.

Right posterior hepatic masses of similar dimensions may produce minor displacement of the intrahepatic portal vein. Primary liver masses should move simultaneously with the liver.

Intraperitoneal Compartments

Perihepatic and upper abdominal compartments. Ligaments on the right side of the liver form the subphrenic and

Figure 13-6   Transverse view of the subphrenic spaces.

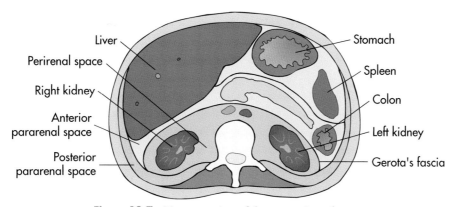

Figure 13-7   Transverse view of the retroperitoneal space.

Figure 13-8   Transverse view of the subhepatic spaces and Morison's pouch.

subhepatic spaces. The falciform ligament divides the subphrenic space into right and left components. The ligamentum teres hepatis ascends from the umbilicus to the umbilical notch of the liver within the free margin of the falciform ligament before coursing within the liver.

The bare area is delineated by the right superior and inferior coronary ligaments, which separate the posterior subphrenic space from the right superior subhepatic space **(Morison's pouch).** Lateral to the bare area and right triangular ligament, the posterior subphrenic and subhepatic spaces are continuous (Figure 13.8).

A single large and irregular perihepatic space surrounds the superior and lateral aspects of the left lobe of the liver, with

the left coronary ligaments anatomically separating the subphrenic space into anterior and posterior compartments (see Figure 13-2).

The left subhepatic space is divided into an anterior compartment (the gastrohepatic recess) and a posterior compartment (the lesser sac) by the lesser omentum and stomach (Figure 13-9). The lesser sac lies anterior to the pancreas and posterior to the stomach.

With fluid in the lesser and greater omental cavities, the lesser omentum may be seen as a linear, undulating echodensity extending from the stomach to the porta hepatis.

Gastrosplenic ligament. The gastrosplenic ligament is the left lateral extension of the greater omentum that connects the

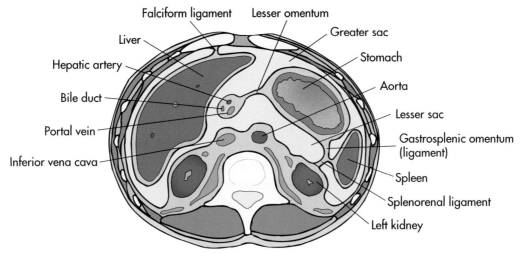

Figure 13-9   Transverse view of the abdomen showing the greater and lesser sac, the falciform ligament, the gastrosplenic ligament, and the splenorenal ligament.

gastric greater curvature to the superior splenic hilum and forms a portion of the left lateral border of the lesser sac (see Figure 13-9).

Splenorenal ligament. The splenorenal ligament is formed by the posterior reflection of the peritoneum of the spleen and passes inferiorly to overlie the left kidney (see Figure 13-9). It forms the posterior portion of the left lateral border of the lesser sac and separates the lesser sac from the renosplenic recess.

The lesser omental bursa. The lesser omental bursa is subdivided into a larger lateroinferior and a smaller mediosuperior recess by the gastropancreatic folds, which are produced by the left gastric and hepatic arteries. The lesser sac extends to the diaphragm. The superior recess of the bursa surrounds the anterior, medial, and posterior surfaces of the caudate lobe, making the caudate a lesser sac structure. The lesser sac collections may extend a considerable distance below the plane of the pancreas by inferiorly displacing the transverse mesocolon or extending into the inferior recess of the greater omentum.

Lower Abdominal and Pelvic Compartments. The supravesical space and the medial and lateral inguinal fossae represent intraperitoneal paravesical spaces formed by indentation of the anterior parietal peritoneum by the bladder, obliterated umbilical arteries, and inferior epigastric vessels.

The retrovesical space is divided by the uterus into an anterior vesicouterine recess and a posterior rectouterine sac (pouch of Douglas) (Figure 13-10).

The peritoneal reflection over the dome of the bladder may have an inferior recess extending anterior to the bladder. Ascites displaces the distended urinary bladder inferiorly but not posteriorly. Intraperitoneal fluid compresses the bladder from its lateral aspect in cases of loculation. Fluid in the extraperitoneal prevesical space has a "dumbbell" configuration, displacing the bladder posteriorly and compressing it from the sides along its entire length.

ABDOMINAL WALL

The paired rectus abdominis muscles are delineated medially in the midline of the body by the linea alba (Figure 13-11). Laterally the aponeuroses of external oblique, internal oblique, and transversus abdominis muscles unite to form a bandlike vertical fibrous groove called the linea semilunaris or spigelian fascia. The sheath of the three anterolateral abdominal muscles invests the rectus both anteriorly and posteriorly. Midway between the umbilicus and symphysis pubis, the aponeurotic sheath passes anteriorly to the rectus (Figure 13-12).

Below the peritoneal line, the rectus muscle is separated from the intraabdominal contents only by the transversalis fascia and the peritoneum. The rectus muscles are seen as a biconvex muscle group delineated by the linea alba and linea semilunaris. The peritoneal line is seen as a discrete linear echogenicity in the deepest layer of the abdominal wall.

PATHOLOGY OF THE PERITONEAL CAVITY

ASCITES

Ascites is the accumulation of serous fluid in the peritoneal cavity. The amount of intraperitoneal fluid depends on the location, volume, and patient position. Factors other than fluid volume that affect the distribution of intraperitoneal fluid include peritoneal pressure, the area from which fluid originates, rapidity of fluid accumulation, presence or absence of adhesions, density of fluid with respect to other abdominal organs, and the degree of bladder fullness.

Sonographic Findings. Serous ascites appears as echo-free fluid regions indented and shaped by the organs and viscera it surrounds or between where it is interposed. The fluid first fills the pouch of Douglas, then the lateral paravesical recesses, before it ascends to both paracolic gutters. The major flow from the pelvis is via the right paracolic gutter. Small volumes of fluid in the supine patient first appear around the inferior

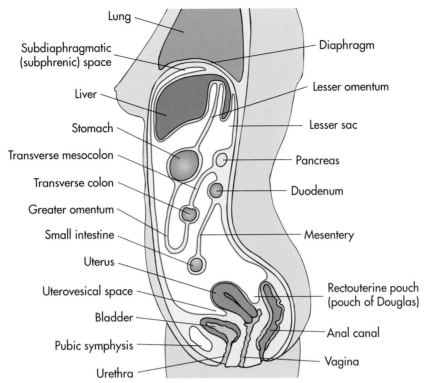

Lung
Subdiaphragmatic (subphrenic) space
Liver
Stomach
Transverse mesocolon
Transverse colon
Greater omentum
Small intestine
Uterus
Uterovesical space
Bladder
Pubic symphysis
Urethra

Diaphragm
Lesser omentum
Lesser sac
Pancreas
Duodenum
Mesentery
Rectouterine pouch (pouch of Douglas)
Anal canal
Vagina

Figure 13-10   Sagittal view of the abdomen delineating the peritoneal cavity.

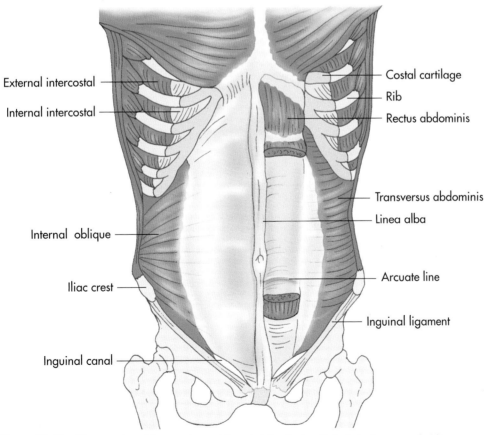

External intercostal
Internal intercostal
Internal oblique
Iliac crest
Inguinal canal

Costal cartilage
Rib
Rectus abdominis
Transversus abdominis
Linea alba
Arcuate line
Inguinal ligament

Figure 13-11   The muscles of the anterior and lateral abdominal walls include the external oblique, internal oblique, transversus, rectus abdominis, and pyramidalis.

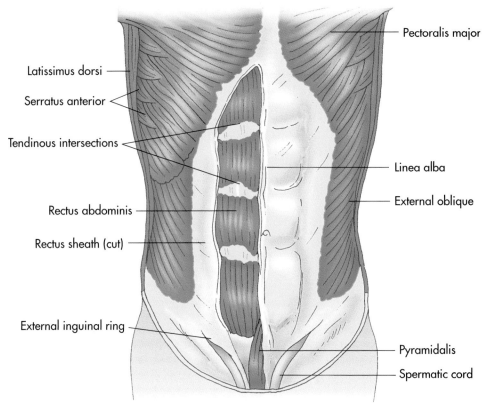

Figure 13-12   The rectus abdominis muscle rises from the front of the symphysis pubis and the pubic crest. On contraction, its lateral margin forms a palpable curved surface, termed the linea semilunaris, that extends from the ninth costal cartilage to the pubic tubercle. The anterior surface of the rectus muscle is crossed by three tendinous intersections, which are firmly attached to the anterior wall of the rectus sheath. The pyramidalis muscle arises by its base from the anterior surface of the pubis and inserts into the linea alba. It lies anterior to the lower part of the rectus abdominis muscle.

tip of the right lobe in the superior portion of the right flank and in the pelvic cul-de-sac, then in the paracolic gutters, before moving lateral and anterior to the liver (Figures 13-13 through 13-15).

The small bowel loops, sinks, or floats in the surrounding ascitic fluid, depending on relative gas content and amount of fat in the mesentery. The middle portion of the transverse colon usually floats on top of fluid because of its gas content, whereas the ascending portions of the colon, which are fixed retroperitoneally, remain in their normal location with or without gas.

Floating loops of small bowel, anchored posteriorly by the mesentery and with fluid between the mesenteric folds, have a characteristic anterior convex fan shape or arcuate appearance. An overdistended bladder may mask small quantities of fluid.

Inflammatory or Malignant Ascites. The sonographer should look for findings within the ascitic fluid that may suggest an inflammatory or malignant process.

Sonographic Findings. In searching for inflammatory or malignant ascites, the sonographer should look for fine or coarse internal echoes; loculation; unusual distribution, matting, or clumping of bowel loops; and thickening of interfaces between the fluid and neighboring structures (Figure 13-16).

Hepatorenal Recess. Generalized ascites, inflammatory fluid from acute cholecystitis, fluid resulting from pancreatic autolysis, or blood from a ruptured hepatic neoplasm or ectopic gestation may contribute to the formation of hepatorenal fluid collections (Figure 13-17). Abdominal fluid collections do not persist 1 week after abdominal surgery as a normal part of the healing process.

Sonographic Findings. Loculated ascites tends to be more irregular in outline, shows less mass effect, and may change shape slightly with positional variation.

ABSCESS FORMATION AND POCKETS IN THE ABDOMEN AND PELVIS

An **abscess** is a cavity formed by necrosis within a solid tissue or a circumscribed collection of purulent material. The sonographer is frequently asked to evaluate a patient to rule out an abscess formation. The patient may present with a fever of unknown origin or with tenderness and swelling from a postoperative procedure. Other clinical signs include chills, weakness, malaise, and pain at the localized site of infection.

Left lobe (medial)   Left lobe (lateral)

Duodenum

Gallbladder

Caudate lobe of liver

Right lobe of liver

Inferior vena cava

Right kidney

Stomach

Aorta

Bowel

A

B   C

D   E

Figure 13-13   **A,** Transverse view of the posterior pararenal space. This space is located between the posterior renal fascia and the transversalis fascia. It communicates with the peritoneal fat, lateral to the lateroconal fascia. The space merges inferiorly with the anterior pararenal space and retroperitoneal tissue of the iliac fossa. Ascites may fill the peritoneal cavity. Small volumes of fluid in the supine position first appear around the inferior tip of the right lobe of the superior portion of the right flank. **B,** Transverse view. *AS,* ascites; *L,* liver; *RK,* right kidney. **C,** Transverse view. **D,** Longitudinal view with fluid in Morison's pouch. **E,** Longitudinal view.

Figure 13-14 Ascites secondary to liver transplant is shown in this sagittal image.

Figure 13-15 Loculated ascites with matted bowel.

Figure 13-16 Malignant ascites. Fine internal echoes are seen in these images of malignant ascites.

Laboratory findings include normal liver function values, increased white blood cell count **(leukocytosis),** generalized **sepsis,** and bacterial cultures (if superficial).

Sonographic Findings. Abscess collections can appear quite varied in their texture depending on the length of time the abscess has been forming and the space available for the abscess to localize. Therefore, many collections appear predominantly fluid-filled with irregular borders; they can also be complex, with debris floating within the cystic mass, or they may show a more solid pattern. If the collection is in the pelvis, careful

analysis of bowel patterns and peristalsis should be made in an attempt to separate the bowel from the abscess collection.

Classically an abscess appears as an elliptical sonolucent mass with thick and irregular margins (Figure 13-18). The margins tend to be under tension and displace surrounding structures. A septated appearance may result from previous or developing adhesions. Necrotic debris produces low-level internal echoes that may be seen to "float" within the abscess. Fluid levels are secondary to layering, probably because of the settling of debris.

Figure 13-17 Fluid in Morison's pouch. Transverse (**A**) and sagittal (**B**) views. *F,* fluid; *GB,* gallbladder; *L,* liver; *RK,* right kidney.

Figure 13-18 Collection of fluid was found posterior to the knee in a patient with a Baker's cyst. Multiple septations are seen within the fluid along with low-level debris echoes.

Figure 13-19 Patient with human immunodeficiency virus *(HIV)* nephropathy showed air with shadowing in the renal collecting system.

Gas-Containing Abscess. Scattered air reflectors may be the sonographer's clue in a gas- or air-filled abscess collection. *Sonographic Findings.* Gas-containing abscesses have varying echo patterns. Generally, they appear as a densely echogenic mass with or without acoustic shadowing and otherwise increased through-transmission (Figure 13-19). A teratoma may mimic the pattern of a gas-containing abscess, but clinical history and x-rays exclude this tumor from the diagnosis. A gas-containing abscess may be confused with a solid lesion because it can be difficult to determine the presence of through-transmission.

Peritonitis. Peritonitis and the resultant abscess formation may be a generalized or localized process. Multiloculated abscesses or multiple collections should be recorded and their size determined as accurately as possible to help plan drainage and improve accuracy in follow-up studies.

Lesser-Sac Abscess. The small slitlike epiploic foramen usually seals off the lesser sac from inflammatory processes extrinsic to it. If the process begins within the lesser sac, such

as with a pancreatic abscess, the sac may be involved along with other secondarily affected peritoneal and retroperitoneal spaces. Differential diagnosis should include pseudocyst, pancreatic abscess, gastric outlet obstruction, and fluid-filled stomach.

Subphrenic Abscess. The left upper quadrant may be difficult to examine because of the air interference. The sonographer may alter the patient's position to a right lateral decubitus position to scan along the coronal plane of the body, or prone, to use the spleen as a window.

Sonographic Findings. A sonographer must be careful of pleural effusions that appear above the diaphragm (Figure 13-20). The sonographer may perform the scan with the patient upright to better demonstrate the pleural and subdiaphragmatic areas.

Subcapsular Collections. Subcapsular collections of fluid within the liver can mimic loculated subphrenic fluid. *Sonographic Findings.* Intraabdominal fluid may be differentiated by its smooth border and its tendency to conform

A   **B**

Figure 13-20   Pleural effusion. **A,** Transverse image shows the pleural effusion posterior to the liver as the transducer is angled in a cephalic direction. **B,** Sagittal images of a patient with a moderate pleural effusion shown superior to the liver.

to the contour of the liver. It displaces the liver medially, rather than indenting the border locally, as subcapsular fluid might. A tense subphrenic abscess can displace the liver.

It may be difficult to distinguish a subphrenic abscess from ascites. To do so, the sonographer can look at the margins of the fluid collection or look for other collections of fluid (in the pelvis) to distinguish ascites from abscess. Preperitoneal fat anterior to the liver may mimic a localized fluid collection.

An abscess collects in the most dependent area of the body; therefore, all the gutters should be examined, including the "pockets" and "pouches" and the spaces above and around the various organs (Box 13-1).

Liver Abscess. There are five major pathways through which bacteria can enter the liver and cause abscess formation:

1. Through the portal system
2. By way of ascending cholangitis of the common bile duct (this is the most common cause in the United States)
3. Via the hepatic artery secondary to bacteremia
4. By direct extension from an infection
5. By implantation of bacteria after trauma to the abdominal wall

Biloma Abscess. Bilomas are extrahepatic loculated collections of bile that may develop because of iatrogenic, traumatic, or spontaneous rupture of the biliary tree.

Sonographic Findings. On ultrasound examination, a biloma abscess may appear cystic with weak internal echoes or a fluid-fluid level if clots or debris are not present. They usually have sharp margins. The extrahepatic bilomas are usually crescentic, surrounding and compressing structures with which they come in contact.

Kidney Abscess. Renal abscesses are classified according to their locations. A renal carbuncle is an abscess that forms within the renal parenchyma. Clinical symptoms vary from none to fever, leukocytosis, and flank pain. Sonography may show a discrete mass within the kidney, which may be cystic, cystic with debris, or solid.

BOX 13-1   SONOGRAPHY OF ABSCESSES

If an abscess is suspected (e.g., the patient has a fever of unknown origin), the sonographer should evaluate the following areas:

- Subdiaphragmatic area (liver and spleen)
- Splenic recess and borders
- Hepatic recess and borders
- Pericolic gutters
- Lesser omentum
- Transverse mesocolon
- Morison's pouch
- Gastrocolic ligament
- Phrenicosplenic ligament
- Recesses between intestinal loops and colon
- Extrahepatic falciform ligament
- Pouch of Douglas
- Broad ligaments (female)
- The area anterior to the urinary bladder

A perinephric abscess is usually the result of a perforated renal abscess that leaks purulent material into the tissue adjacent to the kidney.

Sonographic Findings. Sonographic findings include a fluid collection around the kidney or an adjacent mass, which can vary from a cystic to a more solid appearance.

General Abdominal Abscess. A high percentage of abdominal and pelvic abscesses appear after surgery or trauma. The hepatic recesses and perihepatic spaces are the most common sites for abscess formation. The pelvis is another common site. (Free fluid below the transverse mesocolon often flows into the pouch of Douglas and perivesical spaces.)

Sonographic Findings. An abscess may form in the right subhepatic space. The fluid ascends the right pericolic gutter into Morison's pouch. When the fluid fills Morison's pouch, it spreads past the coronary ligament over the dome of the liver. The presence of a right subhepatic abscess generally implies previous contamination of the right subhepatic space.

Appendiceal Abscess. Acute appendicitis is the most common abdominal pathologic process that requires immediate surgery. The cause of obstruction of the appendix is a fecalith at its origin in the cecum. The appendix becomes distended rapidly after obstruction.

Clinical symptoms include fever and severe pain near McBurney point in the right lower quadrant. (To locate this point, draw a straight line between the umbilicus and the anterior superior iliac spine and then move 2 inches along the line from the iliac spine.) Laboratory findings show an increased white blood cell count. The differential diagnosis includes pelvic inflammatory disease, twisted or ruptured ovarian cyst, acute gastroenteritis, and mesenteric lymphadenitis.

Sonographic Findings. On sonography, a complex mass is found in the right lower quadrant (Figure 13-21). The sonographer should also examine other gutters to rule out differentials. For further information on the appendix, see Chapter 9.

PATHOLOGY OF THE MESENTERY, OMENTUM, AND PERITONEUM

A mass or lesion within the mesentery and omentum may have solid or cystic characteristics, whereas a mass within the peritoneum may show an infiltrative pattern (Table 13-1). With an omental mass, at least one third of these lesions are malignant and secondary neoplasms are more frequent than primary. In the mesentery, a benign primary tumor is more common than a malignant tumor, and secondary neoplasms are more frequent than primary. A cystic mass is more common than a solid mass. Malignant solid tumors are more likely found near the root of the mesentery, whereas benign solid tumors are found in the periphery near the bowel.

CYSTS

Abdominal cysts may have (1) embryologic, (2) traumatic or acquired, (3) neoplastic, or (4) infective and degenerative origins. It is important to determine the organ of origin of the mass. If the mass is adherent to the mesentery or small intestine, it may be very difficult for ultrasound to distinguish the anatomical landmarks necessary to determine the point of origin. Therefore, many patients will have a CT or MRI of the abdomen to better define these borders. Hemorrhage into omental or mesenteric cysts may cause rapid distention and clinically mimic ascites. Peritoneal inclusion cysts are considered in the differential diagnosis when large adnexal cystic structures are identified in a young woman. Fungal infections present as peritoneal cystic lesions.

Sonographic Findings. Mesenteric and omental cysts may be uniloculated or multiloculated with smooth walls and thin internal septations. The internal echoes are correlated with fat globules, debris, superimposed hemorrhage, or infection. They may follow the contour of the underlying bowel and conform to the anterior abdominal wall rather than produce distention.

Urachal Cyst. A urachal cyst is an incomplete regression of the urachus during development. The apex of the bladder is continuous with the allantois, which becomes obliterated and forms a fibrous core, the urachus. The urachus persists throughout life as a ligament that runs from the apex of the bladder to the umbilicus and is called the median umbilical ligament.

Sonographic Findings. On ultrasound examination, the sonographer may see a cystic mass between the umbilicus and the bladder. The mass may be small or giant, multiseptated, and extend into the upper abdomen.

URINOMA

A **urinoma,** an encapsulated collection of urine, may result from a closed renal injury or surgical intervention or may develop spontaneously secondary to an obstructing lesion. The extraperitoneal extravasation may be subcapsular or perirenal: the latter collections are sometimes termed uriniferous pseudocysts. The extravasation may leak around the ureter, where the perinephric fascia is weakest, or into adjoining fascial planes and peritoneal cavity.

Sonographic Findings. Cystic masses are most often oriented inferomedially, with upward and lateral displacement of

A   **B**

Figure 13-21 Appendiceal abscess. **A,** Transverse image of the inflamed appendix with a collection of pus posterior. **B,** Computed tomography scan of the same patient.

TABLE 13-1 DESCRIPTION OF PERITONEAL, OMENTAL, AND MESENTERIC MASSES

Solid	Cystic	Infiltrative
Peritoneal Mass		
• Peritoneal mesothelioma • Peritoneal carcinomatosis	• Cystic mesothelioma • Pseudomyxoma peritonei • Bacterial/mycobacterial infection	• Peritoneal mesothelioma

Solid	Cystic	Infiltrative
Omental Mass		
• Benign: leiomyoma, lipoma, neurofibroma • Malignant: leiomyosarcoma, liposarcoma, fibrosarcoma, lymphoma, peritoneal mesothelioma, hemangiopericytoma, metastases • Infection: tuberculosis	• Hematoma	

Round	Loculated Cystic	Ill-Defined/Stellate
Mesenteric Mass		
• Metastases, especially from colon, ovary • Lymphoma • Leiomyosarcoma • Neural tumor • Lipoma, lipomatosis, liposarcoma • Fibrous histiocytoma • Hemangioma • Desmoid tumor (most common primary)	• Cystic lymphangioma • Pseudomyxoma • Peritonei • Cystic mesothelioma • Mesenteric cyst • Mesenteric hematoma • Benign cystic teratoma • Cystic spindle cell tumor	• Metastases (ovary) • Lymphoma • Fibromatosis • Fibrosing mesenteritis • Lipodystrophy • Mesenteric panniculitis • Stellate: peritoneal mesothelioma, retractile mesenteritis, fibrosis reaction of carcinoid, desmoid tumor, tuberculous peritonitis, metastases, diverticulitis, pancreatitis

the lower pole of the kidney along with medial displacement of the ureter. They usually present on ultrasound as anechoic or contain low-level echoes (Figure 13-22).

PERITONEAL METASTASES
Peritoneal metastases develop from cellular implantation across the peritoneal cavity. The most common primary sites are the ovaries, stomach, and colon. Other less common sites are the pancreas, biliary tract, kidneys, testicles, and uterus. Metastases may arise from tumors, such as sarcomas, melanomas, teratomas, or embryonic tumors.

Sonographic Findings. The metastases form a nodular, sheetlike, irregular configuration. Multiple small nodules are seen along the peritoneal line. The larger masses obliterate the line and cause adhesion to bowel loops.

LYMPHOMAS OF THE OMENTUM AND MESENTERY
Lymphoma presents as a uniformly thick, hypoechoic, band-shaped structure that follows the convexity of the anterior and lateral abdominal wall, creating the omental band.

Sonographic Findings. On ultrasound examination, omental and mesenteric lymphomas present as a lobulated, confluent, hypoechoic mass surrounding a centrally positioned echogenic area. The "**sandwich sign**" represents a mass infiltrating the mesenteric leaves and encasing the superior mesenteric artery.

Figure 13-22 Right lower quadrant pain in young adult with renal transplant shows a fluid collection posterior to the transplanted kidney indenting its posterior wall. This represented a postoperative urinoma.

TUMORS OF THE PERITONEUM, OMENTUM, AND MESENTERY
Secondary tumors and lymphoma are neoplasms that most commonly involve the peritoneum and mesentery.

Peritoneal and Omental Mesothelioma. Peritoneal and omental mesotheliomas most often occur in middle-aged men as the result of exposure to asbestos. The common symptoms are abdominal pain, weight loss, and ascites.

Sonographic Findings. The tumor may present as a large mass with discrete smaller nodes scattered over large areas of the visceral and parietal peritoneum, or it may present as diffuse nodes and plaques that coat the abdominal cavity and envelope and mat together in the abdominal viscera.

PATHOLOGY OF THE ABDOMINAL WALL

ABDOMINAL WALL MASSES

Lesions found within the superficial abdominal wall include inflammatory lesions, hematomas, neoplasms, hernias, and postsurgical lesions. Symmetry of the rectus sheath muscles is a key factor in determining if an abdominal wall mass is present. The higher-resolution transducers may help the sonographer distinguish between the amount of fat and muscle present and an abnormal lesion.

Lymphoceles. A lymphocele is a collection of fluid that occurs after surgery in the pelvis, retroperitoneum, or recess cavities.

Sonographic Findings. Lymphoceles generally look like loculated, simple fluid collections, although they may have a more complex, usually septated, morphology. Differentiation from loculated ascites is usually possible because the mass effect of a lymphocele that is under tension displaces the surrounding organs. Differentiation from other fluid collections is mainly made by aspiration.

EXTRAPERITONEAL HEMATOMA

Extraperitoneal rectus sheath hematomas are acute or chronic collections of blood lying either within the rectus muscle or between the muscle and its sheath. They occur as the result of direct trauma, pregnancy, cardiovascular and degenerative muscle diseases, surgical injury, anticoagulation therapy, steroids, or extreme exercise.

Clinically the patient may present with acute, sharp, persistent nonradiating pain.

Hematomas are caused by surgical injury to tissue or by blunt trauma to the abdomen. Laboratory values may show a decrease in hematocrit and red blood cell count; the patient may go into shock.

Sonographic Findings. On ultrasound examination, the sonographer notices an asymmetry between the rectus sheath muscles. The hematoma may appear as an anechoic mass with scattered internal echoes.

The sonographic appearance depends on the stage of the bleed. Acute bleeds are primarily cystic, with some debris and blood clots; as the blood begins to organize and clot, the mass becomes more "solid" in appearance. Newly formed clots may be very homogeneous. Hematomas can become infected and at any stage may be sonographically indistinguishable from abscesses. They may mimic subphrenic fluid.

Bladder-Flap Hematoma. A bladder-flap hematoma is a collection of blood between the bladder and lower-uterine

segment, resulting from a lower-uterine transverse cesarean section and bleeding from the uterine vessels.

Subfascial Hematoma. A subfascial hematoma is found in the prevesicular space and is caused by a disruption of the inferior epigastric vessels or their branches during a cesarean section.

INFLAMMATORY LESION (ABSCESS)

An abscess or inflammation in the abdominal wall may occur after surgery. The sonogram may show cystic, complex, or solid characteristics. Generally the masses are very superficial and are easy to locate and needle aspirate with ultrasound guidance if necessary. A high-frequency, linear array transducer should be used to image the superficial area.

The patient may present with leukocytosis, **septicemia**, or a previous history of **pyogenic** infection.

Sonographic Findings. On ultrasound examination, an abdominal wall abscess presents as an anechoic or echoic mass with internal echoes from debris. The mass usually has irregular margins and shape. It may have gas bubbles within that show shadowing on the ultrasound image.

NEOPLASM OR PERITONEAL THICKENING

Neoplasms of the abdominal wall include lipomas, desmoid tumors, or metastases. The desmoid tumor is a benign fibrous neoplasm of aponeurotic structures. It most commonly occurs in relation to the rectus abdominis and its sheath (Figure 13-23). The tumor may present as hypoechoic to cystic (except lipomas).

Sonographic Findings. On ultrasound examination, a desmoid tumor presents as anechoic to hypoechoic, with smooth and sharply defined walls.

The peritoneal lining is not seen as a distinct structure during sonography unless it is thickened. This is usually secondary to metastatic implants or to direct extension of the tumor from the viscera or mesentery. Primary mesotheliomas occur rarely.

HERNIA

An abdominal hernia is the protrusion of a peritoneal-lined sac through a defect in the weakened abdominal wall (Figure 13-24). The viscera beneath the weakened tissue may protrude, resulting in a hernia. The most common areas of weakness are the umbilical area and the femoral and inguinal rings. (The inguinal hernia is discussed in Chapter 19.) An incarcerated hernia is one that cannot be "reduced" or pushed back into the abdominal cavity. Complications may arise if edema develops or if the opening constricts so much that the protrusion cannot be placed back into position.

Strangulation (interruption of the blood supply) of the bowel can also occur in an incarcerated hernia that is not surgically repaired in a timely manner. This bowel can become necrotic and require resection.

The abdominal wall hernia consists of three parts: the sac, the contents of the sac, and the covering of the sac. Common locations for hernias are umbilical (congenital or acquired),

Figure 13-23   A and **B,** Gross pathology of a desmoid tumor of the abdominal wall. (From Damjanov I: *Pathology: a color atlas,* St. Louis, 2000, Mosby.)

Figure 13-24   Femoral hernia causing a bulging enlargement of the femoral canal. (From McMinn: *Functional and clinical anatomy,* St. Louis, 1999, Mosby.)

epigastric, inguinal, femoral, and at the separation of the rectus abdominis. The hernia may involve the omentum only or it may mimic other masses. The hernia commonly originates near the junction of the linea semilunaris and arcuate line in the paraumbilical area.

Epigastric hernias are found in the widest part of the linea alba between the xiphoid process and the umbilicus. This hernia is usually filled with fat, which over the years may carry a piece of omentum along with it.

A spigelian hernia is a variant of the ventral hernia, which is found more laterally in the abdominal wall.

Sonographic Findings. Many hernias are palpable and do not require sonographic evaluation. However, if the mass is not well defined on physical examination, ultrasound evaluation may be helpful. If a hernia is suspected, the sonographer will note an interruption of the peritoneal line separating the muscles and abdominal contents.

Sonography may outline the contents of the mass where it is fluid-filled or contains peristaltic bowel or mesenteric fat. If a hernia is suspected, the sonographer should look for a peristalsing bowel within the mass, although the peristalsis may be absent with incarceration. If the hernia is not readily apparent, the patient may be asked to lift the head or to strain (Valsalva maneuver) to see if the mass moves or changes shape.

The sonographic criteria for a hernia include: (1) demonstration of an abdominal wall defect, (2) presence of bowel loops or mesenteric fat within a lesion, (3) exaggeration of the lesion with strain (Valsalva), and (4) reducibility of the lesion by gentle pressure.

BIBLIOGRAPHY

Dahnert W: *Radiology review manual,* ed 3, Philadelphia, 1996, Williams & Wilkins.

Damjanov I, Linder J: *Pathology: a color atlas*, St. Louis, 2000, Mosby.

Diament MJ, Boerhat MI, Kangarloo H: Real-time sector ultrasound in the evaluation of suspected abnormalities of diaphragmatic motion, *J Clin Ultrasound* 13:539, 1985.

Golding RH, Li DKB, Cooperberg PL: Sonographic demonstration of air-fluid levels in abdominal abscesses, *J Ultrasound Med* 1:151, 1982.

Gooding GAW, Cummings SR: Sonographic detection of ascites in liver disease, *J Ultrasound Med* 3:169, 1984.

Gould BE: *Pathophysiology for the health professions*, ed 2, Philadelphia, 2002, WB Saunders Co.

Kawamura DM: *Abdomen and superficial structures*, ed 2, Philadelphia, 1997, Lippincott.

Kordan B, Payne SD: Fat necrosis simulating a primary tumor of the mesentery: sonographic diagnosis, *J Ultrasound Med* 7:345, 1988.

Marchal G and others: Sonographic appearance of normal lymph nodes, *J Ultrasound Med* 4:417, 1985.

McMinn RMH, Gaddum-Rosse P, Hutchings RT and others: *McMinn's functional & clinical anatomy*, St. Louis, 1995, Mosby.

Mittelstaedt CA: *General ultrasound*, New York, 1992, Churchill Livingstone.

Morton MJ, Charboneau JW, Banks PM: Inguinal lymphadenopathy simulating a false aneurysm on color-flow Doppler sonography, *Am J Roentgenol* 151:115, 1988.

O'Neil JD and others: Cystic mesothelioma of the peritoneum, *Radiology* 170:333, 1989.

Savage PE, Joseph AEA, Adam EJ: Massive abdominal wall hematoma: real-time ultrasound localization of bleeding, *J Ultrasound Med* 4:157, 1985.

Wu CC and others: Sonographic features of tuberculous omental cakes in peritoneal tuberculosis, *J Clin Ultrasound* 16:195, 1988.

Yeh HC, Halton KP, Gray CE: Anatomic variations and abnormalities in the diaphragm seen with ultrasound, *Radiographics* 10:1019, 1990.

CHAPTER 14

Abdominal Applications of Ultrasound Contrast Agents

Daniel A. Merton

KEY TERMS

acoustic emission – occurs when an appropriate level of acoustic energy is applied to the tissue, the microbubbles first oscillate and then rupture; the rupture of the microbubbles results in random Doppler shifts appearing as a transient mosaic of colors on a color Doppler display

acute tubular necrosis (ATN) – acute damage to the renal tubules; usually due to ischemia associated with shock

contrast-enhanced sonography (CES) – agent used to reduce or eliminate some of the current limitations of ultrasound imaging and Doppler blood flow detection color flow imaging

first generation agents – agents containing room air (i.e., Albunex)

focal nodular hyperplasia – liver tumors with an abundance of Kupffer cells; sonographically, they are isoechoic to the surrounding normal liver tissue

gray scale harmonic imaging – allows detection of contrast-enhanced blood flow and organs with grayscale ultrasound; in the harmonic-imaging mode, the echoes from the oscillating microbubbles have a higher signal-to-noise ratio than found in conventional ultrasound; regions with microbubbles (e.g., blood vessels and organ parenchyma) are better visualized

harmonic imaging (HI) – in the HI mode, the ultrasound system is configured to receive only echoes at the second harmonic frequency, which is twice the transmit frequency

hepatocellular carcinoma – a common liver malignancy related to cirrhosis; the carcinoma may present as a solitary massive tumor, multiple nodules throughout the liver, or diffuse infiltrative masses in the liver; HCC can be very invasive

induced acoustic emission – after the injection of the tissue-specific UCA Sonazoid, the reflectivity of the contrast-containing tissue increases; when the right level of acoustic energy is applied to tissue, the contrast microbubbles eventually rupture, resulting in random Doppler shifts; these shifts appear as a transient mosaic of colors on the color Doppler display; masses that have destroyed or replaced normal Kupffer cells will be displayed as color-free areas

intravenous injection – a hypodermic injection into a vein for the purpose of injecting a contrast medium

mechanical index (MI) – an index that defines the low acoustic output power that can be used to minimize the destruction of microbubbles by energy in the acoustic field; when the microbubbles in microbubble-based ultrasound contrast agents are destroyed, contrast enhancement is lost

molecular imaging agents – agents include Optison, Definity, Imagent, Levovist, SonoVue

portal hypertension – caused by increased resistance to venous flow through the liver; sonographic findings include dilation of the portal, splenic, and mesenteric veins; reversal of portal venous blood flow; and the development of collateral vessels

renal artery stenosis (RAS) – narrowing of the renal artery; historically, this has been very difficult to evaluate sonographically

second generation agents – agents containing heavy gases (i.e., Optison)

TIPS – transjugular intrahepatic portosystemic shunt

tissue-specific ultrasound contrast agent – a type of contrast agent whose microbubbles are removed from the blood and are taken up by specific tissues in the body; one example is the agent Sonozoid

ultrasound contrast agents (UCAs) – agents that can be administered intravenously to evaluate blood vessels, blood flow, and solid organs

vascular ultrasound contrast agents – a type of ultrasound contrast agent whose microbubbles are contained in the body's vascular spaces; examples of this type of agent include Optison, Definity, Imagent, Levovist, SonoVue

---

The use of contrast media has become a routine part of radiography, computed tomography (CT), and magnetic resonance imaging (MRI). The addition of contrast to these modalities has significantly increased their capabilities to the extent that in many cases contrast is an essential component of the diagnostic imaging examination. However, medical sonography has not benefited to the same degree from the potential of contrast agents. For more than two decades, there has been a sig-nificant amount of research conducted towards the development of **ultrasound contrast agents (UCAs)**.[58] Most of the work has centered on developing agents that can be administered intravenously to evaluate blood vessels, blood flow, and solid organs.

The clinical use of **contrast-enhanced sonography (CES)** is expected to reduce or eliminate some of the current limitations of ultrasound imaging and Doppler blood flow detection. These include limitations of spatial and contrast resolution on grayscale sonography, and the detection of low velocity blood flow and flow in very small vessels using Doppler flow detection modes that include color flow imaging (CFI) and pulsed Doppler with spectral analysis. Advances in ultrasound equipment technology following the development of ultrasound contrast agents have resulted in new "contrast-specific" imaging mode, including grayscale methods, that allow detection of blood flow without the limitations of Doppler. Ultrasound contrast agents hold the promise of improving the sensitivity and specificity of current ultrasound diagnoses and have the potential of expanding sonography's already broad range of clinical applications.

TYPES OF ULTRASOUND CONTRAST AGENTS

VASCULAR ULTRASOUND CONTRAST AGENTS

Sonographic detection of blood flow is limited by many factors, including the depth and size of a vessel, the attenuation properties of intervening tissue, and low-velocity flow. Limitations of ultrasound equipment sensitivity and the operator dependence of Doppler are also factors that may affect the results of a vascular examination. Vascular or blood-pool ultrasound contrast agents enhance Doppler (color and spectral) flow signals by adding more and better acoustic scatterers to the bloodstream (Figures 14-1 and 14-2). This results in improved

A   **B**

Figure 14-1   Color Doppler imaging of a patient's right renal artery before (**A**) and after (**B**) administration of a vascular UCA. Note the increased visualization of flow in the renal artery *(arrows)* after intravenous injection of contrast. In this case no vascular abnormality was detected.

Figure 14-2 Color flow imaging and spectral Doppler analysis of renal artery flow. **A,** Before contrast, the spectral waveforms are weak and there is minimal color flow information. **B,** After intravenous administration of a contrast, the spectral wave forms have a higher signal intensity, and additional color flow information is provided.

Figure 14-3 Power Doppler imaging of a normal right kidney before (**A**) and after (**B**) injection of a vascular UCA. Note the improved demonstration of flow in the renal parenchyma after intravenous injection of contrast.

detection of blood flow from vessels which, without the use of contrast agents, are often difficult to assess, such as the renal arteries, intracranial vessels, and small capillaries within organs (i.e., tissue perfusion) (Figure 14-3). In addition to enhancing Doppler signals, some vascular agents improve grayscale ultrasound visualization of flowing blood and demonstrate changes to the grayscale echogenicity of tissues. Advanced ultrasound modes, such as harmonic imaging, further improve the sonographic detection of contrast within solid organs.

The concept of ultrasound contrast agents was first introduced in 1968 by Gramiak and Shah, who injected agitated saline directly into the ascending aorta and cardiac chambers during echocardiographic examinations.[31] The microbubbles formed by agitation resulted in strong reflections arising from

within the normally echo-free lumen of the aorta and chambers of the heart. Eventually, other solutions were discovered that could produce similar contrast effects. Further investigation found that the microbubbles produced by simple agitation are nonuniform in size and relatively large and unstable, making them unsuitable for sonographic evaluations of the left heart and systemic circulation because the microbubbles do not persist through passage of the pulmonary and cardiac circulation. Furthermore, to provide contrast enhancement, agitated saline required direct injection into the vessel under evaluation (e.g., the aorta) and a more clinically practical administration method, such as intravenous (IV) injection, was desired.

Numerous attempts have been made to encapsulate gas to make a more suitable microbubble-based ultrasound contrast

TABLE 14-1	CONTRAST AGENTS AND MANUFACTURER

Agent	Manufacturer
Optison™	Amersham Health, Oslo
Definity™	Bristol Myers Squibb, N. Billerica, Mass.
Imagent®	Alliance Pharmaceutical Corp., San Diego
Levovist™	Schering AG, Berlin
SonoVue™	Bracco Diagnostics, Milan

agent that can be administered intravenously. For an agent to be clinically useful it should be nontoxic; have microbubbles or microparticles that are small enough to traverse the pulmonary capillary beds (i.e., less than 8 microns in size); and be stable enough to provide multiple recirculations. A number of agents possess these desirable traits, and presently there are several microbubble-based ultrasound agents commercially available worldwide.

Currently, in the United States, the following agents are available and approved by the Food and Drug Administration (FDA) for use in echocardiography: Optison, Definity, and Imagent. Several other transpulmonary agents including Levovist and SonoVue are available in Europe, Asia, and elsewhere. A number of other agents are currently in various stages of clinical trials[40] (Table 14-1).

Described below are several vascular ultrasound contrast agents that have been approved for clinical applications. These details are provided to demonstrate the diversity of approaches used to produce the ultrasound contrast agents. This is not a complete list of all agents that are currently approved for clinical use or in development.

In 1994 Albunex (Mallinckrodt Medical Inc., St. Louis) was the first UCA in the United States to receive FDA approval for use in echocardiography applications. Albunex consists of 5% sonicated human serum albumin (HSA) microspheres containing room air. After IV injection, Albunex reportedly enhanced the detection of blood flow in the heart chambers and improved endocardial border definition (EBD).[14] However, in a large percentage of patients studied, contrast enhancement was limited, particularly in the apex of the left ventricle and during systole. These limitations, combined with the development and availability of more robust agents, eventually led to the removal of Albunex from the market.

The specific type of gas contained within an ultrasound contrast agent microbubble and the composition of its shell influence the microbubble's acoustic behavior (e.g., reflectivity and elasticity), method of metabolism, and its stability within the blood pool.[82] In 1998 Optison (FSO 69) became the second commercially available ultrasound contrast agent in the United States. Like Albunex, the microbubble shell of Optison is 5% human serum albumin. However, unlike the low–molecular-weight, air-filled microbubbles of Albunex, Optison contains a high-molecular weight gas (perfluoropropane), which improves the stability and plasma longevity of the agent. Agents containing room air are commonly

referred to as "first-generation" ultrasound contrast agents, whereas agents containing heavy gases are referred to as "second-generation" agents. Optison has shown potential for use with grayscale harmonic imaging and Doppler modes for echocardiography, systemic vascular, tumor characterization, and abdominal applications.[20,22,42,83]

Levovist (SHU-508A) is another transpulmonary ultrasound contrast agent approved for clinical use in several European countries and Australia. The shell of Levovist consists of 99.9% galactose microparticles with 0.1% palmitic acid. A significant amount of work has been done using Levovist since its European debut in 1996, and there are numerous published reports on its use. Experiments in animals and humans have demonstrated that Levovist can provide contrast enhancement in excess of 3 minutes' duration.[28] Human trials with Levovist have demonstrated its ability to enhance color and spectral Doppler flow signals from both normal and tumor vessels.[5,10,13,64] Temporal measurements of Levovist uptake and washout have been reported in the evaluation of breast masses.[36] This represents a unique quality of contrast-enhanced sonography that may have the potential to help differentiate benign from malignant tumors. Contrast kinetics appears to vary between malignant and benign breast tumors, with a much faster washout seen in malignancies (likely as a result of intratumoral arteriovenous shunts). More research is being conducted to confirm these findings and to evaluate this potential in other applications.

In addition to the more common bolus method of administration, Levovist has also been administered via slow infusion. Albrecht and colleagues have shown that the infusion of Levovist results in contrast enhancement lasting as much as 12 minutes or more compared with slightly more than 2 minutes with a bolus injection.[2] The additional enhancement time provided by the infusion of contrast would likely be useful for difficult and time-consuming evaluations of vessels, such as the renal arteries. Infusion of Definity has also been approved by the FDA and evaluated in clinical trials.[34]

SonoVue (BR-1) is an aqueous suspension of phospholipid-stabilized sulfur hexafluoride (SF-6) microbubbles having a low solubility in blood.[33] SonoVue enhances the echogenicity of blood and provides opacification of the cardiac chambers, resulting in improved left ventricular endocardial border detection. In clinical trials it has been shown to increase ultrasound's accuracy in the detection or exclusion of abnormalities in intracranial, extracranial carotid, and peripheral arteries. SonoVue also increases the quality of Doppler flow signals and the duration of clinically-useful signal enhancement in portal vein assessments. SonoVue improves the detection of liver and breast lesion vascularity, resulting in more specific lesion characterization.[73,74] SonoVue has been approved for use in Europe for echocardiography and macrovascular applications. In the United States, SonoVue has completed clinical trials and its FDA status is pending.

TISSUE-SPECIFIC ULTRASOUND CONTRAST AGENTS

The kinetics of ultrasound contrast agent microbubbles following IV injection are complex, and each agent has its own unique characteristics.[6] In general, after IV administration the agents are contained exclusively in the body's vascular spaces. In general, when a vascular agent's microbubbles are ruptured or otherwise destroyed, the microbubble shell products are metabolized or eliminated by the body, and the gas is exhaled.[82]

Tissue-specific ultrasound contrast agents differ from vascular agents in that the microbubbles are removed from the blood pool and taken up by or have an affinity towards specific tissues (e.g., the reticuloendothelial system in the liver and spleen or a thrombus). Over time, the presence of contrast microbubbles within or attached to the tissue changes its sonographic appearance. By changing the signal impedance (or other acoustic characteristics) of normal and abnormal tissue, these agents improve the detection of abnormalities and permit more specific sonographic diagnoses. Tissue-specific ultrasound contrast agents are typically administered by IV injection. Some tissue-specific agents also enhance the sonographic detection of blood flow and therefore are potentially multipurpose. Because tissue-specific ultrasound contrast agents target specific types of tissue and their behavior is predictable, they can be considered in the category of **molecular imaging agents.**[52]

Sonazoid (NC100100, Amersham Health, Oslo) is a tissue-specific ultrasound contrast agent that contains microbubbles of perfluorobutane gas in a stable lipid shell.[40] After being injected intravenously, Sonazoid behaves as a vascular agent (i.e., it enhances the detection of flowing blood) and over time the microbubbles are phagocytised by the reticuloendothelial system (macrophage Kupffer cells) of the liver and spleen.[6] The intact microbubbles may remain stationary in the tissue for several hours. When insonated after uptake, the stationary contrast microbubbles increase the reflectivity of the contrast-containing tissue. If an appropriate level of acoustic energy is applied to the tissue, the microbubbles first oscillate (emitting harmonic signals that can be detected with grayscale harmonic imaging) and then rupture. The rupture of the microbubbles results in random Doppler shifts appearing as a transient mosaic of colors on a color Doppler display (Figure 14-4). This effect has been termed "induced acoustic emis-sion," "stimulated acoustic emission," or simply "**acoustic emission.**"[25,32] By exploiting the color Doppler depicted acoustic emission phenomenon, masses that have destroyed or replaced the normal Kupffer cells will be displayed as color-free areas and thus become more sonographically conspicuous. These same acoustic emission effects can also be demonstrated using grayscale harmonic imaging (see harmonic imaging discussion)[21,32] (Figure 14-5).

Initial work using VX-2 tumors grown in the livers of rabbits has clearly demonstrated the capability of Sonazoid's acoustic emission characteristics to improve detection of small tumors that were not detectable before the injection of contrast.[21] The acoustic emission effect is not unique to Sonazoid. Other ultrasound contrast agents have been found to demonstrate this effect, including Levovist. However, the effect with Levovist is very short-lived, and it is unclear whether there is true reticuloendothelial system uptake of Levovist microparticles or if they are simply trapped within the vascular sinusoids.[32]

It is important to remember that the acoustic emission effects are independent of contrast motion. In other words, the acoustic emission effect can result from oscillation and eventual rupture of stationary contrast microbubbles, and agents that demonstrate the acoustic emission phenomenon also can be used for nonvascular applications where there is little or no movement of the microbubbles.

Currently, tissue-specific agents that are taken up by the reticuloendothelial system appear to be most useful in the assessment of patients with suspected liver abnormalities, including the ability both to detect and to characterize liver tumors using contrast-enhanced sonography. However, the

Figure 14-5 Gray scale harmonic imaging display of the acoustic emission *(AE)* effect after IV injection of a tissue-specific UCA. As the acoustic energy traverses through the liver parenchyma, it causes the contrast microbubbles to rupture resulting in a characteristic wave of intense echoes *(arrows)*. The normal echogenicity of the liver parenchyma in the near field *(N)* is restored after the microbubbles have ruptured, whereas deep to the AE wave the contrast-enhanced tissue *(CE)* remains echogenic because of the presence of intact microbubbles. This effect is dramatic when visualized in real time.

Figure 14-4 Color Doppler imaging display of acoustic emission *(AE)* after IV injection of a tissue-specific UCA. The rupture of contrast microbubbles present within the RES cells of the liver results in the characteristic random color display.

Figure 14-6   Transverse view of the pancreas after administration of an oral UCA. The contrast-filled stomach *(C)* provides an acoustic window that enhances visualization of the normal pancreatic tail *(PT)*.

properties that permit the microbubbles of one ultrasound contrast agent to be taken up by the reticuloendothelial system while the microbubbles of other agents are not have not been fully identified thus far.[6] Other target or tissue-specific agents are being developed to enhance the detection of thrombi and tumors.

ORAL ULTRASOUND CONTRAST AGENTS

Limitations to the sonographic assessment of the upper abdomen include patient obesity and the presence of gas-filled bowel, which can produce shadowing artifacts. Ingestion of degassed water has been used to improve sonographic examinations of the upper abdominal and retroperitoneal structures such as the pancreas.[50] However, water simply displaces gas and traverses the gastrointestinal tract in an inconsistent and unpredictable manner.

Oral contrast agents have been developed for sonographic applications. SonoRx (Bracco Diagnostics, Princeton, NJ) is an oral UCA that contains simethicone-coated cellulose as its active ingredient.[7,50] Ingestion of SonoRx results in a homogeneous transmission of sound through the contrast-filled stomach (Figure 14-6). Clinical trials have shown that the administration of SonoRx increases the diagnostic capabilities of ultrasound and, at times, obviates the need for additional imaging studies including CT or MRI.[7] Although SonoRx was approved by the United States FDA in 1998 and was commercially available, it is no longer being marketed in the United States.

ULTRASOUND EQUIPMENT MODIFICATIONS

Microbubble-based ultrasound contrast agents enhance the detection of blood flow when used with conventional ultrasound imaging techniques, including gray scale sonography and Doppler techniques (i.e., color flow imaging and Doppler spectral analysis). However, research and experience have led to a better understanding of the complex interactions between acoustic energy (i.e., the ultrasound beam) and ultrasound contrast agent microbubbles, which in turn has led to advances in ultrasound instrumentation. The use of these new "contrast-specific" ultrasound imaging modes can improve the clinical utility of contrast-enhanced sonography. Because current ultrasound system platforms are digital, software-driven changes can be implemented relatively quickly.

Harmonic imaging (HI) uses the same broadband transducers used for conventional sonography. However, in harmonic imaging mode, the ultrasound system is configured to receive only echoes at the second harmonic frequency, which is twice the transmit frequency (e.g., 7.0 MHz for a 3.5 MHz transducer).[18,43] When using a microbubble-based ultrasound contrast agent, the microbubbles oscillate (i.e., they get larger and smaller) when subjected to the acoustic energy present in the ultrasound field. The reflected echoes from the oscillating microbubbles contain energy components at the fundamental frequency and at the higher and lower harmonics (subharmonics). The majority of the development efforts involving harmonic imaging have focused on grayscale harmonic imaging, which allows detection of contrast enhancement of blood flow and organs with grayscale ultrasound. The use of gray scale harmonic imaging contrast-enhanced sonography avoids many of the limitations and artifacts encountered when using Doppler techniques and ultrasound contrast agents, such as angle dependence and "color blooming" artifacts.[19] In the harmonic imaging mode, the echoes from the oscillating microbubbles have a higher signal-to-noise ratio than would be provided by using conventional ultrasound so that regions with microbubbles (e.g., blood vessels and organ parenchyma) are more easily appreciated visually. Although body tissue also generates harmonic signals, compared with those from microbubbles, their contribution to the image is negligible. Recent advances in HI technology (e.g., wide-band HI, phase-inversion HI, and pulse-inversion HI) employ image processing algorithms to subtract echoes arising from stationary tissue, whereas echoes arising from moving scatterers (i.e., microbubbles) are preferentially displayed.[43] Thus wide-band gray scale harmonic imaging provides a way to better differentiate areas with and without contrast and has the potential to demonstrate real-time gray scale blood pool imaging (i.e., "perfusion imaging"). In the author's experience, the benefits of using gray scale harmonic imaging for contrast-enhanced sonography (e.g., higher frame rates, improved contrast resolution, reduced artifacts) are so great that conventional (non-HI) color flow imaging is neither necessary nor advised.

Harmonic Doppler ultrasound modes (e.g., harmonic power Doppler imaging and power modulation imaging) have also been developed. Preliminary investigations with harmonic Doppler modes have identified some potential benefits, including enhanced detection of very low velocity blood flow in organs and suppression of color "flash" artifacts.[15]

When using microbubble-based ultrasound contrast agents, the energy present within the acoustic field can have a detrimental effect on the contrast microbubbles.[9] A significant number of the microbubbles can be destroyed by the acoustic pressure even though the actual pressure contained within the ultrasound field is relatively low. Some ultrasound contrast agents are more prone to this phenomenon than others. Once the microbubble is destroyed, contrast enhancement is no longer provided. This reduces the clinical utility and duration of contrast enhancement. Several approaches have been used to minimize this problem. One relatively easy technique is to use a low acoustic output power as defined by the **mechanical index (MI).**[65] Low-MI ultrasound is a useful technique for a variety of contrast-enhanced sonographic applications, including assessment of liver tumors. However, reducing the MI also limits tissue penetration, so this is not always an adequate solution. Furthermore, the MI may be an imprecise predictor of the effect of acoustic energy on contrast microbubbles.[32]

Equipment manufacturers have recently begun to incorporate intermittent imaging capabilities into their systems to provide an additional option to the user seeking to reduce microbubble destruction during contrast-enhanced examinations.[43,65] In this mode the system is gated to only transmit and receive data at predetermined intervals. The gating may be triggered on a specific portion of the ECG (e.g., the r-wave) or a time interval, such as once or twice per second. Intermittent imaging reduces the exposure of contrast microbubbles to the acoustic energy and allows additional microbubbles to enter the field between signal transmissions. The additional microbubbles then contribute to an even greater increase in reflectivity of the contrast-containing blood or tissue than would be possible by continuous real-time imaging. A disadvantage to intermittent imaging is its lack of a real-time display of data; however, recent advances in instrumentation, such as "flash echocardiography," have begun to address this drawback.[62] This same effect can be obtained by using "frame-one imaging" during contrast-enhanced sonography.[51] Frame-one imaging (also known as *interval delay imaging*) is performed by hitting the freeze control (thus stopping transmission of the ultrasound beam), waiting 5 to 10 seconds for the tissue to fill with contrast, then resuming real-time imaging and quickly freezing the image again. When the cine-loop is reviewed, there will be enhanced echogenicity of contrast-containing tissues on the first one or two frames (Figure 14-7). Intermittent imaging can be combined with wide-band harmonic imaging to further improve the clinical utility of contrast-enhanced sonography.

Moriyasu and others used an intermittent imaging for contrast-enhanced sonography of hepatic tumors.[54] This study showed that the signal intensity is dependent on an interscan delay time during which the acoustic power is lowered under the threshold for passive cavitation of the microbubbles. Another study by Sirlin and others demonstrated that intermittent imaging improves image contrast resolution and that a one-frame-per-second rate has greater contrast resolution than is provided by continuous real-time imaging.[71]

Other system modifications in development include onboard video densitometry, calculation of the integrated backscatter from contrast, and advanced three-dimensional (3-D) imaging (Figures 14-8 and 14-9). Furthermore, the administration of contrast provides the capability to measure the transit time of contrast-containing blood through normal and diseased tissue, blood volume estimates, and tissue perfusion.[4,38,80] Systems will likely be developed that will allow onboard calculation of these unique contrast-specific measurements and calculations provided by the use of ultrasound contrast agents. In the future, additional advancements can be expected, including modifications to the operator interfaces of ultrasound equipment to facilitate routine clinical use of contrast.

CLINICAL APPLICATIONS

HEPATIC APPLICATIONS

Sonographic evaluation of hepatic lesions and other hepatic abnormalities is limited. Although ultrasound is usually sensitive for the detection of medium to large hepatic lesions, it is

A   **B**

Figure 14-7   Enhanced detection of a hypervascular renal tumor using harmonic imaging and interval delay imaging. **A,** A transverse ultrasound image obtained precontrast demonstrates the aorta *(A)* and a suspicious contour defect *(arrow)* near the lower pole of the left kidney. **B,** After IV contrast administration using gray scale harmonic imaging and a manual interval delay, the aorta is filled with contrast and there is increased echogenicity of the suspicious area compared with the normal renal parenchyma. The suspicious area represented a renal cell carcinoma.

Figure 14-8 Contrast-enhanced 3-D PDI of a kidney in an animal model. Note the fine detail of the renal vasculature.

Figure 14-9 The combination of 3-D gray scale harmonic imaging and administration of a vascular UCA results in an "ultrasound angiogram."

limited in its ability to detect small (<10mm), isoechoic, and/or peripherally located lesions, particularly in obese patients or patients with diffuse liver disease. Furthermore, sonography is not as effective as CT or MRI for characterization of hepatic tumors.

Hepatic ultrasound blood flow studies are limited by low velocity blood flow (e.g., in cases of portal hypertension) or for the detection of flow in the intrahepatic artery branches. Ultrasound contrast agents have shown the potential to improve the accuracy of hepatic sonography, including enhanced detection and characterization of hepatic masses and improved detection of intrahepatic and extrahepatic blood flow.

Hepatic Blood Flow. Vascular ultrasound contrast agents have been shown to improve the detection of hepatic blood flow in normal subjects and patients with liver disease and portal hypertension.[1,45,68] Most sonographic examinations for portal hypertension include qualitative assessment of blood flow with color flow imaging to identify the presence and direction of flow in the splenic and superior mesenteric veins, along with the main portal vein and the intrahepatic portal and hepatic veins. When scanning patients with portal hypertension, slow moving portal flow can be difficult to detect. In these cases an ultrasound contrast agent could potentially be used to increase the reflectivity of portal vein blood, thus enhancing its ability to be detected sonographically. The addition of contrast during the ultrasound evaluations of patients with portal hypertension could potentially also improve the detection of portal-systemic collaterals and evaluations of surgically created portosystemic shunts, and improve the confidence of diagnoses in cases of complete or partial portal-system thrombosis.

In a study of both normal volunteers and patients with cirrhosis, Sellars and others found that Doppler flow signals from the portal vein were enhanced in all cases after administration of Levovist.[68] This study compared the duration of enhancement provided by a bolus administration to that of three different infusion rates (slow, medium, and fast). A bolus delivery provided the shortest duration of contrast enhancement, whereas the slow infusion technique provided the longest duration. Contrast enhancement persisted for 113 seconds (mean duration) after a bolus injection compared with as much as 569 seconds (mean duration) following a slow infusion.

Contrast-enhanced sonography has also been used effectively in the assessment of flow through transjugular intrahepatic portosystemic shunts (**TIPS**).[72,78] Uggowitzer and others found that Levovist provided Doppler signal enhancement lasting from 30 seconds to 7 minutes, and Levovist-enhanced scans improved the diagnosis of stent stenosis compared with the conventional ultrasound examinations.[78]

Other studies suggest that contrast-enhanced sonography is useful for evaluation of liver transplant recipients.[49,69,70] Leutoff and others reported their findings of 21 patients (31 examinations) who received orthotopic liver transplants.[49] After Levovist was administered, significantly better arterial flow signals were detected in the porta hepatis and in the right and left lobes of the liver. The authors concluded that the use of contrast-enhanced color flow imaging significantly improved the detection of hepatic arterial flow in transplant recipients. This is a clinically important application of contrast-enhanced sonography because of the frequent use of sonography to evaluate organ recipients in the immediate postoperative period. Although x-ray angiography remains the gold-standard imaging examination to assess patency of the transplanted hepatic artery, it is invasive and not without potential complications. An ultrasound contrast agent used postoperatively could enhance the detection of hepatic artery flow and could potentially reduce the number of unnecessary angiograms.

Published reports have described contrast-enhanced sonography detectable alterations in blood flow transit time through the livers of patients with diffuse hepatic disease when compared with normal controls.[1,46,68] In cases of cirrhosis there is often reduced portal venous flow and a compensatory increase in hepatic artery flow. Albrecht and others reported that after

Figure 14-10   Contrast-enhanced demonstration of the various phases of hepatic blood flow. **A,** Twenty-five seconds after IV injection of an UCA, the first vessels to demonstrate contrast enhancement in the liver are the hepatic arteries *(arrows)* whereas the portal vein *(PV)* remains anechoic in the arterial phase. **B,** In this patient, the portal venous phase occurred 37 seconds after injection with contrast seen in the portal vein. **C,** In the late vascular phase at 71 seconds after injection, the liver parenchyma is becoming echogenic (i.e., contrast-enhanced; *CE*) and there is persistent enhancement of the major hepatic vessels *(arrow heads).*

IV injection of Levovist in patients with cirrhosis the arrival of contrast in the hepatic veins was 24 seconds compared to 49.8 seconds for normal controls.[1] The authors postulated that the increased hepatic artery flow in the cirrhotic patients resulted in the more rapid appearance of contrast in the hepatic veins. While preliminary reports appear promising, additional research in this intriguing application of CES is necessary.

Hepatic Tumors. Many patients who have hepatic tumors first identified sonographically eventually require a CT or MRI examination to better determine the extent of disease and to more accurately characterize the lesions. Using contrast-enhanced sonography, it is possible to distinguish the various phases of blood flow to and within the liver. In normal situations, after IV administration of an ultrasound contrast agent, contrast-enhanced flow in the hepatic artery is identified first (arterial or early vascular phase), followed by enhanced portal venous flow (portal venous phase). Detection of flow in the hepatic capillaries is identified later (late vascular phase) as a parenchymal blush (Figure 14-10). If a reticuloendothelial system-specific agent is used, identification of the delayed

enhancement phase representing the enhancement from the stationary microbubbles that have been phagocytosed by the reticuloendothelial system is possible.

Similar diagnostic criteria currently used for contrast-enhanced CT or MRI, including evaluation of the phase, degree, and pattern of vascularity in and around hepatic tumors, can also be applied to contrast-enhanced sonography.[35,47] In fact, contrast-enhanced sonography, because of its ability to image dynamic events in real-time, may prove to be better than CT or MRI in the evaluation of hemodynamics that occur in the various hepatic vascular phases. Numerous published reports suggest that contrast-enhanced sonography can improve the detection and characterization of liver lesions.*

Goldberg and others used NC100100 (Sonazoid), a tissue-specific agent, for evaluation of solid liver lesions.[27] Using power Doppler imaging in the vascular phase, enhanced detec-

*References 5, 17, 20, 21, 25, 27, 35, 39, 41, 42, 46, 47, 64, 73, 74, 77, 79, 83.

Figure 14-11   Improved detection and characterization of a liver hemangioma. **A,** A conventional ultrasound exam identified a poorly demarcated mass *(arrows)* in the right posterior lobe of the liver. **B,** After contrast administration using GSHI, there is pooling of contrast-containing blood at the periphery of the lesion and increased echogenicity of the normal liver parenchyma. This pattern is characteristic of hemangiomas.

tion of blood flow from vessels in and around hepatic tumors was demonstrated in all patients. In the delayed phase (10 to 30 minutes post UCA injection), there was increased echogenicity of the normal hepatic parenchyma and improved visualization of tumors that were not detected before contrast administration, including detection of tumors as small as 3 mm. Some lesions demonstrated an echogenic rim.

Blomley and others used Levovist to evaluate the detection of tumors using stimulated acoustic emission during ultrasound examinations of patients with known liver metastases.[5] They found that all metastases appeared as areas of reduced or absent acoustic emission on color Doppler imaging scans of the liver. No acoustic emission defects were observed in the livers of three control subjects. The lack of acoustic emission from the hepatic metastases improved the conspicuity of lesions and improved the detection of tumors, including detection of tumors not visualized using conventional sonography.

Cavernous hemangiomas are common benign solid neoplasms of the liver and are frequently detected during hepatic ultrasound examinations. Not all hemangiomas have the "classic" ultrasound appearance of a rounded, homogeneously hyperechoic mass with well-defined margins, nor can they be accurately characterized sonographically (Figure 14-11). Several recent reports have suggested that contrast-enhanced sonography can improve the assessment of hemangiomas.[74,81]

Weskott reported using ultrasound contrast and interval delay gray scale harmonic imaging in an attempt to identify the hemodynamic patterns most consistent with hemangiomas.[81] Fifteen atypical (i.e., hypoechoic) hemangiomas ranging in size from 8 mm to 45 mm were evaluated before and after bolus administration of Levovist. Correlation was made with CT or MRI. All small hemangiomas demonstrated near complete enhancement, with three of the small tumors possessing a central nonenhanced area. The time interval for refill of lesions less than 2 cm in size was under 4 seconds,

whereas larger lesions required up to 3 minutes to enhance. A few larger masses demonstrated areas that did not enhance, which the author suggested was a result of focal intratumoral thrombosis. Weskott[81] concluded that most atypical hemangiomas show rapid refilling of contrast, suggesting that their blood supply was via arteries. Early and late vascular phase imaging provided a means to accurately characterize hemangiomas sonographically.

SonoVue was used in another study of atypical hemangiomas reported by Solbiati and others.[74] Seven atypical hemangiomas (1.5 to 6.5 cm in size) were evaluated with gray scale harmonic imaging before and after bolus administration of contrast. Four lesions appeared hypoechoic or anechoic, whereas the other three were isoechoic and "almost undistinguishable" on baseline (unenhanced) ultrasound. Arterial, portal, and late vascular phase imaging was performed after contrast administration. In the arterial phase, all lesions demonstrated only peripheral enhancement. In the portal phase, and even more so in the late vascular phase, progressive centripetal filling lasting from 5 to 7 minutes was observed in all lesions. The lesions got progressively more echogenic over time, which permitted a confident diagnosis. The authors concluded that multiphase sonography was necessary for accurate diagnosis of atypical hemangiomas and that contrast-enhanced sonography has the potential to obviate the need for CT scans. They also suggested that contrast-enhanced multiphase imaging may be useful to sonographically characterize other hepatic lesions.

Several reports have described the contrast-enhanced sonographic appearance of hepatocellular carcinoma (HCC) as having intense enhancement in the early arterial phase and relatively rapid washout of contrast in the portal phase[37,73,83] (Figure 14-12). In our experience using a reticuloendothelial system-specific agent, HCC lesions can have a similar appearance to focal nodular hyperplasia (FNH) in the early arterial

Figure 14-12   Improved characterization of hepatocellular carcinoma *(HCC)* using a RES-specific UCA. **A,** A conventional ultrasound exam identified a mass *(arrows)* in the right posterior lobe of the liver having mixed echogenicity. **B,** After contrast administration using GSHI, the hepatic artery and portal veins filled with contrast *(arrow heads)* and the mass became brightly echogenic compared with the surrounding liver tissue in the arterial and portal venous phases. **C,** On delayed imaging, the lesion was hypoechoic compared with the surrounding liver tissue. This CES pattern is characteristic of HCC.

phase. However, on delayed phase imaging the HCC tumor will be hypoechoic relative to the surrounding normal liver tissue (because of the lack of Kupffer cells within the tumor), whereas FNH tumors, because they contain an abundance of Kupffer cells, will be isoechoic to the surrounding normal liver tissue (Figure 14-13). The central feeding artery and spoke-wheel radiating branches that are characteristic of FNH on a dynamic CT angio can also be depicted by contrast-enhanced sonography, which may help to differentiate HCC from FNH.[37,79]

Contrast-enhanced sonography has been shown to improve the detection and/or delineation of liver metastases[5] (Figure 14-14). However, accurate characterization of metastatic liver tumors with contrast-enhanced sonography can be problematic because the degree of vascularity in these lesions is related to the primary cancer.[83] Therefore, some metastatic liver lesions will be hypervascular, whereas others are hypovascular. One imaging characteristic of liver metastases that was identified during delayed-phase imaging using a reticuloendothelial system-specific ultrasound contrast agent is an echogenic rim around the tumor.[47] The echogenic rim is thought to reflect the higher concentration of Kupffer cells around metastases and/or a higher degree of contrast which

results from compression of the normal liver parenchyma around the metastases.[47]

By providing a means to detect and differentiate the various vascular enhancement patterns (e.g., degree, architecture, and phasicity) in and around hepatic lesions, contrast-enhanced sonography has the ability to improve characterization of liver lesions, including HCC, FNH, and hemangiomas. In the future, liver lesion characterization may prove to be one of the most clinically valuable radiological applications of contrast-enhanced sonography.

RENAL APPLICATIONS

Published reports have described the use of ultrasound contrast agents in a variety of renal applications, including the evaluation of suspected renal masses and renal artery stenosis.* These reports provide an indication as to what may be expected once vascular ultrasound contrast agents become available for widespread clinical use in the United States.

Renal Artery Stenosis (RAS).   The sonographic evaluation of the main and intrarenal renal arteries in patients with sus-

---

*References 11, 16, 44, 48, 51, 53, 56, 63, 80.

Figure 14-13 Improved characterization of focal nodular hyperplasia (FNH) using a RES-specific UCA.
A, A conventional ultrasound exam identified a hypoechoic mass *(arrow heads)* in the right anterior lobe of
the liver. **B,** After contrast administration using GSHI, the mass became brightly echogenic and
intratumoral vessels having a radiating spokelike pattern could be identified *(arrows)*. A central hypoechoic
area within the mass that did not enhance represents a scar. **C,** On delayed imaging the lesion was isoechoic
compared with the surrounding liver tissue. This CES pattern is characteristic of FNH.

pected **renal artery stenosis (RAS)** is fraught with problems. Because the main renal arteries are retroperitoneal in location, these vessels are typically difficult to evaluate sonographically. Signal attenuation over depth and the overlying bowel often limit sonographic visualization of the main renal arteries, particularly in the obese patient. A significant number of patients will have anatomical variations of the renal vasculature, including duplicate or accessory renal arteries, and these variations can be very difficult to identify using noncontrast ultrasound. Furthermore, there may be limited sonographic windows that can be used to view the renal arteries and these windows may not be in optimal locations from which to obtain adequate Doppler-to-flow angles. Ultrasound examinations for RAS are often time-consuming and are extremely operator dependent. These factors likely contribute to the wide variability reported in the accuracy of sonography when used for RAS examinations.[3,61]

By improving the signal intensity of Doppler flow signals and increasing the likelihood of obtaining adequate Doppler flow information, ultrasound contrast agents hold the promise of improving examinations of patients with suspected RAS[67] (Figure 14-15). Vascular contrast agents significantly increase the ability to visualize blood flow using color flow imaging and improve the intensity of spectral Doppler flow signals. Therefore, in cases where the renal arteries are not visualized or the spectral waveforms are of poor quality, the IV administration of contrast can improve the examination process and potentially reduce the number of technically inadequate or otherwise nondiagnostic examinations (see Figures 14-1 and 14-2).

Needleman reported on the use of contrast in Phase III clinical trials including evaluations of RAS.[56] In this series there were 12 kidneys with dual renal arteries identified with magnetic resonance angiography (MRA). Nine of these were correctly identified with contrast-enhanced sonography, whereas only two cases of dual renal arteries were identified before contrast administration. There were 12 confirmed cases of RAS, three (25%) of which were only detected with contrast-enhanced sonography.

Missouris and colleagues reported on the use of Levovist-enhanced sonography compared with angiography in the evaluation of 21 patients with suspected RAS.[53] Sensitivity and specificity for the detection of RAS improved from 85% and 79%, respectively, on noncontrast studies to 94% and 88% with the addition of Levovist. They also reported that the mean examination time was halved by the addition of Levovist. These studies suggest that the use of ultrasound contrast agents

Figure 14-14   Improved detection and delineation of a colorectal carcinoma liver metastasis. **A,** A transverse conventional ultrasound image at the level of the middle hepatic vein *(arrow)* did not identify the mass, which had been detected on a prior CT examination. **B,** After UCA administration using GSHI in the portal venous phase, there was increased echogenicity of the surrounding liver parenchyma, which resulted in improved delineation of the tumor *(arrow heads)*. Contrast-enhanced blood flow could also be identified in the hepatic vein *(arrow)* and small vessels within the mass *(short arrow)*. In this case, the patient was being evaluated for possible ultrasound-guided radiofrequency ablation of this nonresectable tumor, and the CES results enhanced the ability to identify the location of the tumor and its size and margins.

Figure 14-15   Transverse color Doppler images of the abdominal aorta and proximal left renal artery in a patient with suspected renal artery stenosis. **A,** Before intravenous administration of contrast flow in the aorta *(A)* and proximal-most renal artery *(arrow)* visualized, there is aliasing of the color flow display *(curved arrow)*. **B,** After injection of contrast, the stenotic vessel lumen *(arrows)* can be clearly visualized.

will improve the sonographic evaluations of patients with suspected RAS, while potentially reducing examination time.

Renal Masses.   Diagnostic sonography has been a reliable method of evaluating patients with renal masses, particularly in the differentiation of cystic from solid lesions. Sonography is usually accurate in its ability to identify large (greater than 2 cm) renal cell carcinomas and to identify a tumor thrombus in the renal veins and/or inferior vena cava (IVC). However, in a small percentage of cases sonography cannot identify small neoplasms or differentiate solid hypoechoic renal lesions from hemorrhagic cysts or other benign processes (Figure 14-16). Furthermore, normal anatomical variations, such as a promi-

nent column of Bertin or persistent fetal lobulation, may mimic renal tumors. In these cases other imaging studies, such as CT, MRI, or needle biopsy, may be indicated to make a definitive diagnosis.

By improving the detection of flow in the intrarenal vessels, ultrasound contrast agents may provide a means of identifying and demonstrating the normal renal vasculature and detecting the presence of lesions that distort the vascular architecture[51,63] (see Figure 14-7). Contrast is also likely to improve the detection of abnormal vessels present in renal tumors and to identify flow voids that result from a tumor thrombus in cases of renal vein or IVC involvement (Figures 14-17 and 14-18).

Figure 14-16   Improved characterization of a hypoechoic renal mass. **A,** On the precontrast power Doppler image, a hypoechoic mass *(arrows)* is visualized in the midpole of the right kidney. **B,** After injection of a vascular UCA, blood flow is demonstrated with PDI within the normal renal parenchyma but no flow was detected from within the mass *(arrow)*. The mass was later determined to represent a benign hemorrhagic cyst.

Figure 14-17   Power Doppler imaging *(PDI)* of a suspicious renal mass before and after IV administration of contrast. **A,** On the precontrast image, a subtle hypoechoic mass was identified near the lower pole of the left kidney, but PDI only demonstrates flow around the mass. **B,** After injection of contrast, there are significantly more flow signals detected including intratumoral flow. This was later confirmed as a renal cell carcinoma.

Renal Allografts. Sonography is routinely used to evaluate renal allografts. After renal transplantation, sonography is useful to detect and quantitate postsurgical fluid collections, identify urinary obstruction, and assess blood flow to and from the kidney. Sonography is also useful in the evaluation of intrarenal blood flow. **Acute tubular necrosis (ATN)** and/or acute organ rejection can result from a reduction of flow, which can be detected using conventional Doppler ultrasound techniques. When a vascular abnormality is suspected, angiography can provide a definitive diagnosis. However, angiography is invasive and the use of angiographic contrast can result in additional renal tissue damage.

The enhanced detection of blood flow provided by contrast-enhanced sonography has the potential to improve assess-

ment of the main renal artery and of the vein and iliac vessels to which these vessels are anastomosed. Contrast-enhanced sonography can also be expected to improve the detection and display of flow in the intrarenal vessels, which should enhance sonography's ability to identify areas within the allograft that may have a compromised flow. The use of contrast agents to evaluate intrarenal blood flow may permit better differentiation of regions that have decreased perfusion from true vascular defects resulting from a renal artery branch occlusion or acute rejection.[12]

SPLENIC APPLICATIONS

There are a few reports that describe the use of contrast-enhanced sonography in the evaluation of the spleen.[8,60]

Figure 14-18   Power Doppler imaging of a large renal cell carcinoma before and after IV administration of contrast. **A,** On the precontrast image, blood flow is only detected around the tumor *(T)* periphery. **B,** With contrast enhancement, there are significantly more flow signals detected including intratumoral flow.

Catalano and others studied 55 patients with a variety of suspected splenic abnormalities, including traumatic injuries and tumors.[8] The contrast-enhanced sonography results were compared with baseline (noncontrast) ultrasound, CT, or MRI. In this series, parenchymal injuries were detected with a sensitivity of 63% on baseline ultrasound, whereas the sensitivity improved to 89% after contrast-enhanced sonography. Parenchymal injuries included posttraumatic infarctions that were not identified on baseline ultrasound but were identified with contrast-enhanced sonography. Contrast-enhanced sonography also identified 35 of 39 proven focal lesions in patients with Hodgkin's disease, whereas baseline ultrasound detected only 23 lesions.

In another report, two pediatric patients were evaluated for traumatic splenic injuries.[60] In both cases contrast-enhanced sonography identified splenic hematomas that were not detected on unenhanced ultrasound scans. Contrast-enhanced ultrasound may prove to be a viable alternative to other diagnostic tests for the initial assessment and surveillance of patients with suspected splenic trauma.

PANCREATIC APPLICATIONS

Sonographic visualization of the pancreas is often hampered by the gland's deep location within the retroperitoneum and by the presence of overlying bowel. Although ingestion of water or oral ultrasound contrast agents has been shown to improve the visualization of the pancreas, currently there are no oral ultrasound contrast agents available, and therefore the potential benefits of oral agents will not be discussed here.

Several published reports describe the ability of microbubble-based ultrasound contrast agents to improve pancreatic sonographic evaluations.[55,57,66] Rickes and others compared contrast-enhanced power Doppler imaging to unenhanced grayscale ultrasound and power Doppler imaging in 137 patients suspected of having a pancreatic tumor.[66] Of the 137 patients, a normal pancreas was found in 10; 47 had pancreatic cancer; 41 had lesions associated with pancreatitis; 17 had

neuroendocrine tumors; 12 had cystic lesions of the pancreas; and 10 had other pancreatic diseases. The sensitivity of contrast-enhanced power Doppler imaging for the diagnosis of pancreatic carcinoma was 87% and its specificity was 94%. The corresponding values for chronic pancreatitis were 85% and 99%, respectively. The authors concluded that contrast-enhanced power Doppler imaging had a high sensitivity and specificity in the differential diagnosis of pancreatic tumors.

In Japan Numata and others evaluated the vascularity of autoimmune pancreatitis lesions with contrast-enhanced gray scale harmonic imaging in 6 patients and compared their findings with pathologic conditions.[57] The vascularity of 3 of the 6 lesions studied was also evaluated by contrast-enhanced sonography before and after treatment with corticosteroids. The pancreatic lesions exhibited mild (n = 1), moderate (n = 3), or marked (n = 2) enhancement almost throughout their entirety. The grade of lesion vascularity on the contrast-enhanced sonography images correlated with the pathologic grade of inflammation and inversely correlated with the grade of fibrosis associated with autoimmune pancreatitis. After steroid therapy, the vascularity of all treated lesions decreased. The authors concluded that contrast-enhanced sonography may be useful for evaluating the vascularity of autoimmune pancreatitis lesions and the therapeutic efficacy of steroid therapy.

OTHER APPLICATIONS

Other common abdominal and/or retroperitoneal applications of ultrasound include assessment of flow in the mesenteric arteries for mesenteric ischemia; assessment of flow in the aorta and iliac arteries to evaluate suspected aneurysms, stenoses, or dissections; and assessment of flow in the IVC for evaluation of filters or thromboses. Often these examinations are limited by the presence of overlying bowel and bowel gas or by the effects of signal attenuation due to the deep location of the vessels. Vascular ultrasound contrast agents have been used with success to improve the assessment of the abdominal vasculature and blood flow.[59]

In one published study, contrast-enhanced sonography was used for surveillance of aortic stent grafts.[24] Thirty patients were serially evaluated with contrast-enhanced sonography and the results were compared with either computed tomographic angiography (CTA) or magnetic resonance angiography (MRA) as the gold standard. All CTA- and MRA-detected endoleaks were also detected by contrast-enhanced sonography (yielding a 100% sensitivity for contrast-enhanced sonography). However, contrast-enhanced sonography also detected endoleaks that were not identified by the comparative studies, and therefore the authors considered these to represent false-positives even though some of the leaks may have been true-positives. They concluded that contrast-enhanced sonography may be a useful stent graft surveillance tool by itself or in conjunction with CTA-MRA but that additional studies were necessary.

In the lab at Thomas Jefferson University Hospital, using animal models, we created bleeding sites in the bowel, spleen, and other organs.[26] After IV injection of contrast, the bleeding sites were visualized as areas with the characteristic mosaic color AE display corresponding to the contrast-containing blood pooling in the region of the lacerations. Similar results were obtained using grayscale wide-band HI of bleeding sites.[30] In the future, the use of contrast-enhanced sonography to improve the detection of internal bleeding and for surveillance may prove useful in trauma cases.

Finally, contrast may play a role in the diagnosis and treatment of patients with focal tumors who are going to have or have had chemotherapy, radiofrequency, ethanol, or other focal tumor ablation techniques[29,75] (see Figure 14-14). Ultrasound contrast agents used during the planning stage of an ultrasound-guided ablation can provide a means to better define tumor size and delineate tumor margins, which would help ensure that the entire tumor is ablated while preserving normal tissue. Patients who have had a tumor ablation procedure receive serial imaging examinations to check for a residual viable tumor at the ablation site and to screen for tumor recurrence. Currently, CT and MRI are most commonly used for these serial studies. However, in the future, contrast-enhanced sonography could be used for follow-up examinations. If a radiofrequency ablation procedure is being considered, it is conceivable that if additional ablations are indicated by the contrast-enhanced sonography study they could be performed (under ultrasound guidance) at the time of diagnosis, thus reducing the time between diagnosis and treatment and possibly improving the patient's outcome.

REFERENCES

1. Albrecht T, Blomley MJ, Cosgrove DO and others: Non-invasive diagnosis of hepatic cirrhosis by transit-time analysis of an ultrasound contrast agent, *Lancet* 353:1579-1583, 1999.

2. Albrecht T, Urbank A, Mahler M and others: Prolongation and optimization of Doppler enhancement with a microbubble US contrast agent by using continuous infusion: preliminary experience, *Radiology* 207:339-347, 1998.

3. Berland LL, Koslin DB, Routh WD and others: Renal artery stenosis: prospective evaluation of diagnosis with color duplex US compared with angiography, *Radiology* 174:421-423, 1990.

4. Blomley MJ, Lim AK, Harvey CJ and others: Liver microbubble transit time compared with histology and Child-Pugh score in diffuse liver disease: a cross sectional study, *Gut* 52(8):1188-1193, 2003.

5. Blomley MJK, Albrecht T, Cosgrove DO and others: Improved imaging of liver metastases with stimulated acoustic emission in the late phase of enhancement with the US contrast agent SH U 508A: early experience, *Radiology* 210:409-416, 1999.

6. Blomley MJK, Harvey CJ, Eckersley RJ and others: Contrast kinetics and Doppler intensitometry. In: Goldberg BB, Raichlen JR, Forsberg F, editors: *Ultrasound contrast agents: basic principles and clinical applications,* ed 2, London, 2001, Martin Dunitz.

7. Bree LB, Platt J: Clinical applications of an oral ultrasound contrast agent in the upper abdomen: overview of a phase II clinical trial, *Appl Rad* 28(S);28-32, 1999.

8. Catalano O, Lobianco R, Sandomenico F and others: Realtime contrast-enhanced ultrasound of the spleen: examination technique and preliminary clinical experience, *Radiol Med* 106(4):338-356, 2003.

9. Chomas JE, Dayton PA, Allen J and others: Optical and acoustical observation of contrast-agent destruction. In Goldberg BB, Raichlen JS, Forsberg F, editors: *Ultrasound contrast agents,* ed 2, London, 2001, Martin Dunitz Ltd.

10. Claudon M, Rohban T: Levovist in the diagnosis of renal artery stenosis: results of a controlled multicenter study, *Radiology* 205P:242, 1997.

11. Correas J, Claudon M, Tranquart F and others: Contrast-enhanced ultrasonography: renal applications, *J Radiol* 84:2041-2054, 2003.

12. Correas J, Helenon O, Moreau JF: Contrast-enhanced ultrasonography of native and transplanted kidney diseases, *Eur Radiol* 9 Suppl 3:S394-400, 1999.

13. Cosgrove D, Kedar, R, Bamber JC and others: Color Doppler in the differentiation of breast masses, *Radiology* 189:99-104, 1993.

14. Crouse LJ, Cheirif J, Hanly DE and others: Opacification and border delineation improvement in patients with suboptimal endocardial border definition in routine echocardiography. Results of the phase III Albunex multicenter trial, *J Am Coll Cardiol* 22:1494-1500, 1993.

15. De Jong N, Bouakaz A, Frinking PJA and others: Contrast-specific imaging methods. In Goldberg BB, Raichlen JS, Forsberg F, editors: *Ultrasound contrast agents,* ed 2, London, 2001, Martin Dunitz Ltd.

16. Dowling RJ, House MK, King PM and others: Contrast-enhanced Doppler ultrasound for renal artery stenosis, *Australas Radiol* 43(2):206-209, 1999.

17. Ernst H, Hahn EG, Balzer T and others: Color Doppler ultrasound of liver lesions: signal enhancement after intravenous injection of the ultrasound contrast agent Levovist, *J Clin Ultrasound* 24:31-35, 1996.

18. Forsberg F, Goldberg BB, Liu JB and others: On the feasibility of real-time, in vivo harmonic imaging with proteinaceous microspheres, *J Ultrasound Med* 15:853-860, 1996.

19. Forsberg F, Liu JB, Burns PN and others: Artifacts in ultrasound contrast agent studies, *J Ultrasound Med* 13:357-365, 1994.

20. Forsberg F, Liu JB, Merton DA and others: Tumor detection using an ultrasound contrast agent, *J Ultrasound Med* 4:S8, 1995.

21. Forsberg F, Liu JB, Merton DA and others: Gray scale second harmonic imaging of acoustic emission signals improves detection of liver tumors in rabbits, *J Ultrasound Med* 19:557-563, 2000.

22. Forsberg F, Liu JB, Rawool NM and others: Gray-scale and color Doppler flow harmonic imaging with proteinaceous microspheres, *Radiology* 197(P):403, 1995.

23. Forsberg F, Shi WT, Merritt CRB and others: Does the mechanical index predict destruction rates of contrast microbubbles? *J Ultrasound Med* 20:S12, 2001.

24. Giannoni MF, Palombo G, Sbarigia E and others: Contrast-enhanced ultrasound for aortic stent-graft surveillance, *J Endovasc Ther* 10(2):208-217, 2003.

25. Goldberg BB, Forsberg F, Fitzsch T and others: Induced acoustic emission as a contrast mechanism for detection of hepatic abnormalities, *J Ultrasound Med* 14:S7, 1995.

26. Goldberg BB, Forsberg F, Merton DA and others: Sonographic detection of bleeding sites and other structures with use of a contrast agent, *Radiology* 201(P):197, 1996.

27. Goldberg BB, Leen E, Needleman L and others: Contrast enhanced ultrasound imaging of liver lesions: a phase II study with NC100100, *J Ultrasound Med* 18(S):43, 1999.

28. Goldberg BB, Liu JB, Burns PN and others: Galactose-based intravenous sonographic contrast agent: experimental studies, *J Ultrasound Med* 12:463-470, 1993.

29. Goldberg BB, Liu JB, Merton DA and others: The role of contrast-enhanced US for RF ablation of liver tumor, *Radiology* 217(P):607, 2000.

30. Goldberg BB, Merton DA, Forsberg F and others: Evaluation of bleeding sites with a tissue-specific sonographic contrast agent: preliminary experiences in an animal model, *J Ultrasound Med* 17:609-616, 1998.

31. Gramiak R, Shah PM: Echocardiography of the aortic root, *Invest Radiol* 3:356-366, 1968.

32. Harvey CJ, Blomley MJK, Cosgrove DO: Acoustic emission imaging. In Goldberg BB, Raichlen JS, Forsberg F, editors: *Ultrasound contrast agents,* ed 2, London, 2001, Martin Dunitz Ltd.

33. http://www.astratech.se/Main.aspx/Item/214433/navt/8/navl/46951/nava/46952. Accessed 02/16/04.

34. http://www.definityimaging.com Accessed 2/19/04.

35. Isozaki T, Numata K, Kiba T and others: Differential diagnosis of hepatic tumors by using contrast enhancement patters at US, *Radiology* 229(3):798-805, 2003.

36. Kedar RP, Cosgrove DO, McCready VR and others: Microbubble Doppler angiography of breast masses: dynamic and morphologic features, *Radiology* 189(P):154, 1993.

37. Kim EA, Yoon KH, Lee YH and others: Focal hepatic lesions: contrast-enhancement patterns at pulse-inversion harmonic US using a microbubble contrast agent, *Korean J Radiol* 4:224-233, 2003.

38. Kishimoto N, Mori Y, Nishiue T and others: Renal blood flow measurement with contrast-enhanced harmonic ultrasonography: evaluation of dopamine-induced changes in renal cortical perfusion in humans, *Clin Nephrol* 59(6):423-428, 2003.

39. Kitamura H, Miyagawa Y, Yokoyama T and others: Kupffer cell imaging with ultrasound contrast agent for diagnosis of histological grade of hepatocellular carcinoma, *J Ultrasound Med* 20:S10, 2001.

40. Klein HG: Ultrasound contrast agents: a commercial perspective. In Goldberg BB, Raichlen JS, Forsberg F, editors: *Ultrasound contrast agents,* ed 2, London, 2001, Martin Dunitz Ltd.

41. Koda M, Matsunaga Y, Ueki M and others: Qualitative assessment of tumor vascularity in hepatocellular carcinoma by contrast-enhanced coded ultrasound: comparison with arterial phase of dynamic CT and conventional color/power Doppler ultrasound, *Eur Radiol* 14(6):1100-1108, 2003.

42. Kono Y, Mattrey RF, Pinnell SP and others: Contrast-enhanced B-mode harmonic imaging for the evaluation of HCC viability after therapy in cirrhotic patients, *J Ultrasound Med* 20:S10, 2001.

43. Kono Y, Mattrey RT: Harmonic imaging with contrast microbubbles. In Goldberg BB, Raichlen JS, Forsberg F, editors: *Ultrasound contrast agents,* ed 2, London, 2001, Martin Dunitz Ltd., pp 37-46.

44. Lacourciere Y, Levesque J, Onrot JM and others: Impact of Levovist ultrasonographic contrast agent on the diagnosis and management of hypertensive patients with suspected renal artery stenosis: a Canadian multicentre pilot study, *Can Assoc Radiol J* 53(4):219-227, 2002.

45. Lee KH, Choi BI, Kim KW and others: Contrast-enhanced dynamic ultrasonography of the liver: Optimization of hepatic arterial phase in normal volunteers, *Adbom Imaging* 28(5): 652-656, 2003.

46. Leen E, Anderson WG, Cooke TG and others: Contrast enhanced Doppler perfusion index: detection of colorectal liver metastases, *Radiology* 209(P):292, 1998.

47. Leen E: *Radiological applications of contrast agents in the hepatobiliary system.* In Goldberg BB, Raichlen JS, Forsberg F, editors: *Ultrasound contrast agents,* ed 2, London, 2001, Martin Dunitz Ltd.

48. Lencioni R, Pinto S, Cioni D and others: Contrast-enhanced Doppler ultrasound of renal artery stenosis: prologue to a promising future, *Echocardiography* 16(7, Pt 2):767-773, 1999.

49. Leutoff UC, Scharf J, Richter GM and others: Use of ultrasound contrast medium Levovist in after-care of liver transplant patients: improved vascular imaging in color Doppler ultrasound, *Radiology* 38:399-404, 1998.

50. Lev-Toaff AS, Goldberg BB: *Gastrointestinal ultrasound contrast agents.* In Goldberg BB, editor: *Ultrasound contrast agents,* London, 1997, Martin Dunitz.

51. Merton DA: An easily implemented method to improve detection of ultrasound contrast in body tissues: frame one imaging. *J Diag Med Sonography* 16(1):14-20, 2000.

52. Miller JC and others: Clinical molecular imaging, *JACR* 1:1S, 2004.

53. Missouris CG, Allen CM, Balen FG and others: Non-invasive screening for renal artery stenosis with ultrasound contrast enhancement, *J Hypertens* 14(4):519-524, 1996.

54. Moriyasu F, Kono Y, Nada T and others: Flash echo (passive cavitation) imaging of the liver by using US contrast agents and intermittent scanning sequence, *Radiology* 201(P):196, 1996.

55. Nagase M, Furuse J, Ishii H and others: Evaluation of contrast enhancement patterns in pancreatic tumors by coded harmonic sonographic imaging with a microbubble contrast agent, *J Ultrasound Med* 22(8):789-795, 2003.

56. Needleman L: Review of a new ultrasound contrast agent—EchoGen emulsion, *Appl Rad* 26(S):8-12, 1997.

57. Numata K, Yutaka O, Noritoshi K and others: Contrast-enhanced sonography of autoimmune pancreatitis: comparison with pathologic findings, *J Ultrasound Med* 23(2):199-206, 2004.

58. Ophir J, Gobuty A, McWhirt RE and others: Ultrasonic backscatter from contrast producing collagen microspheres, *Ultrasound Imaging* 2:67-77, 1980.

59. Oka MA, Rubens DJ, Strang JG: Ultrasound contrast agent in evaluation of abdominal vessels, *J Ultrasound Med* 20:S84, 2001.

60. Oldenburg A, Hohmann J, Skrok J and others: Imaging of paediatric splenic injury with contrast-enhanced ultrasonography, *Pediatr Radiol* 34(4):351-354, 2004.

61. Olin JW, Piedmonte MR, Young JR and others: The utility of duplex ultrasound scanning of the renal arteries for diagnosing significant renal artery stenosis, *Ann Intern Med* 122:833-838, 1995.

62. Pelberg RA, Wei K, Kamiyama N and others: Potential advantage of flash echocardiography for digital subtraction of B-mode images acquired during myocardial contrast echocardiography, *J Am Soc Echocardigr* 12:85-93, 1999.

63. Peterson CL, Barr RG: Contrast-enhanced sonography in patients with renal pathology, *J Diag Med Sonography* 16(2):53-56, 2000.

64. Plew J, Sanki J, Young N and others: Early experience in the use of Levovist ultrasound contrast in the evaluation of liver masses, *Australas Radiol* 44:28-31, 2000.

65. Porter TR, Xie F: Accelerated intermittent harmonic imaging. In Goldberg BB, Raichlen JS, Forsberg F, editors: *Ultrasound contrast agents,* ed 2, London, 2001, Martin Dunitz Ltd.

66. Rickes S, Unkrodt K, Neye H and others: Differentiation of pancreatic tumours by conventional ultrasound, unenhanced and echo-enhanced power Doppler sonography, *Scand J Gastroenterol* 37(11):1313-1320, 2002.

67. Robbin ML, Lockhart ME, Barr RG: Renal imaging with ultrasound contrast: current status, *Radiol Clin North Am* 41(5):963-978, 2003.

68. Sellars ME, Sidhu PS, Heneghan M and others: Infusions of microbubbles are more cost-effective than bolus injections in Doppler studies of the portal vein: a quantitative comparison of normal volunteers and patients with cirrhosis, *Radiology* 217(P):396, 2000.

69. Sidhu PS, Marshall MM, Ryan SM and others: Clinical use of Levovist, an ultrasound contrast agent, in the imaging of liver transplantation: assessment of the pre- and post-transplant patient, *Eur Radiol* 10(7):1114-1126, 2000.

70. Sidhu PS, Shaw AS, Ellis SM and others: Microbubble ultrasound contrast in the assessment of hepatic artery patency following liver transplantation: role in reducing frequency of hepatic artery arteriography, *Eur Radiol* 2003.

71. Sirlin CB, Girard MS, Baker K and others: Effect of gated US acquisition on liver and portal vein contrast enhancement, *Radiology* 201(P):158, 1996.

72. Skjoldbye B, Weislander S, Struckmann J and others: Doppler ultrasound assessment of TIPS patency and function—the need for echo enhancers, *Acta Radiol* 39:675-679, 1998.

73. Solbiati L, Cova L, Ierace T and others: Characterization of focal lesions in patients with liver cirrhosis using second generation contrast-enhanced (CE) wideband harmonic sonography (WBHS) in different enhancement phases, *J Ultrasound Med* 20:S10, 2001.

74. Solbiati L, Cova L, Ierace T and others: Diagnosis of atypical hemangioma using contrast-enhanced wideband harmonic sonography (CE-WBHS), *J Ultrasound Med* 20:S9, 2001.

75. Solbiati L, Goldberg SN, Ierace T and others: Radio-frequency ablation of hepatic metastases: post procedural assessment with a US microbubble contrast agent: early experience, *Radiology* 211:643-649, 1999.

76. Strobel D, Krodel U, Martus P and others: Clinical evaluation of contrast-enhanced color Doppler sonography in the differential diagnosis of liver tumors, *J Clin Ultrasound* 28:1-13, 2000.

77. Tanaka S, Kitamra T, Yoshioka F and others: Effectiveness of galactose-based intravenous contrast medium on color Doppler sonography of deeply located hepatocellular carcinoma, *Ultrasound in Med Biol* 21:157-160, 1995.

78. Uggowitzer MM, Hausegger KA, Machan L and others: Echo-enhanced Doppler sonography in the evaluation of transjugular intraheptic portosystemic shunts: clinical applications of a new transpulmonary US contrast agent, *Radiology* 201(P):266, 748, 1996.

79. von Herbay A, Vogt C, Haussinger D: Pulse inversion sonography in the early phase of the sonographic contrast agent Levovist: differentiation between benign and malignant focal liver lesions, *J Ultrasound Med* 21:1191-2000, 2002.

80. Wei K, Le E, Bin JP and others: Quantification of renal blood flow with contrast-enhanced ultrasound, *J Am Coll Cardiol* 15;37(4):1135-1140, 2001.

81. Weskott HP: Contrast-enhanced reperfusion imaging in atypical hepatic hemangiomas, *J Ultrasound Med* 20:S9, 2001.

82. Wheatley MA: Composition of contrast microbubbles: Basic chemistry of encapsulated and surfactant-coated bubbles. In Goldberg BB, Raichlen JS, Forsberg F, editors: *Ultrasound contrast agents,* ed 2, London, 2001, Martin Dunitz Ltd.

83. Wilson SR, Burns PN, Muradali D and others: Harmonic hepatic US with microbubble contrast agent: initial experience showing improved characterization of hemangioma, hepatocellular carcinoma, and metastasis, *Radiology* 215:153-161, 2000.

Ultrasound-Guided Interventional Techniques

M. Robert De Jong

KEY TERMS

alpha fetoprotein (AFP) – a laboratory test that measures levels of alpha fetoprotein in blood serum; an elevated level could indicate a liver lesion

coagulopathy – a defect in blood-clotting mechanisms

fine needle aspiration (FNA) – the use of a fine-gauge needle to obtain cells from a mass

international normalized ratio (INR) – a method developed to standardize prothrombin time (PT) results among laboratories by accounting for the different thromboplastin reagents used to determine PT

pneumothorax – a collection of air or gas in the pleural cavity

prostate specific antigen (PSA) – laboratory test that measures levels of the protein prostate specific antigen in the body; elevated levels could indicate prostate cancer

prothrombin time (PT) – laboratory test used to detect clotting abnormalities of the extrinsic pathway; measured against a control sample, PT tests the time it takes for a blood sample to coagulate after thromboplastin and calcium are added to it

partial thromboplastin time (PTT) – laboratory test that can be used to evaluate the effects of heparin, aspirin, and antihistamines on the blood clotting process; PTT detects clotting abnormalities of the intrinsic and common pathways

thoracentesis – surgical puncture of the chest wall for removal of fluids; usually done by using a large-bore needle

vasovagal – concerning the action of stimuli from the vagus nerve on blood vessels

Ultrasound has been used to assist in interventional procedures since the early days of specially designed A-mode and B-mode transducers (Figure 15-1). Ultrasound-guided interventional techniques are continuing to improve with the new developments in transducer and equipment technology and transducer needle-guide attachments. Ultrasound is being used to perform a variety of invasive procedures on various organs and masses located in the neck, chest, abdomen, retroperitoneum, pelvis, and to drain fluid and abscess collections. Ultrasound is unique as a guidance modality because it combines excellent imaging with real-time visualization and should be the primary guidance technique for percutaneous biopsy whenever possible. It is a true team approach with the radiologist, sonographer, nurse, and cytopathology team all working together for the good of the patient.

ADVANTAGES OF ULTRASOUND-GUIDED PROCEDURES

In recent years, there has been a movement to perform more and more procedures under ultrasound guidance. Retroperitoneal masses, pleural-based masses, deep masses in the liver, and musculoskeletal masses that once typically necessitated a

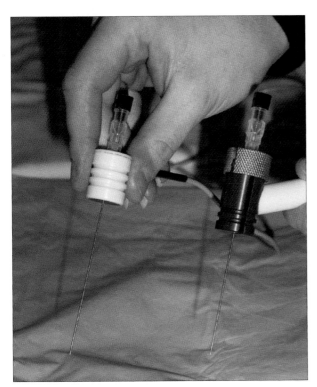

Figure 15-1 A-mode (white) and B-mode (brown) biopsy transducers from the late 1970s.

biopsy under CT guidance or in open surgical biopsies are now being successfully performed using ultrasound guidance.

Ultrasound can be used for the following procedures:

- Obtain biopsy for malignant or benign masses.
- Obtain biopsy of organs for parenchymal disease or transplant rejection.
- Drain fluid collections, such as cysts, ascites, or pleural fluid.
- Drain or obtain samples of abscesses to determine the type of organism on patients who are not responding to antibiotic therapy.
- Assist in placement of drainage tubes or catheters.
- Assist in placement of catheters in arteries and veins.
- Mark spots for biopsies or fluid taps to be performed without direct sonographic guidance.
- Amniocentesis

The main advantage to using ultrasound for guidance is the continuous real-time visualization of the biopsy needle, which allows adjustment of the needle as necessary. Also, as the biopsy specimen is being obtained, the needle tip can be watched in real time to ensure that it does not slip outside the mass. This is especially important in small masses. Ultrasound also has the advantage of allowing different patient positions and approaches to be considered. The patient may be placed in a decubitus or oblique position to allow safe access to the mass (Figure 15-2). Subcostal approaches can allow the use of steep angles with the needle directed cephalad. This can help reduce the risk of a **pneumothorax** or bleeding from an injury to an intercostal artery. Using ultrasound the patient can be placed in a comfortable position and not be made to lie supine or prone. For example, the patient's head may be slightly elevated or he or she may be able to move slightly between passes to relieve back or joint pain. Another benefit is the ability to comfort and reassure the patient because the sonologist, sonographer, and nurse are all near the patient during the procedure. Even the most anxious patients can be coached to cooperate when the team is by their side and not constantly in and out of the room. Other advantages include the ability to perform the biopsy in a single breath hold, portability, lack of radiation, decreased costs, and shorter procedure times.

DISADVANTAGES OF ULTRASOUND-GUIDED PROCEDURES

Despite its many benefits, ultrasound guidance has some limitations, too. Unfortunately, not all masses can be visualized with ultrasound because they may be isoechoic to the normal tissue (Figure 15-3). In the abdomen, bowel gas may move in and obscure the mass before or even during the procedure. The needle tip may be difficult to see or deviate from the projected path because of bending or deflection of the needle. This calls upon the sonographer's scanning skills to maneuver the transducer to find the needle tip or correct for the deviation (Figure 15-4). Other disadvantages of using ultrasound to guide procedures include the inexperience of ultrasound personnel, the comfort level of the radiologist/sonologist with other imaging modalities,

Figure 15-2   A, With the patient supine, the liver mass *(arrow)* is 15 cm deep. **B,** Left lateral decubitus position. The liver has fallen forward and the same mass *(arrow)* is now only 7 cm deep. An easy, successful biopsy showed metastatic disease from a pancreas primary.

Figure 15-3   A, Although a definite mass was seen on a contrast MRI, it was not appreciated by ultrasound. **B,** Using the MRI as a guide and color Doppler to assess for areas of abnormal flow, a successful biopsy was performed on this patient with infiltrative hepatocellular carcinoma.

Figure 15-4   A, The needle *(arrows)* deviated from the projected path of the guide *(dotted line).*
B, Because of the constant deviation of the needle from the projected path, the sonographer had to compensate by moving the transducer laterally so that the needle would pass through the center of the mass. Note that the projected path does not even go through the mass. A diagnosis of hepatocellular carcinoma was obtained.

Figure 15-5 Liver core biopsy in a patient with hepatitis C.

Figure 15-6 A biopsy of a retroperitoneal lymph node could not be performed using ultrasound guidance because of the surrounding vessels.

overlying bowel gas that cannot be displaced, and having to use fixed angles when using needle guides on the transducers.

INDICATIONS FOR A BIOPSY

The most common indication for a biopsy is to confirm malignancy in a mass. The mass may be the primary tumor in a patient with an undiagnosed malignancy or a metastatic mass in a patient with a known primary malignancy. Other indications may include the need to differentiate between a metastatic mass or a second primary in a patient with a known malignancy, determine the cause of metastases in a patient with multiple primaries, differentiate recurrent tumor from postoperative or therapy scarring or changes, differentiate malignancy from inflammatory or infectious disease, and characterize a benign mass. Another common reason is to obtain a sample of the parenchyma in an organ to determine the severity of a disease process. Some examples include hepatitis, renal failure, and rejection in a transplanted organ (Figure 15-5).

CONTRAINDICATIONS FOR A BIOPSY

Contraindications of ultrasound-guided procedures are few mainly due to its minimally invasive nature. Contraindications may include an uncorrectable bleeding disorder, the lack of a safe needle path (Figure 15-6), and an uncooperative patient. Patient cooperation is necessary so that a safe biopsy may be obtained of the mass. If the patient will not hold still, is jumpy, or cannot control his or her breathing, the risk of a complication increases significantly as does the danger to the sonographer or sonologist of being stuck by a dirty needle.

LABORATORY TESTS

Blood or urine tests are typically not requested before a procedure, with the exception of bleeding times. Usually an abnormal laboratory test will be part of the work-up before a procedure is requested. Some examples of what the tests seek to determine include: elevated **alpha fetoprotein (AFP)** with a liver lesion; elevated **prostate specific antigen (PSA)** as an indication of prostate cancer; changes in thyroglobulin levels in patients with a history of thyroid cancer; and increased white blood cells to determine if a lesion is an abscess or hematuria with a renal mass.

One lab test that should be reviewed before a procedure is the patient's bleeding times. These tests measure the time it takes the blood to form a clot. This is especially important for patients who are on "blood thinners," such as Coumadin, heparin, or aspirin therapy. Since vitamin K is essential in the blood clotting process, patients with liver disease are also at risk for prolonged bleeding or the formation of hematomas. To eliminate patient rescheduling or cancellation, test results should be obtained as close to the date of the procedure as possible, although results may be acceptable up to 3 to 4 weeks before the scheduled procedure. These simple blood tests can be performed the morning of the procedure, as results can usually be obtained in 2 to 3 hours.

There are at least a dozen factors that are necessary to form a blood clot to stop bleeding. Clotting occurs through a complex series of reactions called the *coagulation cascade.* There are three pathways in the blood clotting process: intrinsic, extrinsic, and common. To evaluate all three pathways, both **prothrombin time (PT)** and **partial thromboplastin time (PTT)** are assessed. PTT can be used to evaluate the effects of heparin, aspirin, and antihistamines on the blood clotting process. PTT evaluates factors found in the intrinsic and common pathways. PTT values may vary depending on the method and activators used, with normal values typically between 60 and 70 seconds. PT is used to evaluate factors found in the extrinsic pathway, which may be affected by patients on Coumadin. Normal values are typically between 10 and 13 seconds.

Because of the variability of PT results among laboratories, a standard method was developed called **international normalized ratio (INR).** The INR was created in 1983 by the World Health Organization to account for the various thromboplastin reagents used to determine PT that caused fluctuations in normal values. The INR is a calculation that adjusts for the variations in PT processing and values so that test results from different laboratories can be compared. The INR is expressed as a number. Values of less than 1.4 are necessary to ensure a safe procedure. The INR-PT is not used on patients with liver disease or on heparin. It is evaluated for patients taking anticoagulants, especially Coumadin.

TYPES OF ULTRASOUND-GUIDED PROCEDURES

Ultrasound is used in the following interventional procedures: biopsies, core biopsies, needle placement for draining ascitic fluid or pleural effusions, needle placement for collecting fluid or abscesses, placement of catheters, placement of nephrostomy tubes in obstructed kidneys, and transjugular intrahepatic portosystemic shunt (TIPS).

Biopsies are used to confirm if a mass is benign, malignant, or infectious. Most biopsies are easily and safely performed as an outpatient procedure. Biopsy success rates have been reported to have sensitivities of greater than 85% and specificities of greater than 95%. Cell type is often needed to determine treatment type and options because specific tumors respond better to certain types of chemotherapy or to radiation therapy.

Fine needle aspiration (FNA) or cytologic aspiration uses thin-gauge needles to obtain cells from the mass. FNAs are performed using a 20- to 25-gauge needle, preferably with a cutting tip, such as a Franseen needle (Figure 15-7). These types of needles have the least risk associated with their use, allowing multiple passes as necessary. The specimen is obtained by using a capillary action technique. This involves a fine up-and-down motion of the needle, which obtains the necessary cells through a scraping or cutting action. An FNA technique reduces the trauma to the cells and decreases the amount of background blood. If the sample is scant, suction techniques can be used. Suction technique involves using a syringe and tubing attached to the needle. As the needle is being moved up and down, suction is applied to draw up the cells. Because of its thin size, the needle can safely go through a large or small bowel and near vascular structures. FNA in conjunction with onsite cytopathology can help ensure that the procedure is diagnostic and help minimize the number of passes.

A core biopsy uses an automated, spring-loaded device, termed a biopsy gun, to provide a core of tissue for histologic analysis. The biopsy device is cocked and the needle tip is placed just inside the mass. The button is then pushed and the cutting needle is thrown, obtaining a core of tissue, which is

deposited into a slot on the inner needle (Figure 15-8). There are various throw lengths available, ranging from 10 to 23 mm, with 20 mm being the most common. The snapping sound that the device makes can be startling to patients, and it is advised to let them hear the sound before the specimen is obtained. This also ensures that the device is not defective. Core biopsy needles are larger in diameter and range in size from 14 to 20 gauge. A core biopsy provides tissue for histologic analysis and can also be used in conjunction with FNA techniques, especially if a definitive diagnosis could not be determined from just the FNA or if the cytopathologist requires more tissue for a more accurate diagnosis or special stains. Core biopsies are also used to diagnosis diffuse parenchymal disease of the liver and kidney, in transplanted organs, and in breast and prostate biopsies.

Ultrasound is routinely used to guide needle placement to drain or obtain samples from ascitic fluid or pleural effusions. Usually these procedures are performed without the use of a needle guide. If just a small amount of fluid is necessary, a 22- or 20-gauge needle is used. If the fluid is viscous, an 18- or 16-gauge needle may be required. If the goal is to drain as much fluid as possible, a special needle, called a centesis needle, is used (Figure 15-9). After the needle is properly placed, it is removed, leaving a catheter with side holes to safely drain the fluid. For large volume drainage, 1-L vacuum bottles are used to remove the fluid. Ultrasound can be used periodically to check the amount of fluid remaining or to help reposition the

Figure 15-8 Needles used for core biopsies.

Figure 15-7 Needles used for FNA biopsies.

Figure 15-9 A centesis catheter with the arrow pointing to the side hole.

Figure 15-10 **A,** Bowel is sucked up against the catheter *(arrows)* obstructing the flow of fluid. **B,** By having the patient roll into an oblique position, the fluid collected to the dependent portion and the bowel loop floated away from the catheter allowing drainage to resume.

catheter to free it from the bowel, which may be sucked against the wall of the catheter (Figure 15-10). Usually the sonographer can scan outside the sterile field. Small fluid pockets or multilocular collections are usually best performed using a needle guide.

Fluid or abscess collections are usually performed using a needle guide. Abscess or fluid collections may be located in or around the liver, pancreas, kidney, abdominopelvic cavities, or prostate. Ultrasound can also be used to provide guidance to drain the gallbladder in patients who have cholecystitis, especially in acalculous cholecystitis or in very sick patients for whom surgery would be contraindicated. The needle gauge used will depend on the thickness of the fluid. For pelvic collections, depending on their location, an endovaginal approach should be considered in women, and endorectal approaches in men and women. Catheters may be left in place to drain the collection. Patients may receive follow-up examinations to ensure that the cavity is getting smaller and to ensure that the catheter is still in the correct position. These follow-up examinations are usually performed under fluoroscopy in a procedure called a sinogram, although ultrasound can also be used.

Ultrasound can also be used to guide placement of catheters in the subclavian, jugular, or femoral vessels; in nephrostomy tube placement in obstructed kidneys; and to assist in TIPS procedures.

ULTRASOUND GUIDANCE METHODS

Free Hand Technique. There are currently two main ways to perform ultrasound-guided procedures. One method is called the free hand technique and is performed without the use of a needle guide on the transducer. The person who performs the biopsy will also usually hold the transducer. The transducer is still placed in a sterile cover. Care must be taken to align the needle with the transducer and the sound beam (Figure 15-11). A variation of this technique allows the sonog-

rapher to scan outside the sterile field while the physician performs the biopsy (Figure 15-12). Again, to see the needle tip, the transducer must be aligned to the needle path. If the needle becomes lost on the image, the transducer should be repositioned in alignment with the needle to see the needle tip. The free hand technique allows more flexibility in choosing the needle path. However, it is more technically challenging, especially for deep lesions (Figure 15-13).

Needle Attached to Transducer. The second method involves using a needle guide that is attached to the transducer (Figure 15-14). The predicted needle path is displayed on the screen and the mass is lined up along the path. Some transducers offer a choice of angles, usually a steep angle and a shallower angle (Figure 15-15). This gives some flexibility around vessels or other structures. Benefits of using a needle guide include a faster learning curve, faster placement of the needle, and assurance of the needle going through the anesthetized area when multiple passes are necessary. Needle guides have been shown to be invaluable when taking a biopsy of deep or small masses.

ULTRASOUND BIOPSY

CYTOPATHOLOGY

Whenever possible, biopsies should be performed with a cytopathology team present to ensure that enough diagnostic material is obtained to minimize the number of passes. Additional material may also be requested by the cytopathologist for special stains and flow cytometry. (Flow cytometry may be necessary when lymphoma is suspected.) The cytopathologist may also request that a core sample be obtained to enhance the chances of obtaining a diagnosis for the patient. However, although it does increase the percentage of successful biopsies, having someone from cytopathology present may increase the overall procedure time and cost.

A   **B**

Figure 15-11   **A,** One-person free hand technique with the needle in plane to the transducer. **B,** One-person free hand technique. Notice that the needle is not in plane with the transducer.

Figure 15-12   Two-person free hand technique with the sonographer scanning outside the sterile field.

Figure 15-14   Biopsy using a needle guide.

Figure 15-13   This paracentesis was performed without the use of a guide since it was a superficial collection.

BIOPSY TECHNIQUES: STEP BY STEP

A PT, PTT, and platelet count are required before most procedures. Some departments may not require a hemostatic evaluation for fluid aspirations and superficial or low-risk biopsies, such as of the thyroid or prostate gland. Anticoagulants should be discontinued before the biopsy to reduce the risk of post-procedural bleeding. The wait times for various drugs are 4 to 6 hours for heparin, 3 to 4 days for Coumadin, and 5 to 7 days for aspirin. A patient with a problem **coagulopathy** may need to be given a platelet transfusion just before and during the procedure.

Before beginning the procedure, the patient's medical history, lab values, and imaging studies should be reviewed and blood work checked. If the PT, PTT, and INR are normal, then the procedure can safely begin.

The next step is to explain the procedure to the patient. A well-informed patient is usually more relaxed and cooperative. The patient must be informed of the potential risks, alternate methods of obtaining the same information, and the potential course of the disease if the biopsy were not performed and the correct treatment could not be planned. The benefits of the procedure and what to expect during the procedure, especially the necessity for multiple passes, should also be discussed, along with any potential complications that may lead to inconclusive specimens. The patient's role in the procedure should be explained, including how they need to keep still and follow breathing instructions. Identification of all personnel in the

A　　　　　　　　　　　　　**B**

Figure 15-15　**A,** Needle guide attachment that offers a choice of two angles. The guide is in position for angle B. **B,** Needle guide attachment that offers a choice of a 15- or 30-degree angle. The transducer is set up for the 30-degree angle. This patient was determined to have metastatic disease from a lung primary.

room should be given because the room can become quite crowded with attendance by the sonographer, attending physician, fellow and/or resident, nurse, and cytopathology team, if they are used. At this time, the psychological needs of the patient should be determined and sedatives ordered if necessary. The patient needs to be awake for the procedure so that he or she can stay in the necessary position and control breathing. Time should also be allowed for the patient to ask questions.

After obtaining the patient's consent for the procedure, the next step in the process is to review any diagnostic imaging studies, such as an ultrasound, CT, MRI, or PET scan. If possible, the film demonstrating the mass should be hung in the room. If there are no view boxes in the room, the film should be accessible in the room. In this filmless era of PACS, if there are no viewing monitors in the room, a film with the necessary images should be printed, if possible—especially for chest, retroperitoneal masses, and other challenging masses. While the sonographer is reviewing the images, the nurse should be getting the patient in the scanning/procedure room, performing the preprocedural checklist, placing the patient into a gown, and taking vital signs. If necessary, the ECG and pulse oximeter machine should be connected to the patient. These are necessary whenever there is a chance of a pneumothorax.

Next, a limited ultrasound is performed to localize the mass and to choose the optimal approach and best transducer type and frequency (Figure 15-16). The sonographer should determine multiple approaches, if necessary, and review them with the radiologist and/or sonologist. An x or a dot is marked on the skin with a marker at the site where the needle will pierce the skin. The distance to the mass also needs to be measured to determine the needle length necessary to reach the mass. This is done by placing the caliper at the bottom of the mass. This should be performed with the needle guide lines on the screen because the machine will now take into account the

length of the needle inside the needle guide, which is typically 2 to 4 cm. Common needle lengths are 6, 9, 15, and 20 cm (Figure 15-17). Usually, it is best to have the sonographer on one side of the patient, preferably next to the ultrasound machine, and the physician on the other side of the patient. Sometimes the best path requires that the sonographer and physician be on the same side of the patient. If this is the situation, then the physician should be in front of the sonographer. If the sonographer cannot see the screen, then he or she may try being in front of the physician. If that obstructs the physician's view of the screen, then the sonographer may need to be on the side of the patient away from the machine. If both are on the same side and the sonographer's position interferes with the biopsy, then they should go to the other side of the stretcher. This may mean that someone else will need to document the needle tip or adjust controls as necessary, such as the nurse or other available personnel. The sonographer should consider rearranging the relationship of the stretcher and machine to accommodate both the sonographer and physician on the same side of the patient. Also, the sonographer could sit on a stool or even a footstool in front of the physician. Remember to always consider scanning ergonomics.

The new national patient safety standards set by the Joint Commission on Accreditation of Healthcare Organizations (JCAHO) mandate that a "time-out" be performed before beginning any procedure. A member of the biopsy team should ask the patient to recite his or her full name. The patient's ID or history number is confirmed, along with the type and location of the procedure. This is usually recorded at the bottom of the consent form. The words "time-out" may also be typed on the screen and an image documented to be part of the ultrasound examination. This is helpful because there will then be the preprocedural image; the "time-out" image, which documents date and time; and the needle tip documentation images (Figure 15-18).

A   **B**

Figure 15-16   **A,** A large mediastinal mass seen with a 5-MHz curved array transducer. **B,** Here, using a 7-MHz linear array transducer because the hypoechoic area in the mass was better appreciated. Adenocarcinoma was diagnosed *(arrow).*

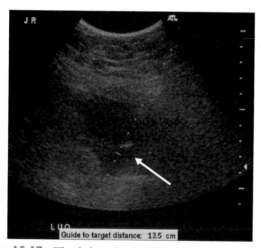

Figure 15-17   The dash in the dotted line represents the needle length necessary to reach a depth of 13.5 cm; therefore, a 15-cm length needle is necessary for this ascites drainage.

The radiologist and/or sonologist may start prepping the skin while the sonographer preps and bags the transducer. Prepping the transducer requires the assistance of another person, such as a nurse, a student, a radiologist, or another sonographer, to maintain sterility of the transducer. Transducer preparation is quick and simple and consists of covering the transducer with a sterile cover and attaching the needle guide to the transducer. Depending on the transducer, the needle guide may be covered by the sterile bag, or it may also be sterile and placed over the sterile bag. Please note that the use of sterile bags and sterile guides may vary among institutions. For example, one institution may bag the transducer and guide keeping it sterile for a thyroid biopsy, whereas another may use the transducer and guide in a clean but not sterile fashion.

After the transducer guide is attached, the correct size needle guide is attached or inserted into the transducer guide. These guides are based on the gauge of the needle or catheter being used. These may need to be changed during the procedure. For example, the 22-gauge guide may be needed during the FNA, but changed to an 18-gauge guide for the core. Also, on a deep lesion, a 22-gauge needle may start the procedure, but, because it keeps deviating, it may be necessary to switch to a sturdier 20-gauge needle (Figure 15-19).

After the patient and transducer are prepped, sterile gel is used to rescan and check the mark. Once the area of the biopsy has been rechecked, local skin anesthetic is given, usually with a 25-gauge needle.

Deeper numbing can be given along the needle path using the needle guide. This is important for patient comfort, especially on deep masses and liver masses, as the liver capsule is very sensitive. If at all possible, the transducer should stay on the anesthetized area to ensure that the needle is always passing through the numbed tissue. Typically, a 9-cm, 22-gauge spinal needle is used for the deeper numbing. It is important that the physician squirt the lidocaine or numbing agent through the needle before inserting the needle into the patient. This is done so that air is not introduced into the patient's tissue, obscuring the mass and the needle path. The patients should be reminded that they should not feel any sharp pain, but that they may feel pressure. Also, it is a good idea to let patients know that they may feel some pressure from the transducer as it is held in place.

The sonographer holds the transducer as the radiologist and/or sonologist performs the biopsy. In some institutions, the radiologist and/or sonologist may be the person who holds the transducer while they perform the biopsy. When a free hand technique is used, the radiologist and/or sonologist will usually hold the transducer. The needle should be advanced in a swift motion while the needle is being tracked. Echogenic tip

Figure 15-18 **A,** Preprocedural image demonstrating the iliac node and needle path. **B,** "Time out" to verify patient's name and procedure. **C,** The procedure has begun. The arrow is pointing to the needle tip. This patient had lymphoma.

Figure 15-19 **A,** The transducer and sterile kit, which includes the bag, guide attachment, needle gauge inserts, rubber bands, and sterile gel. **B,** Prepped transducers.

needles should be used because the tip of the needle has been scored to produce an increase in scattered echoes, causing it to be echogenic. The shaft of the needle is echogenic because it is a specular reflector, whereas the tip of the needle is more echogenic due to its being scored. Some needles have the stylet scored to enhance visualization of the needle (Figure 15-20). For neck, chest, abdominal, and retroperitoneal biopsies, the patient is asked to stop breathing while the needle is inserted. A typical FNA pass lasts between 20 and 40 seconds. If patients cannot hold their breath for this long, they should be instructed to breathe shallowly until the needle is removed because deep breaths may cause the needle to bend. When a sonographer assists with the procedure, he or she will have one sterile hand, which is holding the transducer, while the other hand will be dirty because it will be manipulating the controls on the ultrasound machine.

After the procedure is finished, the patient's skin is cleaned and a bandage placed over the biopsy site. The dirty bag and guide are removed from the transducer. Care should be taken not to accidentally throw the reusable guide in the garbage. The sonographer may scan the area to look for any postprocedural complications, such as a hematoma. Color or power Doppler can be used to ensure that there is no active bleeding. This is especially useful in renal biopsies. If an active bleed is discovered, the sonographer can use the transducer to apply pressure over the area to stop the bleeding. Usually the bleeding can be stopped within 5 to 10 minutes. If the bleeding cannot be stopped, the interventional radiology department should be contacted immediately (Figure 15-21).

Before the patient leaves the room, the nurse will assess the patient's pain level and take vital signs. The sonographer should take the transducer and guide, clean the gel and blood off them, and soak them in a disinfectant solution, according to the hospital's infection control policies and the recommendations of the transducer manufacturer.

The patient is then taken to a holding or observation area. Depending on the type of procedure, the patient may remain

Figure 15-20 Needle with an echogenic stylet *(arrows)* allowing easy visualization of the needle. This hypoechoic mass was a metastatic lesion from a colon primary.

in this area from 15 to 120 minutes. If the patient's pain or discomfort increases, the sonographer should rescan to look for a hematoma. Patients who remain stable can be discharged with appropriate instructions or sent back to their units. Patients who have had chest procedures or procedures near the lungs will be sent to radiology for a chest x-ray to ensure that there is no pneumothorax.

Typically, a follow-up phone call is made by the nurse within the next 24 to 72 hours to ensure that the patient did not experience any complications.

Biopsy Complications. Complications from an ultrasound-guided biopsy are usually minor and may include postprocedural pain or discomfort, **vasovagal** reactions, and hematomas. Serious complications, although rare, include bleeding, hemorrhage, pneumothorax, pancreatitis, biliary leakage, peritonitis, infection, and death. Seeding of the needle track by malignant cells is very rare, with an estimated occurrence of 1 in 20,000 patients (Figure 15-22).

Inconclusive Biopsy Specimens. Unfortunately, not all biopsies yield sufficient material to provide a diagnosis. Causes of a poor specimen include insufficient material, necrotic lesion, and failure to sample the mass. If this occurs, a repeat biopsy may be required. If the first biopsy was performed without the presence of a cytopathology team, they should be present for the repeat procedure.

THE SONOGRAPHER'S ROLE IN PROCEDURES

Interventional procedures can be very challenging for everyone involved. A sonographer who has an interest in interventional ultrasound can be a valuable asset to the interventional team. Sonographers may work closely with a radiologist or sonologist or with other physicians, such as a nephrologist in native kidney biopsies, surgeons in kidney transplant or liver biopsies, or other clinicians in ascites taps or in a **thoracentesis.**

Involvement of sonographers has many benefits. They can locate the pathologic condition and determine various approaches, offering their recommendation of the best and safest needle path to the mass. Using their scanning skills, they can optimize the image to locate subtle masses and use Doppler to ensure that there are no vessels in the needle path. The sonographer can place the patient in a variety of positions to determine the best approach. For example, by placing the patient in a left posterior oblique or left lateral decubitus position, the liver may drop into a more subcostal position or a mass may roll away from a vessel. Placing the patient in a prone position may give better access to a renal mass. The sonographer's knowledge of new technologies, such as harmonic and compound imaging, may facilitate finding the mass (Figure 15-23).

TRANSDUCER SELECTION

The sonographer's choice of the proper transducer is very important. This means choosing not only the right frequency but also the correct transducer type. Sometimes it may be

Figure 15-21   **A,** Perinephric bleed *(arrow)* and hematoma after native renal biopsy. **B,** After pressing over the area of the bleed with the curved linear array transducer for 5 minutes, the bleeding stopped. **C,** Patient with a 5 cm bleed after a native renal biopsy. **D,** After 35 minutes of applied transducer pressure, the hematoma keeps increasing in size and is now 12.5 cm. Interventional radiology was called in for this patient.

Figure 15-22   **A,** Pleural-based lung lesion. **B,** The needle nicked the lung causing a small pneumothorax *(arrow)*. Fortunately an adequate specimen was obtained, which proved to be adenocarcinoma of the lung.

Figure 15-23 **A,** Cystic renal cell carcinoma *(arrow)* that was better visualized using harmonic imaging (*Gen* = normal image, *Harmon* = harmonic image). **B,** Image of a pancreatic head mass *(arrow)* using normal imaging parameters. **C,** Same patient, but now using compound imaging, which better defined the borders of the mass, leading to a successful biopsy and a diagnosis of adenocarcinoma.

better to use a transducer not normally associated in a routine examination of that area, for example, using an endocavitary transducer for a mediastinal or subclavicular mass or a phased array transducer to get to masses that require an intercostal approach in the chest (Figure 15-24). Because of the angle provided, a linear array may provide a safer choice in a pelvic node than may a curved array. In the abdomen and pelvis, both a curved array and a phased array transducer should be evaluated.

PATIENT BREATHING

Another aspect of the sonographer's preparation for the procedure is determining the effects of the patient's breathing on the mass. It is important to determine how much the mass moves with respiration and also how well and how long the patient can hold his or her breath. This will also give the sonographer and the patient a chance to practice breathing so that the patient knows what to expect. The sonographer can also point out the mass to the patient on the screen and show how breathing affects the location of the mass. They can then work together so that the patient can watch the screen and know how deep of a breath to take so that the mass lines up on or between the dotted lines on the screen. Besides abdominal and chest masses, neck and thyroid masses can also move with respiration.

Figure 15-24 Using an endocavitary transducer gave better access and resolution on this metastatic supraclavicular node in a patient with a history of thyroid cancer. The node was positive.

ASSISTING THE PHYSICIAN

Sonographers can assist with probe preparation and cleaning up. They can be scanning the next patient while the physician signs up the following patient or checks and dictates other studies. With a sonographer involved, a second physician may not be required, thus allowing patient flow to continue in the department.

During procedures, the sonographer should not be afraid to dialogue with the physician. For example, if they realize that the needle is approaching a major vessel, they should calmly and professionally tell the physician to stop (Figure 15-25). Also, they may need to discuss and determine solutions to problems, such as needle deviation. If a hematoma is forming, the sonographer may want to alert the physician so that they can decide whether to proceed with or stop the procedure (Figure 15-26). Patients tend to talk to the sonographer more, and their questions or fears can then be relayed to the physician. The sonographer can also gently remind the physician that the patient is holding his or her breath when they are taking a longer time than usual to obtain the specimen or can catch the patient's signal that they need to breathe and let the physician know.

The sonographer can also assist the physician by being a second set of hands during the procedure. The sonographer can adjust imaging controls, freeze and unfreeze the image, and track the needle tip. When using biopsy guides, the sonographer can hold the transducer. This can be especially helpful when aspiration techniques are used. The sonographer can use the transducer to press the bowel out of the way, allowing the mass to be seen. Because this increased transducer pressure needs to be maintained during the procedure, another set of hands is necessary. This technique can also be used to minimize the distance between the skin and the mass on deep lesions (Figure 15-27).

ASSISTING THE PATIENT

The sonographer can assist and encourage the patient during the procedure. This can be valuable in helping the patient

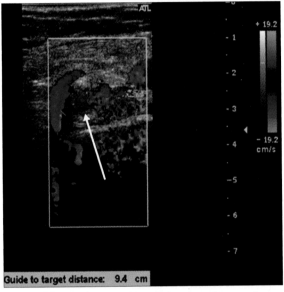

Figure 15-25 The sonographer must communicate to the physician if the needle deviates toward any of the vessels around this 1-cm node *(arrow)* in an HIV patient.

Figure 15-26 After the first pass on this liver core biopsy, a small subcapsular hematoma formed, thus canceling the second pass.

A   **B**

Figure 15-27 **A,** These deep retroperitoneal lymph nodes are difficult to see with normal scanning techniques. There is 5.4 cm of tissue between the abdominal wall and the anterior surface of the nodes. **B,** By applying pressure with the transducer, the distance from the abdominal wall and the nodes has decreased to 1.2 cm and now allows visualization of the nodes. This amount of pressure was applied during the biopsy, allowing a successful biopsy and a diagnosis of lymphoma.

control his or her breathing and giving the patient someone to talk to as necessary. The sonographer can coach and support the patient emotionally, thus allowing the physician to concentrate on the procedure or discuss the specimen with the cytopathologist, if present.

The sonographer's specialized knowledge also benefits patients. Using their Doppler skills, sonographers can locate vessels that may potentially traverse the needle path or be in close proximity to the mass. They can help guide the needle safely to deep retroperitoneal masses that may be near major vessels. Also, by using color or power Doppler, the sonographer can locate vessels in a mass that may represent viable tumor tissue. This can be very beneficial in masses that have necrotic areas (Figure 15-28).

FINDING THE NEEDLE TIP

The needle tip should appear as an echogenic dot on the ultrasound image. Visualizing the needle tip depends on several factors, including the type of needle, because specially designed echogenic needles are better seen than normal needles; the gauge of the needle, because larger gauge needles cause brighter reflections; the transducer frequency, using the highest frequency possible; the placement of the focal zone, which should be at or just below the level of the mass; using only one focal zone, because multiple focal zones may decrease the frame rate; and the echogenicity of the mass, because hypoechoic masses allow easier visualization of the needle than more echogenic masses (Figure 15-29). The needle should be inserted quickly and steadily and the tip followed as it advances towards the mass. The needle may deviate out of the projected path and away from the ultrasound beam, making it impossible to see the needle tip. This deviation of the needle can be caused by the physician bending or tilting the needle as it is being advanced or by the tissue and muscle planes it is traversing (Figure 15-30). Echogenic needle tips or scored stylets help to see the needle and needle tip better.

Tricks to try to see the needle tip include the following:

- Moving the needle up and down in a bobbing motion.
- Bobbing or jiggling the stylet inside the needle.
- Angling the transducer in a superior or inferior motion.

A **B** **C**

Figure 15-28 **A,** After several specimens only showed necrotic tissue, color Doppler was used to locate flow within the mass. Viable tissue was found in this location, and a diagnosis of a mediastinal adenocarcinoma was made. **B,** Transverse image of the upper abdomen in a patient with a suspected hepatic flexure tumor. **C,** Using color Doppler, the colon mass was defined and an ultrasound-guided biopsy was performed.

Figure 15-29 A, The needle tip is easily seen *(arrow)* in this patient with a hypoechoic metastatic lesion. **B,** The needle tip is harder to see *(arrow)* in this patient with a hyperechoic metastatic lesion.

Figure 15-30   Notice that the needle is being inserted with bending, which caused the needle to deviate out of the plane of the needle path and lose visualization of the needle tip.

Figure 15-31   This needle *(arrow)* deviated because a larger needle guide was placed in the attachment. This allowed a lot of play in the needle guide. After the needle guide size was corrected, an uneventful thyroid biopsy was performed in this benign nodule.

This is helpful when the needle is bent out of the plane of the sound beam.

- Using harmonics or compound imaging.
- As a last resort, removing the needle and starting again, closely watching the displacement of the tissue as the needle advances.

WHAT TO DO WHEN THE NEEDLE DEVIATES

Deviation of the needle from the projected path can be an issue. The tissue between the skin and the mass is usually the cause of this problem. If it is a constant problem, the sonographer can overcorrect (i.e., the sonographer can move the transducer more lateral or medial so that the path the needle is following will intersect the mass). It is important that the sonographer verify the correct size of needle guide because if the guide is too big, there is some play within it that can cause

this problem (Figure 15-31). Also the sonographer should make sure that the transducer is perpendicular to the lesion and that the needle guide touches the patient's skin. It is important that the sonographer become familiar with the various transducers and guides, how they should be placed on the body, and how to correct or adjust their scanning as necessary. If the problem persists, sometimes using a 20-gauge needle as opposed to a 22-gauge needle may correct the situation. In extreme cases, another pathway may need to be determined.

Another problem is when the mass is small and is pushed out of the way by the needle, as can happen with small nodes. Again, the sonographer needs to know how to counter these situations. Applying firm pressure with the transducer against the mass or trying to get the needle to approach the center of the mass so that it does not push the mass left or right can stabilize the mass and allow the needle to enter. Sometimes another approach may be necessary to break down the sterile field and start again. When these situations arise, the sonographer should be thinking of possible solutions to suggest.

COMMON BIOPSIES AND PROCEDURES

LIVER BIOPSY

The liver is one of the most common organs for biopsy, either for specific areas or masses or for diffuse parenchymal abnormalities. Liver masses are amenable to ultrasound-guided biopsy in the majority of cases. These include metastatic masses, suspected hepatocellular carcinoma (HCC) in patients with elevated AFP, or atypical benign lesions, such as adenomas, focal nodular hyperplasia, or hemangiomas. A biopsy is necessary for a hypoechoic area in a cirrhotic liver, although it may turn out to be a regenerating liver nodule. The inability to take a biopsy of a liver mass can be caused by the failure either to visualize the mass or to find a safe approach to the mass. Whenever possible, a subcostal approach should be used to avoid the possibility of a pneumothorax or damage to the intercostal arteries (Figure 15-32). Obtaining a biopsy in masses at the dome of the liver is easier under ultrasound than CT, although a steep-angle approach is often required. In some cases scanning and taking a biopsy in a sagittal plane are helpful. Core biopsies may be obtained on patients with hepatitis, cirrhosis, or increased liver function tests. The left lobe of the liver is biopsied using a subcostal approach. This is easier to perform and is more comfortable for the patient than the traditional blind approach through the ribs of the right lobe. Specific complications of liver biopsies include pneumothorax for masses near the dome of the liver, bile leak, and hematomas (Figure 15-33). With small masses, zoom techniques should be used to allow easier visualization of the mass (Figure 15-34).

PANCREATIC MASS BIOPSY

Most pancreatic mass biopsies are performed to confirm the diagnosis of adenocarcinoma, unresectable adenocarcinoma, or pancreatitis in patients with unusual imaging studies. The needle has to traverse the stomach or colon, but complications are rare. Color Doppler is useful to map out vessels, especially if there is encasement of them by the mass. Good specimens can usually be obtained near the biliary drainage tube, if the patient has one. A curved linear array transducer is preferred because it can help display bowel gas with its large footprint. Pancreatic biopsies can be very challenging because gas can move into the field obstructing visualization of the mass, even after the biopsy has started. Other challenges include finding a safe path around the various vessels, deflection or bending of the needle as it goes through the stomach, and patient breathing, which can cause the pancreas to move with respirations (Figure 15-35). Specific complications of pancreatic biopsies include pancreatitis.

RENAL MASS BIOPSY

Most solid renal tumors are surgically resected without obtaining a biopsy. However, a biopsy of a renal mass may be requested to differentiate an incidental renal cell carcinoma from a renal metastasis in a patient with a known primary cancer or if the patient has a prior history of renal cell carcinoma. Atypical cysts, especially those with thick septations, necessitate a biopsy to differentiate between a cystic renal cell carcinoma and a benign complex cyst. Renal parenchymal biopsies are requested on patients with proteinuria or in renal failure. They are performed with the patient prone, using the lower pole of the left kidney. The sonographer should guide the needle through the parenchymal tissue, such as through the upper or lower pole (Figure 15-36). Specific complications of renal biopsies include perinephric hematoma and hematuria. The sonographer should perform a color Doppler scan

A   **B**

Figure 15-32   **A,** This liver lesion *(arrow)* was only seen intercostally with the patient supine. **B,** With the patient in a right posterior oblique position, the liver fell below the ribs allowing better visualization and a subcostal approach on this metastatic mass.

Figure 15-33 **A,** Hematoma *(arrow)* in Morison's pouch after a liver core biopsy. **B,** The hematoma extended into the scrotal sac. Color Doppler verified that there was flow present in the testicle.

Figure 15-34 **A,** Small, 1 cm hypoechoic metastatic lesion *(arrow)* at normal scale size. **B,** The same small 1-cm metastatic lesion using a write zoom.

immediately after a biopsy to ensure that there is no active bleeding.

RENAL TRANSPLANTS

Ultrasound is used to guide biopsies when there is elevation of the BUN or creatinine or when the cause of rejection needs to be determined for treatment. Using color Doppler, the main renal vessels should be located. Typically, a biopsy of the upper pole of the kidney is taken to avoid possible lacerations of the main renal vessels and ureter. It is also recommended that a color Doppler image of the kidney be obtained to use as a baseline in case there are complications, such as an arteriovenous fistula (AVF) or pseudoaneurysm formation. Ultrasound can also be used to direct drainage of perinephric fluid collections, such as lymphoceles. Specific complications include hematomas, hematuria, and AVF (Figure 15-37).

ADRENAL BIOPSY

The most common indication for an adrenal biopsy is to differentiate an adenoma from a metastatic mass, particularly in

Figure 15-35 On this pancreatic head mass, the biopsy path was determined to avoid the mesenteric vessels.

Figure 15-36 Renal core biopsy through the lower pole of the left kidney.

Figure 15-37 After biopsy, image of this renal transplant demonstrates an arteriovenous fistula.

tally probably represents an adenoma, and a biopsy is not required. This is especially true if the mass is less than 3 cm in diameter, there is no known primary tumor, and there is no evidence of an endocrine abnormality. Also, it is important to exclude a pheochromocytoma with clinical and laboratory data, since a biopsy can cause a hypertensive crisis. Specific complications can include a pneumothorax and hematomas.

SPLEEN BIOPSY

Masses in the spleen are rare. Most lesions are metastatic in origin or are from lymphoma involvement. Since the spleen is highly vascular, there is an increased risk for bleeding or hemorrhage.

RETROPERITONEAL LYMPH NODE BIOPSY

Most retroperitoneal masses, including paraaortic and paracaval lymph nodes, are amenable to ultrasound guidance. These can be very technically challenging, especially with small masses and in large patients; therefore, the use of a needle guide is essential. Usually an anterior approach is preferred, and, by applying a firm and steady pressure with the curved linear array transducer, overlying bowel loops and intraabdominal fat can be displaced. This technique also reduces the depth at which the needle needs to be placed. Vascular structures are identified with color Doppler. Real-time monitoring of the needle tip ensures that the needle excursions during the biopsy stay within the node. For patients with suspected lymphoma, tissue needs to be obtained not only to diagnose lymphoma but also to determine the subtype, since this is critical for treatment. Usually part of the sample is sent for flow cytometric studies and a core may also be necessary. Specific complications include retroperitoneal hematomas.

LUNG BIOPSY

Ultrasound guidance has been shown to be a safe alternative to CT for biopsy of pleural, parenchymal, or mediastinal masses abutting the chest wall. This technique is associated with a high success rate and lower complications than CT. It is particularly valuable for small peripheral masses in close proximity to a rib and diaphragmatic masses, where slight respiratory excursion can affect the position of the mass. The transducer is placed parallel to the intercostal space and the needle is advanced in a single breath hold, minimizing trauma to the pleura. The tip is monitored to ensure that it does not slip out of the mass into normal, aerated lung. Intraparenchymal tumors are generally not amenable to ultrasound guidance, unless they are within an area of consolidation or the patient has a large pleural effusion that can be used as an acoustic window. Lung lesions can be very challenging using ultrasound, and it is always helpful to have the CT films present for guidance. These lesions are usually small and mobile with respiration. Creative positioning may be necessary to get between ribs and around the scapula. The patient may need to be placed in an oblique, decubitus, or prone position. A pillow or sponges may be placed under the patient to spread the ribs apart. The patient's arm may also need to be adjusted to get the scapula out of the way in apical lesions.

patients with a known malignancy, especially melanoma. The right adrenal gland is usually more accessible and can be reached via a transhepatic approach. Left adrenal mass biopsies can be more difficult, and the patient may need to have a biopsy in an oblique, a decubitus, or even a prone position. A solid, homogeneous adrenal mass that is discovered inciden-

A   **B**

Figure 15-38   A, Pleura-based lung lesion *(arrow)* that was difficult to access with this vector array transducer. **B,** Using this curved array transducer, which has the biopsy guide through the middle of the transducer, this lung mass was better defined and offered a safe approach. The arrow is pointing to the needle tip.

Transducer type also must be evaluated, because sometimes a phased array transducer provides better access than a linear array transducer (Figure 15-38). Fortunately, resolution is not as much as an issue as is accessibility. Start with a small foot print phased array transducer because it helps get between the ribs and allows the sonographer to angle through the rib space. Once the lesion is located, the linear array transducer can be evaluated for path access. Specific complications include pneumothorax.

THYROID BIOPSY

Thyroid biopsies can be helpful in distinguishing malignant masses from goiters or adenomas. Also, new masses may be assessed for recurrence in patients with known thyroid cancers. Biopsies should be taken in various portions of the mass to confirm colloid or abnormal cells and should be obtained in areas where small calcifications are noted because there is a higher percentage of positive cells in these areas (Figure 15-39). Large masses seen in a superclavicular location may not be amenable using a linear array transducer. High-frequency curved arrays or even an endocavitary transducer may give more access to the mass. Specific complications include neck pain and hematomas.

BIOPSY OF NECK NODES AND MASSES

Biopsies of neck masses can easily be performed with ultrasound guidance. In a patient with a history of thyroid cancer, it is important to differentiate between malignant and infectious nodes. Round, homogeneous nodes are usually suspicious for cancer as opposed to more oval nodes with echogenic centers from a fatty hilum. Other causes of neck masses include lymphoma and submandibular gland tumors (Figure 15-40).

Figure 15-39   After several negative passes in this large thyroid nodule, positive cells were obtained in the area of the small calcifications *(arrow).*

MUSCULOSKELETAL BIOPSY

Ultrasound has also proven successful in biopsies of masses in the extremities. These may be muscular in origin, such as a leiomyosarcoma or rhabdomyosarcoma, or from nerves, such as a schwannoma or neurofibroma. If it is a bony lesion that has broken through the cortex, ultrasound can be used. Ewing's sarcoma, osteosarcoma, and metastatic spread from prostate cancer are examples.

PELVIC MASS BIOPSY

A biopsy can be obtained for a variety of pelvic masses using ultrasound guidance. Pelvic lymph nodes can be seen and color

A   **B**

Figure 15-40 **A,** This lymph node exhibits the characteristics of a benign lymph node: oval in shape with a fatty hilum. **B,** Even though this node had the characteristics of a benign node, a biopsy was still performed. Surprisingly, the specimen came back positive for metastatic disease.

Doppler used to identify the iliac vessels. Perisacral masses may be seen with the patient supine, using a curved linear array transducer. If unable to see the mass with the patient supine, a prone approach should be used. In women, pelvic masses or fluid collections should be evaluated with both a transabdominal approach and an endovaginal approach. Endovaginal biopsies are usually performed with the patient in stirrups.

PROSTATE GLAND BIOPSY

A biopsy can be taken for men with elevated PSA levels, palpable nodules, or lesions seen in the peripheral zone using an endorectal transducer. The biopsy is obtained while the patient is in the left lateral decubitus position. Since the biopsy is through the rectal wall, the patient should be placed on a broad-spectrum antibiotic the day before and usually for two days after the biopsy to reduce the chance of an infection. Random samples can be taken as follows: one from the apex, middle, and base of the peripheral zone on both the right and left sides of the gland. Some clinicians also advocate taking a sample from the central gland on both sides. Endorectal transducers and their biopsy planes may vary between machines. In coronal-based biopsies, it may be necessary to turn the transducer 180 degrees to biopsy the left side to reduce the risk of injury to the prostatic urethra. (Remember to hit the left/right invert button if this is the case.) On the patient where a rectal approach is not feasible due to rectal surgery, a transperineal biopsy can be performed. The best transducer is typically a phased array transducer. The patient is placed in stirrups with the perineum exposed. The penis and

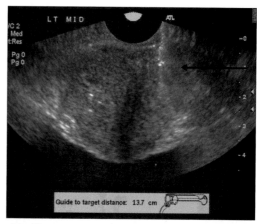

Figure 15-41 Prostate biopsy of a patient with an elevated PSA. Although no discrete mass was seen, adenocarcinoma of the prostate was found in one of the biopsy specimens.

scrotum need to be positioned out of the biopsy field and held in place with towels and tape. The patient is usually given intravenous sedation in addition to plenty of local anesthesia. Because of the lack of resolution, random specimens are obtained from the right and left sides of the prostate gland (Figure 15-41).

PLEURAL FLUID

Patients may be marked for a thoracentesis or have the procedure performed under sonographic guidance. Patients should be scanned in the same position that the procedure will be performed in, which is usually in an upright position, through the back. In cases of loculated fluid, it is beneficial to review the chest x-ray before scanning (Figure15-42). Care should be taken to identify the diaphragm and examine above the diaphragm so that the spleen or liver is not accidentally mistaken for a collection. This may happen as a result of an air artifact and the reduced overall gain that is typically used. A guide may not be necessary if the fluid is not complicated and the pocket large enough. When marking the patient, it is important not to press too hard on the skin because this will change the depth of the fluid and may cause the clinician not to advance the needle far enough to reach the fluid. The distance to the fluid and the distance to midpocket are usually measured. To scan between the ribs, a phased array transducer is preferred (Figure 15-43). If no fluid is visible, the patient should be scanned in the supine position to see if there are any fluid layers above the diaphragm.

ASCITES

Patients may be marked for an ascites tap or have the procedure under sonographic guidance. The entire abdomen and pelvis should be evaluated for the extent of the fluid and to locate the biggest pocket of ascites. To pool the fluid in the pelvis, the patient may be scanned with their abdomen elevated 30 to 45 degrees. A guide may be used if the fluid is septated or if the pocket is small or there are organs or bowel loops in the way. During the procedure, the patient may be rolled into an oblique position so that the fluid drains to the dependent portion where the needle is located. Again, when marking the fluid, care should be taken to apply just enough pressure with the transducer to make contact with the skin because this will influence the measurement of the fluid (Figure 15-44). The distance to the fluid and the distance to midpocket are measured (Figure 15-45). A postprocedural image can be taken to document the remaining amount of fluid (Figure 15-46).

Figure 15-42 Because of the loculations in the fluid, an ultrasound-guided thoracentesis was performed to remove some fluid for cytology.

Figure 15-43 Example of a marking for a thoracentesis to be performed without ultrasound guidance. The distance to the fluid is 1.27 cm and to the midpocket is between 4.16 and 7.21 cm.

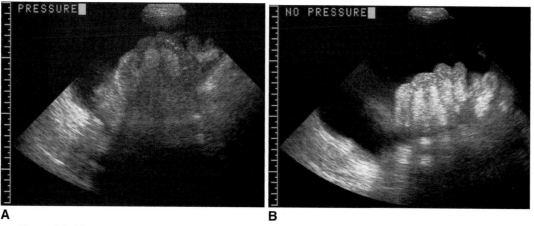

A   **B**

Figure 15-44 **A,** There is too much pressure from the transducer, giving the appearance that there is only a minimal amount of ascitic fluid in this area. **B,** Now, using minimal transducer pressure, a pocket of ascites is demonstrated.

Figure 15-45   An example of marking for a paracentesis. The distance to the fluid is 1.08 cm, and it is 7.11 cm to the fluid back wall.

Figure 15-46   Image documenting the residual fluid after a paracentesis.

SELECTED BIBLIOGRAPHY

Bernadino ME: Automated biopsy devices: significance and safety, *Radiology* 176:615-616, 1990.

Charboneau JW, Reading CC, Welch TJ: CT and sonographically guided needle biopsy: current techniques and new innovations, *AJR* 154:1-10, 1990.

Cronan JJ: Percutaneous biopsy, *Radiol Clin North Am* 34(6):1207-1223, 1996.

Hopper KD: Percutaneous, radiographically guided biopsy: a history, *Radiology* 196:329-333, 1995.

Ljung B-ME, Geller DA: Fine-needle aspiration techniques for biopsy of deep-seated impalpable targets: a primer for radiologists, *AJR* 171:325-328, 1998.

Middleton WD, Hiskes SK, Teefey SA and others: Small (1.5 cm or less) liver metastases: US-guided biopsy, *Radiology* 205:729-732, 1997.

Moore EH: Technical aspects of needle aspiration lung biopsy: a personal perspective, *Radiology* 208:303-318, 1998.

Sheafor DH, Paulson EK, Simmons CM and others: Abdominal percutaneous interventional procedures: comparison of CT and US guidance, *Radiology* 207:705-710, 1998.

Ward SC, Carey BM, Chalmers AG and others: The role of immediate cytological evaluation in CT-guided biopsy, *Clin Radiol* 49:531-534, 1994.

Wood BJ, Khan MA, McGovern F and others: Imaging guided biopsy of renal masses: indications, accuracy, and impact on clinical management, *J Urol* 161(5):1470-1474, 1999.

www.healthatoz.com Last accessed 3/18/05.

www.heartcenteronline.com Last accessed 3/18/05.

CHAPTER *16*

Emergent Abdominal Ultrasound Procedures

Sandra L. Hagen-Ansert

OBJECTIVES

- Name the most frequent reasons why people go to the emergency room
- List the complications of peritoneal lavage
- Name the reasons why ultrasound is a good screening tool for the trauma patient
- Define the goal of ultrasound in the assessment of blunt trauma
- Describe the sonographic findings of free fluid in the abdomen and/or pelvis
- Define the pitfalls and limitations of using ultrasound in the trauma patient
- Identify the most common modalities used to evaluate acute flank pain
- Describe the sonographic findings in aortic dissection
- Name the three types of abdominal hernias
- Describe the sonographic findings of a hernia

ASSESSMENT OF ABDOMINAL TRAUMA
PERITONEAL LAVAGE
COMPUTED TOMOGRAPHY
ULTRASOUND

FOCUSED ASSESSMENT WITH SONOGRAPHY FOR TRAUMA
ASSESSMENT OF BLUNT TRAUMA WITH ULTRASOUND
PARENCHYMAL INJURY

RIGHT UPPER QUADRANT PAIN: ACUTE CHOLECYSTITIS

EPIGASTRIC PAIN: PANCREATITIS

FLANK PAIN: UROLITHIASIS
CLINICAL FINDINGS FOR UROLITHIASIS
RADIOGRAPHIC EXAMINATION FOR UROLITHIASIS

AORTIC DISSECTION
CAUSES OF AORTIC DISSECTION
CLINICAL FINDINGS FOR AORTIC DISSECTION

RIGHT LOWER QUADRANT PAIN: APPENDICITIS

PARAUMBILICAL HERNIA
CAUSES OF HERNIATION

KEY TERMS

extracorporeal shock-wave lithotripsy (ESWL) – a procedure that breaks up kidney stones; shock waves are focused on the stones, disintegrating them and permitting their passage in the urine

focused assessment with sonography for trauma (FAST) – limited examination of the abdomen or pelvis to evaluate free fluid or pericardial fluid

hemoperitoneum – collection of bloody fluid in the abdomen or pelvis secondary to trauma or surgical procedure

incarcerated hernia – imprisonment or confinement of a part of the bowel; the visceral contents cannot be reduced

intravenous urography (IVU) – procedure used in radiography wherein contrast is administered intravenously to help visualize the urinary system

peritoneal lavage – invasive procedure that is used to sample the intraperitoneal space for evidence of damage to viscera and blood vessels

pseudodissection – condition seen in a patient with aortic dissection; there is no intimal flap seen, only hypoechoic thrombus near the outer margin of the aorta with echogenic laminated clot

reducible hernia – capable of being replaced in a normal position; the visceral contents can be returned to normal intraabdominal location

strangulated hernia – an incarcerated hernia with vascular compromise

The assessment of the abdomen for possible sustained intraabdominal injury caused by blunt abdominal trauma is a common clinical challenge for surgeons and emergency medicine physicians. The physical findings may be unreliable because of the state of patient consciousness, neurologic deficit, medication, or other associated injuries. The health care staff in emergency departments in the United States has used ultrasound for over a decade now with great success.

The most common reasons people go to the emergency room include problems in the following areas: lower gastrointestinal system, genitourinary system, cardiac concerns, orthopedics, respiratory complaints, nervous system complaints, lacerations, limb and joint problems, skin problems, and upper gastrointestinal problems.

The primary focus of this chapter is to cover the more common emergent abdominal procedures that the sonographer is likely to encounter in a "call back" situation from the emergency department.

ASSESSMENT OF ABDOMINAL TRAUMA

PERITONEAL LAVAGE

Peritoneal lavage is used to sample the intraperitoneal space for evidence of damage to the viscera and blood vessels. It is usually used as a diagnostic technique in certain cases of blunt abdominal trauma. This technique has been used as a surgical tool for the diagnosis of **hemoperitoneum** since 1965. A sensitivity of 95% has been found with this tool in the evaluation of intraperitoneal hemorrhage. However, this invasive procedure carries a complication risk of bowel perforation, bladder penetration, vascular laceration, and wound complications. It also is limited to injuries of the retroperitoneum and pancreas or contained injuries to solid intraperitoneal organs. It is inappropriate for alert patients in stable condition (who represent the majority of patients with blunt abdominal trauma).

The patient is placed in the supine position and the urinary bladder is emptied by catheterization. The stomach is emptied by a nasogastric tube because a distended stomach may extend to the anterior abdominal wall. The skin is anesthetized and a small vertical incision is made. The incision is made either in the midline or at the paraumbilical site with multiple layers of tissue penetrated before the parietal peritoneum is located (Figure 16-1).

Although peritoneal lavage has been used successfully to assess abdominal injuries, it is an invasive procedure. Peritoneal lavage carries a risk of organ injury and decreases the specificity of subsequent ultrasonography or computed tomography (CT) because of the introduction of intraperitoneal fluid and air.

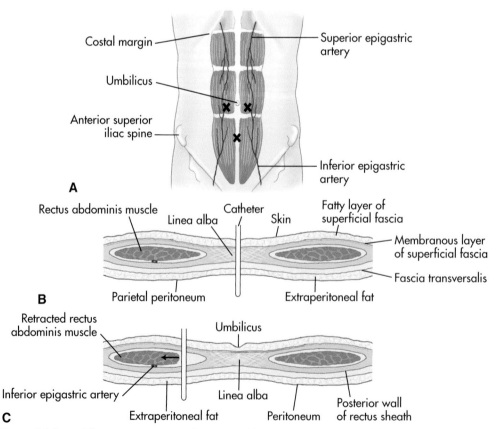

Figure 16-1 A, The two common sites for peritoneal lavage. **B,** Cross section of the anterior abdominal wall in the middle. Note the structures pierced by the catheter. **C,** Cross section of the anterior abdominal wall just lateral to the umbilicus.

COMPUTED TOMOGRAPHY

CT remains the radiology standard for investigating the injured abdomen, but requires patient transfer and inevitable delay (bowel preparation). CT is usually performed in patients in whom intraabdominal injury is strongly suspected. Other indications for CT include equivocal findings of abdominal examination in stable patients, persistent abdominal pain, and decreasing hematocrit. CT is unsuitable for patients who are clinically unstable.

ULTRASOUND

The clinical use of ultrasound in the evaluation of blunt trauma has existed in Europe and Asia for more than 20 years. Using ultrasound as a screening procedure involves many factors. The clinicians are looking for a screening tool that will be fast, accurate, portable, and easy to perform. Ultrasound is now well established as a noninvasive and easily repeatable tool to image many areas of the body.

FOCUSED ASSESSMENT WITH SONOGRAPHY FOR TRAUMA

Focused assessment with sonography for trauma is also known as the "**FAST**" scan in the emergency department. This is a limited examination of the abdomen or pelvis to evaluate free fluid or pericardial fluid. In the context of traumatic injury, free fluid is usually due to hemorrhage and contributes to the assessment of the circulation.

The FAST scan area of evaluation is widespread, extending from the pericardial sac to the urinary bladder and includes the perihepatic area (including Morison's pouch), perisplenic region (including splenorenal recess), paracolic gutters, and cul-de-sac (Figure 16-2). The visceral organs are assessed for heterogeneity and evaluated with color Doppler if necessary.

Accessibility and speed of performance are critical in the trauma setting. On-site personnel who are educated in performing the ultrasound examination provide the highest success rate. Limitations of ultrasound include its dependence on operator skill, which becomes particularly important if surgeons or emergency physicians with limited training perform the studies. Although CT remains the standard of reference for intraperitoneal and retroperitoneal assessment, this application is not readily available at the bedside.

ASSESSMENT OF BLUNT TRAUMA WITH ULTRASOUND

Ultrasound of the abdomen and pelvis is performed simultaneously with the physical assessment, resuscitation, and stabilization of the trauma patient. The length of time of the examination is usually about 5 minutes. The goal is to scan the four quadrants, pericardial sac, and cul-de-sac for the presence of free fluid or hemoperitoneum. Ultrasound has been found to be highly sensitive for the detection of free intraperitoneal fluid, but not sensitive for the identification of organ injuries. If the patient is hemodynamically stable, the value of ultrasound is limited by the large percentage of organ injuries that are not associated with free fluid.

Protocol for Focused Assessment with Sonography for Trauma. The ultrasound examination is performed with the proper transducer according to the patient size. The patient is usually in the supine position. The right and left upper quadrants of the abdomen, epigastrium, paracolic gutters, retroperitoneal space, and pelvis are evaluated with ultrasound (Box 16-1). If there is no contraindication to catheterization, the empty bladder is filled with 200 to 300 ml of sterile saline through a Foley catheter to ensure bladder distention to allow adequate visualization of the pelvic cavity. The examination is focused to look for the presence of free fluid, the texture of the visceral organs, and the pericardial sac around the heart.

The initial survey is directed in the subcostal plane with the transducer angled in a cephalic direction towards the four-chamber view of the heart to image the pericardial sac (Figure 16-3). The right upper quadrant is then evaluated, including the diaphragm, dome of the liver, subhepatic space (Morison's pouch), right kidney, and right flank (Figure 16-4). The liver is quickly scanned to look for texture abnormalities (Figure 16-5). The epigastrium is briefly examined (Figure 16-6). The transducer is then moved to the left upper quadrant to observe the diaphragm, spleen, left kidney, and left flank and to search for the presence of fluid (Figure 16-7). The pelvic cavity (with the bladder distended) is evaluated for the presence of free fluid in the cul-de-sac (Figure 16-8).

Sonographic Findings. In the trauma setting, free fluid usually represents hemoperitoneum, although it may also represent bowel, urine, bile, or ascitic fluid. Hemorrhage in the peritoneal cavity collects in the most dependent area of the abdomen (Figure 16-9). The fluid is usually hypoechoic or hyperechoic, with a few internal echoes and conforms to the anatomic site it occupies. The most common site of fluid accumulation is the subhepatic space (Morison's pouch), regardless of the site of the injury (Figure 16-10). The next most common space is the pelvis. The blood in the pelvis may collect centrally in the pouch of Douglas or laterally in the

Text continued on p. 462

BOX 16-1　FAST SCAN PROTOCOL

- Fill urinary bladder
- Scan subxiphoid to look for pericardial effusion
- Evaluate RUQ: diaphragm, subhepatic space/Morison's pouch, right kidney, right flank
- Evaluate liver for texture abnormalities
- Evaluate epigastrium
- Evaluate LUQ: diaphragm, spleen, left kidney, left flank
- Evaluate RLQ
- Evaluate LLQ

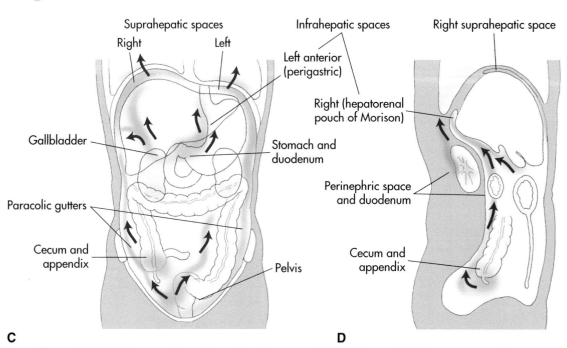

Figure 16-2 **A,** Transverse view of the perihepatic space and Morison's pouch. **B,** Transverse view of the perisplenic area and the splenorenal ligament. **C,** Anterior view of the collection of fluid in the abdomen and pelvic cavities. **D,** Sagittal view of the right abdomen shows how the fluid collects in the most dependent areas of the abdomen and pelvis.

Figure 16-3 **A,** Subcostal view of the four chambers of the heart. The transducer is angled sharply in a cephalic direction in the subcostal area. Cardiac pulsations are noted and the four chambers of the heart should be seen. **B,** Normally, there is no significant fluid that separates the outer layer of the heart (epicardium) within the pericardial sac. **C,** Subcostal four-chamber view shows a tip of the left lobe of the liver anterior to the large pericardial effusion that fills the pericardial cavity.

Figure 16-4 Gross anatomy **(A)** and transverse **(B)** images of the right upper quadrant and normal liver.

Figure 16-5 Gross anatomy (**A**) and sagittal (**B**) images of the right upper quadrant and normal liver demonstrates a good border between the liver and right kidney with no fluid in Morison's pouch. **C,** Sagittal image of the dome of the normal homogeneous liver. **D,** Sagittal image of the pleural cavity, the dome of the liver with the transducer along the lateral or axillary right upper quadrant.

Figure 16-6 Gross anatomy (**A**) and transverse (**B**) images of the epigastric area of the abdomen. The horseshoe shape of the spine is the most posterior reflection with the aorta and inferior vena cava directly anterior. The celiac axis arises from the anterior wall of the aorta. The left lobe of the liver is identified anterior to the pancreas, which lies directly anterior to the prevertebral vessels (aorta, inferior vena cava, celiac axis, and splenic vein).

Figure 16-7 A, Gross anatomy of the left upper quadrant. **B,** Sagittal image of the normal pleural cavity, diaphragm, spleen, and upper pole of the left kidney. **C,** Sagittal image of the normal left kidney without evidence of surrounding fluid or inhomogeneity.

Figure 16-8   A, Normal sagittal pelvic image with a distended urinary bladder and uterus posterior. It is not uncommon to see a small amount of fluid in a female of menstrual age. **B,** Transverse image of the distended urinary bladder as it provides a window for the uterus and adnexal area.

paravesical space (Figure 16-11). When fluid is present, the poorly visualized loops of bowel are separated by triangular collections of fluid. If there is a massive hemoperitoneum, the intraperitoneal organs will float in the surrounding fluid.

If the collection of fluid is small, the surgeon may not want to do an immediate laparotomy. Close monitoring of the patient with either ultrasound or CT imaging may help to define the further extent of the injury after the patient stabilizes.

PARENCHYMAL INJURY

The ultrasound appearance of hepatic and splenic injury will vary with both the type and time of injury. Liver lacerations or contusions are more easily detected with ultrasound than any other visceral abdominal injury. Such injuries appear as heterogeneous or hyperechoic. Hematomas and localized lacerations will appear echogenic or hypoechoic, which over time will become anechoic with the onset of hemolysis (Figure 16-12). Pitfalls of abdominal ultrasound include failure to show contained solid-organ injuries; injuries to the diaphragm, pancreas, and adrenal gland; and some bowel injuries. Therefore a negative ultrasound does not exclude an intraperitoneal injury, and close clinical observation or CT is warranted.

A brisk intraparenchymal hemorrhage may be identified as an anechoic region within the abnormal parenchyma; whereas a global parenchymal injury may project in the liver as a widespread architectural disruption with absence of the normal vascular pattern. An extensive splenic injury presents as a diffusely heterogeneous parenchymal pattern with both hyperechoic and hypoechoic regions.

The early diagnosis of parenchymal injury can affect patient treatment. The clinically stable patient with a hemoperitoneum and an obvious splenic injury seen on ultrasound can be taken directly to surgery. However, if extensive hepatic disruption is demonstrated, the surgeon may want further investigation with CT or even angiography before the surgery is performed.

Free Pelvic Fluid in Women. In female patients of reproductive age with trauma, free fluid isolated to the cul-de-sac is likely physiologic and clinical follow-up should suffice. Female patients with fluid elsewhere usually have a clinically important injury and require further evaluation.

Pitfalls and Limitations. As in other ultrasound procedures, obesity may prevent adequate visualization of the anatomical structures. In some cases the presence of subcutaneous emphysema precludes adequate ultrasound views. The presence of subcutaneous air from a pneumothorax that dissects into the abdominal cavity may collect over the liver or spleen.

An intraperitoneal clot is usually hyperechoic relative to the neighboring structures; occasionally, though, it is isoechoic, and intraperitoneal bleeding or parenchymal injury may go unrecognized.

Figure 16-9   Transverse image of a patient with pleural effusion as seen posterior to the right lobe of the liver. Fluid will collect in the most dependent area of the abdomen and should not be confused with pleural fluid.

Figure 16-10   RUQ fluid is present in a patient after trauma. There is a small amount of fluid seen in Morison's pouch anterior to the kidney. *F,* fluid; *IVC,* inferior vena cava; *L,* liver; *RK,* right kidney.

Figure 16-11   **A** and **B,** Endovaginal images of fluid in the pouch of Douglas.

Figure 16-12   Splenic hematoma secondary to splenic trauma from an automobile accident.
A, Ultrasound demonstration of the somewhat hypoechoic mass with low-lying echoes adjacent to the spleen. **B,** Perinephric hematoma in a patient after a renal biopsy procedure.

Contained parenchymal injuries of the liver and spleen, as well as bowel injuries, may not be accompanied by hemoperitoneum and may therefore be missed if screening ultrasound alone is used to evaluate for blunt trauma. Ultrasound may not depict injuries to the diaphragm, the pancreas, the adrenal gland, and bone.

RIGHT UPPER QUADRANT PAIN: ACUTE CHOLECYSTITIS

One of the most frequent complaints in the emergency department is the onset of severe right upper quadrant pain. If the patient is female with symptoms of right upper quadrant pain, fever, and leukocytosis, acute cholecystitis should be ruled out. The most common cause of acute cholecystitis is cholelithiasis with a cystic duct obstruction. Sonographic findings include a thickened gallbladder wall, a positive sonographic Murphy's sign, sludge, pericholecystic fluid, and a very dilated gallbladder.

EPIGASTRIC PAIN: PANCREATITIS

Midepigastric pain that radiates to the back is characteristic of acute pancreatitis. Pancreatitis occurs when the toxic enzymes escape into the parenchymal tissue of the gland, causing

obstruction of the acini, ducts, small blood vessels, and fat with extension into the peripancreatic tissue. Clinical findings of fever and leukocytosis are found along with elevated enzymes. The serum amylase levels increase within the first 24 hours of onset, but fall rather quickly, whereas the lipase levels take longer to elevate (as much as 72 hours) and remain elevated for a longer period of time. Sonographic findings in acute pancreatitis show a normal to edematous gland that is somewhat hypoechoic to normal texture. The borders are irregular secondary to the inflammation. Increased vascular flow may be apparent because of the inflammatory nature of the disease.

FLANK PAIN: UROLITHIASIS

Flank pain caused by urolithiasis is a common problem in patients coming to the emergency department. Radiology plays a vital role in the evaluation of these patients through the use of ultrasonography, nuclear medicine, intravenous urography, conventional radiography, and the unenhanced CT.

Traditional evaluation of the patient with flank pain consisted of conventional radiography followed by **intravenous urography (IVU)** with noniodinated contrast. In those patients unable to undergo IVU safely (i.e., patients with acute renal failure and pregnant patients), ultrasound was used to evaluate for secondary signs of obstruction, namely hydronephrosis. In patients with acute renal failure, nuclear medicine examinations may be used to provide information on renal function. Computerized unenhanced tomography has largely replaced these other modalities with the ability to identify calculi and their location, determine the size, and guide the management.

CLINICAL FINDINGS FOR UROLITHIASIS

Acute ureteral obstruction usually manifests as renal colic, a severe pain that is often spasmodic, that increases to a peak level of intensity, and then decreases before increasing again. The pain can also manifest as steady and continuous. The pain usually begins abruptly in the flank and increases rapidly to a level of discomfort that often requires narcotics for adequate pain control. Over time, the pain may radiate to the lower abdomen and into the scrotum or labia as the stone moves into the more distal portion of the ureter.

Urinalysis is the initial laboratory examination. Hematuria is the common finding in 85% of the patients. However, if the stone completely obstructs the ureter, no hematuria will be present. Clinical symptoms, such as fever, leukocytosis, and urine gram staining, can help identify a superimposed urinary tract infection.

Stone size is important in treatment. More than 90% of stones smaller than 4 mm and 50% of stones 4 to 7 mm in diameter will pass spontaneously. The primary method for treatment of symptomatic urolithiasis is **extracorporeal shock-wave lithotripsy (ESWL)**.

RADIOGRAPHIC EXAMINATION FOR UROLITHIASIS

Intravenous urography (IVU) is the least expensive initial examination for the patient suspected of having urolithiasis, since the majority of urinary calculi are radiopaque. The IVU has been the traditional modality of chooce for evaluation of patients suspected of having urolithiasis. After the IV administration of contrast material, the classic signs of ureteral obstruction include delayed opacification of the collecting system and a persistent delayed nephrogram that increases in intensity with time.

Sonographic Findings. The calculi seen by ultrasound are highly echogenic foci with distinct acoustic shadowing. Stones as small as 0.5 mm may be seen with ultrasound. When obstruction occurs, ultrasound is very effective in demonstrating the secondary sign of hydronephrosis (Figure 16-13). The evaluation of the distal ureters may be obscured by overlying bowel gas in the pelvis. With the bladder distended, color Doppler is an excellent tool to image the presence of ureteral jets in the bladder. The transducer should be angled in a cephalic presentation through the distended urinary bladder. Color Doppler is turned on and the probe is held stationary to watch for the appearance of ureteral jets. The PRF (pulse repetition frequency) should be decreased to assess the low velocity of the ureteral jet flow. The color gain should be turned up just enough to barely see color in the background. Usually within 2 to 3 minutes the jet will light up with color as the urine drains into the bladder (Figure 16-14). Be sure to look for the presence of both the right and left ureteral jet with this technique. Power Doppler may also be used to image the ureteral jets and is very effective.

The presence of hydronephrosis in a pregnant patient may be more problematic because it is not uncommon for the kidneys to become slightly hydronephrotic during the latter stage of pregnancy because the uterus enlarges and causes pressure on the ureter. This is seen especially in the right kidney because it lies lower than the left and is more likely to show minimal hydronephrosis. Therefore, the appearance of ureteral jets may help to rule out the presence of obstruction secondary to calculi.

AORTIC DISSECTION

A dissecting aortic aneurysm is a condition in which a propagating intramural hematoma actually dissects along the length of the vessel, stripping away the intima and, in some cases, part of the media (Figure 16-15). The resultant aortic dissection is

Figure 16-13 Ultrasound demonstration of hydronephrosis secondary to a stone in the urinary system.

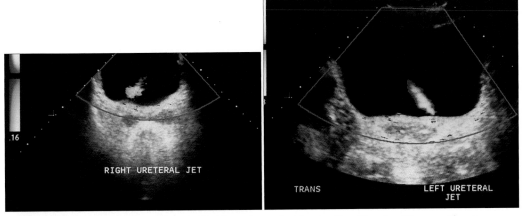

Figure 16-14 Normal ureteral jets in bladder as imaged with color flow Doppler. (Courtesy Shpetim Telegrafi, New York University.)

Figure 16-15 Gross pathology of a dissecting aortic aneurysm demonstrates the layers of the aortic wall separated by the blood. (From Damjanov I, Linder J: *Pathology: a color atlas,* St Louis, 2000, Mosby.)

a defect or tear in the aortic intima with concomitant weakness of the aortic media. At this point, blood surges into the media, separating the intima from the adventitia. This channel is called the "false lumen." This blood in the false lumen can reenter the true lumen anywhere along the course of the dissection. Most aortic dissections will occur at one of three sites: (1) at the root of the aorta with possible extension into the arch, descending aorta, and abdominal aorta; (2) at the level of the left subclavian artery, with extension into the descending aorta or abdominal aorta; and (3) only at the level of the ascending aorta.

Approximately 70% of dissections are located in the ascending aorta, 10% to 20% in the aortic arch, and 20% in the abdominal aorta. Most often, the dissection will propagate distally in the aorta into the iliac vessels, although proximal extension can occur.

CAUSES OF AORTIC DISSECTION

Systemic hypertension is nearly always associated with aortic dissection (Box 16-2). The age of most patients affected ranges

> ### BOX 16-2 CAUSES OF AORTIC DISSECTION
>
> - Hypertension (70%-90%)
> - Marfan's syndrome (16%)
> - Pregnancy
> - Acquired or congenital aortic stenosis
> - Coarctation of the aorta
> - Trauma
> - Iatrogenic (cardiac catheterization, aortic valve replacement)

from 50 to 70 years, with a higher prevalence in males than females. In the under age 40 group, the incidence is equal. In women, 50% of dissections occur during pregnancy. (Hormonal imbalance, associated hypertension, and sclerosis and necrosis of both the medial layer and the vasa vasorum all play a contributory role.) Without treatment, a dissecting aorta may result in death if the dissection obstructs the blood flow to the brain or the tear is so great that volumes of blood loss occur.

CLINICAL FINDINGS FOR AORTIC DISSECTION

The most typical presentation is that of a sudden onset of severe, tearing chest pain radiating to the arms, neck, or back. Syncope occurs in a small percentage of patients. The complexity of the symptoms will depend upon the extension of the dissection, the specific branches of the aorta involved, and the location of external rupture if present (Table 16-1). If the carotid artery is affected, hemiplegia may result. Involvement of the subclavian or iliac vessels will appear with decreased or absent pulses in the arms or legs.

The location of the pain may be a clue to the site of the dissection. If the pain centers in the anterior thorax, a proximal dissection may be present; severe pain in the interscapular area is more common with distal involvement. However, the majority of patients with distal dissection of the aorta have

TABLE 16-1	COMMON EMERGENCY CONDITIONS	
Clinical Findings	**Sonographic Findings**	

RUQ Pain: Cholecystitis

RUQ pain	Thickened GB wall
Fever	+ Murphy's sign
Nausea, vomiting	Pericholecystic fluid
Leukocytosis	Dilated GB

Epigastric Pain: Pancreatitis

Midepigastric pain	Normal to edematous gland
Radiating to back	Hypoechoic texture
Fever	Irregular borders
Leukocytosis	Increased vascular flow
↑ Amylase	
↑ Lipase	

Flank Pain: Urolithiasis

Spasmodic flank pain	Echogenic foci with shadowing
Pain may radiate into pelvis	Hydronephrosis may be present
Hematuria	Look for ureteral jets in bladder
Fever	
Leukocytosis	

Thoracic Or Abdominal Pain: Aortic Dissection

Sudden onset of severe chest pain with radiation to arms, neck, or back	Aneurysm Look for flap at site of dissection
Syncope may be present	Look for false lumen

RLQ PAIN: Appendicitis

Intense RLQ pain	Distended, noncompressible
Nausea, vomiting	appendix
Fever	↑ Color flow
Leukocytosis	McBurney sign

Lower Abdominal Pain: Paraumbilical Hernia

Asymptomatic to mild discomfort	Lower abdominal mass; look for peristalsis of bowel in hernia
Palpable mass	
Valsalva: shows exaggeration of mass	
Reduce sac with gentle pressure	

Figure 16-16   Surgical revelation of a large abdominal aortic aneurysm that has dissected and ruptured into the abdominal cavity.

On ultrasound examination, the classic finding is the visualization of the flap at the site of the dissection. An echogenic intimal membrane within the aorta and/or the iliac arteries may be seen to move freely with arterial pulsations on sonography if both the true and false lumen are patent (Figure 16-16). However, if the membrane is thick and the lumen is thrombosed, the membrane may not move. Color Doppler may demonstrate slow flow in both the true and false lumen. The flow is decreased or reversed in the false lumen. The sonographer should look for the presence of the intimal membrane with concomitant clotting in the iliac, celiac, and superior mesenteric arteries.

A **"pseudodissection"** on color flow demonstrates a turbulent blood flow pattern, indicating a hypoechoic thrombus near the outer margin of the aorta with an echogenic laminated clot. No intimal flap is seen with a pseudodissection.

RIGHT LOWER QUADRANT PAIN: APPENDICITIS

Acute appendicitis is one of the most common diseases that necessitates emergency surgery and is the most common atraumatic surgical abdominal disorder in children 2 years of age and older. The early diagnosis of acute appendicitis is essential in the prevention of perforation, abscess formation, and postoperative complications. The classic clinical symptoms include exquisite lower abdominal pain, nausea, vomiting, fever, and leukocytosis. The quick release is performed by applying pressure with the fingertips directly over the area of the appendix and then quickly letting go. With appendicitis, the patient will usually have rebound tenderness, "McBurney's sign," associated with peritoneal irritation. Ultrasound examination uses a graded compression technique over the right lower quadrant. Gradual pressure with the transducer is

back pain. Occlusion of the visceral arteries may appear with abdominal pain.

Sonographic Findings. In the acute aortic dissection, time is of the essence and therefore MRI and/or contrast-enhanced CT are the imaging modalities of choice for evaluating aortic dissections. In the stabilized patient with a suspected dissection, sonography may be performed. Since most dissections are seen in the ascending aorta, a transesophageal echocardiogram will be performed in the cardiology division. If the dissection is suspected in the abdomen, an abdominal ultrasound may be requested. The size of the aorta may be somewhat enlarged, but not necessarily aneurysmal.

Figure 16-17   Right inguinal hernia that causes a bulging enlargement of the inguinal canal. (From McMinn RMH: *Functional and clinical anatomy,* St Louis, 1995, Mosby.)

Figure 16-18   Ultrasound evaluation in real time shows the peristalsis of the multiple bowel loops in the swollen scrotal sac.

placed over the point of tenderness in an effort to displace the bowel and to image the area of the inflamed appendix (see Table 16-1).

PARAUMBILICAL HERNIA

A common cause of abdominal pain and intestinal obstruction is the presence of an abdominal wall hernia. The hernia may be classified into one of three types: (1) **reducible hernia** is one in which the visceral contents can be returned to the normal intraabdominal location; (2) **incarcerated hernia** means the visceral contents cannot be reduced; and (3) **strangulated hernia** is an incarcerated hernia with vascular compromise.

A hernia forms when the abdominal wall muscles are weakened, thus allowing the viscera to protrude into the weakened abdominal wall. The weakest area of the abdomen is the site of the umbilicus and this paraumbilical hernia occurs more often in females (Figure 16-17).

CAUSES OF HERNIATION

Common causes of herniation include congenital defect or weakening of the abdominal wall; increased abdominal pressure secondary to ascites, abdominal mass, bowel obstruction, obesity, and repeated pregnancy. Strangulation of the colon and omentum is a complication of the hernia. Another complication of a hernia is rupture of the abdominal wall in severe chronic ascites.

Sonographic Findings. The real-time visualization of the bowel within the hernia provides critical information for the clinician. Sonography allows visualization of the peristaltic movement of the bowel during Valsalva maneuvers and determines the presence or absence of vascular flow within the defect.

The sonographic criteria for a paraumbilical hernia include (1) demonstration of an anterior wall defect, (2) presence of

bowel loops within the sac, (3) exaggeration of the sac during the Valsalva maneuver, and (4) reducibility of the sac with gentle pressure (Figure 16-18). Most paraumbilical hernias contain colon, omentum, and fat. The large intestine will display a complex pattern of fluid, gas, and peristalsis. Of course, the mesenteric fat is very echogenic.

The high-frequency linear array transducer allows the sonographer to demonstrate a wide area of the abdominal wall. Reduced gain to demonstrate the layers of the abdominal wall will be useful to see the distinction between the hernia, bowel, and muscular layers of tissue. Color flow will be necessary to determine the vascular flow within the hernia sac. The patient should be instructed to perform a Valsalva maneuver to determine the site of wall defect and confirm the presence of the protruding hernia. It is important to visualize the peristalsis of the bowel loops within the hernia to confirm the diagnosis (see Table 16-1).

SELECTED BIBLIOGRAPHY

Brown MA, Casola G, Sirlin CB and others: Blunt abdominal trauma: screening US in 2,693 patients, *Radiology* 218:352-358, 2001.

Chambers JA, Pilbrow WJ: Ultrasonography in abdominal trauma: an alternative to peritoneal lavage, *Arch Emerg Med* 5:26-33, 1998.

Cramer MM: Color flow duplex examination of the abdominal aorta: atherosclerosis, aneurysm, and dissection, *JVT* 19(5-6):249-260, 1995.

Harrison LA, Keesling CA, Martin NL and others: Abdominal wall hernias: review of herniography and correlation with cross sectional imaging, *Radiographics* 15:315-332, 1995.

Henningsen C: *Clincal guide to ultrasonography,* St Louis, 2004, Mosby.

Hoffman R, Nerlich M, Muggia-Sullam M and others: Blunt abdominal trauma in cases of multiple trauma evaluated by ultrasonography: a prospective analysis of 291 patients, *J Trauma* 32:452-458, 1992.

John W, Kefer MP: Ultrasound detection of free intraperitoneal fluid associated with hepatic and splenic injuries, *South Med J* 1:94, 54-57, 2001.

Leonhardt WC: Ultrasound classics—just when you thought it was safe to go home, SDMS Annual Meeting, 2003.

Lingawi SS, Buckely AR: Focused abdominal US in patients with trauma, *Rad* 217:426-429, 2000.

McGahan JP, Wang L, Richards JR: Focused abdominal US for trauma, *Radiographics* 21:S191-S199, 2001.

McKenney KL: Role of ultrasound in the diagnosis of intraabdominal catastrophes, *Radiographics* 19:1332-1339, 1999.

Poletti PA, Kinkel K, Vermeulen B and others: Blunt abdominal trauma: should US be used to detect both free fluid and organ injuries? *Radiology* 227:95-103, 2003.

Sirlin CB, Casola G, Brown MA and others: US of blunt abdominal trauma: importance of free pelvic fluid in women of reproductive age, *Radiology* 219:229-235, 2001.

Snell RS: *Clinical anatomy,* Philadelphia, 2004, Lippincott, Williams & Wilkins.

Tamm EP, Silverman PM, Shuman WP: Evaluation of the patient with flank pain and possible ureteral calculus, *Radiology* 228:319-329, 2003.

PART III

Superficial Structures

CHAPTER 17

The Breast

Sandra L. Hagen-Ansert, Tamara L. Salsgiver, and M. Elizabeth Glenn

KEY TERMS

acinus (acini) – glandular (milk-producing) component of the breast lobule; the breast contains hundreds of lobules, each containing several small glands (acini)

adenosis – overgrowth of the acini within the terminal ductal lobular unit (TDLU) of the breast; one component of a fibrocystic condition

anechoic – without echoes; simple cyst on ultrasound should be anechoic

antiradial – plane of imaging on ultrasound of the breast that is perpendicular to the radial plane of imaging; the radial plane of imaging uses the nipple as the center point of an imaginary clock face imposed on the breast, such that the radial 12 o'clock plane is a line extending upward toward the top of the breast; similarly the radial 9 o'clock plane extends straight out to the right aspect of the breast, and so on; three-dimensional measurements of a breast mass can be recorded using sagittal/transverse or radial/antiradial planes

apocrine metaplasia – form of fibrocystic change in which the epithelial cells of the acini undergo alteration (metaplasia); the epithelial cells assume a columnar shape similar to sweat (apocrine) glands. This process can lead to cyst formation, hyperplasia, and other changes of fibrocystic condition.

areola – the pigmented skin surrounding the breast nipple.

asymptomatic – without symptoms; in the case of breast cancer screening, only those women without any symptoms of possible breast cancer (i.e., asymptomatic) are eligible for a screening mammogram, which is a fast, low-cost mammogram examination; a screening mammogram is different from a diagnostic mammogram in that it is a more extensive examination for evaluation of a specific symptom or an abnormal finding

atypical ductal hyperplasia (ADH) – see atypical hyperplasia

atypical hyperplasia – abnormal proliferation of cells with atypical features involving the TDLU, with an increased likelihood of evolving into breast cancer; in atypical ductal hyperplasia (ADH), the pathologist recognizes some, but not all, of the features of ductal carcinoma in situ (DCIS); atypical lobular hyperplasia (ALH) shows some, but not all, the features of lobular carcinoma in situ (LCIS); ALH and LCIS are now grouped by some authors under the term lobular neoplasia

atypical lobular hyperplasia (ALH) – see atypical hyperplasia and lobular neoplasia

axilla – armpit; the axilla contains the lymph nodes that drain the majority of the breast tissue; in the case of invasive breast cancer, the lymph nodes are generally sampled to accurately stage the breast cancer and direct further treatment

breast – differentiated apocrine sweat gland with a functional purpose of secreting milk during lactation

breast cancer (breast carcinoma) – breast cancer involves two main types of cells (ductal and lobular); ductal cancer, accounting for approximately 85% of the breast cancer cases, also includes many subtypes, such as medullary, mucinous, tubular, apocrine, or papillary types; in addition, very early or preinvasive breast cancer is generally ductal in type; this preinvasive breast cancer is also called in situ, non-invasive, or intraductal breast cancer; another commonly used term for this early type of cancer is *ductal carcinoma in situ*, or DCIS

breast cancer screening – screening for breast cancer involves annual screening mammography (starting at age 40), monthly breast self-examination (BSE), and regular clinical breast examination (CBE)

breast imaging reporting and data system (BI-RADS) – trademark system created by the American College of Radiology (ACR) to standardize mammographic reporting terminology, categorize breast abnormalities according to the level of suspicion for malignancy, and to facilitate outcome monitoring; this system of classification of breast imaging results has now been made a mandatory part of mammogram reports by federal legislation (Mammography Quality Standards Act of 1994)

breast self-examination (BSE) – part of breast cancer screening; every woman is encouraged to perform breast self-examination monthly starting at age 20; BSE is usually best performed at the end of menses

clinical breast examination (CBE) – part of breast cancer screening; every woman is encouraged to have a thorough CBE in conjunction with her routine health care assessment; between ages 20 and 40, CBE is advised every 3 years; from age 40 on, CBE should be performed by the woman's regular health care provider annually

Cooper's ligaments – connective tissue septa that connect perpendicularly to the breast lobules and extend out to the skin; are considered to be the fibrous "skeleton" supporting the breast glandular tissue

cyst – fluid-filled sac; cysts in the breast result usually either from obstruction of the terminal duct draining the normal fluid secretions from the acinar units of the lobule, or from overproduction of fluid from the acini; cysts can vary in size from a millimeter to several centimeters; cysts are typically simple (anechoic, sharply marginated) or complex (thick irregular wall, internal debris, internal echoes, intracystic mass)

cyst aspiration – common breast procedure (both diagnostic and interventional), involves placing a needle through the skin of the breast into a cystic mass and pulling fluid out of the cystic mass through the needle; in the case of a palpable cyst, this procedure can be performed in a physician's office; in the case of a small, complex, or nonpalpable cyst, image guidance (usually with ultrasound) can be used to facilitate the aspiration

diagnostic breast imaging – also called "consultative," "work-up," or "problem-solving" mammography or breast imaging; this type of breast imaging examination is more intensive than routine screening mammography; diagnostic breast imaging is usually directed toward a specific clinical symptom of possible breast cancer, or an abnormal finding on a screening mammogram; the goal of diagnostic breast imaging is to categorize the abnormality according to the level of suspicion for cancer (see BI-RADS)

epitheliosis – overgrowth (hyperplasia) of the cells lining the small ducts of the TDLU; epitheliosis is one of the common components of most varieties of fibrocystic condition

fibroadenoma – most common benign solid tumor of the breast, consisting predominantly of fibrous and epithelial (adenomatous) tissue elements. These masses tend to develop in young women (even teenagers), tend to run in families, and can be multiple. The usual appearance of a fibroadenoma is a benign appearing mammographic mass (round, oval, or gently lobular and well circumscribed) with a correlating sonographic mass that is well defined and demonstrates homogeneous echogenicity.

fibrocystic condition (FCC) – also called *fibrocystic change* or *fibrocystic breast,* this condition represents many different tissue processes within the breast that are all basically normal processes that in some patients become exaggerated to the point of raising concern for breast cancer. The main fibrocystic tissue processes are adenosis, epitheliosis, and fibrosis. These processes can cause symptoms, such as lumps and pain, and changes on the mammogram that mimic cancer. These processes can cause mammographic changes, such as cysts, microcalcifications, distortion, and masslike densities. Common pathologic changes of FCC include apocrine metaplasia, microcystic adenosis, sclerosing adenosis, and many others. Only a few fibrocystic tissue processes are associated with an increased risk of subsequent development of breast cancer. See atypical hyperplasia.

fremitus – refers to vibrations produced by phonation and felt through the chest wall during palpation; a technique used in conjunction with power Doppler to identify the margins of a lesion

gynecomastia – hypertrophy of residual ductal elements that persist behind the nipple in the male. There is generally no lobular (glandular) tissue in the male patient, causing a palpable, usually tender lump. A breast mass resulting from gynecomastia must be distinguished from male breast cancer.

hyperechoic – echo texture that is more echogenic than the surrounding tissue. Hyperechoic masses in the breast are nearly always benign.

hypoechoic – echo texture that is less echogenic than the surrounding tissue. Most solid breast masses (including cancer) are hypoechoic.

infiltrating (invasive) ductal carcinoma – cancer of the ductal epithelium; most common general category of breast cancer, accounting for around approximately 85% of all breast cancers. This cancer usually arises in the terminal duct in the TDLU. If the cancerous cells remain within the duct without invading the breast tissue beyond the duct wall, this is ductal carcinoma in situ (DCIS). If the cancerous cells invade breast tissue (i.e., invasive ductal carcinoma or IDC), the cancer may spread into the regional lymph nodes and beyond. Of the many subtypes of IDC, the most common is infiltrating ductal carcinoma, not otherwise specified (IDC-NOS).

infiltrating (invasive) lobular carcinoma (ILC) – cancer of the lobular epithelium of the breast, arises at the level of the TDLU; accounts for 12% to 15% of all breast cancers

isoechoic – echo texture that resembles the surrounding tissue. In the breast, isoechoic masses can be difficult to identify.

juxtathoracic – near the chest wall (thorax)

lobular carcinoma in situ (LCIS) – see lobular neoplasia

lobular neoplasia – a term preferred by many authors to replace LCIS (not considered a true cancer nor treated as such) and atypical hyperplasia

mammary layer – middle layer of the breast tissue (one of three layers recognized on breast ultrasound between the skin and the chest wall) that contains the ductal, glandular, and stromal portions of the breast

multicentric breast cancer – breast cancer occurring in different quadrants of the breast and are at least 5 cm or more apart; multicentric cancers are more likely to be of different histologic types than is a multifocal cancer

multifocal breast cancer – breast cancer occurring in more than one site within the same quadrant or the same ductal system of the breast

nonpalpable – cannot be felt on clinical examination; nonpalpable breast mass is one that is usually identified on screening mammogram and is too small to be felt as a breast lump on BSE or CBE

Paget's disease – surface erosion of the nipple (reddened area with flaking and crusty areas) that results from direct invasion of the skin of the nipple from underlying breast cancer

palpable – can be felt on clinical examination; palpable breast lump is one that is identified on CBE or BSE

peau d'orange – French term that means "skin of the orange;" descriptive term for skin thickening of one breast that, on clinical breast examination, resembles the skin of an orange. The thickening is caused by the pores of the skin opening to allow edema to directly evaporate through the skin since inflammatory disease has blocked the lymphatic drainage of fluids building up in those tissues. Such an appearance can result from an inflammatory breast condition (mastitis), simple edema, or skin involvement from underlying breast cancer.

radial – plane of imaging on ultrasound of the breast, see antiradial

retromammary layer – deepest of the three layers of the breast noted on breast ultrasound. The retromammary layer is predominantly fatty and can be thin. The retromammary layer separates the active breast glandular tissue from the pectoralis fascia overlying the chest wall muscles.

sentinel node – represents the first lymph node along the axillary node chain. This is the node chain the surgeon identifies for evidence of metastasis.

spiculation – fingerlike extension of a malignant tumor; usually appears as a small line that radiates outward from the margin of a mass

subcutaneous layer – most superficial of the three layers of the breast identified on breast ultrasound, the subcutaneous layer is mainly fatty; it is located immediately beneath the skin and superficial to the mammary layer. The subcutaneous layer can be very thin and difficult to recognize.

tail of Spence – a normal extension of breast tissue into the axillary or arm pit region

terminal ductal lobular unit (TDLU) – smallest functional portion of the breast involving the terminal duct and its associated lobule containing at least one acinus (tiny milk-producing gland). The TDLU undergoes significant monthly hormone-induced changes and radical changes during pregnancy and lactation. The TDLU is the site of origin of nearly all significant pathologic processes involving the breast, including all elements of fibrocystic condition, fibroadenomas, and in situ and invasive breast cancer (both lobular and ductal).

One out of eight American women will develop **breast cancer**. It is the most common type of cancer among women in the United States and is the leading cause of cancer death among women between the ages of 40 and 59. Early detection of breast cancer is vital, since cancer can be difficult to eradicate once it has spread. Delays in early detection and treatment can be particularly tragic because the survival rate for localized breast cancer adequately treated is 98% after 5 years and 95% after 10 years, whereas metastatic cancer shows survival rates of only 30% to 50% after 10 years. Ultrasound evaluation of the **breast** plays a vital role in the early detection and characterization of breast masses and provides real-time guidance during interventional breast procedures.

This chapter presents an overview of breast anatomy, physiology, sonographic evaluation techniques, and breast pathology with emphasis on breast cancer diagnosis and staging.

HISTORICAL OVERVIEW

John Wild published the first paper on breast ultrasound in 1951. This early paper described the A-mode technique of ultrasound imaging. Advancements in ultrasound equipment design allowed increased tissue characterization and by 1970, gray scale ultrasound technique had significantly improved diagnostic accuracy. Dedicated whole breast ultrasound units were tested as a potential screening method for the detection of breast cancer. This effort, unfortunately, failed. Whole breast ultrasound imaging units gave way to smaller units with hand-held transducers for breast evaluation. Although ultrasound was not an effective primary tool in **breast cancer screening,** its usefulness as an adjunctive tool to mammography for breast lesion characterization became increasingly evident. Screening mammograms have long been considered the gold standard for breast cancer screening, although accumulating evidence suggests that ultrasound screening in conjunction with mammography may be beneficial in patients with very dense tissue, complicated mammograms, or very high risk factors for breast cancer.

Most clinical laboratories today use high-resolution, real-time sonography as an adjunct to mammographic screening. Although screening the entire breast with ultrasound is not routinely done, most ultrasound laboratories currently perform the breast examination within a localized area to characterize palpable lesions or suspicious areas seen on a mammogram. High frequency 10 to 15 MHz transducers have the optimum resolution and the short-to-medium focus necessary for obtaining high-quality images of the breast parenchyma. The high frame-rates available with real-time ultrasound systems in use today facilitates ultrasound guidance during interventional procedures of the breast to include **cyst aspirations,** core biopsies, preoperative localization techniques, and vacuum-assisted biopsies for small lesion diagnosis and removal.

ANATOMY OF THE BREAST

NORMAL ANATOMY

The breast is a modified sweat gland located in the superficial fascia of the anterior chest wall. The major portion of the breast tissue is situated between the second or third rib superiorly, the sixth or seventh costal cartilage inferiorly, the anterior axillary line laterally, and the sternal border medially. In many women, the breast extends deep toward the lateral upper margin of the chest and into the **axilla.** This extension is referred to as the axillary tail of the breast or **tail of Spence** (Figure 17-1).

The surface of the breast is dominated by the nipple and the surrounding areola. A few women may have ectopic breast

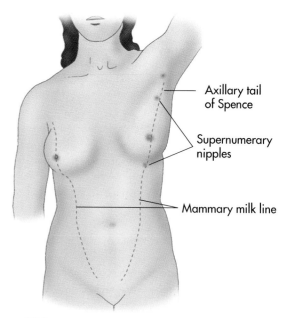

Figure 17-1 The mammary milk line is the anatomic line along which breast tissue can be found in some women. The axillary tail of Spence is an extension of breast tissue into the axilla that is present in some women.

BOX 17-1 **BREAST ANATOMY**

- Subcutaneous layer: thin layer
  Fatty tissue
  Cooper's ligaments
- Mammary: functional portion of the breast
  15 to 20 lobes radiate from the nipple
  Lactiferous ducts carry milk from acini to the nipple
  Terminal ductal lobular unit (TDLU) made up of acini and terminal ducts
  Fatty tissue interspersed between lobes
  Cooper's ligaments extend from the retromammary fascia to the skin and provide support
- Retromammary layer: thin layer
  Fatty tissue
  Cooper's ligaments
- Pectoralis major muscle
- Pectoralis minor muscle
- Ribs
- Chest wall

---

tissue or accessory (supernumerary) nipples. Ectopic breast tissue and accessory nipples are usually located along the mammary milk line, which extends superiorly from the axilla downward and medially in an oblique line to the symphysis pubis of the pelvis.

Sonographically, the breast is divided into three layers located between the skin and the pectoralis major muscle on the anterior of the chest wall. These layers include the subcutaneous layer, the mammary (glandular) layer, and the retromammary layer (Figure 17-2, Box 17-1). The subcutaneous

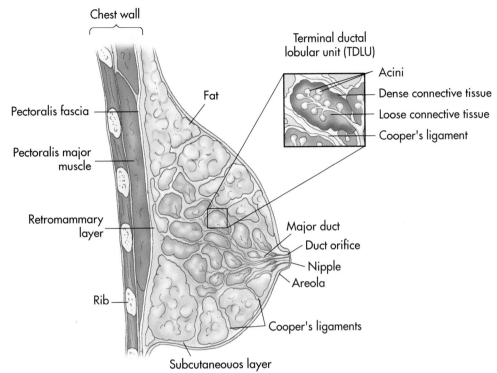

Figure 17-2   Breast anatomy. There are 15 major ductal systems within the breast. Each gives rise to many separate terminal ductal lobular units (TDLUs) containing the terminal ducts, at least one lobule, and the separate acinar units (milk-producing glands) within each lobule. Each TDLU is surrounded by varying amounts of loose and dense connective tissue. The TDLU represents the site of origin of nearly all pathologic processes of the breast. The Cooper's ligaments surround and suspend each of the TDLUs within the surrounding fatty tissue. The ligaments extend to the subcutaneous layer of the skin and the deep retromammary layer next to the pectoralis fascia overlying the chest wall.

and retromammary layers are usually quite thin and consist of fat surrounded by connective tissue septa. Although fat is often quite echogenic in other parts of the body, it is the least echogenic tissue within the breast. The fatty tissue appears hypoechoic, while the ducts, glands, and supporting ligaments appear echogenic (Figure 17-3).

The mammary/glandular layer includes the functional portion of the breast and the surrounding supportive (stromal) tissue. The functional portion of the breast is made up of 15 to 20 lobes, which contain the milk-producing glands, and the ductal system, which carries the milk to the nipple. The lobes emanate from the nipple in a pattern resembling the spokes of a wheel. The upper, outer quadrant of the breast contains the highest concentration of lobes. This concentration of lobes in the upper-outer quadrant of the breast is the reason a majority of tumors are found here, as most tumors originate from within the ducts. The lobes of the breast resemble a grapevine branch; the major duct branches into smaller branches called lobules. Each lobule contains acini (milk-producing glands), which are clustered on the terminal ends of the ducts like grapes on a vine. There are literally hundreds of acini within each breast (Figures 17-4 and 17-5). The terminal ends of the duct and the acini form small lobular units referred to as **terminal ductal lobular units (TDLU)**, each of which is surrounded by both loose and

Figure 17-3   Sonographic layers of breast tissue. The three layers of breast tissue are bordered by the skin and chest wall muscles *(arrows)*. The subcutaneous fat layer and the retromammary fat layer are usually very thin *(arrowheads)*. The mammary layer *(asterisks)* varies remarkably in thickness and in echogenicity, depending on location within the breast (most glandular tissue is located in the upper outer quadrant) and the patient's age, hormonal status (e.g., pubertal, mature, gravid, lactating, or postmenopausal), and inherited breast parenchymal pattern.

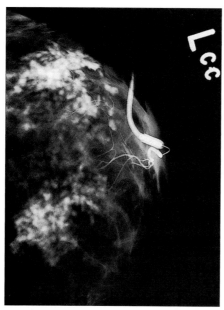

Figure 17-4 Galactogram (contrast injected retrograde into a single ductal system) showing opacification of individual glands (terminal ductal lobular units, or TDLUs). Normally, TDLUs are 2 mm or less in diameter. The TDLU is the site of origin of most pathologic processes within the breast. (Courtesy Lynn W. Gayden, MD, Chief Radiologist, Women's Health Center, Memphis, Tenn.)

Figure 17-5 Three-dimensional histology showing normal terminal ductal lobular units (TDLUs) and dilated TDLUs. Normal TDLUs are usually no larger than 2 mm. Fibrocystic condition and other pathologic processes can cause marked enlargement of the TDLU. Note the difference between the normal TDLU within the black box and the dilated TDLU filling the right half of the image. The white box shows a single dilated acinus within the enlarged TDLU, showing cellular changes of apocrine metaplasia (one of the tissue changes of fibrocystic condition recognized by pathologists), and causing the lining cells to enlarge and overproduce fluid. (Courtesy Laszlo Tabar, MD, Professor of Radiology, University of Uppsala, Sweden.)

dense connective tissue. The TDLUs are invested within the connective tissue skeleton of the breast (see Figures 17-2, 17-4, and 17-5). The normal TDLUs are 1 to 2 mm in size and are not usually differentiated sonographically. The TDLU is significant in that nearly all pathologic processes that occur within the breast originate here. The space between the lobes

Figure 17-6 The hypoechoic pectoralis muscle *(arrows)* is seen between the retromammary layer and the ribs.

is filled with connective and fatty tissue known as stroma. These stromal elements are located both between and within the lobes and consist of dense connective tissue, loose connective tissue, and fat. The connective tissue septa within the breasts form a fibrous "skeleton," which is responsible for maintaining the shape and structure of the breast. These connective tissue septa are collectively called **Cooper's ligaments;** they connect to the fascia around the ducts and glands and extend out to the skin.

The pectoralis major muscle lies posterior to the retromammary layer. It originates at the anterior surface of medial half of clavicle and anterolateral surface of sternum and inserts into the intertubercular groove on the anteromedial surface of the humerus (see Figure 17-2). The lower border of the pectoralis major muscle forms the anterior margin of the axilla. The pectoralis minor muscle lies superolateral and posterior to the pectoralis major. The pectoralis minor courses from its origin near the costal cartilages of the third, fourth, and fifth ribs to where it inserts into the medial and superior surface of the coracoid process of the scapula. These muscles sonographically appear as a hypoechoic interface between the retromammary layer of the breast and the ribs (Figure 17-6). Although a majority of lesions are found within the glandular tissue of the breast, it is important to evaluate tissue all the way to the chest wall.

SONOGRAPHIC APPEARANCE

The boundaries of the breast are the skin line, nipple, and retromammary layer. These generally give strong, bright echo reflections. The areolar area may be recognized by the slightly lower echo reflection as compared with the nipple and skin. The internal nipple may show low to bright reflections with posterior shadowing, and it has a variable appearance (Figure 17-7).

Subcutaneous fat generally appears hypoechoic, whereas Cooper's ligaments and other connective tissue appear echogenic and are dispersed in a linear pattern (Figure 17-8). Cooper's ligaments are best identified when the beam strikes them at a perpendicular angle and compression of the breast often enhances the ability to visualize them.

Figure 17-7   Shadow from the areolar area prevents imaging directly posteriorly to the nipple. The transducer should be moved away from the nipple area to image the mammary and retromammary layers.

BREAST DUCTAL ECTASIA
PANORAMIC SonoCT™ IMAGING

Figure 17-8   Subcutaneous fat is hypoechoic, whereas Cooper's ligaments appear echogenic within the subcutaneous layer *(arrows)*.

BREAST FIBROADENOMA

Figure 17-9   Mammary-glandular layer lies between the subcutaneous fatty layer anteriorly and retromammary layer posteriorly as seen in this patient with a fibroadenoma.

SOLID BREAST MASS

Figure 17-10   The retromammary layer is similar in echogenicity and echo texture to the subcutaneous layer. This patient had a solid breast mass anterior to the retromammary layer.

The mammary/glandular layer lies between the subcutaneous fatty layer anteriorly and the retromammary layer posteriorly (Figure 17-9). The fatty tissue interspersed throughout the mammary/glandular layer dictates the amount of intensity reflected from the breast parenchyma. If little fat is present, there is a uniform architecture with a strong echogenic pattern (because of collagen and fibrotic tissue) throughout the mammary/glandular layer. When fatty tissue is present, areas of low-level echoes become intertwined with areas of strong echoes from the active breast tissue. The analysis of this pattern becomes critical to the final diagnosis, and one must be able to separate lobules of fat from a marginated lesion.

The retromammary layer is similar in echogenicity and echotexture to the subcutaneous layer, although the boundary echoes resemble skin reflections (Figure 17-10). The pectoral muscles appear as low-level echo areas posterior to the retromammary layer. The ribs sonographically appear as hyperechoic rounded structures with dense posterior shadowing. They are easily identified by their occurrence at regular intervals along the chest wall.

There are several normal structures within the breast that can appear abnormal, unless care is taken during the sonographic examination. The ducts immediately behind the nipple frequently cause acoustic shadowing and can be mistaken for a suspicious breast mass. Angling of the transducer in the retroareolar tissue will usually improve visualization and eliminate doubt. The distinction of a subtle isoechoic or hypoechoic sonographic mass from normal fibroglandular tissue can sometimes be troublesome in the breast. The adipose or fatty tissue can situate itself in and among the areas of glandular tissue and, in some scanning planes, mimic isoechoic or hypoechoic masses. It is helpful to turn on the structures to see if they are consistent or lengthen out within the scanning plane. To see if a structure will lengthen out geometrically, rotate the transducer 90 degrees during real-time. In the case of a true sonographic mass, a mass will maintain its shape in both dimensions, confirming its three-dimensional character, whereas glandular tissue elements will elongate and appear less like a mass.

PARENCHYMAL PATTERN

The size and shape of the breasts vary remarkably from woman to woman. Some women have more glandular tissue, some

Figure 17-11   Dense breast. **A,** Example of dense breast tissue on mammogram. Mammographic technique emphasizes tissue contrast. As a result, the skin is often not visible on routine images. The skin is separated in this case by nearly 2 cm from the outer margins of the dense mammary layer. **B,** Example of ultrasound appearance of dense breast tissue. **C,** Example of variation in breast tissue pattern at different locations even within the same breast.

have less. Some have more fatty tissue than others, while some have more connective tissue so their breasts are firmer. Some women have very little breast tissue and appear flat-chested. The size and shape of the breasts also varies over time because of the changes that occur during the menstrual cycle, with pregnancy and breast-feeding, and during menopause. Most of the differences in breast sizes between women are due to the amount of fatty tissue within the breasts.

The involutional changes that occur in the breast throughout life affect the appearance and pattern of the breast parenchyma. Involution is hallmarked in breast imaging by the remodeling process that causes glandular tissue to be slowly replaced by fatty tissue. This accounts for the differences in size, shape, and architecture of breast tissue.

Generally, in a young woman, fibrous tissue elements predominate and the resulting appearance on mammography and ultrasound is a dense echogenic pattern of tissue (Figure 17-11). In a pregnant or lactating woman, the glandular portions of the breast proliferate remarkably in both density and volume creating interfaces that are less echogenic. As a woman ages, the glandular breast tissue undergoes cell death and is remodeled by the indecision of fatty tissue. The tissue is progressively replaced by fat and, with the onset of menopause, the ducts atrophy, resulting in a mammographic and sonographic pattern with less fibrous tissue elements (Figure 17-12). This fatty breast is the one most difficult to image by sonography as all three layers of the breast appear hypoechoic, with less distinction between the layers. Sonographically, cancers can be difficult to differentiate in the fatty breast because most cancers appear hypoechoic and can be difficult to differentiate from the normal breast tissue. Although sonography of the fatty breast is difficult, mammography images this type of breast very well.

VASCULAR SUPPLY

The main arterial supply to the breast comes from the internal mammary and the lateral thoracic artery. Over half of the

Figure 17-12   Fatty breast. **A,** Example of predominantly fatty tissue on mammogram. **B,** Example of ultrasound appearance of predominantly fatty tissue. Note the loss of sonographic detail in the deeper layers of the breast and chest wall. Fat deflects the ultrasound beam and degrades detail. **C,** Example of improved visualization of skin and subcutaneous tissues with a standoff pad.

breast, mainly the central and medial portions, is supplied by the anterior perforating branches of the internal mammary artery. The remaining portion, the upper outer quadrant, is supplied by the lateral thoracic artery; intercostals, subcapsular, and thoracodorsal arteries contribute in lessor ways to the blood supply.

Venous drainage is mainly provided by superficial veins that can be seen sonographically just under the skin. These surface veins are often enlarged with superior vena caval syndrome, chronic venous thrombosis of the subclavian vein, and in cases of arteriovenous shunts placed in patients with chronic renal insufficiency. Figure 17-13 shows an example of a grossly dilated surface vein in the breast. When there is doubt concerning the vascular nature of a long, tubular, **anechoic** structure on breast ultrasound, such as the distinction between a dilated duct and a vessel, color flow vascular imaging or Doppler ultrasound techniques can easily resolve this situation.

LYMPHATIC SYSTEM

Lymphatic drainage from all parts of the breast generally flows to the axillary lymph nodes. The flow of lymph is promoted by valveless lymphatic vessels that allow the fluid to mingle and proceed unidirectionally from the superficial to the deep nodes of the breast. The flow of lymph moves from the intramammary nodes and deep nodes centrifugally toward the axillary and internal lymph node chains. It has been estimated that only about 3% of lymph is eliminated by the internal chain, whereas 97% of lymph is removed by the axillary chain.

Part of the standard surgical therapy of invasive breast cancer involves axillary lymph node dissection. This is vital in the staging and management of breast cancer because nodal status affects the patient's prognosis and is important in guiding adjunctive therapy. Although most tumors can infiltrate and spread via the axillary lymph nodes, they may begin their infiltration by using alternative lymph channels, such as the internal mammary chain within the chest, across the midline to the contralateral breast, deep into the interpectoral (Rotter's) nodes, or into the supraclavicular nodes (Figures 17-14, 17-15, and 17-16).

THE MALE BREAST

In males, the nipple and areola remain relatively small. The male breast normally retains some ductal elements beneath the nipple, but does not develop the milk-producing lobular and

Figure 17-13   Dilated veins in the breast. **A,** Mammographic image of a breast showing markedly dilated surface veins in an elderly woman. **B** and **C,** Ultrasound images of veins just under the skin of the breast in the same patient. In cases in which there is doubt, color flow mapping or Doppler techniques will easily confirm the vascular nature of these dilated tubular structures and distinguish them from dilated ducts.

BOX 17-2   **MALE PATIENTS AT INCREASED RISK FOR BREAST CANCER**

- Klinefelter's syndrome
- Male-to-female transsexual
- History of prior chest wall irradiation (especially for Hodgkin's lymphoma)
- History of orchitis or testicular tumor
- Liver disease
- Genetic predisposition (BRCA2 gene mutation, breast cancer in female relatives, p53 mutation)

acinar tissue. The ductal elements usually remain small, but can hypertrophy during puberty and later in life under the influence of hormonal fluctuations, disease processes, or medications. This condition, in which the ductal elements hypertrophy, is called benign **gynecomastia** (Figure 17-17). Imaging with mammography and ultrasound is often requested in order to exclude breast cancer as a cause.

Although breast cancer is uncommon in males, it does occur. Approximately 1300 new cases are diagnosed each year within the United Sates. The occurrence approximates 1% of the incidence in women. Box 17-2 lists male patients at an increased risk for breast cancer.

PHYSIOLOGY OF THE BREAST

The primary function of the breast is fluid transport. The breast includes the fat, ligaments, glandular tissue, and ductal system that work together to provide a fluid transport, and only one entity in this group produces milk. The ductal system is critical in the transport of fluids within the breast and it is also a source for ductal pathologic conditions. Ducts consist of epithelium cells, which line the interior of the ducts, and a myoepithelium set of cells, which controls the contracts of the ducts. It is these cells that promote the transport of milk and fluids, but they also can be the cause of early changes that indicate disease.

An important function of the breast during the reproductive years is to make milk from nutrients and water taken from the bloodstream. Milk is produced within the acini and carried to the nipple by the ducts.

The female breast is remarkably affected by changing hormonal levels during each menstrual cycle and is further affected by both pregnancy and lactation (breast-feeding). Breast development begins before menarche and continues until the female is approximately 16 years old. During this time, the ductal system proliferates under the influence of estrogen. During pregnancy, acinar development is accelerated to enable milk production by estrogen, progesterone, and prolactin. Prolactin is a hormone produced by the pituitary gland, which stimu-

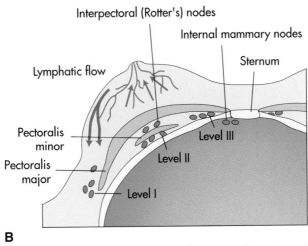

Figure 17-14 Lymphatic drainage of the breast. **A,** General position of the major axillary lymphatic groups I, II, and III in relation to the pectoralis major and minor muscles of the chest wall. On the right side of the figure, the major lymphatic flow from the periareolar plexus toward the axilla is shown. Alternative routes of lymphatic flow include (1) retromammary nodes, (2) contralateral flow to the opposite breast, (3) interpectoral (Rotter's) nodes located between the pectoralis major and minor muscles, (4) supraclavicular nodes, and (5) diaphragmatic nodes. **B,** Same information in cross section.

lates the acini to produce and excrete milk. Prolactin levels usually rise during the latter part of pregnancy, but the effects on milk production are suppressed by high levels of progesterone. The expulsion of the placenta after the birth of a baby causes a drop in circulating progesterone, initiating milk production within the breasts. The physical stimulation of suckling by the baby initiates the release of oxytocin (produced by the hypothalamus and released by the pituitary gland), which further incites prolactin secretion, stimulating additional milk production. Full maturation of the acini occurs during lactation and is thought to be mildly protective against the development of breast cancer. At the end of lactation, the breast tissue parenchyma involutes. Breast evaluation by mammography can be difficult in a dense, lactating breast; therefore, mammographic screening of the breast is usually not performed until at least 6 months after cessation of lactation.

BREAST EVALUATION OVERVIEW

BREAST SCREENING

The primary purpose of breast screening is the detection and diagnosis of breast cancer in its earliest and most curable stage. The accurate identification of benign breast lesions during cancer screening is also important to good care because it can save the patient from unnecessary surgical procedures and resultant tissue scarring.

There are three general categories of **diagnostic breast imaging,** two of which involve breast ultrasound. These three categories include breast cancer screening (generally performed by physical breast evaluation and with mammography), diagnostic interrogation (consultative, problem solving, work-up), and interventional breast procedures (histologic diagnosis and/or localization).

Figure 17-15   Normal and abnormal lymph nodes. **A** and **B,** Ultrasound images of a normal lymph node showing a smooth homogeneously hypoechoic cortex and echogenic fatty internal hilum. **A,** Lymph node "en face." **B,** Lymph node in profile, with the fatty hilum (containing the afferent and efferent vascular and lymphatic vessels) extending out to the left *(arrowhead)*. **C, D,** and **E,** Ultrasound images of abnormal lymph nodes. Signs of suspicion for metastatic involvement of lymph nodes include an irregular, inhomogeneous cortex and loss of the fatty hilum. **C,** Lymph node that has nearly lost the fatty hilum and has a poorly defined but relatively homogeneous cortex. This may be either a reactive lymph node or one with early metastatic involvement. **D,** Similar lymph node that has completely lost its fatty hilum but has a smooth homogeneous cortex. **E,** Large hypoechoic mass that has no sonographic characteristics of a normal lymph node. This mass was sampled by ultrasound-guided core biopsy, confirming a low axillary lymph node nearly completely replaced with metastatic cancer.

Figure 17-16 Metastatic spread of breast cancer to the opposite breast. **A,** Mammogram showing several moderate- to low-density, relatively benign appearing masses *(arrows)* in a patient with history of mastectomy for cancer in the opposite breast. **B,** Ultrasound image of one of the masses shows a solid mass with an irregular, poorly defined margin and heterogeneous echogenicity. These lesions were all metastatic lesions from the opposite breast, likely from an alternative route of lymphatic spread across the midline.

Figure 17-17 Two male patients with palpable breast masses. **A,** Mammographic appearance of benign gynecomastia. This condition is nearly as often unilateral as bilateral. **B,** Ultrasound example of the frequently masslike appearance of gynecomastia. **C,** Mammography example of male breast cancer. **D,** Ultrasound image with standoff pad of palpable suspicious breast mass in elderly male. Note the heterogeneous echogenicity and the elevation of the skin over the mass. (*B,* Courtesy Anna E. Mize, MD, Women's Health Center, Memphis, Tenn.)

BOX 17-3　BREAST CANCER SCREENING

BREAST SELF-EXAMINATION (BSE)
- Monthly beginning at age 20

CLINICAL BREAST EXAMINATION (CBE) BY A HEALTH CARE PROVIDER
- Ages 20 to 39: Every 3 years
- Ages 40 on: Yearly

SCREENING MAMMOGRAPHY
- Yearly starting at age 40

Exceptions: Personal history of breast cancer, first-degree relative (mother or sister) with premenopausal breast cancer, atypical hyperplasia or LCIS on a prior breast biopsy, or known breast cancer gene mutation (BRCA1 or BRCA2)

BOX 17-5　SIGNS OF BREAST CANCER ON MAMMOGRAPHY

PRIMARY SIGNS

Common:
- Irregular (spiculated), high-density mass
- Clustered pleomorphic microcalcifications
- Focal distortion (with no history of prior biopsy, infection, or trauma)

Less Common:
- Focal asymmetric density (with associated palpable lump or solid sonographic mass)
- Developing density

SECONDARY SIGNS

Common:
- Nipple or skin retraction
- Skin thickening
- Lymphedema pattern
- Increased vascularity

BOX 17-4　CLINICAL SIGNS AND SYMPTOMS OF POSSIBLE BREAST CANCER

- New or growing dominant, discrete breast lump
  Hard, gritty, or irregular surface
  Usually (not always) painless
  Does not fluctuate with hormonal cycle
  Up to 5% can occur outside the reach of mammography
  Distinguish from "lumpy" breast texture
- Unilateral single duct nipple discharge
  Spontaneous, persistent; serous or bloody
- Surface nipple lesions
  Nonhealing ulcer
  Focal irritation
- New nipple retraction
- New focal skin dimpling or retraction
- Unilateral new or growing axillary lump
- Hot, red breast

Note: Although these clinical signs and symptoms may indicate the presence of breast cancer, it is important to understand that in the majority of cases the cause is not cancer but rather a benign condition.

Breast cancer screening is recommended in women without clinical signs of breast cancer (see Box 17-3). According to the American Cancer Society, breast cancer screening involves monthly **breast self-examination (BSE),** regular **clinical breast examination (CBE)** by a physician or other health care provider, and annual screening mammography. Monthly BSE is best performed at the end of menses and should begin at age 20. CBE should be performed once every 3 years from ages 20 to 39 and at least yearly from age 40 on. Screening mammography should be performed yearly starting at age 40. BSE and CBE are important steps in breast cancer screening because 70% of cancers are found through lumps felt during BSE and CBE. BSE and CBE may also identify other signs or symptoms of possible breast cancer that require further evaluation by diagnostic breast imaging (Box 17-4).

Mammography, sonography, and MRI are the primary imaging tools used for diagnostic breast evaluation. Mammography provides a sensitive method of screening for breast cancer, whereas ultrasound and MRI are used to provide additional characterization and further interrogation of breast lesions that are not well visualized by mammography. The mammographic signs of breast cancer are listed in Box 17-5. Because ultrasound examination is performed by scanning in cross-sectional planes, it is difficult to adequately screen the entire breast in most patients. Ultrasound may be used for screening purposes in young, dense breasts, which are difficult to penetrate by mammography, to evaluate palpable masses that are not visible on a mammogram and to image the deep **juxtathoracic** tissue not normally visible by mammography. Ultrasound is also useful in differentiating structures within uniformly dense breast tissue where mammography is limited (e.g., in differentiating solid, round masses from fluid-filled **cysts** and visualizing tissue adjacent to implants or other structures that limit visualization by mammography). MRI is also a useful tool in breast imaging, but is prohibitively expensive for screening purposes. Because a strong magnetic field is used to create images, not all patients are good candidates for MRI (e.g., patients with pacemakers or artificial joints). Patients who suffer from uncontrolled claustrophobia are also not good candidates for MRI.

BREAST EVALUATION

The overall goal of breast evaluation is the proper classification of a breast lesion according to the level of suspicion for breast cancer. Thorough evaluation takes into account the results of both the breast imaging assessment and the clinical assessment. The appropriate next step in patient management is dictated by the level of suspicion for cancer in any breast lesion and takes into account the age and individual risk factors for each particular patient. Risk factors for breast cancer are listed in Box 17-6.

BOX 17-6   RISK FACTORS FOR BREAST CANCER

- Female gender
- Increasing age
- Family history of breast cancer
- Personal history of breast cancer
  First-degree relative (mother, sister, daughter)
  Premenopausal breast cancer
  Multiple affected first- and second-degree relatives
  Associated cancers (ovarian, colon, prostate)
- Biopsy-proven atypical proliferative lesions
  Lobular neoplasia (lobular carcinoma in situ)
  Atypical epithelial hyperplasia
- Prolonged estrogen effect
  Early menarche
- Late menopause
- Nulliparity
- Late first pregnancy

BOX 17-7   CLINICAL EVALUATION OF THE PATIENT WITH A BREAST PROBLEM

HISTORY
- Patient age
- Risk factors for breast cancer
- Onset and duration of mass
- Relation to menstrual cycle

BREAST EXAMINATION (FOR PALPABLE MASS)
- Location of mass
  Clock face or quadrant
- Characteristics of mass
  Size
  Shape (round, oval, lobular, irregular)
  Surface contour (smooth, irregular)
  Consistency (soft, rubbery, firm, hard, gritty)
  Mobility (moveable, fixed)

TABLE 17-1 ACR* BI-RADS CLASSIFICATION OF MAMMOGRAPHIC MASSES	
BI-RADS Category	Action Required
1 Normal	Routine follow-up
2 Benign	Routine follow-up
Examples:	
Simple cyst	
Fibroadenoma	
Intramammary lymph node	
3 Probably benign	Short-term follow-up
Example:	(to document
Round or oval solid mass	stability)
4 Suspicious	Biopsy should be
Examples:	considered
Irregular solid mass	
Clustered pleomorphic microcalcifications	
Focal distortion	
Growing noncystic mass	
5 Highly suggestive of malignancy	Appropriate action
Examples:	should be taken
Spiculated mass	
Spiculated mass with microcalcifications	
Spiculated mass with secondary signs	
(nipple retraction, skin thickening, etc.)	

*Adapted, as modified, with permission of the American College of Radiology. No other representation of these documents is authorized without express, written permission of the American College of Radiology.

Clinical Assessment. It is important to recognize clinical signs or symptoms of possible breast cancer (see Box 17-4). These patients with clinical indications of breast cancer generally undergo diagnostic breast interrogation. Diagnostic imaging of the breast is tailored to the patient's age and specific clinical problem. Clinical history and examination of the patient with a breast problem (Box 17-7) help determine the next diagnostic step. In the patient with no signs or symptoms of possible breast cancer, screening mammography is typically the first diagnostic test performed.

Screening Mammography. In women ages 40 and over who are **asymptomatic** (without clinical signs of possible breast cancer), annual screening by mammography is recommended. Usually less than 10% of these women will have abnormalities detected on the screening examination that require further work-up. When a breast lesion is identified by

mammography, it is normally described using guidelines contained within the **breast imaging reporting and data system (BI-RADS)**. The BI-RAD system was developed by the American College of Radiology (ACR). A key component of this system is an overall outcome assessment category that indicates the suspicion of malignancy (Table 17-1). Figures 17-18, 17-19, 17-20, and 17-21 present mammographic and sonographic examples of various BI-RADS category masses.

Diagnostic Breast Interrogation. Diagnostic (consultative, work-up, problem solving) breast interrogation is performed on all patients who present with any clinical signs of possible breast cancer found on CBE or BSE, and patients who are recalled for additional evaluation because of an abnormal screening mammogram. Diagnostic mammography involves specialized detail views to analyze specific areas of the breast in question. In at least one third of cases, adjunctive ultrasound of the breast is used to further evaluate questionable mammographic or clinical findings (see later discussion).

Interventional Breast Procedures. In some breast lesions, interventional procedures are necessary for definitive diagnosis. A common example is a smooth, benign appearing mass identified by mammography that correlates with a hypoechoic sonographic lesion, but does not meet the criteria for interpretation as a simple cyst. Cyst aspiration can be performed to determine whether the lesion is a complex cyst or truly a solid

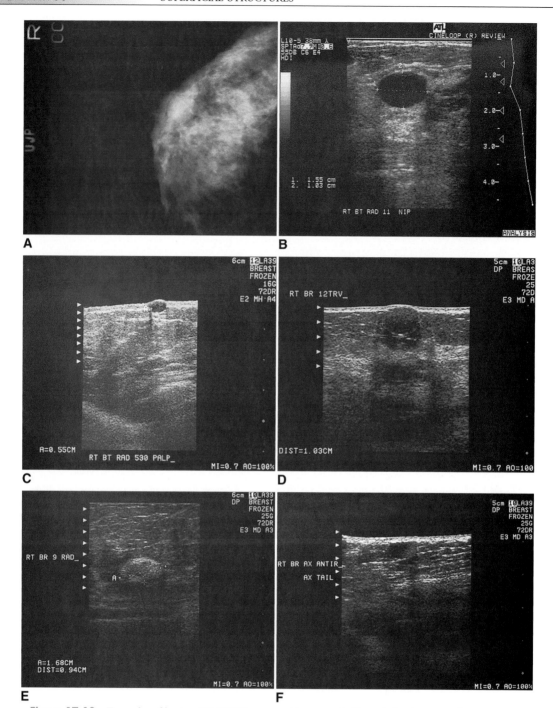

Figure 17-18 Examples of benign (BI-RADS category 2) masses. **A,** Smooth, benign appearing mammographic mass. **B,** Same mass on ultrasound showing classic features of a simple cyst. **C,** Ultrasound example of a sebaceous cyst. Note the smooth, hypoechoic appearance and classic location within the skin. **D,** Ultrasound example of an isoechoic mass abutting the dermis. This is an epidermal inclusion cyst, often indistinguishable from a sebaceous cyst. These lesions appear within the skin or at the junction of the dermis and the subcutaneous fatty layer. **E,** Vague, low-density mammographic mass correlated to this echogenic mass on ultrasound. Echogenic masses are nearly always benign, but the level of suspicion should be determined by the mammographic appearance. **F,** Small mass on mammogram in this hospitalized patient on warfarin appears as a small, superficial complex cyst with a "fluid-fluid" level consistent with a small, resolving hematoma (a galactocele in a lactating patient has a similar appearance, but is located within the mammary layer). This superficial hematoma may resolve completely or may evolve into an oil cyst.

Figure 17-18, cont'd **G,** Mammographic mass with mixed fatty and soft tissue elements, surrounded by a thin capsule *(arrowheads).* This is a breast hamartoma. **H,** Ultrasound appearance of the same hamartoma. Note that its high fat content makes differentiation from surrounding fatty tissue difficult.

Figure 17-19 Example of probably benign (BI-RADS category 3) mass. **A,** Ultrasound appearance of a smooth, benign appearing mass with homogeneous echogenicity, wider than tall, showing low-level posterior acoustic enhancement. This image is taken without applied compression. **B,** Same mass with applied compression, showing the decreased anteroposterior dimension. Most benign masses are soft and compressible.

mass. Under real-time sonographic guidance, a needle is guided into the lesion in an attempt to aspirate fluid. Successful fluid aspiration is diagnostic of a complex cyst. The same approach can be used to guide fine-needle aspiration for cytology, core-needle biopsies for histology, preoperative needle wire localization of masses for surgery, and for the injection of radioactive tracers for **sentinel node** identification and mapping.

In some cases, a patient will have a clinical sign or symptom of possible breast cancer, and yet diagnostic breast imaging shows no abnormality. The most common clinical problem is the patient with a breast lump and negative breast imaging. If no imaging correlation can be identified to explain the patient's breast lump, the patient must be managed clinically, which means that she is examined sequentially through at least one menstrual cycle. In the overwhelming majority of cases, the breast lump will improve or resolve completely, confirming the diagnosis of clinical fibrocystic condition. If the breast lump does not improve or continues to grow, surgical biopsy is performed.

SONOGRAPHIC EVALUATION OF THE BREAST

INDICATIONS FOR SONOGRAPHIC EVALUATION

The sonographer must have basic clinical information regarding any patient who is referred for breast ultrasound. Pertinent clinical information includes the patient's age, risk factors for breast cancer (see Box 17-6), symptoms, and the location and clinical impression of any breast lumps. Any history of trauma to the breast or previous breast surgeries is also helpful. Inspection of the breast during the ultrasound examination will often reveal pertinent findings. For example, the examiner should make note of any surface nipple erosion (possible **Paget's disease**), nipple or skin retraction, skin thickening (edema, scarring, or **peau d'orange**), scars, signs of inflammation (induration and erythema), or contusion. Sonography is normally used as an adjunct to mammography, but may be the initial method of imaging when there is a palpable breast lump,

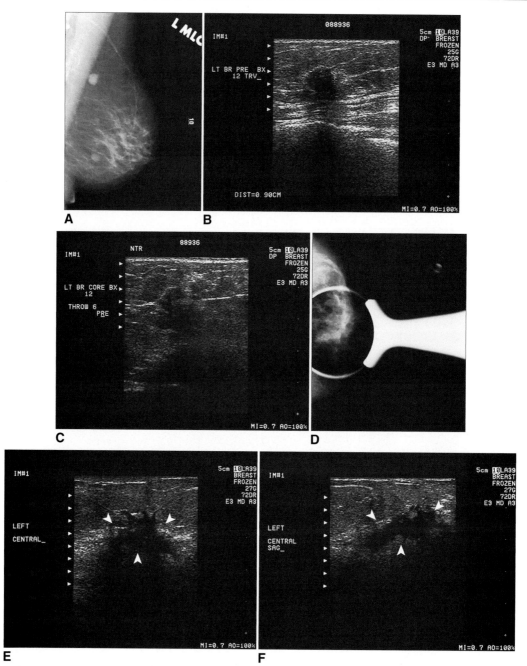

Figure 17-20   Example of suspicious (BI-RADS category 4) masses. **A,** Irregular mammographic mass that had shown interval growth. **B,** Ultrasound appearance of the same mass, with a heterogeneous echogenicity but only a slightly irregular margin. There is weak posterior acoustic shadowing. **C,** Fourteen-gauge core biopsy needle traversing the mass. Pathologic condition confirmed an infiltrating ductal carcinoma. **D,** Mammographic area of focal distortion that persisted with detail imaging. Transverse (**E**) and sagittal (**F**) ultrasound images confirm a three-dimensional area of focal distortion. The patient had no history of previous surgery, injury, or infection in this breast to explain the distortion.

in a young patient with dense breasts, in a pregnant or lactating patient, in a patient with breast augmentation, or in a patient with a difficult or compromised mammogram.

Palpable Breast Lump.   Patients are often referred for breast ultrasound because of a **palpable** breast lump. Pertinent clinical information that should be provided by the referring physi-

cian includes size and location of the lump, when it was noticed, and its relation to the menstrual cycle. The physician's clinical impression (e.g., suspicion of cancer, probable fibrocystic condition, or possible abscess) can help focus the sonographer's examination. The sonographer can often feel the mass of concern while scanning the breast. This can help guide the examination and over time will lead to improved expertise on

Figure 17-21   Example of highly suspicious (BI-RADS category 5) mass. **A,** Magnification view of a palpable lump showing a spiculated, highly suspicious mammographic mass. **B,** Ultrasound image of the same mass. Note the heterogeneous echogenicity, poorly defined and irregular margin, and "higher than wide" appearance, which does not change with most cancers even with applied compression. **C,** Spot compression mammogram of a small spiculated mass. **D,** Ultrasound image showing a small mass with similar features as those in B.

the part of the sonographer in differentiating lesions. For example, a dominant cyst is frequently round or oval (long axis toward nipple), smooth, soft (some cysts under tension can be firm and are usually very tender), and easily movable. Fibroadenomas are usually similar in shape, but are often quite firm and rubbery in consistency, and homogeneously solid on ultrasound. Breast cancer, by contrast, will generally be painless (although some cancers are associated with focal pain), lobular or irregular in shape, uneven in surface contour (sometimes gritty in texture), and fixed or poorly movable (Box 17-8).

Young Patient with Dense Breasts. Ultrasound is the primary tool in breast imaging in all women under age 30, according to most authors. Mammography is added as necessary on a limited basis between ages 20 and 30, mainly to rule out microcalcifications (a sign of possible breast cancer that may not be visible by ultrasound). Mammography is rarely indicated for patients under age 20 and, in some centers, under age 25. The three main reasons for this are that breast cancer is rare in women under age 25, that breast tissue at this age is generally denser and more difficult to analyze by mammogra-

phy, and that young breast tissue is more sensitive to damage from radiation.

Most breast masses that arise during the teen years are fibroadenomas (Figure 17-22). Other common causes of breast lumps include the developing breast bud immediately behind the nipple (which must never be mistaken for an abnormal mass and surgically removed) or a dominant cyst. Less commonly, a hyperplastic lymph node, abscess, hematoma, or giant fibroadenomas can present before age 20. Malignant breast lesions in patients under age 20 are extremely rare. When they do occur, they are generally not of breast origin, but rather metastatic or of soft tissue origin (such as soft tissue sarcomas). If a young patient has a rapidly enlarging or a painful mass, surgical excision should be considered.

Pregnant or Lactating Patient. Sonography is the primary tool for breast imaging in a pregnant patient. Mammography is added (with abdominal shielding) to allow accurate characterization of a breast mass as necessary. Diagnostic evaluation of a breast mass (including biopsy if indicated) should not be delayed because of the pregnancy.

Figure 17-22   Smooth, solid mass (fibroadenoma). **A,** Ultrasound image of a growing palpable mass in a teenage female. This was one of several similar masses. Fibroadenomas are frequently multiple and often run in families. Please note the hypoechoic, homogeneous echogenicity of the mass, and the low-level posterior acoustic enhancement and the edge refraction. **B,** The patient was referred for large-core needle biopsy for diagnosis. This ultrasound image shows the 14-gauge core biopsy needle in postfire position traversing the superficial portion of the mass. The approximate area of the sample notch where tissue is obtained is indicated by the arrows. Multiple passes are made to ensure adequate sampling and a reliable tissue diagnosis. **C,** Note the echogenic core biopsy tract within the mass *(arrows)*. Fresh hemorrhage along the needle tract caused the echogenic appearance. The prefire position of the needle adjacent to the mass, in preparation for the next tissue sampling, is also visible *(arrowhead)*.

Most masses that present in a pregnant or lactating patient are benign fibroadenomas. These can often enlarge rapidly because of the marked increase in circulating hormone levels during pregnancy and lactation. The increase in circulating hormones, however, can have a similar effect on breast cancers. In patients who develop breast cancer during pregnancy, the cancers are often diagnosed at a later stage than in the non-pregnant patient.

Other breast problems that may arise during pregnancy or lactation include mastitis, abscesses, cysts, or galactoceles (a cyst containing milk). In the case of a galactocele, a fat-fluid level may be visible both by mammography and by ultrasound, but more commonly this lesion appears as a complex cyst. Galactoceles or cysts can be easily aspirated under ultrasound guidance.

Patient with Breast Augmentation.   Sonographic evaluation of the breast in a patient who has had breast augmentation or reconstruction with silicone implants has shown to be

of benefit. Mammography is often limited in its ability to image beyond the implant, whereas ultrasound has the ability to evaluate the tissue surrounding the implant, search for the presence of defects in the membrane, and look for leakage into the breast parenchyma. An intracapsular implant rupture occurs when there is a breach of the membrane surrounding an implant, but the silicone that leaks out is still confined within the fibrous scar tissue, which forms a "capsule" around the implant. As the implant collapses and the membrane folds inward, a series of discontinuous echogenic lines parallel to the face of the transducer may be seen and are referred to as the "stepladder sign" or "linguine sign" (Figure 17-23). Caution must be used when evaluating internal echoes within an implant because the internal architecture of an implant may appear heterogeneous as a result of reverberation artifacts and or a mixture of the gel with other fluids that may have been injected into the implant during surgery, giving a false-positive stepladder sign. An implant rupture allowing an extracapsular leakage of silicone into the tissue sonographically appears as an

Figure 17-23   Seroma. This chronic seroma (noninfected fluid collection) has been repeatedly aspirated in this patient with previous silicone implants that ruptured. Note the thick septations (synechiae) within the seroma. (Courtesy Lynn W. Gayden, MD, Chief Radiologist, Women's Health Center, Memphis, Tenn.)

BOX 17-8

DIFFERENTIAL DIAGNOSIS LISTS

SMOOTH MASS
Common:	Simple cyst
	Complex cyst
	Fibroadenoma
	Lymph node
	Oil cyst
Less common:	Galactocele
	Seroma
	Hematoma
	Phyllodes tumor
	Cancer

FOCAL DISTORTION
Common:	Postsurgical scar
	Fibrocystic condition
	Cancer
Less common:	Prior infection
	Old hematoma
	Degenerating fibroadenoma
Uncommon:	Fibrocystic condition

PALPABLE BREAST LUMP WITH NEGATIVE BREAST IMAGING
Common:	Fibrocystic condition
Less common:	Resolving trauma
Uncommon:	Cancer

---

indistinctly marginated area of increased echogenicity along the margin of the implant, with a dirty posterior acoustic shadowing and the presence of noise. The depiction of an extracapsular rupture has been described as having a "snowstorm" appearance. Ultrasound is often the first choice of imaging procedures to examine the implant. If the image is unclear, magnetic resonance imaging (MRI) may be used to further define the area in question.

Patient with a Difficult or Compromised Mammogram. There are some patients for whom breast imaging by mammography is limited in its sensitivity (as in the case of very dense breast tissue) or in its ability to visualize the breast tissue (as in the case of retroglandular breast implants) (Figure 17-24). Mammography has difficulty in distinguishing between scar tissue and breast cancer. With more women having breast reduction surgeries, these reduction scars, along with previous open biopsy scars, form tissue that is distorted and is difficult to distinguish from breast cancer distortion of normal tissue.

There are also patients for whom examination of breast tissue is compromised because of postsurgical or postradiation changes (Figures 17-25 and 17-26). This is a common situation in the patient who has had breast-conserving therapy for early-stage breast cancer located close to the chest wall or in the axillary tail near the armpit. As technologic advances in ultrasound continue to improve its sensitivity and specificity, the routine use of adjunctive breast ultrasound and mammogram in certain high-risk or complicated patients is being advocated (Box 17-9). Although sonography is an invaluable aid to breast imaging, it should not be used as a substitute for a mammogram because microcalcifications and focal distortion, two of the three principal signs of breast cancer seen by mammography, are often difficult to visualize with ultrasound.

TECHNIQUE
Scanning is performed using the real-time technique. In most laboratories and clinics, hard copy images are produced to document the examination. The image must first be optimized using electronic focusing, overall gain, and time gain compensation (TGC) adjustment. The goal is to balance the image from the low-level echoes of the subcutaneous fat to the low-level echoes of the retromammary fat. This should result in an image that clearly shows all levels of the breast from the skin level through the echogenic breast core and the deeper echogenic chest wall layers. Moderate compression applied with the transducer during scanning will improve detail and decrease the depth of tissue the ultrasound beam must traverse. In the case of a negative breast ultrasound examination, the usual practice is to record representative images of each quadrant, the subareolar ducts, or specific radial images of the breast, depending on the protocol of the imaging center.

Positioning. Patients are usually scanned in the supine position using a handheld, high-resolution transducer. The patient is positioned with her arm behind her head on the side of the breast to be examined. This will spread the breast tissue more evenly over the surface of the chest and provide a more stable scanning surface and easier access to the axilla. When scanning the medial portion of the breast, a supine position works well. For the lateral margin of the breast, the patient can be rolled slightly toward the opposite side (approximately 30 to 45 degrees) and stabilized with a cushion under her shoulder and hips.

If a lesion identified on a mammogram cannot be located sonographically, it may be helpful to sit the patient upright and position the breast in the same positions used to obtain the

Figure 17-24   Ruptured silicone breast implants. **A,** Mammogram showing retroglandular implant with extracapsular silicone *(arrow)*. **B,** Ultrasound image of the same case showing typical "snowstorm" appearance of free extracapsular silicone *(arrowheads)*. **C,** Ultrasound image of normal intact silicone implant. Note the anechoic appearance of the silicone and the double echogenic margin of the implant perpendicular to the incident sound waves *(small arrows)*. **D** and **E,** Two ultrasound images of the same silicone breast implant taken at separate times showing intracapsular rupture. **D,** Note the echogenic fibrous capsule *(arrowheads)* that is no longer a double line, but only a single line. Note the nonparallel echogenic interfaces *(arrows)* within the silicone. These interfaces represent portions of the collapsed and ruptured envelope surrounded by silicone still contained within the fibrous capsule. Compare this appearance with **(E),** the same patient at an earlier time, showing the double echogenic interface *(arrowheads)*. Note the faint parallel lines under the echogenic capsule *(arrows)* representing reverberation artifact.

Figure 17-25 Postsurgical breast scar causes interruption in the ultrasound beam at the site of the scar (area of the shadowing).

Figure 17-26 Lumpectomy site after radiation demonstrates irregular area that appears to be "masslike" without defined borders in the breast.

mammogram. This will allow easier localization and a similar frame of reference.

Scanning Technique. When examining for a palpable mass or for correlation with an abnormal mammogram, some centers scan only the area of interest. For example, if a mass in the upper inner quadrant of the right breast is seen on the mammogram, then only the upper inner quadrant of the right breast will be scanned by ultrasound. This is a more specific approach to lesion evaluation, results in fewer cases of false-positive sonographic findings, and is more cost effective than scanning the entire breast. Other centers, however, routinely scan the entire breast. Breast scanning points to remember are listed in Box 17-10.

When a patient is being evaluated for a palpable breast mass or for a specific abnormality seen on a mammogram, the abnormality is first located with a preliminary scan. It is helpful to mark the external skin over the mass. The transducer orientation should remain the same as with conventional ultrasound examinations (i.e., the patient's right side is oriented to the left of the screen on transverse images, and the notch of the transducer is directed cephalad on longitudinal images.

The mass is then thoroughly scanned in orthogonal planes (90 degrees apart) to evaluate the lesion in three dimensions. This can be recorded using sagittal and transverse images or using radial/antiradial transducer positions (Figure 17-27). The use of the radial/antiradial positions is unique to the breast and can often pick up subtle abnormalities extending toward the nipple along the ductal system from the mass. All dominant solid masses are generally recorded with three-dimensional measurements (length, width, and height) to facilitate management decisions and future follow-up and measure the distance of the mass from the mass.

Annotation. Labeling sonographic images of the breast is extremely important in the identification and correlation of breast images with images from other modalities. Most imaging centers have traditionally used the quasigrid pattern. This views the breast as a clock face. Directly above the nipple on either breast is 12 o'clock. Right medial breast and left lateral breast are 3 o'clock. Directly below the nipple bilaterally is 6 o'clock, and right lateral breast and left medial breast are 9 o'clock, respectively (Figure 17-28).

Many imaging centers will further subdivide the breast with three concentric circles, with the center being the nipple (Figure 17-29). The first ring circles one third of the breast tissue, encompassing the area just outside the nipple, or zone 1. The second ring is about two thirds of the breast surface from the nipple, or zone 2. The final ring is to the breast periphery, or zone 3. Lesions located close to the nipple are labeled "A." Lesions in the middle of the breast are labeled "B," and lesions located at the outer margin of the breast are labeled "C" (Box 17-11).

Finally, depth of any pathologic condition is documented. The breast is again divided into thirds from skin to the pectoralis major. Depth A is the most superficial third of the breast. Depth B is the middle layer. And depth C is the deepest third of the breast. Superficial lesions located close to the skin surface are labeled as "1," lesions in the middle of the breast are labeled "2," and deeper lesions located toward the chest wall are labeled "3."

With solid lesions, it is important to document the orientation of the mass in addition to identifying its location. The orientation of a lesion is determined by aligning the transducer with the longest axis of a lesion and identifying whether the long axis is oriented in a **radial** or **antiradial** plane. This is

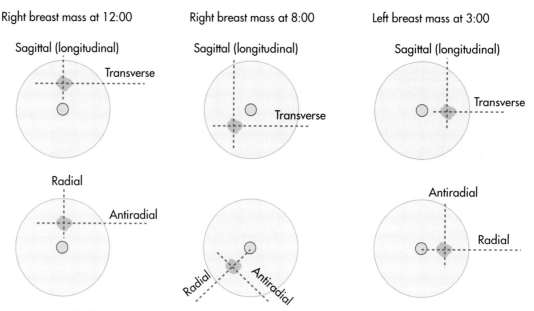

Figure 17-27   Examples of sagittal and transverse, plus radial and antiradial, transducer positions.

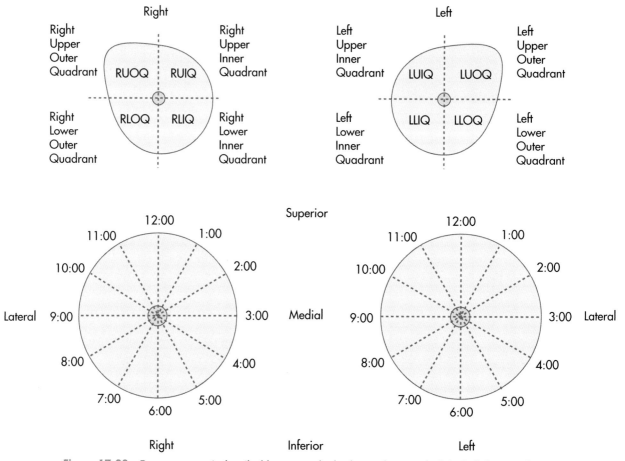

Figure 17-28   Breast anatomy is described by two methods: the quadrant method (right/left, upper/lower, and inner/outer quadrants) and the clock face method.

Figure 17-29 **A** and **B**, Zones of the breast are shown. **B**, Documentation of depth of tissue. **C**, Localization of mass in the right breast. **D**, Anterior and posterior mammogram of the breast. **E**, Longitudinal view of the breast mass. **F**, Medial to lateral mammogram acquisition. (Adapted from Henningsen C: *Clinical guide to ultrasonography*, St Louis, 2004, Mosby.)

important because malignancies tend to grow within the ducts and will often follow the ductal system in a radial plane towards the convergence at the nipple. The various methods of annotation described above can be combined to relay a specific location and orientation of a lesion. For example, a lesion labeled "RT BREAST 2:00 B3 RAD" can easily be relocated for follow-up; this lesion in the right breast is deeply situated towards the chest wall in the 2 o'clock position approximately midway between the nipple and the outer margin of the breast, and its long axis is oriented radially towards the nipple.

SONOGRAPHIC CHARACTERISTICS OF BREAST MASSES

Sonographic evaluation of a breast lesion normally begins with the determination of whether a lesion is cystic or solid (Box

17-11). The distinction between a cyst and a solid mass is extremely important for management purposes; a cyst that meets the criteria of a simple cyst on ultrasound is universally considered benign. Solid masses, however, have a malignant potential. Although the vast majority of solid masses are benign, further characterization of a solid lesion is necessary.

To be considered a simple cyst, a lesion must meet several criteria on ultrasound: it must be devoid of internal echoes (anechoic), show smooth inner margins with an imperceptible capsule, and demonstrate posterior acoustic enhancement (Table 17-2). Cysts within the breast can be multilocular with thin internal septations. In the case of simple cysts, no further work-up is usually necessary. In some cases, however, these cysts will be painful or disturbing to the patient. Aspiration

BOX 17-10 **BREAST SCANNING POINTS TO REMEMBER**

- Image optimization (image tissue from skin through chest wall equally)
- Lesion location and annotation methods
  Clock face
  Quadrant
  Distance from nipple
  "1,2,3 . . . A,B,C" method
- Three-dimensional measurement methods
  Sagittal/transverse
  Radial/antiradial
- Ultrasound pitfalls
  Pseudomass
  Infiltrative pattern
  Large, fatty breast

BOX 17-11 **SONOGRAPHIC CHARACTERISTICS OF BREAST LESIONS**

SIMPLE CYST
- Smooth walls
- Anechoic
- Posterior enhancement

COMPLICATED CYST
- Wall thickening or irregularities
- Septations
- Internal echoes

SOLID MASS
- Margins
  Benign: smooth, rounded
  Malignant: indistinct, fuzzy, spiculated
- Disruption of breast architecture
  Benign: grow within tissue causing compression of the tissue adjacent to the mass
  Malignant: grow through tissue without compressing adjacent tissue and may cause retraction of the nipple or dimpling of the skin
- Shape
  Benign: rounded or oval, large lobulations (<3)
  Malignant: sharp, angular, microlobulations (>3)
- Orientation
  Malignant: taller-than-wide highly suspicious, radial growth suspicious for intraductal lesions
- Internal echo pattern
  Benign: isoechoic, hyperechoic
  Malignant: hypoechoic, weak internal echoes, clustered microcalcifications
- Attenuation effects
  Benign: posterior enhancement
  Malignant: strongly attenuating
- Mobility
  Benign: some mobility
  Malignant: firmly fixed
- Compressibility
  Benign: fatty tumors are usually compressible
  Malignant: rigid, noncompressible
- Vascularity
  Malignant: hypervascular, feeder vessel may be identified

can be performed quickly and easily under ultrasound guidance (Figure 17-30).

If the cyst has internal echoes, wall irregularity, mural nodularity or septation, shadowing, nonuniform internal echoes, or any other feature not associated with a simple cyst, it is by definition a complex cyst, and aspiration and/or biopsy should be considered. Complex cysts are often indistinguishable from homogeneous solid sonographic masses because of their thick proteinaceous fluid content. Other complex cysts have thick or irregular capsules, a possible intracystic mass, or dependent debris. Cysts with layering calcifications or floating crystals (these can be seen moving on real-time scanning) are benign, although careful ultrasound technique is required to distinguish these cysts from those requiring further evaluation.

The usual approach to a small, smooth, round or oval, benign appearing solid mass in low-risk patients favors close-interval follow-up breast imaging. Color Doppler has been successfully used to interrogate solid masses to check for increased vascular flow. The demonstration of increased vascular flow could accelerate the need for biopsy of these masses.

Figure 17-30   Symptomatic cyst. **A,** Simple cyst on ultrasound (notice the lack of internal echoes, the smooth internal margin, imperceptible capsule, strong posterior acoustic enhancement, and edge refraction) is large enough to create a painful lump in the patient's breast. **B,** Aspiration was done under sonographic guidance. Note the echogenic needle tip in the cyst *(arrow).*

TABLE 17-2 SONOGRAPHIC CHARACTERISTICS OF COMMON LESIONS

Mass	Characteristics
Simple cyst	Oval or round, anechoic, imperceptible capsule, posterior acoustic enhancement, edge refraction shadowing, often compressible
Fibrocystic changes	Multiple cysts, well circumscribed, thin walls, increased fibrous stroma
Complex cyst	Irregular or thickened wall, mural nodule, fluid levels, debris, particulate echoes, variable degrees of shadowing
Benign	
Fibroadenoma	Oval or gently lobular, hypoechoic, uniform echogenicity, smooth, distinct margins, wider-than-tall, posterior acoustic enhancement, edge refraction shadow
Lipoma	May be large, smooth walls, hypoechoic (isoechoic with fat), posterior acoustic enhancement, easily compressible
Fat necrosis	Irregular, complex mass with low-level echoes; may have posterior acoustic shadow, separate from breast parenchyma
Abscess	Hypoechoic, complex lesion, posterior enhancement, thick walls, fluid levels
Cystosarcoma phyllodes	Large, hypoechoic tumor, well-defined margins, decreased through-transmission, fine or course internal echoes, variable amounts of shadowing
Intraductal papilloma	Intracystic lesion with fibrovascular stalk
Malignant	Irregular, spiculated, indistinct, or angular margins, hypoechoic, heterogeneous echogenicity, taller-than-wide, posterior acoustic shadowing, noncompressible, hypervascular with feeder vessel
Ductal carcinoma in situ (DCIS)	Calcifications and ductal enlargement with extension within the ducts
Invasive ductal carcinoma (IDC)	Begins in the ducts, invades the fatty tissue of the breast
Lobular carcinoma in situ (LCIS)	Confined to the gland, difficult to distinguish sonographically
Invasive lobular carcinoma (ILC)	Begins in the lobule, extends into the fatty tissue; often bilateral, multicentric, or multifocal

Modified from László Tabár, MD, Professor of Radiology, Uppsala, Sweden.

Tissue diagnosis is suggested in high-risk patients or patients with larger masses. The size cutoff for tissue diagnosis versus follow-up varies. In a low-risk patient with a single, dominant, smooth, solid mass, follow-up is offered for masses with a diameter of up to 1 cm. Some physicians will recommend following lesions up to 1.2 or even 1.5 cm in size, especially in the case of multiple bilateral masses. In a high-risk patient or in a patient who is not comfortable waiting on follow-up for an answer, tissue diagnosis can be pursued more aggressively. Options include fine-needle aspiration cytology, large-core needle biopsy, vacuum-assisted biopsy, and surgical excisional biopsy (Figure 17-31). High-quality sonographic imaging of a solid breast mass is quite accurate at characterizing a lesion as probably benign or probably malignant in a majority of cases (see Table 17-2). It is important, however, to realize that there is significant overlap in the appearance of benign and malignant lesions; ultrasound cannot be used as a substitute for tissue diagnosis when sonographic findings are indeterminate or a biopsy is indicated by clinical examination or patient history.

Margins. The margins of a mass should be investigated carefully. A technique called **fremitus** can be used to identify and confirm the margins of a mass. Fremitus is a palpable tremor or vibration of the chest wall. Using power Doppler, have the patient hum. The vibrations of the chest wall will carry through to the breast tissue, creating a power Doppler signal. The lesion is normally void of signal, making it easier to identify its margins. This technique can be useful in confirming the presence of a mass when in doubt, identifying multifocal masses, differentiating diffuse masses, and locating palpable masses that are isoechoic with the breast parenchyma.

Benign lesions usually have smooth, rounded margins (Figure 17-32, A-C). Malignant tumors are aggressive and tend to grow through tissue via finger-like extensions called **spiculation** (Figure 17-32, D). Spiculated margins are the ultrasound finding with the highest positive predictive value of malignancy and correlate with mammographic spiculation. Sonographic spiculations appear as small lines that radiate outward from the surface of a mass. They are typically alternating hypoechoic and hyperechoic lines. Ductal extensions project radially from the tumor and are oriented towards the nipple. Small extensions may not be visible sonographically, but may make the margins of a lesion appear indistinct or fuzzy.

Disruption of Breast Architecture. Benign tumors are usually slow growing and do not invade surrounding tissue. They tend to grow horizontally within the tissue planes, parallel to the chest wall. Larger benign lesions will often cause compression of the tissue adjacent to the mass, implying that the mass is pushing against adjacent breast tissue, as opposed to infiltrating it.

Malignant lesions, on the other hand, tend to grow right through the normal breast tissue. As malignant masses enlarge, they may cause retraction of the nipple or dimpling of the skin as the spiculations pull on the Cooper's ligaments (Figure 17-33).

Shape. A rounded or oval shape is usually associated with benign lesions, while sharp, angular margins are associated with malignancy. Mild undulations in contour can be seen in benign masses such as fibroadenomas; however, microlobulations (very small 1 to 2 mm lobulations) are more often associated with malignancy. Lobulations associated with benign fibroadenomas are usually large, rounded lobulations and do not exceed three in number. Microlobulations associated with malignancy are usually smaller, sharper, and more numerous.

Figure 17-31   Core biopsy of isoechoic mass close to chest wall. **A,** Ultrasound image of an isoechoic mass *(arrowheads)* located immediately adjacent to the pectoralis muscle *(arrows).* **B,** Core biopsy needle *(arrowheads)* is directed parallel to the chest wall. Note the loss of information posterior to the needle caused by acoustic shadowing and reverberation echoes *(asterisks).*

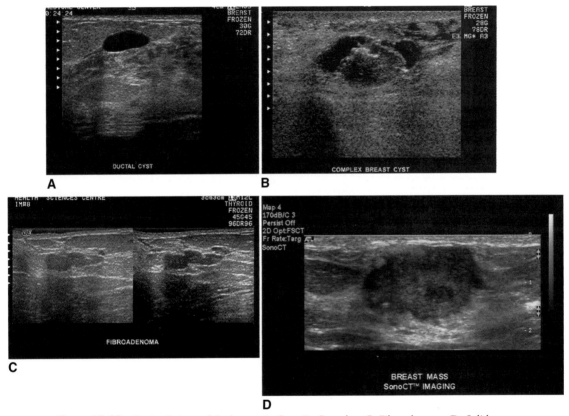

Figure 17-32   Benign lesions of the breast. **A,** Cyst. **B,** Complex. **C,** Fibroadenoma. **D,** Solid mass.

Orientation. The normal tissue planes of the breast are horizontally oriented. Benign lesions tend to grow within the normal tissue planes and their long axis lies parallel to the chest wall. Malignant lesions are able to grow through the connective tissue and may have a vertical orientation when imaging the breast from anterior to posterior. If a mass measures longer in the anteroposterior dimension (height) than in either transverse or sagittal planes (width), the mass has a vertical orientation is usually described as being "taller-than-wide" and is suspicious for malignancy.

Internal Echo Pattern. Lesions that appear isoechoic with the breast parenchyma or have echoes equivalent to or brighter than that of fat are most often benign. A solid lesion that is hypoechoic relative to the normal breast parenchyma is more suspicious for malignancy. Malignant lesions tend to be very

Figure 17-33 Malignant lesions interrupt the normal breast architecture as they spread throughout the tissue.

hypoechoic relative to fat and usually have weak internal echoes. They are often associated with a dense posterior shadowing, making the lesion difficult to penetrate.

Microcalcifications within a solid mass are associated with a breast malignancy. Ultrasound is less sensitive than mammography in the detection of microcalcifications due to the heterogeneous appearance of the normal breast tissue. Microcalcifications seen with ultrasound are typically very small echogenic foci, which do not create shadows because of their small size. While calcifications are not frequently visualized by sonography, their detection in a hypoechoic mass is suspicious for malignancy.

Attenuation Effects. Enhancement behind a lesion is normally caused by a weakly attenuating structure and usually indicates the lesion is made up of fluid and is a characteristic associated with benign lesions. Most solid lesions will not enhance, with the exception of a fibroadenoma.

Shadowing behind a solid breast mass is another suspicious sonographic sign for malignancy because malignant tumors tend to be very attenuating. Posterior shadowing should not be confused with edge or refraction shadowing, where shadowing occurs at the curved edge of a smooth, benign mass.

Mobility. Benign lesions will normally demonstrate a limited degree of mobility or may roll away as they are palpated. Because of the spiculations associated with malignancy, malignant lesions are normally very fixed or rigid in their position.

Compressibility. If pressure applied by the transducer causes the lesion to compress or change shape, the lesion is probably benign and most likely represents a fat lobule. Malignant lesions are normally very hard and noncompressible.

Vascularity. Doppler interrogation of a breast lesion is an essential element of the study. Although breast lesions are not associated with consistent resistance patterns on Doppler ultrasound, malignant masses will often demonstrate increased vascularity within the lesion and often have a feeder vessel, which can be identified with careful evaluation. Vessels that penetrate

a mass are very suspect for malignancy and should be checked using color or power Doppler to ascertain the number and also to look for intratumoral vessels.

PATHOLOGY

The most common pathologic lesions of the female breast are, in order of decreasing frequency, fibrocystic disease, carcinoma, fibroadenoma, intraductal papilloma, and duct ectasia. Benign lesions are the most common breast lesions, occurring in 70% of proved lesions in biopsies or removed. Several parameters must be considered when a dominant mass has been palpated including the patient's age, physical characteristics of the mass, and previous medical history. Lesions more common to younger women are fibrocystic disease and fibroadenomas. Older or postmenopausal women are more likely to have intraductal papillomas, duct ectasia, and cancer.

DIFFERENTIAL DIAGNOSIS OF BREAST MASSES

Symptoms of breast masses include pain, a palpable mass, spontaneous or induced nipple discharge, skin dimpling, ulceration, or nipple retraction. Benign processes are usually associated with pain, tumor, and nipple discharge. Skin dimpling or ulceration and nipple retraction nearly always result from cancer. Benign tumors are rubbery, mobile, and well defined (as seen in a fibroadenoma), whereas malignant tumors are often stone hard and irregular with a gritty feel. Soft tumors usually represent a lipoma (fat tissue). Cystic masses are like a balloon of water, well delineated but not as mobile as fibroadenomas because they form part of the breast parenchyma, whereas a fibroadenoma has a capsule.

BENIGN CONDITIONS

Cysts. Cysts are commonly seen in women 35 to 55 years of age. Symptoms include history of changing with the menstrual cycle, pain (especially when the cyst is growing rapidly), recent lump, and tenderness. Small cysts may not regress completely and may persist from one cycle to the next.

Fibrocystic Condition. Fibrocystic changes produce histologic alterations in the terminal ducts and lobules of the breast in both the epithelial and the connective tissue. Fibrocystic changes are usually accompanied by pain or tenderness in the breast and represent normal physiologic processes of breast tissue that fluctuate under the influence of the normal female hormonal cycles. These processes become magnified in some patients to the point of causing symptoms that are upsetting to the patient (mainly pain and tenderness or recurrent cysts). In some cases, **fibrocystic condition (FCC)** causes changes that are frankly worrisome for breast cancer. In all age groups, the most common diagnosis at breast biopsy is FCC. These biopsies are prompted by a growing or dominant clinically suspicious breast lump.

The terms fibrocystic condition or fibrocystic change (use of the term fibrocystic disease is discouraged) actually encompass many different processes under one term. There is abundant inaccuracy and confusion that results from using the term fibrocystic condition. In some cases FCC may refer to the normal hormonal fluctuation of breast texture. At the other end of the spectrum, a surgical biopsy may be undertaken because of a growing suspicious breast lump. In a few cases, a biopsy reveals tissue changes that mean the patient is at increased risk for subsequent development of breast cancer.

Clinical signs and symptoms of FCC include the lumps and pain that the patient feels that fluctuate with every monthly cycle. In most cases, both breasts are equally involved. In some cases, FCC may affect just one area of one breast. This can be frightening for the patient and is a frequent cause of referral for diagnostic breast imaging.

There are imaging signs of FCC that may be visible on the mammogram or breast ultrasound. On mammogram, FCC may cause diffuse benign microcalcifications, **adenosis,** and multiple round masses. Ultrasound of the breast will show the round masses as multiple cysts (Figure 17-34).

There are many separate tissue processes of FCC recognized by the pathologist in reviewing breast tissue under a microscope, including **apocrine metaplasia,** fibrosis, epithelial ductal hyperplasia, sclerosing adenosis. In correlating the pathologic results of a breast biopsy to the indication for biopsy (i.e., palpable breast lump, suspicious mammographic or sonographic mass, or clustered microcalcifications), it is very important for the physician to document that the pathologic results are concordant with the targeted lesion. If a breast biopsy was performed because of suspicious microcalcifications, for example, the pathology report should state that microcalcifications were seen. If there were no microcalcifications seen on pathology slides, then this is a discordant result and will require further investigation.

In an attempt to create a more clinically relevant classification of tissue processes under the enormous and confusing heading of fibrocystic condition, these processes have been separated into three categories. These include (1) nonproliferative lesions (no increased risk of subsequent development of breast cancer); (2) proliferative lesions without atypical cells (mildly elevated risk of subsequent breast cancer); and (3) proliferative lesions with atypical cellular changes (moderately increased risk of subsequent breast cancer). Any woman with an atypical pro-

liferative breast lesion (especially lobular neoplasia) who also has a family history of a first-degree relative with breast cancer will have double the risk of subsequent breast cancer compared with the patient with an atypical proliferative lesion alone (Table 17-3).

Fibroadenoma. The most common benign breast tumors are **fibroadenomas,** and they occur primarily in young women. They may be found in one breast or both breasts. The growth of a fibroadenoma is stimulated by estrogen. Under normal circumstances, hormonal influences on the breast (estrogen) result in the proliferation of epithelial cells in lactiferous ducts and in stromal tissue during the first half of the menstrual cycle. During the second half this condition regresses, allowing breast tissue to return to its normal resting state. In certain disturbances of this hormonal mechanism, the regression fails to occur and results in the development of fibrous and epithelial nodules that become fibroadenomas, fibromas, or adenomas, depending on the predominant cell type. They may also be related to pregnancy and lactation.

Clinically a fibroadenoma is firm, rubbery, freely mobile, and clearly delineated from the surrounding breast tissue (Figure 17-35). It is round or ovoid, smooth or lobulated, and usually does not cause loss of contour of the breast unless it develops to a large size. It rarely causes mastodynia, and it does not change size during the menstrual cycle. Fibroadenomas tend to grow very slowly. A sudden increase in size with acute pain may be a result of hemorrhage within the tumor.

TABLE 17-3	FIBROCYSTIC CONDITION: COMMON BREAST LESIONS—RISK OF SUBSEQUENT BREAST CANCER
Classification	Description
Nonproliferative lesions: no increased risk	Cyst Apocrine metaplasia Fibroadenoma Ductal ectasia Mild epithelial ductal hyperplasia Benign microcalcifications
Proliferative lesions without atypical features: mildly increased risk (1.5 to 2×)	Moderate or florid epithelial ductal hyperplasia Sclerosing adenosis Radial scar (complex sclerosing lesion) Intraductal papilloma
Proliferative lesions with atypical features: moderately increased risk (4 to 6×)	Atypical ductal hyperplasia Atypical lobular hyperplasia Lobular neoplasia (alternative term for lobular carcinoma in situ [LCIS])

Note: Patients with an atypical proliferative lesion and a first-degree relative with breast cancer are at even greater risk for subsequent breast cancer.

Map 4
170dB/C 4
Persist Off
2D Opt:FSCT
Fr Rate:Surv
SonoCT™
XRes™

BREAST CYSTS
SonoCT™ IMAGING WITH XRES™ TECHNOLOGY

Figure 17-34 Fibrocystic condition shows two sonolucent structures within the breast.

Figure 17-35   Fibroadenoma. Smooth, ovoid, solid mass with a low-level internal echo pattern.

Figure 17-36   Lactating breast abscess shows a diffuse mottled appearance of the breast with irregular margins and posterior enhancement.

Calcification may follow hemorrhage or infarction, and thus the tumor may have calcifications and may mimic the appearance of a carcinoma on mammography. Sonographically, fibroadenomas have benign characteristics with smooth, rounded margins and low-level homogeneous internal echoes and may demonstrate intermediate posterior enhancement. Fibroadenomas are normally hypoechoic, but are occasionally **hyperechoic** to the fat within the breast.

Lipoma. A pure lipoma consists entirely of fatty tissue. Other forms of lipoma consist of fat with fibrous and glandular elements interspersed (fibroadenolipoma). A lipoma may grow to a large size before it is clinically detected. It is usually found in middle-aged or menopausal women. Clinically on palpation a large, soft, poorly demarcated mass is felt that cannot be clearly separated from the surrounding parenchyma. There is no thinning or fixation of the overlying skin. Sonographically, it may be difficult or impossible to detect a lipoma in a fatty breast. Lipomas typically have smooth walls, are hypoechoic, and appear similar to fat. They will often demonstrate posterior enhancement and are easily compressible.

Fat Necrosis. Fat necrosis may be caused by trauma to the breast, surgery, radiation treatments, or plasma cell mastitis or may be related to an involutional process or other disease present in the breast, such as cancer. It is more frequently found in older women. Clinical palpation reveals a spherical nodule that is generally superficial under a layer of calcified necrosis. A deep-lying focus of necrosis may cause scarring with skin retraction and thus mimic carcinoma. Sonographically, fat necrosis appears as an irregular, complex mass with low-level echoes, may mimic a malignant lesion, and may appear as fat, but is separate and different from the rest of the breast parenchyma. Acoustic shadowing may or may not be present.

Acute Mastitis. Acute mastitis may result from infection, trauma, mechanical obstruction in the breast ducts, or other conditions. It often occurs during lactation, beginning in the lactiferous ducts and spreading via the lymphatics or blood. Acute mastitis causes an enlarged, reddened, tender breast, and

is often confined to one area of the breast. Diffuse mastitis results from the infection being carried via the blood or breast lymphatics and thus affecting the entire breast. These patients are treated initially with antibiotics and are referred for breast imaging when the acute inflammatory symptoms are sufficiently reduced to allow good quality mammography and breast ultrasound to rule out inflammatory breast cancer as a cause.

Chronic Mastitis. An inflammation of the glandular tissue is considered to be chronic mastitis. It is very difficult to differentiate by ultrasound; the echo pattern is mixed and diffuse with sound absorption. It usually is found in elderly women. There is a thickening of the connective tissue, which results in narrowing of the lumen of the milk ducts. The cause is inspissated intraductal secretions, which are forced into the periductal connective tissue. Clinically the patient usually has a nipple discharge, and frequently the nipple has retracted over a period of years. Palpation reveals some subareolar thickening but no dominant mass.

Abscess. An abscess may be single or multiple. Acute abscesses have a poorly defined border, whereas mature abscesses are well encapsulated with sharp borders. A definite diagnosis cannot be made from a mammogram alone. Aspiration is necessary. Clinical findings show pain, swelling, and reddening of the overlying skin. The patient may be febrile, and swollen painful axillary nodes may be present. Sonographic findings may show a diffuse, mottled appearance of the breast, irregular margins, posterior enhancement, and low-level internal echoes (Figure 17-36). If associated with mastitis, skin thickening is almost always present and edema leads to diffusely increased echogenicity of the breast tissue. Color or power Doppler of the breast may be helpful to document hyperemia associated with increased vascularity and tip the scales toward abscess rather than hematoma.

Cystosarcoma Phyllodes. Cystosarcoma phyllodes is a rare, predominantly benign breast neoplasm. It comprises less than 1% of all breast neoplasms, yet it is the most frequent sarcoma of the breast. It is more commonly found in women in their 50s and usually is unilateral. It may arise from a fibroadenoma. Many patients may notice that a small breast mass that has been present for a long time suddenly begins to grow rapidly. Although it is considered a benign lesion, 27% of these tumors are malignant; 12% metastasize.

When the tumor is small, it is well delineated, firm, and mobile, much like a fibroadenoma. As it enlarges, the surface may become irregular and lobulated. Skin changes can develop from increasing pressure. Edema may produce a skin change. As pressure increases, it causes trophic changes and eventual skin ulcerations. Infection and abscess formation may be a secondary complication. The tumor never adheres to the adjacent soft tissue or underlying pectoral muscle; therefore, dimpling of the skin or fixation of the tumor is not observed. Sonographic findings include a large, hypoechoic tumor with well-defined margins and decreased through-transmission. Internal echoes may be fine or coarse with variable amounts of shadowing.

Intraductal Papilloma. An intraductal papilloma is a small, benign tumor that grows within the acini of the breast. It occurs most frequently in women 35 to 55 years of age. The predominant symptom is spontaneous nipple discharge arising from a single duct. When the discharge is copious, it is usually preceded by a sensation of fullness or pain in the areola or nipple area and is relieved as the fluid is expelled. It has a "raspberry-like" configuration on the mammogram and in this way helps to promote correlation between the mammogram and the sonogram.

Papillomas are usually small, multiple, and multicentric. They consist of simple proliferations of duct epithelium projecting outward into a dilated lumen from one or more focal points (Figure 17-37), each supported by a vascular stalk from which it receives the blood supply. Trauma may rupture the stalk, filling the duct with blood or serum. Papillomas may also grow to a large size and thus become palpable lesions. They are somewhat linear, resembling the terminal duct, and are usually benign.

Figure 17-37   Complex cyst with debris and intracystic mass. **A,** Ultrasound image of a complex cyst with irregular dependent debris *(arrows)*. **B,** Another image of the same complex cyst showing an intracystic mass *(arrowhead)* and thickened septations *(small arrows)*. **C,** Postaspiration pneumocystogram (air in cyst cavity) showing the intracystic mass *(arrow)* and the septations *(small arrows)*. Intracystic masses are usually benign papillomas, but may sometimes be papillary carcinomas. (Courtesy Lynn W. Gayden, MD, Women's Health Center, Memphis, Tenn.)

MALIGNANT CONDITIONS

Malignancies generally develop over a long time period. It is not unusual for several years to pass from the first appearance of **atypical hyperplasia** to the final diagnosis of in situ cancer. Malignant cells grow along a line of least resistance, such as in fatty tissue. In fibrotic tissue, most cancer growth occurs along the borders. Lymphatics and blood vessels are frequently used as pathways for new tumor development. If the tumor is encapsulated, it continues to grow in one area, compressing and distorting the surrounding architecture. When the carcinoma is contained and has not invaded the basal membrane structure, it is considered in situ. Most cancer originates in the terminal ductal lobular units, whereas a smaller percentage originates in the glandular tissue. The breast lobules are concentrated in the upper outer quadrant of the breast and so it is not surprising that a majority of breast cancers (50%) are found there, followed by a lesser incidence in the retroareolar area (17%), upper inner quadrant (15%), lower outer quadrant (10%), and lower inner quadrant (5%). Multifocal masses are least common and occur in approximately 3% of cases.

Cancer of the breast is of two types: sarcoma and carcinoma. Sarcoma refers to breast tumors that arise from the sup-portive or connective tissues. Sarcomas tend to grow rapidly and invade fibrous tissue. Carcinoma refers to breast tumors that arise from the epithelium, in the ductal and glandular tissue, and usually has tentacles. Other malignant diseases affecting the breast are a result of systemic neoplasms, such as leukemia or lymphoma.

Breast carcinomas are generally categorized by two factors: where the cancer cells originate (ductal or lobular) and whether the cancer is prone to spreading (noninvasive or invasive). Most breast carcinomas begin within the ducts of the breast and are called ductal or intraductal carcinomas. Breast cancers that form in the lobules are called lobular carcinomas. Carcinomas that do not normally spread outside of the duct or lobule are called noninvasive, noninfiltrating, or in situ cancers, whereas cancers that spread into nearby tissue are said to be invasive or infiltrating.

Ductal Carcinoma In Situ (DCIS). DCIS is also known as intraductal carcinoma. DCIS is characterized by cancer cells that are present inside the ducts, but they have not yet spread through the walls of the ducts into the fatty tissue of the breast (Figure 17-38). Because these are confined to the duct and have not spread, they usually have a 100% cure rate.

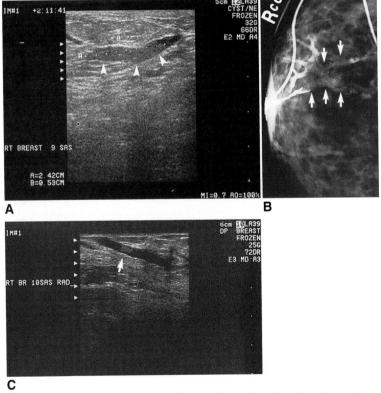

Figure 17-38   Intraductal masses. **A,** Ultrasound image shows a large intraductal mass in a patient with a unilateral single-duct discharge *(arrowheads).* **B,** Magnification view from a galactogram, in which contrast was injected retrograde into the duct orifice from which the discharge was expressed. Note the large filling defect *(arrows).* **C,** Ultrasound image from another patient showing a small intraductal mass *(arrow).* The majority of intraductal masses are benign papillomas. It is generally difficult, however, to distinguish an intraductal papilloma from an early intraductal cancer. (**B,** Courtesy Lynn W. Gayden, MD, Chief Radiologist, Women's Health Center, Memphis, Tenn.)

A

B   **C**

Figure 17-39 Suspicious microcalcifications (DCIS) and occult infiltrating ductal carcinoma.
A, Magnification mammogram image of pleomorphic (irregular shapes) suspicious microcalcifications
identified on screening mammogram in this asymptomatic young woman. No mass was visible on the
mammogram. **B,** Ultrasound demonstration of echogenic microcalcification within a dilated duct *(arrows).*
C, Ultrasound image of the same breast showing an unsuspected sonographic mass with suspicious features
(note the mass is taller than wide, shows an irregular indistinct margin, and shows asymmetric posterior
shadowing and heterogeneous echogenicity). Ultrasound-guided, large-needle core biopsy-proved infiltrating
malignancy. This altered the patient's management, requiring a mastectomy and axillary node dissection for
staging.

Calcifications and ductal enlargement with extension within
the ducts are common (Figure 17-39).

Invasive Ductal Carcinoma (IDC). IDC accounts for
nearly 80% of breast cancers. Like DCIS, these cancers begin
in the ducts, but unlike DCIS, they invade the fatty tissue of
the breast and have the potential to metastasize via the bloodstream or lymphatic system. It is important to get a definitive
diagnosis and begin treatment before it spreads to other organs.

Lobular Carcinoma In Situ (LCIS). LCIS is not considered a "cancer" because it has a low malignant potential. LCIS
is often referred to as lobular neoplasia and is classified as a
precancerous growth that begins in the lobule. LCIS is confined to the gland and does not penetrate through the wall of
the lobule. LCIS does not usually form a distinct mass and can
therefore be difficult to pick up using mammography and
ultrasound screening. Women with LCIS are at a higher risk
of developing invasive breast cancer later on.

Invasive Lobular Carcinoma (ILC). ILC begins in the
lobule, where it extends into the fatty tissue of the breast.
Similar to IDC, invasive lobular carcinoma has the potential
to metastasize and spread to other parts of the body. ILC is the
second most common type of invasive tumors, accounting for
10% to 15% of all breast cancers. ILC is often bilateral,
multicentric, or **multifocal** (Figure 17-40).

Breast cancers are considered multifocal when more than
one tumor is identified and they are located within the same
quadrant or ductal system and are within 5 cm of each other.
Breast cancers are considered multicentric when they are
located in different quadrants and are located at least 5 cm
apart. Multifocal lesions tend to be of the same cell type histologically, whereas multicentric lesions are more likely to be
of two different cell types.

The more favorable cancers remain localized to the breast
longer, and treated patients have a 75% survival rate after 10
years. They represent only 10% to 12% of all breast cancers.
This group includes medullary, intracystic papillary, papillary,

Figure 17-40 Infiltrating lobular carcinoma. **A,** Craniocaudal view of both breasts shows portion of nodular density *(arrow)* in posterior central right breast. **B,** Spot compression magnification view shows wispy area *(arrow)* of parenchymal density in the inframammary fold corresponding to the nodule on the craniocaudal view. **C,** Sonogram of area of mammographic abnormality shows hypoechoic, ill-defined area of architectural distortion *(AD)* with infiltration *(arrow)* into the adjacent fibroglandular parenchyma *(F)* ultrasound-guided biopsy confirmed the diagnosis of infiltrating lobular carcinoma. **D,** In another patient with vague thickening on self-examination, a mammogram showed dense glandular tissue but no focal mass. Ultrasound demonstrates an extensive hypoechoic angular mass *(M)* occupying nearly two thirds of the breast. Fibroglandular tissue *(F)*. (From Rumack C, Wilson S, Charboneau W: *Diagnostic ultrasound,* ed 3, St Louis, 2005, Mosby.)

colloid, adenoid cystic, and tubular carcinoma. Other malignant tumors that have a better than average prognosis after treatment include malignant cystosarcoma phyllodes and stromal sarcomas because they rarely metastasize to regional nodes.

Definitive identification of a tumor type can only be made by histologic tissue examination. Although many solid lesions have definite malignant characteristics, many lesions have a crossover of benign and malignant characteristics on ultrasound and their nature is indeterminate by sonographic evaluation alone. It is also not uncommon for malignant lesions to have a benign appearance on ultrasound, therefore making it extremely important to consider the patient's risk factors and clinical history when considering the differential diagnosis. The following is a brief description of the more common malignancies affecting the breast.

Figure 17-41   Papillary carcinoma. **A,** Mediolateral oblique view of the left breast shows well-circumcised mass containing area of increased density. Slight marginal irregularity is seen *(arrows)*. **B,** Circumscribed complex mass with anterior protuberance *(curved arrow)*. Central area of echogenicity is surrounded circumferentially by what most likely represents the cystic component *(C)* of this in situ papillary carcinoma with stromal invasion. (From Rumack C, Wilson S, Charboneau W: *Diagnostic ultrasound,* ed 3, St Louis, 2005, Mosby.)

Comedocarcinoma.   Intraductal solid carcinoma in which the lactiferous ducts are filled with a yellow pastelike material that looks like small plugs (comedones) when sectioned is called **comedocarcinoma.** Histologically the ducts are filled with plugs of an epithelial tumor that have a central necrosis, giving rise to the pastelike material. Both invasive and noninvasive forms exist.

Noninvasive forms may lack any clinical or palpatory findings. If there is a nipple discharge, it is more frequently clear than bloody (unlike papillary carcinoma, in which bloody discharge is typical). The patient may complain of pain or the sensation of insects crawling on the breast. With early invasion, minimal thickening of the surrounding breast tissue may be palpated. In the advanced stage the clinical signs are nipple retraction, dominant mass, and fixation.

Microcalcifications are commonly seen on mammography and may be picked up sonographically. Intraductal carcinomas have malignant characteristics, including irregular margins, a diffuse internal echo pattern, and attenuation with shadowing.

Juvenile Breast Cancer.   Juvenile breast cancer is similar to the ductal carcinoma in situ and invasive ductal carcinoma found in adults. Generally, it occurs in young females, between 8 and 15 years of age, and has a good prognosis when treated early.

Papillary Carcinoma.   Papillary carcinoma is a tumor that initially arises as an intraductal mass. It may also take the form of an intracystic tumor, which is rare. The early stage of papillary carcinoma is noninvasive. The tumor occasionally arises from a benign ductal papilloma. It is associated with little fibrotic reaction.

Both intraductal and intracystic forms exist, and these represent 1% to 2% of all breast carcinomas. The earliest clinical sign of intraductal papillary carcinoma is bloody nipple discharge. Occasionally a mass can be palpated as a small, firm, well-circumscribed area and may be mistaken for a fibroadenoma (Figure 17-41). There may be nodules of blue or red discoloration under the skin with central ulceration. A diffusely nodular appearance overlying the skin is a special variant of multiple intraductal papillary carcinoma. Intracystic papillary carcinoma is clinically indistinguishable in its early stages from a cyst or fibroadenoma. When the tumor has invaded through the cyst wall, it is palpable as a poorly circumscribed mass. Papillary carcinoma typically has a more favorable prognosis than other kinds of carcinoma.

Paget's Disease.   Paget's disease arises in the retroareolar ducts and grows in the direction of the nipple, spreading into the intraepidermal region of the nipple and areola, and has a rashlike appearance that may be confused with a melanoma. Any ulceration, enlargement, or deformity of the nipple and areola should suggest Paget's disease. This is a relatively rare tumor, accounting for 2.5% of all breast cancers. It typically occurs in women over 50 years of age. Differential diagnosis includes benign inflammatory eczematous condition of the nipple, because palpatory findings are frequently not present. The primary ductal cancer may be quite deep or embedded in fibrotic tissue. Sonographically, Paget's disease will present as a retroareolar mass with irregular margins, heterogeneous internal echoes, and attenuation with posterior shadowing.

Scirrhous Carcinoma. Scirrhous carcinoma is a type of intraductal tumor with extensive fibrous tissue proliferation (very dense fibrosis). Focal calcification may also be present. Histologically the cells are found in narrow files or strands, clusters, or columns and may form lumina with varying frequency.

Scirrhous is the most common form of breast cancer and often has no specific histologic findings or patterns and is therefore often classified as ductal carcinoma that is not otherwise specified (NOS). The classic clinical signs are a very firm nodular, frequently nonmovable mass often with fixation and flattening of overlying skin and nipple retraction. The retraction is a result of an infiltrative shortening of Cooper's ligaments because of productive fibrosis (see Figure 17-22). Fixation and retraction of the nipple may be the result of a subareolar carcinoma, but may also be caused by benign fibrosis of the breast. It is important to note that some patients normally have inverted nipples. The size of the cancer may vary from a few millimeters to involvement of nearly the entire breast. The deep-lying scirrhous carcinoma may grow into and become fixed to the thoracic wall. A bloody discharge is rare in this tumor.

Medullary Carcinoma. Medullary carcinoma is a densely cellular tumor containing large, round, or oval tumor cells. It usually is a well-circumscribed mass, with the center frequently necrotic, hemorrhagic, and cystic (Figure 17-42). Medullary carcinomas are relatively rare, comprising less than 5% of breast cancers. The age of occurrence is slightly lower than for the average breast cancer, with a majority of cases occurring in women younger than 50. Medullary carcinomas are usually well circumscribed, often large, and resemble a fibroadenoma with a fairly benign appearance. Discoloration of the overlying skin is often seen as a clinical finding, and bilateral occurrence is more frequent with medullary carcinoma than in other cancers.

Colloid Carcinoma. Colloid carcinoma (mucinous) is a relatively rare type of ductal carcinoma accounting for approximately 3% of breast carcinomas. The cells of the tumor produce secretions that fill lactiferous ducts or the stromal tissues in which the tumor cells are invading. Clinically they present in older women as a slow-growing, smooth, and not particularly firm mass upon palpation. The sonographic appearance is often similar to a fibroadenoma with smooth margins and posterior enhancement. The echotexture has been described as having a "salt and pepper" appearance (Figure 17-43).

Tubular Carcinoma. Tubular carcinoma represents an extremely well differentiated form of **infiltrating** (invasive) **ductal carcinoma** usually less than 2 cm in dimension. Tubular carcinoma occurs in women with an average age of 50 and has a favorable prognosis with a low rate of recurrence or metastasis. Death is rare. Tubular carcinoma typically has poorly circumscribed margins and a hard consistency (Figure 17-44).

ULTRASOUND-GUIDED INTERVENTIONAL PROCEDURES

Ultrasound is an important guide to many diagnostic and interventional procedures in the breast. These include cyst aspiration, fine-needle aspiration cytology (FNAC), abscess or

Figure 17-42 Medullary carcinoma. Sonogram depicts lobulated mass (*arrows*) with ill-defined margins, low-level internal echoes, and a small amount of posterior acoustic enlargement. (From Rumack C, Wilson S, Charboneau W: *Diagnostic ultrasound,* ed 3, St Louis, 2005, Mosby.)

BOX 17-12   ULTRASOUND-GUIDED INTERVENTIONAL PROCEDURES

- Cyst aspiration
- Fine-needle aspiration cytology (FNAC)
- Drainage procedures
- Preoperative needle (wire) localization
- Large-core needle biopsy
- Vacuum-assisted needle biopsy
- Sentinel node biopsy

seroma drainage, large-core needle biopsy, vacuum-assisted needle biopsy, ultrasound-guided preoperative needle wire localization for surgical excision, and injection of a radiopharmaceutic agent for sentinel node identification and biopsy (Box 17-12). Sterile coupling gel is available commercially, as are sterile plastic transducer sleeves. It is possible and more cost effective to use isopropyl alcohol as a coupling agent during procedures.

When using ultrasound to guide any diagnostic or interventional procedure in the breast, the high-frequency, narrow-beam linear array transducer is a valuable tool. Even narrow-gauge needles (22 or 25 gauge) can be seen and accurately guided into cysts or masses. The key to visualizing the needle is to keep it oriented as nearly parallel to the transducer

Figure 17-43   Mucinous (colloid) carcinoma. **A,** Spot compression mammographic view of palpable (denoted by radiopaque marker) circumscribed mass. A satellite nodule suggestive of diverticulum is seen laterally *(curved arrow).* **B,** Sonography of a portion of the mass responds well with the mammogram margins are well defined, and the diverticulum-like satellite *(curved arrow)* is easily seen. This homogeneous mass shows posterior acoustic enhancement. (From Rumack C, Wilson S, Charboneau W: *Diagnostic ultrasound,* ed 3, St Louis, 2005, Mosby.)

Figure 17-44   Tubular carcinoma. **A,** Magnified mammographic view shows mass with central radiolucent areas and very long radiating spiculations, suggesting radial scar. **B,** Sonogram depicts 0.7-cm, solid, hypoechoic mass with irregular, poorly defined margins *(arrows)* and posterior acoustic attenuation, common features of carcinoma. (From Rumack C, Wilson S, Charboneau W: *Diagnostic ultrasound,* ed 3, St Louis, 2005, Mosby.)

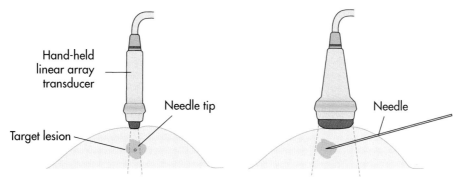

Figure 17-45 Placement of the needle tip is facilitated by keeping it in the field of vision and as parallel as possible to the transducer surface.

face as possible. Accuracy in placing the needle tip within the target lesion is also aided when the lesion is kept in the field of vision along with the needle (Figure 17-45). This protects the patient, because the main hazard for the patient is inadvertent piercing of the chest wall. Puncture of the lung resulting in a pneumothorax can occur in some cases with asthenic patients (especially those with emphysema, in which case the lung may protrude between ribs). If care is taken to maintain the needle parallel to the transducer face, the needle tip will remain parallel to the chest wall and help prevent potential complications.

Another important consideration in planning needle procedures in the breast is the approach. When dealing with any breast lesion that has the potential of malignancy, selection of the needle approach can have consequences in future therapeutic and reconstructive surgical procedures. Although the shortest approach from skin to target lesion has been advocated in the past for preoperative needle wire localizations and is often the favored route for ultrasound-guided core biopsy, a more horizontal approach will often facilitate a better cosmetic outcome for the patient if a mastectomy is necessary. Preprocedure consultation with the referring surgeon concerning the approach for needle wire localizations and core biopsies will ensure the best final outcome for the patient.

Cyst Aspiration. Cyst aspiration is a common interventional technique employed in the breast. The cystic fluid is usually "straw-colored" when it is withdrawn unless it is tinged with blood. The two main indications are a symptomatic cyst (one large enough to create a palpable lump or cause a patient pain) and a hypoechoic lesion on ultrasound that does not meet criteria for a simple cyst (Figure 17-46). In the latter situation, aspiration determines whether the lesion is simply a complex cyst or a solid mass. This distinction is important for patient management. Occasionally, cyst aspiration will be undertaken because cysts are so large or so numerous that visualization of breast tissue by mammogram is significantly compromised.

Fine-Needle Aspiration Cytology (FNAC). The FNAC procedure uses a fine needle (usually 25 gauge) and an aspiration technique intended to harvest individual cells for diagnosis. The technique is used in the United States and many

other countries. It is fast, easy for the patient, and generally very cost effective. The single greatest problem in FNAC is an inadequate specimen. Another limitation in FNAC is the requirement for a specially trained and experienced pathologist (cytopathologist), not available in many centers. This technique has not been as popular in the United States in part because of the somewhat greater inaccuracy of FNAC diagnosis (especially in fibrous malignant lesions and in proliferative benign lesions) and because of the greater availability of the more accurate (although more invasive) large-core needle biopsy.

Drainage Procedures. When clinically indicated, most cases of breast abscess, seroma, or hematoma will be easily palpated and drained in a simple office procedure by a breast surgeon or other physician. In some cases, the physician or surgeon may request ultrasound guidance. These lesions differ from simple cysts in that they typically require a larger needle (at least 18 gauge); have thicker, more fibrous capsules; have thicker fluid, often with abundant cellular debris; and frequently have numerous fibrous synechiae within the lesion that can interfere with complete evacuation of contents. The goal in therapy of a breast abscess is complete eradication of the abscess, usually accomplished with a combination of drainage and antibiotic therapy. Seromas and hematomas are fluid accumulations within the breast that are not infected. These lesions have similar imaging characteristics (smooth mammographic mass, complex cyst on ultrasound). They differ in the amount of blood and blood by-products within the fluid. They usually are encountered during healing from surgical procedures and are not infrequently seen after lumpectomy or following a large-core needle biopsy. In some cases, blunt trauma may lead to a hematoma, and occasionally, foreign body reaction or implant rupture may cause a seroma.

Preoperative Needle Wire Localization. Ultrasound offers a quick method for placement of a percutaneous needle wire assembly for preoperative localization of a **nonpalpable** breast lesion for surgical excision (Figure 17-47). Ultrasound guidance offers a significant advantage in complicated cases, such as localization of a lesion adjacent to a breast implant (Figure 17-48), a lesion close to the chest wall, or a lesion in other areas not easily approached under mammographic guidance.

Figure 17-46 Complex cyst. **A,** Mammogram shows a smooth, benign appearing dominant mass. **B,** Ultrasound shows a lobular, smooth, hypoechoic lesion with weak posterior acoustic enhancement. Cyst aspiration attempt under ultrasound guidance was done to assess this lesion as cystic or solid. Benign cyst fluid was obtained, and a pneumocystogram (air injected through the aspiration needle into the cyst cavity with a postaspiration mammogram) was performed. **C,** Postaspiration view of a normal pneumocystogram *(arrowheads)* after successful aspiration of a complex cyst. Pneumocystography can be used to exclude the possibility of an intracystic mass and may prevent or retard cyst recurrence.

Figure 17-47 Preoperative needle wire localization of spiculated cancerous mass. **A,** Ultrasound image shows a sonographic mass with suspicious features. **B,** Ultrasound image shows the echogenic wire through the center of the mass. **C,** Mammogram taken after wire placement shows the hook wire through the center of the cancerous mass. This wire placement aids the surgeon in identifying and removing tissue around the target mass.

Figure 17-48   Preoperative needle wire localization of sonographic mass adjacent to saline breast implant. **A,** Ultrasound image shows a small, solid mass *(arrows)* near the anterior margin of the patient's intramammary saline implant. **B,** Under ultrasound guidance, the needle wire assembly can be guided carefully through the mass, avoiding inadvertent piercing of the implant. **C** and **D,** Mammogram and ultrasound performed after wire placement shows the position of the wire adjacent to the implant. The wire *(arrowheads)* did not pierce the implant. The arrow identifies the approximate position of the target mass (not visible on mammogram).

Large-Core Needle Biopsy.   Ultrasound offers a fast and easy method for guiding large-core needle biopsy of solid masses. Patient comfort is enhanced, procedure time is often shorter, and ultrasound guidance is more cost effective in general than prone stereotactic procedures. It should be noted, however, that stereotactic guidance is still the preferred method for evaluation of clustered pleomorphic microcalcifications, which are difficult to see by ultrasound. An exception to this rule is illustrated in Figure 17-49, in which ultrasound scanning of a patient with multiple suspicious microcalcifications noted on a screening mammogram revealed an unsuspected solid mass. Ultrasound-guided core biopsy of the solid mass revealed infiltrating malignancy, which altered the patient's management.

Vacuum-Assisted Needle Biopsy.   A relatively new breast biopsy technique is a vacuum-assisted breast biopsy. The biopsy is a percutaneous procedure that relies on stereotactic mammography or ultrasound imaging for guidance. Stereotactic mammography is performed using computers to pinpoint the exact location of a breast mass taken from two different angles. The computer coordinates help the physician guide the needle to a position posterior to the mass. Ultrasound may also be used to guide the needle and allows the physician to observe the biopsy procedure in "real time." Vacuum-assisted biopsy is a minimally invasive procedure that allows the removal of multiple larger tissue samples with a single insertion of the needle. A special biopsy probe and needle are used. The needle used in a vacuum-assisted biopsy is generally a larger gauge than the needles used for core biopsies and has a special cutting blade at the tip to make the needle easier to insert. The opening of the needle (aperture) is located along the side of the needle on the distal end. Using ultrasound guidance, the needle is inserted immediately posterior to the tumor. Once sampling is initiated, a vacuum pulls the tumor into the opening on the needle and a rotating cutting blade slices the tissue. The tissue sample is sent to a special chamber in the biopsy probe where it can be retrieved without removing the needle. This technique allows multiple tissue samples to be taken with minor rotations of the needle. It is also possible to completely remove smaller masses by taking multiple samples.

Figure 17-49   Suspicious microcalcifications (DCIS) and occult infiltrating ductal carcinoma.
A, Magnification mammogram image of pleomorphic (irregular shapes) suspicious microcalcifications identified on a screening mammogram in this asymptomatic young woman. No mass was visible on mammogram.
B, Ultrasound demonstration of echogenic microcalcification within a dilated duct *(arrows).* **C,** Ultrasound image of the same breast showing an unsuspected sonographic mass with suspicious features (note the mass is taller than wide, shows an irregular indistinct margin, and shows asymmetric posterior shadowing and heterogeneous echogenicity). Ultrasound-guided large-needle core biopsy-proved infiltrating malignancy. This altered the patient's management, requiring a mastectomy and axillary node dissection for staging.

Sentinel Node Biopsy.   Standard surgical therapy of breast cancer has, for many years, involved a full level I and at least a partial level II axillary lymph node dissection. This results in a small but significant rate of morbidity from lymphedema, nerve damage, or in severe cases loss of arm and shoulder function. An important step forward in surgical therapy for breast cancer involves sentinel node biopsy (SNB). In this procedure, the superficial subcutaneous tissues around the tumor bed and/or the areola are injected with methylene blue dye and/or radioactive-labeled solution (usually technetium-labeled filtered sulfur colloid). Both of these substances are taken up by the lymphatics and transported to the first, or "sentinel," lymph node along the axillary node chain. This lymph node is then identified in surgery and carefully analyzed for evidence of metastasis. This is generally followed by a limited axillary node dissection. Early experience with this procedure shows an excellent accuracy rate for detecting lymph node metastases and results in a reduced rate of morbidity and a faster recovery for the patient (Figure 17-50).

Figure 17-50   Injection of radiopharmaceutic agent around tumor for sentinel lymph node identification. Ultrasound image showing echogenic fluid *(arrow)* being injected in the superficial tissue around a mass *(arrowhead).* The needle is visible *(small arrow).* Injection of radioactive tracer in a saline solution can be done around the tumor, in the subcutaneous tissue over the tumor, and/or in the periareolar tissue. Over several hours, the radioactive tracer will move through the breast lymphatic system and into the first or "sentinel" lymph node, usually the lowest node in the level I axillary lymph node chain.

SELECTED BIBLIOGRAPHY

American Cancer Society: Breast cancer: detection and symptoms, revised 9/20/99. http://www3.cancer.org/cancerinfo/ load_cont.asp.

American College of Radiology: Breast imaging reporting and data system (BI-RADS™), ed 3, Reston, Va, 1998, American College of Radiology.

Andolina L and others: *Mammographic imaging: a practical guide,* ed 2, Philadelphia, 1999, Lippincott, Williams, & Wilkins.

Handel ER, Jackson VP: Sonographically guided interventional procedures. In Bassett LW, Jackson VP, editors: *Diagnosis of diseases of the breast,* Philadelphia, 1997, WB Saunders.

Harris JR, Lippman ME, Morrow M, and others. *Diseases of the breast,* ed 2, Philadelphia, 1999, Lippincott, Williams, & Wilkins.

Ikeda D: *Breast imaging: the requisites,* St Louis, 2004, Mosby.

Kopans DB: *Breast imaging,* ed 2, Philadelphia, 1998, Lippincott-Raven.

Lanfranchi ME: *Breast ultrasound,* London, 2000, Marban Publishers (out of print).

Nwariaku FE: Sentinel lymph node biopsy, an alternative to elective axillary dissection for breast cancer, *Am J Surg* 176:529, 1998.

Romrell LJ, Bland KI: Anatomy of the breast, axilla, chest wall, and related metastatic sites. In Bland KI, Copeland EM, editors: *The breast: comprehensive management of benign and malignant diseases,* Philadelphia, 1998, WB Saunders.

Seymour MT and others: Ultrasound assessment of residual abnormalities following primary chemotherapy for breast cancer, *Br J Cancer* 76(3):371, 1997.

Veronesi U and others: Sentinel lymph node biopsy and axillary dissection in breast cancer: results in a large series, *J Natl Cancer Inst* 91:368, 1999.

Wilhelm MC, Langenburg SE, Wanebo HJ: Cancer of the male breast. In Bland KI, Copeland EM, editors: *The breast: comprehensive management of benign and malignant diseases,* Philadelphia, 1998, WB Saunders.

CHAPTER 18

The Thyroid and Parathyroid Glands

Sandra L. Hagen-Ansert

KEY TERMS

adenoma – benign thyroid neoplasm characterized by complete fibrous encapsulation

adenopathy – enlargement of the lymph nodes

anaplastic carcinoma – rare, undifferentiated carcinoma occurring in middle age

branchial cleft cyst – remnant of embryonic development that appears as a cyst in the neck

calcitonin – a thyroid hormone that is important for maintaining a dense, strong bone matrix and regulating the blood calcium level

cystic hygroma – cystic neck mass caused by malformations of the cervical thoracic lymphatic system

de Quervain's thyroiditis – viral infection of the thyroid that causes inflammation

diffuse nontoxic goiter (colloid goiter) – occurs as a compensatory enlargement of the thyroid gland resulting from thyroid hormone deficiency

euthyroid – refers to a normal functioning thyroid gland

fine-needle aspiration – invasive procedure used to obtain a small specimen from a specific lesion

follicular carcinoma – occurs as a solitary malignant mass within the thyroid gland

goiter – enlargement of the thyroid gland that can be focal or diffuse; multiple nodules may be present

Graves' disease – autoimmune disorder of diffuse toxic goiter characterized by bulging eyes (exophthalmos)

Hashimoto's thyroiditis – chronic inflammation of the thyroid gland caused by the formation of antibodies against normal thyroid tissue

hyperparathyroidism – disorder associated with elevated serum calcium level, usually caused by a benign parathyroid adenoma

hyperthyroidism – oversecretion of thyroid hormones

hypophosphatasia – low phosphatase level, which can be seen with hyperparathyroidism

hypothyroidism – underactive thyroid hormones

isthmus – small piece of thyroid tissue that connects the right and left lobes of the gland

longus colli muscle – wedge-shaped muscle posterior to the thyroid lobes

medullary carcinoma – neoplastic growth that accounts for 10% of thyroid malignancies

microcalcifications – tiny echogenic foci within a nodule that may or may not shadow

multinodular goiter – nodular enlargement of the thyroid associated with hyperthyroidism

nodular hyperplasia – degenerative nodules within the thyroid

papillary carcinoma – most common form of thyroid malignancy

parathyroid hormone (PTH) – a hormone that is secreted by parathyroid glands, which regulate serum calcium levels

parathyroid hyperplasia – enlargement of multiple parathyroid glands

primary hyperparathyroidism – oversecretion of parathyroid hormone, usually from a parathyroid adenoma

pyramidal lobe – present in small percentage of patients; extends superiorly from the isthmus

secondary hyperparathyroidism – enlargement of parathyroid glands in patients with renal failure or vitamin D deficiency

serum calcium – laboratory value that is elevated with hyperparathyroidism

sternocleidomastoid muscles – large muscles anterolateral to the thyroid

strap muscles – group of three muscles (sternothyroid, sternohyoid, and omohyoid) that lie anterior to the thyroid

thyroglossal duct cysts – congenital anomalies that present in midline of the neck anterior to the trachea

thyroiditis – inflammation of the thyroid

thyroid-stimulating hormone (TSH) – a hormone secreted by the pituitary gland that stimulates the thyroid gland to secrete thyroxine and triiodothyronine

---

The thyroid gland is the part of the endocrine system that maintains body metabolism, growth, and development through the synthesis, storage, and secretion of thyroid hormones. These hormones include triiodothyronine (T_3), thyroxine (T_4), and calcitonin. Disorders of the thyroid may result from pituitary or thyroid gland dysfunction.

Unless the thyroid gland is enlarged, it is not easily palpated by physical examination. A general enlargement of the gland is called a **goiter** with obvious swelling in the neck area. A localized enlargement is a nodular goiter. Both deficient and excessive secretion may cause enlargement.

High-resolution ultrasound is used to evaluate the thyroid gland as it lies superficially within the neck. The examination is easy to perform and well tolerated by patients. Ultrasound of the thyroid is used to define the texture of a palpable lesion (i.e., solid or cystic, complex or calcified) and to determine if the lesion is single or multiple. The size and location of the nodule and the evaluation of the adjacent lymph node adenopathy may be imaged with ultrasound. Ultrasound is used to define the anatomic structures within and surrounding the thyroid gland rather than to determine the physiology of the gland. The functional state is better determined by nuclear scintigraphy and laboratory measurements of the thyroid hormone present in the blood. Interventional procedures under ultrasound guidance, including **fine-needle aspiration** and alcohol ablation of parathyroid adenomas, is an important application of ultrasound. The evaluation of the parathyroid gland and other lesions of the neck will also be presented in this chapter.

ANATOMY OF THE THYROID GLAND

The thyroid is located in the anterior neck at the level of the thyroid cartilage. The thyroid gland consists of right and left lobes in the lower neck. These two lobes are connected across the midline by the thin bridge of thyroid tissue called the **isthmus**. The thyroid straddles the trachea anteriorly, whereas the paired lobes extend on either side of the trachea, bounded laterally by the carotid arteries and jugular veins (Figure 18-1). When present, the **pyramidal lobe** arises from the isthmus and tapers superiorly just anterior to the thyroid cartilage.

SIZE

The size and shape of the thyroid gland varies with gender, age, and body surface area, with females having a slightly larger gland than males (Table 18-1). In tall individuals, the lateral lobes of the thyroid have a longitudinally elongated shape on sagittal scans, whereas in shorter individuals the gland is more oval. As a result, the normal dimensions of the gland have a wide range of variability. The lobes are normally equal in size. In the newborn, the gland measures 18 to 20 mm long, with an anteroposterior (AP) diameter of 8 to 9 mm. By age 1, the mean length is 25 mm and the AP diameter is 12 to 15 mm. The normal adult thyroid measures 40 to 60 mm in length, 20 to 30 mm in AP diameter, and 15 to 20 mm in width. The isthmus is the smallest part of the gland and has a 2 to 6 mm AP diameter. A pyramidal lobe that extends superiorly from the isthmus is present in 15% to 30% of patients.

RELATIONAL ANATOMY

Anterior. Along the anterior surface of the thyroid gland lie the **strap muscles,** including the sternothyroid, omohyoid, sternohyoid, and **sternocleidomastoid muscles** (Figure 18-2). The sternohyoid and omohyoid muscles are seen on ultrasound as thin, hypoechoic bands anterior to the gland. The

TABLE 18-1	**SIZE OF THE THYROID**	
Dimension	Adults	Children
Length	40-60 mm	20-30 mm
Anteroposterior	20-30 mm	12-15 mm
Width	15-20 mm	10-15 mm

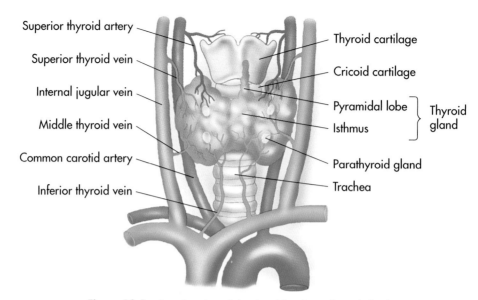

Superior thyroid artery

Superior thyroid vein

Internal jugular vein

Middle thyroid vein

Common carotid artery

Inferior thyroid vein

Thyroid cartilage

Cricoid cartilage

Pyramidal lobe ⎫ Thyroid

Isthmus ⎭ gland

Parathyroid gland

Trachea

Figure 18-1   Anterior view of the thyroid and parathyroid glands.

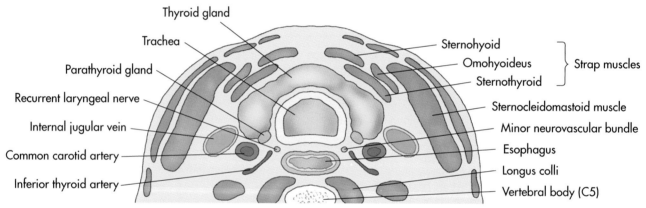

Thyroid gland

Trachea

Parathyroid gland

Recurrent laryngeal nerve

Internal jugular vein

Common carotid artery

Inferior thyroid artery

Sternohyoid

Omohyoideus ⎫ Strap muscles

Sternothyroid ⎭

Sternocleidomastoid muscle

Minor neurovascular bundle

Esophagus

Longus colli

Vertebral body (C5)

Figure 18-2   Cross-section of the thyroid region showing the thyroid gland, vascular, and muscular relationships to one another.

sternocleidomastoid muscle is seen as a larger oval band that lies anterior and lateral to the gland.

Posterior. Posterolateral anatomy includes the carotid sheath with the common carotid artery, internal jugular vein, and vagus nerve. The **longus colli muscle** is posterior and lateral to each thyroid lobe and appears as a hypoechoic triangular structure adjacent to the cervical vertebrae (see Figure 18-2).

Medial. Medial anatomy consists of the larynx, trachea, inferior constrictor of the pharynx, and esophagus. The esophagus, primarily a midline structure, may be found to the left of the trachea (see Figure 18-2). It is identified by the target appearance in the transverse plane and by its peristaltic movements when the patient swallows. The posterior border of each thyroid lobe is related to the superior and inferior parathyroid glands and the anastomosis between the superior and inferior thyroid arteries.

BLOOD SUPPLY

Blood is supplied to the thyroid by four arteries. Two superior thyroid arteries arise from the external carotids and descend to the upper poles. Two inferior thyroid arteries come from the thyrocervical trunk of the subclavian artery and ascend to the lower poles. Doppler peak systolic velocities reach 20 to 40 cm/sec in the major thyroid arteries and 15 to 30 cm/sec in the intraparenchymal arteries. Corresponding veins drain into the internal jugular veins (see Figure 18-1).

THYROID PHYSIOLOGY AND LABORATORY DATA

As part of the endocrine system, the role of the thyroid is to maintain normal body metabolism, growth, and development by the synthesis, storage, and secretion of thyroid hormones. The mechanism for producing thyroid hormones is iodine metabolism. The thyroid gland traps iodine from the blood and, through a series of chemical reactions, produces the thyroid hormones triiodothyronine (T3) and thyroxine (T4). These are stored in the colloid of the gland. When thyroid hormone is needed by the body, it is released into the bloodstream by the action of thyrotropin, or **thyroid-stimulating hormone (TSH),** which is produced by the pituitary gland.

The secretion of TSH is regulated by thyrotropin-releasing factor, which is produced by the hypothalamus (located in the brain). The level of thyrotropin-releasing factor is controlled by the basal metabolic rate. A decrease in the basal metabolic rate, a result of a low concentration of thyroid hormones, causes an increase in thyrotropin-releasing factor. This causes increased secretion of TSH and a subsequent increase in the release of thyroid hormones. When the blood level of hormones is returned to normal, the basal metabolic rate returns to normal and TSH secretion stops.

Calcitonin decreases the concentration of calcium in the blood by first acting on bone to inhibit its breakdown. With less bone being resorbed, less calcium moves out of bone into blood, decreasing the concentration of calcium in the blood. Calcitonin secretion increases after any concentration of blood calcium increase. Thus calcitonin helps to maintain homeostasis of blood calcium. It helps prevent an excess of calcium in the blood (hypercalcemia) from occurring.

EUTHYROID, HYPOTHYROIDISM, AND HYPERTHYROIDISM

Euthyroid. When the thyroid is producing the right amount of thyroid hormone, it is considered to be normal, or **euthyroid.** Abnormal secretions of the thyroid hormone may result in hypothyroidism (undersecretion) or **hyperthyroidism** (oversecretion).

Hypothyroidism. The undersecretion of thyroid hormones is **hypothyroidism.** This condition may be caused by low intake of iodine (goiter) in the body, inability of the thyroid to produce the proper amount of thyroid hormone, or a problem in the pituitary gland that does not control the thyroid production.

Clinical signs and symptoms of hypothyroidism include myxedema, weight gain, hair loss, increased subcutaneous tissue around the eyes, lethargy, intellectual and motor slowing, cold intolerance, constipation, or a deep husky voice. Treatment with thyroid hormone can reverse the condition.

Hyperthyroidism. The oversecretion of thyroid hormones is **hyperthyroidism** (Box 18-1). This occurs when the entire gland is out of control or if a localized neoplasm (such as an adenoma) causes overproduction of the thyroid hormone.

Hyperthyroidism dramatically increases the metabolic rate; clinical signs include weight loss, increased appetite, high degree of nervous energy, tremor, excessive sweating, heat intolerance, and palpitations, and many patients show signs of exophthalmos (protruding eyes).

TESTS OF THYROID FUNCTION

Nuclear medicine is used to determine the function of the thyroid. A small amount of radioactive iodine is injected into

---

BOX 18-1　COMMON DISORDERS ASSOCIATED WITH HYPERTHYROIDISM (ACCOUNTS FOR 99% OF CASES)

DIFFUSE TOXIC HYPERPLASIA (GRAVES' DISEASE)
Toxic multinodular goiter
Toxic adenoma

UNCOMMON
Acute or subacute thyroiditis
Hyperfunctioning thyroid cancer
Choriocarcinoma or hydatidiform mole
TSH-secreting pituitary adenoma
Neonatal thyrotoxicosis associated with maternal Graves'
　disease

---

the bloodstream. In normal individuals, a certain percent of the amount injected will be taken into the thyroid gland within 24 hours. In patients with hyperthyroidism, a greater percent is taken up; in patients with hypothyroidism, a smaller percent is taken up. The amount taken up by the thyroid is determined by measuring the radioactivity accumulated in the gland with a gamma camera.

The laboratory tests for thyroid can measure the amount of T3 or T4 in the blood. This amount is elevated in patients with hyperthyroidism and decreased in patients with hypothyroidism.

SONOGRAPHIC EVALUATION OF THE THYROID

The sonographer should obtain a patient history before the ultrasound examination. Pertinent information regarding the patient's general health, thyroid medications, previous imaging studies (i.e., scintigraphy), family history of hyperparathyroidism or thyroid cancer, or prior history of radiation or surgery to the neck should be noted in the examination record.

The patient is placed in the supine position with a pillow under both shoulders to provide a moderate hyperextension of the neck. This position allows the lower lobes of the gland to be more readily visualized with ultrasound.

A high-resolution linear 7.5- to 10-MHz (or higher) transducer should be used. Each lobe requires careful scanning in both the longitudinal and transverse planes. The lateral, mid, and medial parts of each lobe are examined in the longitudinal plane (Figure 18-3) and so labeled.

The superior, mid, and inferior portions of each gland are examined individually and labeled in the transverse plane (Figure 18-4). If possible, the patient's head should be turned to the opposite side to enable better visualization of each lobe. Having the patient swallow allows visualization of the lower pole of the thyroid gland. Swallowing raises the entire gland and brings the lower pole into the field of view.

Landmarks for the transverse image include the common carotid artery, the trachea, and the jugular vein (Figure 18-5). The common carotid artery is a circular, pulsatile structure

Figure 18-3　Longitudinal images of the normal thyroid gland. **A,** Long, lateral. *C,* Carotid; *T,* thyroid. **B,** Long, mid. Measurement of the length and AP dimension of the gland. **C,** Long, medial. *T,* Thyroid.

directly adjacent to the gland. The oval-shaped jugular vein is lateral to the carotid artery. The trachea is noted in the middle of the neck with posterior shadowing.

Transverse and longitudinal images of the isthmus must also be obtained (Figure 18-6). The examination should also extend laterally to include the region of the carotid artery and jugular vein to identify enlarged cervical lymph nodes.

The normal thyroid gland has a fine homogeneous echotexture that is more echogenic than the surrounding muscle structure. The vascular structures may be seen as tubular anechoic structures within the gland. Color Doppler with a low pulse repetition frequency (PRF) will distinguish these structures as blood-filled. The muscles surrounding the gland (infrahyoid, sternocleidomastoid, and longus colli) are hypoechoic compared with the thyroid tissue. The esophagus may be seen to the left of the midline, next to the trachea, with a hypoechoic rim surrounding an echogenic center.

If an abnormality is encountered, all sonographic characteristics (i.e., cystic areas, calcification, or a halo) should be demonstrated. It is not uncommon for sonography to demonstrate multiple nodules in a gland previously suspected of having only a solitary lesion.

PATHOLOGY OF THE THYROID GLAND

The most common cause of thyroid disorders worldwide is iodine deficiency, leading to goiter formation and hypothyroidism. In areas not deficient in iodine, autoimmune processes are believed to be the basis for most cases of thyroid disease, which ranges from hyperthyroidism to hypothyroidism. Enlargement of the thyroid gland is termed goiter. See Table 18-2 for clinical findings, sonographic findings, and differential considerations.

NODULAR THYROID DISEASE

Goiter is an enlargement of the thyroid gland, which is often visible on the anterior neck. The enlargement is due to compensatory hypertrophy and hyperplasia of the follicular epithelium caused by a derangement that hampers hormone secretion. A goiter may become very large, compressing the esophagus and interfering with swallowing, or it can cause pressure on the trachea. Other causes of goiter include Graves' disease, thyroiditis, neoplasm, or a cyst.

Endemic goiter may affect large groups of people in a specific geographic area. This usually occurs in areas where there

C

Figure 18-4 Transverse images of the normal thyroid gland. **A,** Trans, superior. *O,* Omohyoid muscle; *S,* sternohyoid muscle; *SC,* sternocleidomastoid. **B,** Trans, mid. Measurement of the width of the gland. **C,** Trans, inferior.

Figure 18-5 Normal image of both lobes of the thyroid are made to show the comparable homogeneity of each lobe. *C,* Carotid; *T,* thyroid; *is,* isthmus; *Tr,* trachea.

Figure 18-6 The isthmus *(arrows)* is shown in the transverse view at the inferior border of the thyroid gland.

are low iodine levels in the soil and food (e.g., mountainous areas or around the Great Lakes). Normally the iodine is trapped by the thyroid gland and used to synthesize the T3 and T4 hormones. This dietary deficiency leads to low T3 and T4 production and a compensatory increase in thyroid-

stimulating hormone (TSH) from the pituitary, producing hyperplasia and hypertrophy in the thyroid gland. For the most part, the use of ionized salt has solved this problem.

There are certain types of foods that may block the synthesis of T3 and T4 but increase the TSH secretion. Thus TSH

TABLE 18-2   THYROID FINDINGS: NODULAR THYROID DISEASE

Clinical Findings	Sonographic Findings	Differential Considerations
Nontoxic Simple Goiter		
Thyroid enlargement Hypothyroidism	Sometimes smooth, sometimes nodular; possible compression of surrounding structures	Thyroiditis Neoplasm
Toxic Multinodular Goiter		
Thyroid enlargement	Enlarged inhomogeneous gland; can have focal scarring, focal ischemia, necrosis, and cyst formation	Neoplasm Cyst
Graves' Disease		
Diffuse toxic goiter Ophthalmopathy Cutaneous manifestations Hyperthyroidism	Diffusely homogeneous and enlarged	Neoplasm
Thyroiditis		
Swelling and tenderness of the thyroid; later, hypothyroidism	Homogeneous enlargement with nodularity; later, inhomogeneous enlargement	Neoplasm
Benign Lesions		
Cysts		
Solitary nodules or multiple nodules	Anechoic areas, echogenic fluid, or moving fluid levels	Toxic multinodular goiter
Adenoma		
Usually euthyroid or hyperthyroid	Compression of adjacent structures; fibrous encapsulation; range from anechoic to hyperechoic; may have halo	Graves' disease

causes hyperplasia of the gland and can promote goiter formation when such food (i.e., cabbage, turnips, and other related vegetables) is ingested in large quantities.

A toxic goiter is a hyperthyroid condition resulting from hyperactivity of the thyroid gland, perhaps caused by excessive stimulation from TSH, which produces a large nodular gland.

Nodular hyperplasia, multinodular goiter, and **adenomatous hyperplasia** are some of the terms used to describe goiter, which is the most common thyroid abnormality. Goiters can be diffuse and symmetric or irregular and nodular. Goiters may result from hyperplasia, neoplasia, or an inflammatory process. Normal thyroid function, hyperfunction, or hypofunction can also cause enlargement of the gland.

Sonographic Findings. Sonography shows that the goitrous gland is usually enlarged, nodular, and sometimes heterogeneous. Sonography can be helpful in the evaluation of nodular thyroid disease to determine the location and characterization of palpable neck masses.

Nontoxic (Simple) Goiter. Nontoxic (simple) goiter occurs as a diffuse thyroid enlargement not resulting from a neoplasm or inflammation. It is not initially associated with hypothyroidism or hyperthyroidism. The goiter is formed when the gland is unable to provide an adequate supply of thyroid hormone. This deficiency may be the result of iodine shortage (dietary) or malfunction of the gland itself. The gland

becomes diffusely and uniformly enlarged in an attempt to trap and use every atom of iodine. Often the gland is able to keep up with the demand and provides normal release of hormones. However, in some cases the gland lags behind the demand and the patient develops hypothyroidism. In the first stage, hyperplasia occurs; in the second stage, colloid involution occurs. Progression of this process leads to an asymmetric and multinodular gland with hemorrhage and calcification (Figure 18-7). Laboratory data reveal evidence of hypothyroidism.

Sonographic Findings. Clinical findings show enlargement of the thyroid gland, sometimes smooth, sometimes nodular; one side may enlarge more than the other. Compression of the surrounding structures may be noted on ultrasound.

Toxic Multinodular Goiter. Multinodular goiter (adenomatous hyperplasia) is one of the most common forms of thyroid disease. Approximately 80% of nodular thyroid disease is caused by hyperplasia of the gland. It occurs in up to 5% of any population. Nodularity of the gland can be the end stage of **diffuse nontoxic goiter (colloid goiter).** Although some cases of multinodular goiter arise spontaneously, many are believed to begin as nontoxic goiters that have overtaken the gland.

Sonographic Findings. Ultrasound examination shows an enlarged, inhomogeneous gland. As the disease progresses, areas of focal scarring and ischemia, as well as necrosis and cyst formation, may appear within the gland (Figure 18-8).

Fibrosis or calcifications may also manifest. Some of the nodules are poorly circumscribed; others appear to be encapsulated (Figure 18-9). Enlargement can involve one lobe to a greater extent than the other and sometimes causes difficulty in breathing and swallowing (Figure 18-10).

Figure 18-7 The heterogeneous appearance is well seen within the adenoma with well-defined, discrete borders. The hypoechoic halo is shown surrounding the lesion *(arrows)*.

Figure 18-8 Increased vascularity is shown on the left image in a patient with a multinodular goiter (shown with arrows on the right).

Lesions in a multinodular goiter have many sonographic features of true adenomas. The multiple nodules of adenomatous hyperplasia may demonstrate halos and may have clear or nondiscrete borders (Figure 18-11). The solid portion of the lesions may have the same echo texture as the normal thyroid tissue. Calcifications and cystic areas may be present within the nodules.

Graves' Disease. Graves' disease occurs more frequently in women over 30 years of age and is related to an autoimmune disorder. It is characterized by thyrotoxicosis and is the most frequent cause of hyperthyroidism. Graves' disease is characterized by a triad of the following findings: hypermetabolism, diffuse toxic goiter, exophthalmos (inflammatory infiltration of the orbital tissue resulting in proptosis, or bulging of the eyes), and cutaneous manifestations (thickening of the dermis of the pretibial areas and the dorsum of the feet). Hyperthyroidism associated with a diffuse hyperplastic goiter is present (Figure 18-12). Clinically the thyroid gland is diffusely homogeneous and enlarged.

The exophthalmos is characterized by the presence of protruding, staring eyes with decreased movements. This results from increased tissue mass in the orbit pushing the eyeball forward and from increased sympathetic stimulation affecting the eyelids.

Thyrotoxic crisis, or thyroid storm, is an acute situation in a patient with uncontrolled hyperthyroidism, usually precipitated by infection or surgery. It may be life threatening because of resulting hyperthermia, tachycardia, heart failure, and delirium.

Sonographic Findings. On ultrasound examination, the gland appears hypoechoic with diffuse enlargement without palpable nodules. The overactivity of Graves' disease is manifested sonographically by increased vascularity on color Doppler imaging leading to the term "thyroid inferno" (Figure 18-13).

Thyroiditis. Swelling and tenderness of the thyroid is called **thyroiditis.** Thyroiditis is caused by infection or can be related to autoimmune abnormalities. There are two types of thyroiditis: de Quervain's and Hashimoto's.

Figure 18-9 **A,** A patient with an asymmetric, multinodular goiter on the right shows a complex sonographic pattern. The left lobe is normal. **B,** Increased vascularity is seen surrounding the heterogeneous lesion.

Figure 18-10   Multinodular goiter shows inhomogeneous pattern. Right lobe is more than twice the size of the left lobe.

Figure 18-11   Gross pathology of a nodular goiter. The thyroid is enlarged with nodules that vary in size and shape. (From Damjanov I, Linder J: *Pathology: a color atlas,* St Louis, 2000, Mosby.)

Figure 18-12   Gross pathology of a patient with Graves' disease shows symmetrical enlargement of the thyroid gland. (From Damjanov I, Linder J: *Pathology: a color atlas,* St Louis, 2000, Mosby.)

de Quervain's thyroiditis is probably caused by a viral infection of the thyroid, which results in diffuse inflammation of the thyroid with enlargement and tenderness. The disease has a gradual or fairly abrupt onset, and the pain may be severe. de Quervain's thyroiditis may cause transient hyperthyroidism, but in a period of weeks or months the swelling and pain subside and the gland functions normally.

Hashimoto's thyroiditis is the most common form of thyroiditis characterized by a destructive autoimmune disorder, which leads to chronic inflammation of the thyroid. The outstanding feature is a painless, diffusely enlarged gland in a young or middle-aged female. The entire gland is involved with an inflammatory reaction; enlargement is not necessarily symmetric (Figure 18-14). Homogeneous enlargement initially occurs with nodularity; as the disease progresses, the gland shows inhomogeneous enlargement. Mild to moderate tenderness is present. Eventually, the gland becomes severely damaged with resultant hypothyroidism.

Sonographic Findings. The gland may appear hypoechoic compared with a normal thyroid texture. The texture is coarse and homogeneous. Multiple ill-defined hypoechoic areas separated by thickened fibrous strands are noted. Discrete thyroid nodules are less commonly seen. Color Doppler shows increased vascularity. Over time, the gland becomes fibrotic, ill-defined, and heterogeneous. There is an increased risk for malignant disease associated with Hashimoto's disease.

BENIGN LESIONS

A discrete nodule of the thyroid gland is the most common reason for an ultrasound examination. Nodular thyroid disease is frequently encountered in the adult population, with up to 7% found to have a benign nodule, with women more frequently affected than men. Nodules can be imaged with ultrasound and described to help determine whether the nodule is benign or malignant. Confirmation of the complex or solid lesion may be made through fine-needle biopsy.

Cysts. Cysts are thought to represent cystic degeneration of a follicular adenoma.

Figure 18-13   Increased color Doppler indicates increased vascularity in the thyroid gland in a patient with Graves' disease.

Figure 18-14 Gross pathology of a patient with Hashimoto's thyroiditis. The enlarged gland is multinodular with multiple lymphoid infiltrates. (From Damjanov I, Linder J: *Pathology: a color atlas*, St Louis, 2000, Mosby.)

Figure 18-15 A large, anechoic cyst *(cy)* is seen to displace the normal thyroid gland.

Sonographic Findings. The degenerative changes of nodules correspond to their sonographic appearance. Purely anechoic areas result from serous or colloid fluid, echogenic fluid, or moving fluid; fluid levels correspond to hemorrhage. Approximately 20% of solitary nodules are cystic. Blood or debris may be present within them (Figure 18-15). As with all simple cysts, the sonographic appearance of a simple thyroid cyst must be anechoic and have sharp, well-defined walls and distal acoustic enhancement.

Adenoma. An **adenoma** is a benign thyroid neoplasm characterized by complete fibrous encapsulation. Adenomas represent only 5% to 10% of all nodular disease of the thyroid and are seven times more common in females than in males. The benign follicular adenoma is a true thyroid neoplasm that is characterized by compression of adjacent tissue and fibrous encapsulation (Figure 18-16).

Adenomas are homogeneous with variable size. Usually the lesion is solitary with areas of hemorrhage or necrosis. The adenoma is slow growing unless hemorrhage occurs, which causes sudden and painful enlargement. Most patients are euthyroid or hyperthyroid. Some nodules produce a thyroid hormone; if they do, they may or may not be controlled by the usual hormonal controls.

Figure 18-16 Gross pathology of follicular adenoma. The nodule is well circumscribed with a fibrous capsule separating it from the normal parenchyma. (From Damjanov I, Linder J: *Pathology: a color atlas*, St Louis, 2000, Mosby.)

Sonographic Findings. Adenomas have a broad spectrum of ultrasound appearances. They range from anechoic to completely hyperechoic and commonly have a peripheral halo. The halo, or thin echolucent rim surrounding the lesion, may represent edema of the compressed normal thyroid tissue or the capsule of the adenoma (Figure 18-17). In a few instances, blood may surround the lesion. Although the halo is a relatively consistent finding in adenomas, additional statistical information is necessary to establish its specificity. Hyperfunction of the adenoma can exhibit increased blood flow patterns as seen on Doppler along the peripheral borders or within the lesion.

Adenomas that contain anechoic areas are a result of cystic degeneration (probably from hemorrhage) and usually lack a well-rounded margin. This lack of a discrete cystic margin is helpful in differentiation from a simple cyst. Calcification along the rim can also be associated with adenomas. Its acoustic shadow may preclude visualization posteriorly. Color Doppler has not been found to add specific additional information to the examination in an effort to separate a benign from a malignant process.

MALIGNANT LESIONS

Carcinoma of the thyroid is rare. A solitary nodule may be malignant in a small percentage of cases, but the risk of malignancy decreases with the presence of multiple nodules. A solitary thyroid nodule in the presence of cervical adenopathy on the same side suggests malignancy.

Sonographic Findings. The ultrasound appearance of thyroid cancer is highly variable. The neoplasm can be of any size, single or multiple, and can appear as a solid, partially cystic, or largely cystic mass. Occasionally, thyroid cancer presents as a small, solid nodule. Thyroid cancer is usually hypoechoic relative to normal thyroid, but thyroid carcinomas with the same echo texture as normal thyroid have been reported.

Figure 18-17   Sonographic variations of adenomas. **A,** A well-defined adenoma with a hypoechoic halo is seen on the right lobe. **B,** Thyroid adenoma demonstrating a halo. **C,** Large calcification within a thyroid adenoma *(black arrow).* Shadowing from the calcification *(white arrows).* **D,** Large, echogenic mass within the hemorrhagic adenoma *(arrows).*

Calcifications are present in 50% to 80% of all types of thyroid carcinoma. Increased vascularity may be present.

Papillary Carcinoma. The most common of the thyroid malignancies is called **paillary carcinoma** and is the predominant cause of thyroid cancer in children. Females are affected more often than males. Round, laminated calcifications are seen in 25% of the cases (Figure 18-18). The major route of spread of papillary carcinoma is through the lymphatics to the nearby cervical lymph nodes. Approximately 20% of patients with papillary thyroid cancer have metastatic cervical adenopathy.

Sonographic Findings. Sonographic characteristics of papillary carcinoma include hypoechogenicity (90% of cases), **microcalcifications** that appear as tiny, punctate hyperechoic foci (with or without acoustic shadowing), hypervascularity (90% of cases), and cervical lymph node metastasis (in approximately 20% of cases) (Figure 18-19).

Follicular Carcinoma. Follicular **carcinoma** of the thyroid is usually a solitary mass of the thyroid. This type of thyroid cancer is more aggressive than papillary cancer (Figure 18-20).

Sonographic Findings. An irregular, firm, nodular enlargement is characteristic.

Medullary Carcinoma. Medullary **carcinoma** accounts for 10% of thyroid cancers. It presents as a hard, bulky mass that causes enlargement of a small portion of the gland and can involve the entire gland (Figure 18-21).

Sonographic Findings. In patients with medullary thyroid carcinoma, thyroid lesions appear as punctuated, bright, echogenic foci within solid masses (Figure 18-22). These correspond pathologically to deposits of calcium surrounded by amyloid. Ultrasound is highly sensitive in detecting metastatic lymphadenopathy in these patients; thus careful evaluation of the entire neck area surrounding the thyroid is important.

Anaplastic Carcinoma. Anaplastic carcinoma (*anaplastic* means undifferentiated) is rare and accounts for less than 10% of thyroid cancers. It usually occurs after age 50. This lesion presents as a hard, fixed mass with rapid growth. Its growth is

Figure 18-18   Gross pathology of papillary carcinoma. Large solid tumor mass nearly replaced one lobe of the thyroid gland. (From Damjanov I, Linder J: *Pathology: a color atlas,* St Louis, 2000, Mosby.)

Figure 18-19   Solitary lesion representing a papillary carcinoma upon biopsy *(arrows).*

locally invasive in surrounding neck structures, and it usually causes death by compression and asphyxiation because of invasion of the trachea.

Sonographic Findings. The sonographic appearance of this type of thyroid cancer is as a hypoechoic mass, with invasion of the surrounding muscles and vessels of the neck.

Lymphoma. Lymphoma in the thyroid is primarily the non-Hodgkin's type. The tumor affects older females and accounts for 4% of all thyroid malignancies. Clinically the patient has a rapidly growing mass in the neck area. In many cases of lymphoma, the patient has a preexisting chronic lymphocytic thyroiditis (Hashimoto's disease).

Figure 18-20   Gross pathology of follicular carcinoma shows a well-circumscribed tumor. (From Damjanov I, Linder J: *Pathology: a color atlas,* St Louis, 2000, Mosby.)

Figure 18-21   Gross pathology of medullary carcinoma shows a well-defined mass in the thyroid gland. (From Damjanov I, Linder J: *Pathology: a color atlas,* St Louis, 2000, Mosby.)

Figure 18-22   Arrows indicate a medullary carcinoma causing enlargement of the inferior pole of the right thyroid gland. *IP,* inferior pole; *SP,* superior pole.

Sonographic Findings. The sonographic appearance of lymphoma is characterized by a nonvascular hypoechoic and lobulated mass. There may be large areas of cystic necrosis within the tumor. The adjacent thyroid parenchyma may be heterogeneous secondary to associated chronic thyroiditis.

ANATOMY OF THE PARATHYROID GLAND

The parathyroid glands are normally located on the posterior medial surface of the thyroid gland. Most people have four parathyroid glands, but to have three to five parathyroid glands is not uncommon. Parathyroid glands have been found in different places, such as in the neck and mediastinum. The four parathyroid glands are paired. Two lie posterior to each superior pole of the thyroid, and the other two lie posterior to the inferior pole (see Figure 18-1).

Each gland is flat and disc shaped. The echo texture is similar to that of the overlying thyroid gland. For this reason, normal-size glands (less than 4 mm) are usually not seen by ultrasound, but occasionally a single gland may be imaged and appear as a flat hypoechoic structure posterior and adjacent to the thyroid. Enlarged glands (greater than 5 mm) have a decreased echo texture and appear sonographically as elongated masses between the posterior longus coli and the anterior thyroid lobe.

PARATHYROID PHYSIOLOGY AND LABORATORY DATA

The parathyroid glands are the calcium-sensing organs in the body. They produce **parathyroid hormone (PTH)** and monitor the **serum calcium** feedback mechanism. The stimulus to PTH secretion is a decrease in the level of blood calcium. When the serum calcium level decreases, the parathyroid glands are stimulated to release PTH. When the serum calcium level increases, parathyroid activity decreases. PTH acts on bone, kidney, and intestine to enhance calcium absorption. Patients with unexplained hypercalcemia detected on routine blood chemistry screening are the most common referrals for parathyroid echography. Symptomatic renal stones, ulcers, and bone pain are other indications.

SONOGRAPHIC EVALUATION OF THE PARATHYROID GLAND

For successful sonographic detection of parathyroid abnormalities, a high-resolution (7.5- to 15-MHz) transducer must be used. The patient is placed supine with the neck slightly hyperextended. From the upper neck, just under the jaw, to the sternal notch, transverse and longitudinal planes must be examined and the observations recorded. To detect any inferiorly located parathyroid glands, the patient is asked to swallow to elevate the thyroid gland during real-time scanning. Normal parathyroid glands are seldom identified.

Under normal circumstances it is not common to be able to visualize the parathyroid glands because they are closely attached to or embedded in the thyroid glands and therefore

Figure 18-23 Parathyroid hyperplasia shows enlargement of all four parathyroid glands. (From Damjanov I, Linder J: *Pathology: a color atlas,* St Louis, 2000, Mosby.)

lack acoustical differences. This anatomic relationship, coupled with the small size of the parathyroid glands, makes visualization a challenge. However, with high-resolution technology and 3-D and harmonic imaging, visualization of the parathyroid glands is not as difficult as it once was.

In many cases a prominent **longus colli muscle** (Figure 18-23) appears as a discrete area posterior to the thyroid; it is important not to confuse this normal anatomy with a mass. Longitudinal sections can usually solve the problem. A linear appearance of the muscle is evident in this plane. The minor neurovascular bundle, consisting of the inferior thyroid artery and recurrent laryngeal nerve, may also be a source of confusion. Longitudinal scans can often eliminate this confusion by identifying the bundle's tubular appearance.

PATHOLOGY OF THE PARATHYROID GLAND

PRIMARY HYPERPARATHYROIDISM

Primary hyperparathyroidism is a state of increased function of the parathyroid glands. Women have primary hyperparathyroidism two to three times more frequently than men; it is particularly common after menopause. Primary hyperparathyroidism is characterized by hypercalcemia, hypercalciuria, and low serum levels of phosphate (**hypophosphatasia**).

Most patients are asymptomatic at the time of diagnosis and have no manifestations of **hyperparathyroidism,** such as nephrolithiasis and osteopenia. Primary hyperparathyroidism occurs when increased amounts of PTH are produced by an adenoma, primary hyperplasia, or rarely carcinoma located in the parathyroid gland.

Primary Hyperplasia. Of the patients with hyperparathyroidism, approximately 10% have **parathyroid hyperplasia.** Primary hyperplasia is defined as hyperfunction of all parathyroid glands with no apparent cause. Only one gland may significantly enlarge, with the remaining glands only mildly affected, or all glands may be enlarged (Figure 18-23). In any case, they rarely reach more than 1 cm in size.

Pitfalls to be aware of in diagnosing parathyroid enlargement include recognition of normal cervical structures (veins, arteries, esophagus, muscles), which can simulate adenomas and produce false-positive results.

Adenoma. Adenoma is the most common cause of primary hyperparathyroidism (80% of cases). A solitary adenoma may involve any one of the four glands with equal frequency. Adenomas are benign and are usually less than 3 cm. The most common shape of a parathyroid adenoma is oval (Figure 18-24). *Sonographic Findings.* Parathyroid adenomas are hypoechoic (Figure 18-25), and the vast majority are solid. Superior parathyroid adenomas are located adjacent to the posterior aspect of the mid portion of the thyroid. The location of inferior thyroid adenomas is more variable, but they may be found close to the caudal tip of the lower pole of the thyroid. The parathyroid gland may also be ectopic, making it difficult to locate with ultrasound or for the surgeon. Common ectopic locations are mediastinal, retrotracheal, intrathyroid, and carotid sheath/undescended.

Adenomas are encapsulated and have a discrete border. Differentiation of adenomas and hyperplasia is difficult on histologic and morphologic grounds. Color Doppler may show a hypervascular pattern or a peripheral vascular arc that may aid in the differentiation from hyperplastic regional lymph nodes, which have hilar flow.

Carcinoma. Histologic differentiation of adenoma and carcinoma is very difficult. Metastases to regional nodes or distant organs, capsular invasion, or local recurrence must be present for cancer to be diagnosed. Most cancers of the parathyroid glands are small, irregular, and rather firm masses. The mass may adhere to surrounding structures.

SECONDARY HYPERPARATHYROIDISM

Secondary hyperparathyroidism is a chronic hypocalcemia caused by renal failure, vitamin D deficiency (rickets), or malabsorption syndromes. These abnormalities induce PTH secretion, which leads to secondary hyperparathyroidism. The hyperfunction of the parathyroids is apparently a compensatory reaction; renal insufficiency and intestinal malabsorption cause hypocalcemia, which leads to stimulation of PTH. All four glands are usually affected.

MISCELLANEOUS NECK MASSES

The role of ultrasound in evaluating palpable neck masses is to determine the site of origin and assess lesion texture.

DEVELOPMENTAL CYSTS

Thyroglossal Duct Cysts. Congenital anomalies that appear in the midline of the neck anterior to the trachea are called **thyroglossal duct cysts** (Figure 18-26). They are oval or spherical masses rarely larger than 2 or 3 cm. A remnant of the tubular development of the thyroid gland may persist between the base of the tongue and the hyoid bone. This narrow, hollow tract, which connects the thyroid lobes to the floor of the pharynx, normally atrophies in the adult. Failure to atrophy creates the potential for cystic masses to form anywhere along it.

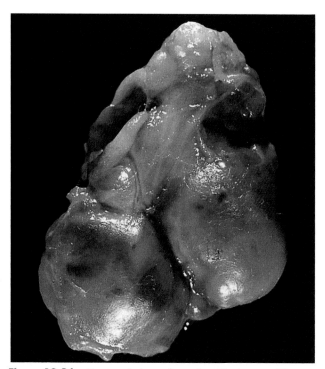

Figure 18-24   Gross pathology of parathyroid adenoma. The gland is enlarged and nodular. (From Damjanov I, Linder J: *Pathology: a color atlas,* St Louis, 2000, Mosby.)

Figure 18-25   Transverse image of an enlarged parathyroid gland. Parathyroid *(arrow)*; C, carotid; *LC,* longus colli; *T,* trachea; *TT,* thyroid tissue.

Figure 18-26 Transverse image at the level of the thyroid gland *(TG)*, demonstrating a thyroglossal duct cyst *(C)* in the midline anterior to the trachea *(TR)*. *CA,* Carotid artery; *IS,* isthmus of thyroid gland.

Branchial Cleft Cysts. Branchial cleft cysts are cystic formations usually located lateral to the thyroid gland. During embryonic development, the branchial cleft is a slender tract extending from the pharyngeal cavity to an opening near the auricle or into the neck. A diverticulum may extend either laterally from the pharynx or medially from the neck. Although primarily cystic in appearance, these lesions may present with solid components, usually of low-level echogenicity, particularly if they have become infected.

ABSCESS

Abscesses can arise in any location in the neck.

Sonographic Findings. The sonographic appearance of an abscess ranges from primarily fluid-filled to completely echogenic. Most commonly, it appears as a mass of low-level echogenicity with rather irregular walls. Chronic abscess may be particularly difficult to demonstrate because the indistinct margins blend with surrounding tissue. The role of ultrasound in evaluating abscess is localization for percutaneous needle aspiration and follow-up examination during and after treatment.

ADENOPATHY

Sonographic Findings. In the neck, the shape of the node is important. A normal lymph node is oval in shape with a homogeneous texture with a central core echo complex. The more rounded the node, the more likely the node is malignant. Low-level echogenicity of well-circumscribed masses is the classic sonographic appearance of enlarged lymph nodes. However, in some cases the node appears echo-free. Inflammatory processes may also exhibit a cystic nature. Differentiation of inflammation from neoplastic processes is not always possible by sonographic criteria alone. To confirm a neoplastic process, a fine-needle biopsy is performed.

SELECTED BIBLIOGRAPHY

Barreda R, Kaude JV, Fagein M and others: Hypervascularity of non-toxic goiter as shown by color-coded Doppler sonography, *AJR Am J Roentgenol* 156:199, 1991.

Brander A, Viikinloski P, Nichels J and others: Thyroid gland: US screening in a random adult population, *Radiology* 181:683-687, 1991.

Brkljacic B and others: Ultrasonic evaluation of benign and malignant nodules in echographically multinodular thyroids, *J Clin Ultrasound* 22:71, 1994.

Chang DG, Yang PC, Yu CJ and others: Differentiation of benign and malignant cervical lymph nodes with color Doppler sonography, *AJR Am J Roetgenol* 162:956-960, 1994.

Clark KJ, Cronan JJ, Scola FH: Color Doppler sonography: anatomic and physiologic assessment of the thyroid, *J Clin Ultrasound* 23:215-223, 1995.

Gladziwa U and others: Secondary hyperparathyroidism and sonographic evaluation of parathyroid gland hyperplasia in dialysis patients, *Clin Nephrol* 38:162, 1992.

Gooding G: Thyroid and parathyroid. In Mittlestaedt C, editor: *General ultrasound,* New York, 1992, Churchill Livingstone.

Hennemann G: Non-toxic goiter, *Clin Endocrinol Metab* 8:167, 1999.

Holmes EC, Morton DL, Ketcham AS: Parathyroid carcinoma: a collective review, *Ann Surg* 169:631, 1999.

Hopkins CR, Reading CC: Thyroid and parathyroid imaging, *Semin Ultrasound CT MR* 16: 279-295, 1995.

Kerr L: High-resolution thyroid ultrasound: the value of color Doppler, *Ultrasound Q* 12:21, 1994.

Kohri K, Ishikawa Y, Kodama M and others: Comparison of imaging methods for localization of parathyroid tumors, *Am J Surg* 164: 140-145, 1992.

Kuntz KM: "Neck mass." In Henningsen C, editor: *Clinical guide to ultrasonography,* St Louis, 2004, Mosby.

Meola M and others: Color-Doppler in the imaging work-up of primary hyperparathyroidism, *J Nephrol* 12(4):270, 1999.

Rosai J: *Ackerman's surgical pathology,* ed 8, St Louis, 1996, Mosby.

Solbiati L, Cioffi V, Ballarati E: Ultrasonography of the neck, *Radiol Clin North Am* 30:941, 1992.

Takashima S and others: Primary thyroid lymphoma: comparison of CT and US assessment, *Radiology* 171:439, 1995.

Turnbridge WM, Caldwell G: *The epidemiology of thyroid diseases,* Philadelphia, 1991, JB Lippincott.

Van Herle AJ and others: The thyroid nodule, *Ann Intern Med* 196:221, 1992.

The Scrotum

Cindy A. Owen

KEY TERMS

centripetal artery – terminal intratesticular arteries arising from the capsular arteries

cremasteric artery – small artery arising from the inferior epigastric artery (a branch of the external iliac artery), which supplies the peritesticular tissue, including the cremasteric muscle

cremasteric muscle – an extension of the internal oblique muscle that descends to the testis with the spermatic cord; contraction of the cremasteric muscle shortens the spermatic cord and elevates the testis

cryptorchidism – (undescended testes) testicles remain within the abdomen or groin and fail to descend into the scrotal sac

dartos – layer of muscle underneath the scrotal skin

deferential artery – arises from the vesicle artery (a branch of the internal iliac artery) and supplies the vas deferens and epididymis

ejaculatory ducts – connect the seminal vesicle and the vas deferens to the urethra at the verumontanum

epididymal cyst – cyst filled with clear, serous fluid located in the epididymis

epididymis – anatomic structure formed by the network of ducts leaving the mediastinum testis that combine into a single, convoluted epididymal tubule; located on the posterolateral aspect of the testis; the epididymis consists of the head, the body, and the tail; spermatozoa mature and accumulate within the epididymis

epididymitis – inflammation of the epididymis

hematocele – blood located between the visceral and parietal layers of the tunica vaginalis

hydrocele – fluid formed between the visceral and parietal layers of the tunica vaginalis

mediastinum testis – central linear structure formed by the convergence of multiple thin septations within the testicle, the septations are invaginations of the tunica albuginea

pampiniform plexus – plexus of veins in the spermatic cord that drain into the right and left testicular veins; when a varicocele is present, dilation and tortuosity may develop

pudendal artery – the internal and external pudendal arteries partially supply the scrotal wall and epididymis and occasionally the lower pole of the testis

pyocele – pus located between the visceral and parietal layers of the tunica vaginalis

recurrent rami – terminal ends of the centripetal (intratesticular) arteries that curve backward toward the capsule

rete testis – network of the channels formed by the convergence of the straight seminiferous tubules in the mediastinum testis; these channels drain into the head of the epididymis.

scrotum – sac containing the testes and epididymis

seminal vesicles – reservoirs for sperm located posterior to the bladder

septa testis – multiple septa formed from the tunica albuginea that course toward the mediastinum testis and separate the testicle into lobules

spermatic cord – structure made up of vas deferens, testicular artery, cremasteric artery, and pampiniform plexus that suspends the testis in the scrotum

spermatocele – cyst in the vas deferens containing sperm

testicle – male gonad that produces hormones that induce masculine features and spermatozoa

testicular artery – artery arising from the aorta just distal to each renal artery; it divides into two major branches supplying the testis medially and laterally

testicular vein – the pampiniform plexus forms each testicular vein; the right testicular vein drains directly into the inferior vena cava, whereas the left testicular vein drains into the left renal vein

tunica albuginea – inner fibrous membrane surrounding the testicle

tunica vaginalis – membrane consisting of a visceral layer (adherent to the testis) and a parietal layer (adherent to the scrotum) lining the inner wall of the scrotum; a potential space between these layers is where hydroceles may develop

urethra – tubular structure that extends from the bladder to the end of the penis

varicocele – dilated veins in the pampiniform plexus

vas deferens – tube that connects the epididymis to the seminal vesicle

verumontanum – junction of the ejaculatory ducts with the urethra

---

Ultrasound is the imaging modality of choice for evaluation of the scrotum. High-frequency ultrasound imaging, combined with color and spectral Doppler, quickly and reliably provide valuable information in the assessment of scrotal pain or mass. In particular, color Doppler has a central role in the evaluation of suspected testicular torsion by demonstrating an absence of flow in the affected testis. Additionally, color Doppler plays a key role in the evaluation of testicular infection by demonstrating hyperemic flow on the affected side. Ultrasound imaging accurately differentiates intratesticular and extratesticular masses and cystic versus solid masses. Advances in the development of ultrasound equipment have provided improved spatial and contrast resolution, reduced speckle artifact, and increased sensitivity to the display of scrotal perfusion. This steady progress in ultrasound image quality has enhanced our ability to clearly define the scrotal anatomy and to more accurately depict and differentiate

abnormalities. This chapter covers the pertinent anatomy of the scrotum and its contents, including the vascular supply. The ultrasound scanning protocol is discussed with tips on scanning techniques and potential pitfalls. A review of the disease processes affecting the scrotum is provided, including a description of sonographic findings.

ANATOMY OF THE SCROTUM

The testes are symmetric, oval-shaped glands residing in the scrotum. In adults, the testis measures approximately 3 to 5 cm in length, 2 to 4 cm in width, and approximately 3 cm in height. Each testis is divided into more than 250 to 400 conical lobules containing the seminiferous tubules. These tubules converge at the apex of each lobule and anastomose to form the rete testis in the mediastinum. The rete testis drains into the head of the epididymis through the efferent ductules (Figure 19-1). Sonographically, the testes appear as smooth, medium gray structures with a fine echo texture.

The epididymis is a 6- to 7-cm tubular structure beginning superiorly and then coursing posterolateral to the testis. It is divided into a head, body, and tail. The head is the largest part of the epididymis, measuring 6 to 15 mm in width. It is located superior to the upper pole of the testis (Figure 19-2). It contains 10 to 15 efferent ductules from the rete testis, which converge to form a single duct in the body and tail. This duct is known as the ductus epididymis. It becomes the vas deferens and continues in the spermatic cord. The body of the epididymis is much smaller than the head. It is difficult to see with ultrasound on normal individuals. It follows the posterolateral aspect of the testis from the upper to the lower pole. The tail of the epididymis is slightly larger and is positioned posterior to the lower pole of the testis. The appendix of the epididymis is a small protuberance from the head of the epididymis. Postmortem studies have shown the appendix epididymis in 34% of testes unilaterally and 12% of testes bilaterally. The normal epididymis usually appears as isoechoic or hypoechoic compared with the testis, although the echo texture is coarser.

At the upper pole of the testis, the appendix testis is attached. It is located between the testis and epididymis. Post-

Figure 19-1 Transverse ultrasound scan of the normal rete testis. With the use of high resolution imaging and transducer frequencies of 10 MHz or greater, the normal rete testis can sometimes be depicted with ultrasound. It appears as tiny tubules adjacent to the epididymal head and testis mediastinum *(arrow)*.

Figure 19-2 Sagittal ultrasound scan of a normal epididymis and testis. The head of the epididymis is seen superior to the upper pole of the testis *(white arrow)*. The body of the epididymis is seen posterior to the testis *(black arrow)*. Note the coarse echo texture of the epididymis compared with the fine texture of the testis.

Figure 19-3 Sagittal ultrasound scan of the normal testis demonstrates the appendix testis as a small structure superior to the testis *(arrow)*. The appendix testis is isoechoic to the testis. A small hydrocele improves the visibility of the appendix testis.

mortem studies have shown the appendix testis to be present in 92% of testes unilaterally and 69% bilaterally (Figure 19-3).

The testis is completely covered by a dense, fibrous tissue termed the **tunica albuginea.** The posterior aspect of the tunica albuginea reflects into the testis to form a vertical septum known as the mediastinum testis. Multiple septa **(septa testis)** are formed from the tunica albuginea at the mediastinum. They course through the testis and separate it into lobules. The mediastinum supports the vessels and ducts coursing within the testis. The mediastinum is often seen on ultrasound as a bright hyperechoic line coursing craniocaudad within the testis (Figure 19-4, *A, B*). The **tunica vaginalis** lines the inner walls of the scrotum, covering each testis and epididymis. It consists of two layers: parietal and visceral. The parietal layer is the inner lining of the scrotal wall. The visceral layer surrounds the testis and epididymis. There is a small bare area, which is posterior. At this site, the testicle is against the

scrotal wall, preventing torsion. Blood vessels, lymphatics, nerves, and spermatic ducts travel through the area (see Figure 19-1). The space between the layers of the tunica vaginalis is where hydroceles form. It is normal to see a small amount of fluid in this space.

The **vas deferens** is a continuation of the ductus epididymis. It is thicker and less convoluted. The vas deferens dilates at the terminal portion near the seminal vesicles. This portion is termed the ampulla of the deferens. The vas deferens joins the duct of the seminal vesicles to form the **ejaculatory duct,** which in turn, empties into the **urethra.** The junction of the ejaculatory ducts with the urethra is termed the **verumontanum.** The urethra courses from the bladder to the end of the penis. In men, the urethra transports both urine and semen outside the body.

The vas deferens, testicular arteries, venous pampiniform plexus, lymphatics, autonomic nerves, and fiber of the cremaster form the **spermatic cord.** The cord extends from the scrotum through the inguinal canal and internal inguinal rings to the pelvis. The spermatic cord suspends the testis in the scrotum.

VASCULAR SUPPLY

Right and left **testicular arteries** arise from the abdominal aorta just below the level of the renal arteries. They are the primary source of blood flow to the testis. The testicular arteries descend in the retroperitoneum and enter the spermatic cord in the deep inguinal ring. Then they course along the posterior surface of each testis and pierce the tunica albuginea forming the capsular arteries, which branch over the surface of the testis. With high-frequency ultrasound imaging, the capsular artery is sometimes seen as a hypoechoic linear structure on the surface of the testis. Color Doppler can be used to confirm its identity (Figure 19-5). The capsular arteries give rise to centripetal arteries, which course from the testicular surface toward the mediastinum along the septa. Before reaching the mediastinum, they curve backward forming the **recurrent rami** (centrifugal arteries) (Figure 19-6). These further branch into arterioles and capillaries. With sensitive color Doppler settings, the recurrent rami may be seen giving a candy cane appearance (Figure 19-7).

In approximately one half of normal testes, a transmediastinal (or transtesticular) artery is visualized coursing through the mediastinum toward the testicular capsule. A large vein is often identified adjacent to the artery (Figure 19-8). On color Doppler, the transmediastinal artery will have a different color than the centripetal arteries because its flow is directed away from the mediastinum and toward the capsule. Upon reaching the testicular surface opposite the mediastinum, the transmediastinal artery courses along the capsule as capsular arteries. Spectral Doppler waveforms obtained from the capsular, centripetal, or transmediastinal arteries show a low-resistance waveform pattern in normal individuals (Figure 19-9). Box 19-1 diagrams arterial branching in the testicles.

The **cremasteric** and **deferential arteries** accompany the testicular artery within the spermatic cord to supply the

A   **B**

Figure 19-4 **A,** Transverse ultrasound scan through the midtestis showing a cross-sectional view of the mediastinum testis. The mediastinum appears as a brightly echogenic focus in transverse views. **B,** Sagittal ultrasound scan through the mid testis showing a long axis view of the mediastinum testis. The mediastinum is seen as a hyperechoic linear structure *(arrow).*

Figure 19-5 Transverse ultrasound view of the testis depicting the capsular artery in a patient with orchitis. The capsular artery is seen as an anechoic structure coursing along the surface of the testis *(arrow).*

Figure 19-6 Color Doppler image of the testis depicting the capsular artery giving rise to centripetal arteries. A transmediastinal artery is seen coursing from the mediastinum to the testicular surface. It then branches across the top of the testis as capsular arteries. The flow direction in the transmediastinal artery (blue) is opposite that of the centripetal arteries (red). The centripetal arteries rise from the capsular arteries with a flow direction through the testis toward the mediastinum, whereas the blood flow in the transmediastinal artery courses from the mediastinum to the testicular capsule.

extratesticular structures. They also have anastomoses with the testicular artery and may provide some flow to the testis. The cremasteric artery branches from the inferior epigastric artery (a branch of the external iliac artery). It provides flow to the cremaster muscle and peritesticular tissue. The deferential artery arises from the vesicle artery (a branch of the internal iliac artery). It mainly supplies the epididymis and vas deferens. The scrotal wall is also supplied by branches of the pudendal artery.

Venous drainage of the scrotum occurs through the veins of the **pampiniform plexus.** The pampiniform plexus exits from the mediastinum testis and courses in the spermatic cord. It converges into three sets of anastomotic veins: the testicular, deferential, and cremasteric. The right **testicular vein** drains into the inferior vena cava and the left testicular vein joins the left renal vein. The deferential vein drains into the

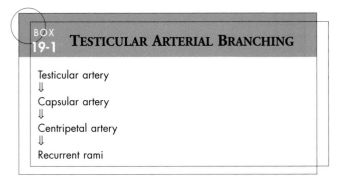

BOX 19-1   **TESTICULAR ARTERIAL BRANCHING**

Testicular artery
⇓
Capsular artery
⇓
Centripetal artery
⇓
Recurrent rami

Figure 19-7 Color Doppler image of the testis depicting the recurrent rami. A centripetal artery is seen coursing from the testicular capsule. Before reaching the mediastinum, it turns backward in a candy cane pattern, forming recurrent rami.

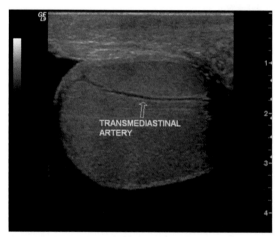

Figure 19-8 Transverse US image shows a normal transmediastinal artery coursing from the mediastinum to the testicular capsule. It appears as an anechoic or hypoechoic tube. Transmediastinal arteries are seen in approximately 50% of testes.

pelvic veins, and the cremasteric vein drains into tributaries of the epigastric and deep pudendal veins.

PATIENT POSITIONING AND SCANNING PROTOCOL

Ultrasound examination of the scrotum is performed with the patient in the supine position. The penis is positioned on the abdomen and covered with a towel. The patient is asked to place his legs close together to provide support for the scrotum. Alternatively, a rolled towel placed between the thighs can support the scrotum. It is often unnecessary to place a towel for support if the legs are positioned close together. This may be more comfortable for the patient in pain.

A generous amount of warmed gel is applied to the scrotum to ensure adequate probe contact and eliminate air between the probe and skin surface. Rarely, a stand-off pad may be nec-

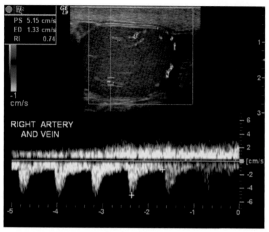

Figure 19-9 Spectral Doppler image showing the normal low resistance waveform pattern of the intratesticular arteries. A low-resistance waveform demonstrates forward flow during both systole and diastole. In this image, the Doppler sample volume includes both a transmediastinal artery and its accompanying vein. The venous and arterial flow signals are on opposite sides of the Doppler baseline, as their flow is in opposite directions.

essary to improve imaging of very superficial structures, such as a tunica albuginea cyst. However, with the use of high-frequency probes (10 to 14 MHz), this is usually not necessary. Instead of a stand-off pad, an extra thick mound of gel may be adequate to improve near field imaging.

Before beginning the scrotal ultrasound, it is necessary to determine clinical findings. Was this patient referred because of a palpable mass, scrotal pain, swollen scrotum, or other reason? It is important to ask the patient to describe his symptoms, including history, location, and duration of pain. Can he feel a mass? If so, ask the patient to find the lump. Then place the probe exactly over this location to examine the site. Did the patient experience trauma? When did the trauma occur? Ask him to describe what happened. Has he had a vasectomy? When? This information is not only helpful in guiding the exam, but it is important to the interpreting physician and gives confidence to the patient in the quality of the ultrasound study. Box 19-2 lists important tips when performing an ultrasound examination of the scrotum.

Scrotal ultrasound is always a bilateral exam, with the asymptomatic side used as a comparison for the symptomatic side. To begin, it is best to perform a brief survey scan to determine what abnormalities, if any, are present. Each testis is scanned from superior to inferior and carefully examined to determine if abnormal findings are present. The size, echogenicity, and structure of each testis are evaluated. The testicular parenchyma should be uniform with an equal echogenicity between sides. Think of these questions as you scan: Is the parenchyma homogeneous or heterogeneous? Is there a mass? If so, is it cystic or solid? Is it intratesticular or extratesticular? Is one testis much larger than the other? Which side is swollen or is one side shrunken? Each testis should appear similar in size and shape. Is the epididymis normal? Is the skin thickened? Turn on color Doppler to assess the flow. Is there an absence of flow in the testis or is it hyperemic? How

Figure 19-10   Transverse ultrasound image in a normal patient demonstrating both testes at the same time. The size, echogenicity, and texture are similar between sides. It is advisable to obtain an image like this in all cases to allow comparison between the testes.

does the color Doppler compare between sides? They should show about the same amount of flow when using the same color Doppler setup. Check the flow in each epididymis. Again, compare between sides. They should be similar. After the survey scan, images are obtained that demonstrate the findings.

Representative images are obtained in at least two planes, transverse and sagittal, with additional imaging planes scanned as needed to demonstrate the findings. In transverse, images are taken that show the superior, mid, and inferior portion of each testis. The width of the testis is measured in the mid transverse view. A transverse view of the head of the epididymis is included. Superior to the epididymal head, an image is obtained to demonstrate the area of the spermatic cord. In the sagittal plane, images are taken to show the medial, mid, and lateral portions. A long axis measurement of testicular length is obtained in the midsagittal image. Again, additional images may be taken to demonstrate abnormal areas. An image is obtained of the epididymal head superior to the **testicle.** The body and tail of the epididymis can be demonstrated coursing posteriorly on each side. Scrotal skin thickness is evaluated and compared from side to side. At least one image is taken to show both testes at the same time so the interpreting physician can compare size and echogenicity (Figure 19-10). Additional views may be taken in patients with suspected varicocele. These include upright positioning and the Valsalva maneuver. Color and spectral Doppler are used in all examinations with representative images taken to demonstrate both arterial and venous flow in each testis. Table 19-1 lists the scanning protocols for scrotal ultrasound.

TECHNICAL CONSIDERATIONS

High-frequency linear array transducers are preferred for scrotal imaging because they provide the best spatial resolution. However, the field of view is limited with linear arrays. Occasionally, a larger field of view is required to measure the anatomy or display anatomic relationships. Ultrasound systems provide numerous methods to meet this need. They include virtual convex imaging, panoramic imaging, stitching images together, or using a curved array transducer.

Real-time imaging of the scrotum is performed with a high-frequency linear array probe of at least 7.5 MHz. Since high-

TABLE 19-1	ULTRASOUND SCROTAL SCAN PROTOCOL	
Transverse Image	**Sagittal Image**
Spermatic cord area	Spermatic cord area
Epididymal head	Epididymal head with superior testis
Superior testis	Long axis mid with measurement
Mid testis with measurement	Medial long axis
Inferior testis	Lateral long axis
Transverse view showing both testes	
Color Doppler of epididymal head	
Color Doppler of mid testis	
Spectral Doppler of artery	
Spectral Doppler of vein	

Note: In patients with suspected varicocele, additional views include upright view of spermatic cord with and without Valsalva maneuver.

frequency transducers have better spatial and contrast resolution compared with lower frequency transducers, they are preferred for scrotal imaging. Probes with frequencies of 10 to 15 MHz are usually best. As there is a tradeoff between frequency and penetration, the highest frequency providing adequate penetration should be used. In patients with considerable wall edema and thickening, frequencies as low as 5 to 7.5 MHz may be necessary to adequately penetrate through the testis.

Many ultrasound systems have a trapezoid or virtual convex feature that can be selected with the linear array probes. This is very helpful for measuring the long axis of the testis or when an abnormal area cannot be entirely imaged with the standard linear format (Figure 19-11, *A*). It is best to use this feature selectively instead of routinely since steering the beam to create the wider format negatively impacts image quality. The steering widens the distance between scan lines and degrades lateral resolution.

In cases of large hydroceles, hematomas, or swelling, an even larger field of view may be required. In these cases, a

Figure 19-11   A, Transverse ultrasound scan of a scrotal hematoma using a virtual convex to create a sector or trapezoidal format using a linear array probe. The field of view is enlarged to allow better depiction of the size and location of the hematoma compared with the testes. This feature is useful for measuring testicular length and showing abnormal areas that are too large to view with the standard linear format. However, since the scan lines are steered to create this image, lateral resolution is decreased compared with the standard format. **B,** Transverse ultrasound view of the same scrotal hematoma using a panoramic setting. This feature allows the image to build as the transducer is moved across the anatomy. It is very useful for showing large masses and anatomic relationships. **C,** Sagittal ultrasound image in a patient with epididymitis and hydrocele. The image was obtained by stitching together two images in a combined mode. This is another useful tool when a larger field of view is necessary to demonstrate anatomy. **D,** Sagittal ultrasound image of the testis surrounded posteriorly by a large hydrocele. The linear array format could not display the entire hydrocele, so a 7-MHz curved array transducer was used to better demonstrate a pathologic condition.

panoramic tool may be useful. This tool allows the image to build as the probe is moved over the skin surface. A very long image can be obtained that shows anatomic relationships (Figure 19-11, *B*). Images may also be stitched together in a combined mode. The first image is obtained in one window, and then the probe is moved and another image is obtained attempting to match the boundaries of the first image (Figure 19-11, *C*). Another way to obtain a larger field of view is to use a 5- to 7.5-MHz curved array transducer for a portion of the exam to demonstrate the entire scrotal contents. Again, this should be done selectively to obtain the necessary images, then returning to the high-frequency linear array probe for further evaluation of each testis (Figure 19-11, *D*).

Most modern ultrasound scanners offer additional features that enhance the quality of the ultrasound image. These features include, but are not limited to, compound imaging, harmonics, extended field of view imaging, virtual convex, speckle reduction algorithms, and use of multiple focal zones (Table 19-2). All of these controls may be adjusted to improve image quality.

Color and spectral Doppler play an important role in scrotal ultrasound. The typical color/spectral Doppler frequencies used for scrotal ultrasound are between 4 to 8 MHz. The upper frequency range is used to improve sensitivity to slow flow. This is important in evaluation of testicular torsion or tumor vascularity. Penetration is decreased with higher frequencies, so it is

TABLE 19-2 SCANNING FEATURES

Feature	What Is It?	Advantage	Disadvantage
Harmonics	Selective reception of harmonic frequencies generated within the tissue	• Improve contrast resolution • Improved visibility of low-level echoes • Reduction of artifacts	Less penetration (uses higher frequency)
Compound imaging	Uses multiple-angled firings to create one image	• Improved border definition • Reduced speckle • Less angle dependence	• Slows frame rate • Loss of some beneficial artifacts (i.e., shadowing, refraction, and enhancement)
Speckle reduction algorithms	Sophisticated algorithms applied to the image to reduce speckle (salt and pepper appearance of ultrasound image)	• Improves contrast resolution • Improved conspicuity of masses	None
Extended field of view imaging	Image builds up as probe is moved across anatomy	Improved ability to show anatomic relationships of structures too large to fit in linear array format	May be difficult to perform on uncooperative patient or over sharply curving interface
Trapezoid or virtual convex imaging	Steering of linear array probe to create sector format	Gives larger field of view with linear array probes	Reduces lateral resolution
Multizone focus	Use of multiple focal zones to create an extended area of focus on one image	Improves lateral resolution	Slows frame rate

TABLE 19-3 COLOR/POWER DOPPLER PARAMETERS

Parameter	What Is It?	How To Adjust
Gain	Amplification of selected frequency shift signal	Turn up until noise is present and then decrease until noise goes away
PRF (Pulse repetition frequency)	PRF is the number of pulses transmitted per second; sets the Nyquist limit; main control affecting sensitivity to flow	Adjust on the asymptomatic side so that flow is visible without too much flash or motion artifact; decrease to improve sensitivity to slow flow; increase to reduce aliasing
Wall filter	Color signals received below the wall filter setting do not appear on the image	Decrease to improve sensitivity and to reduce flash/motion artifact
Line density	Density of scan lines contained within the color box	Turn up to improve lateral resolution of vessels; turn down to increase frame rate
Threshold	Level of grayscale brightness that is allowable to be overwritten by color when both grayscale and color information are obtained for the same pixel location within the image	Turn up so that color information is prioritized compared with grayscale information; if the threshold (also known as color/write priority) is set too low, small intratesticular vessels will not be filled with color
Packet size	Number of pulses on each color scan line	Turn up to improve signal to noise ratio and sensitivity; turn down to improve frame rate
Color box size	Region of interest that is color encoded within the image	Set just over the area of interest; increasing color box size or depth will slow frame rate

important to make sure that the color penetrates to the depth of interest. Color and spectral Doppler findings in the symptomatic side are always compared with the asymptomatic side.

Power Doppler is often used as a way to quickly get to a sensitive setting that will demonstrate slow flow. Power Doppler is showing the amplitude or power of the moving signal, whereas color Doppler is showing the frequency shift. Power Doppler does not demonstrate flow direction or aliasing and to some offers a more straightforward display of blood flow. Presets for power Doppler are often set at a lower PRF than color Doppler since aliasing is not an issue. So pushing

the power Doppler button may show more flow with less adjustment of controls. This often provides a quick way to get to a more sensitive flow setting. Persistence is usually much greater with power Doppler requiring a steady hand and slower movement of the probe. To further enhance power Doppler, the same parameters are adjusted as for color Doppler.

Familiarity with color Doppler controls is very important when performing scrotal ultrasound. The sonographer may need to adjust some of the following color Doppler parameters throughout the study to enhance the visibility of scrotal perfusion (Table 19-3):

Figure 19-12   **A,** Transverse color Doppler image of a normal testis. Almost no color signal is apparent in the testis because of the high PRF setting. The velocity scale values adjacent to the color bar show a velocity sensitivity of 25 cm/sec. **B,** Image of the same testis, using a much lower PRF setting. The velocity scale shows a flow sensitivity of 2 cm/sec. Many intratesticular vessels can now be seen with color Doppler.

- **Gain**—The color gain control is used to amplify the reflected color Doppler signal. Whenever the expected amount of color is not visible in the image, the color gain should be increased until noise is present. Once color noise is visible, the gain can be decreased until it just disappears. At this point the color gain setting is optimized.
- **Scale/pulse repetition frequency (PRF)**—The PRF is the number of pulses transmitted in one second. This important color parameter affects the sensitivity of the system to display slow flow. It also sets the point at which color aliasing occurs (Nyquist limit). The control has different names depending on the ultrasound equipment being used. It is variably named scale, PRF, or flow rate. The PRF is reduced to improve sensitivity to slow flow. This is critical when ruling out testicular torsion. If the PRF is set too high, slow flow may not be visible. When the PRF is set too low, excessive color aliasing occurs. This makes it impossible to determine flow direction or assess flow quality. Neither of these factors is significant in scrotal ultrasound, so it is common to use low PRF settings. However, flash artifact from patient motion is more apparent with very low PRF's and may make scanning difficult. It is recommended to adjust the PRF so that the asymptomatic testicular flow is well demonstrated without excessive flash artifact. Then compare the same settings on the contralateral side (Figure19-12).
- **Wall filter**—The wall filter acts as an electronic eraser. Color echoes that lie below the filter cutoff do not appear on the image display. The wall filter is adjusted downward to enhance flow sensitivity. It is turned up to reduce flash artifact. On most ultrasound systems, the wall filter is automatically adjusted with the PRF. But in some instances, it may be beneficial to make further adjustments.
- **Line density**—The line density is the number or density of the scan lines contained within the color box. It affects the lateral resolution of the color display. As line density is increased, lateral resolution is improved. The size of the intra-

testicular arteries is displayed more accurately when line density is high. Frame rate becomes slower as the line density is increased because more transmitted pulses are required to create each image frame. If the frame rate becomes too slow, the line density can be decreased. The user must choose the tradeoff between resolution and frame rate (Figure 19-13).

- **Threshold**—The B/Color threshold is used to determine whether a gray scale or color pixel is displayed in any given location on the image. Color and power Doppler images are color overlays on top of an existing grayscale image. A problem arises when both grayscale and color information are received for the same pixel location. The threshold control allows the user to prioritize either grayscale or color. For ultrasound of most small parts, including scrotal imaging, it is best to set the threshold so that color is prioritized. Based on the setting, when both color and grayscale information are received for the same pixel location, the one displayed is based on the brightness (amplitude) of the grayscale dot and the frequency shift and/or power level of the color signal. This feature is not as important when looking at large vessels, such as the common carotid artery, because the vessel lumen typically does not contain grayscale information and color can be freely displayed in those pixels. But in small parts imaging, most vessels are so small that the lumen is either not seen or filled with grayscale echoes because of volume averaging. In these instances, color will not be displayed unless the threshold control is set to a level that prioritizes color.
- **Packet size**—The packet size is the number of sound pulses transmitted on each scan line within the color box. The packet size is usually set between 8 and 16 pulses on each scan line. The packet size affects the signal-to-noise ratio, improving color sensitivity when more pulses are used. As the number of packets (pulses) is increased on each scan line, the frame rate gets slower. The packet size can be reduced to raise the frame rate when necessary, or increased to

Figure 19-13   A, This image was obtained at a low line density setting. The vessels appear wider than expected (poor lateral resolution). **B,** When the line density is increased, the vessel size is more accurately displayed. Frame rate is slower because there are more scan lines within the same sized color box.

improve color sensitivity. The key factor affecting color sensitivity, however, is the PRF.

• **Color box/region of interest**—The color box or region of interest is the area within the grayscale image where flow is color encoded. The width of the color box affects the frame rate. If the color box is very wide, more scan lines are required to complete each image frame. This means that a greater number of pulses must be transmitted. This takes more time, so the frame rate is reduced. Color box depth also affects frame rate. When the color box is placed deep in the image, the round-trip time for the sound is increased. This slows down the frame rate.

Understanding the factors affecting color frame rate, sensitivity, and resolution allow the sonographer to optimize the color parameters for each clinical situation. Most systems have specific presets for each ultrasound application. Selection of the scrotal preset will set the color parameters near an optimal setting for a typical, normal exam. However, the user must further adjust the controls to enhance visibility of scrotal perfusion in abnormal states.

SCROTAL PATHOLOGY

Table 19-4 lists the pathology and sonographic appearance associated with scrotal trauma, infection, and fluid collections. Although the sonographer is not responsible for the interpretation of the ultrasound images, an understanding of the various differential considerations is useful to fully evaluate the lesion. Table 19-5 lists many of the common and uncommon masses or fluid collections found within or surrounding the testes.

ACUTE SCROTUM

Scrotal Trauma. Scrotal trauma presents a challenge to the sonographer because the scrotum is often painful and swollen. Trauma may be the result of motor vehicle accident, athletic

injury, direct blow to the scrotum, or a straddle injury. The most important goal of the ultrasound exam in testicular trauma is to determine if a rupture has occurred. Rupture of the testis is a surgical emergency requiring a prompt diagnosis. If surgery is performed within 72 hours following injury, up to 90% of testes can be saved, but only 45% can be saved after 72 hours. Hydrocele and hematocele are both complications of trauma. However, neither is specific to trauma. Hematoceles contain blood and are also found in advanced cases of epididymitis or orchitis.

Sonographic Findings. The sonographic findings associated with scrotal rupture include a focal alteration of the testicular parenchymal pattern, interruption of the tunica albuginea, irregular testicular contour, scrotal wall thickening, and **hematocele.** These findings may also be associated with abscess, tumor, or other clinical conditions. When combined with a history of trauma, they suggest rupture.

The sonographic appearance of hematoceles varies with age. An acute hematocele is echogenic with numerous, highly visible echoes that can be seen to float or move in real time. With time, hematoceles show low-level echoes and develop fluid-fluid levels or septations. The presence of a hematocele does not confirm rupture. The hematoceles result from bleeding of the pampiniform plexus or other extratesticular structure.

Hematomas associated with trauma may be large and cause displacement of the associated testis. Hematomas appear as heterogeneous areas within the scrotum. They tend to become more complex with time, developing cystic components. Hematomas may involve the testis or epididymis, or they can be contained within the scrotal wall. Since hematomas are avascular, color Doppler is helpful in identifying them as areas with no flow (Figure 19-14).

Other uses of color Doppler in testicular trauma include identification of blood flow disruption across the surface of the testis. This is an indication of rupture. Color Doppler can aid in separating a normally vascularized testis from one that is disrupted by hematoma. Epididymitis may result from trauma,

TABLE 19-4	SCROTAL INFECTION, TRAUMA, AND FLUID COLLECTIONS
Pathology	Sonographic Appearance

Infection

Epididymitis	Enlarged epididymis
	Heterogeneous texture
	Hypoechoic, may contain hyperechoic areas
	↑ Blood flow in the epididymis
Focal orchitis	Hypoechoic area within testis
	↑ Blood flow in the testis
Diffuse orchitis	Enlarged, hypoechoic testis
	↓ Echogenicity of the whole testis

Trauma

Rupture	Irregular contour
	Focal alteration in echogenicity
Hematoma	Heterogeneous area
	Becomes hyperechoic as the blood clot ages
	Avascular
Torsion	Grayscale image of testis normal when duration <4 hours
	Testis enlarged and hypoechoic 4-12 hours
	Testis heterogeneous after 24 hours
	Absence of testicular flow

Fluid Collections

Hydrocele	May be anechoic, but often contains low-level echoes
	Surrounds anterolateral aspect of testis
Spermatocele	Located in head of epididymis
	May contain internal echoes and/or septations
	Smooth walls
	Posterior acoustic enhancement
Epididymal cyst	May be located anywhere in epididymis
	Usually small, anechoic
	Ultrasound cannot differentiate between spermatocele and epididymal cyst
	Posterior acoustic enhancement
Varicocele	Tortuous, dilated veins
	Increased size with Valsalva maneuver or patient standing
	Dilated veins fill with color on Valsalva maneuver
	Spectral Doppler confirms venous flow
Hematocele	Contains low-level echoes
	May contain septations and loculations

TABLE 19-5	DIFFERENTIAL CONSIDERATIONS: EXTRATESTICULAR FLUID COLLECTIONS OR MASSES
Common:	Hydrocele
	Varicocele
	Ascites
	Hematocele
	Spermatocele
	Epididymitis
Uncommon:	Cysts
	Pyoceles
	Herniated bowel
	Metastasis
	Polyorchidism
	Extratesticular
	Seminoma
Extratesticular Cystic Mass	
Common:	Hematocele
	Spermatocele
Uncommon:	Pyocele
	Epididymal cyst
	Herniated bowel
Hypoechoic Lesion	
Common:	Seminoma
	Embryonal cell carcinoma
	Choriocarcinoma
	Mixed cell tumor
	Lymphoma
	Leukemia
Uncommon:	Teratoma
	Torsion
	Metastasis
	Epididymal tumor
	Abscess
Enlarged Testicle	
Common:	Tumor
	Edematous testis caused by trauma
	Torsion
Uncommon:	Myeloma of testicle
	Idiopathic macroorchidism
Enlarged Epididymis	
Common:	Epididymitis
	Sperm granuloma
Uncommon:	Polyorchidism
	Lipoma
Hypoechoic Band in Testis	
Common:	Normal mediastinum testis
	Normal vessels

and color Doppler imaging can be used to identify the associated increased vascularity in the **epididymis.** Torsion may also be associated with trauma. Color Doppler is used to confirm an absence of flow in the testis with torsion.

Epididymo-Orchitis. Epididymo-orchitis is infection of the epididymis and testis. It most commonly results from the spread of a lower urinary tract infection via the spermatic cord. Less common causes include mumps, syphilis, tuberculosis, viruses, trauma, or chemical causes. Epididymo-orchitis represents the most common cause of acute scrotal pain in adults. The epididymis is the organ primarily involved with infection,

spreading to the testis in about 20% to 40% of cases. Orchitis almost always occurs secondary to epididymitis. Patients typically have increasing scrotal pain over 1 or 2 days. The pain may be mild or severe. Symptoms may also include fever and urethral discharge.

Sonographic Findings. **Epididymitis** appears as an enlarged, hypoechoic gland. If secondary hemorrhage has occurred, the epididymis may contain focal hyperechoic areas. Hyperemic flow is confirmed with color Doppler (Figure 19-15). The normal epididymis shows little flow with color

Doppler. The amount of color flow signal should be compared between sides. The affected side shows significantly more flow than the asymptomatic epididymis. It is important to use the same color Doppler settings when comparing the amount of flow between sides.

With epididymitis, Doppler waveforms demonstrate increased velocities in both systole and diastole. A low-resistance waveform pattern is present (see Figure 19-15). If the infection is isolated to the epididymis, the testis will appear normal. When orchitis has developed, ultrasound imaging will show an enlarged testis. The infection may be focal or diffuse with the affected areas appearing hypoechoic compared with the surrounding tissue. Focal areas of infection within the testis will result in a heterogeneous appearance on ultrasound. A diffusely infected testis will appear enlarged and homogeneous with a hypoechoic echogenicity (Figure 19-16). Up to 20% of

cases will have a normal appearing epididymis and testis on ultrasound. Ultrasound gray scale findings associated with epididymo-orchitis are not specific and may also be seen with torsion or tumor. Color and spectral Doppler are key tools in differentiating between epididymo-orchitis and torsion in the patient with acute scrotal pain.

Epididymo-orchitis causes hyperemic flow with significantly more visible vessels on color Doppler compared with the asymptomatic side. The hyperemic flow is seen in the epididymis and testis when both are involved but isolated to the epididymis if the testis is normal. Documentation of the findings with ultrasound must include an image showing both testes so the size and echogenicity can be compared. It is also recommended to obtain an image with the color box opened wide enough to show portions of both testes so that the amount of flow between sides can be easily compared.

Other findings associated with epididymitis and epididymo-orchitis include scrotal wall thickening and **hydrocele.** Hydroceles are found around the anterolateral aspect of the testis. They may appear anechoic or contain low-level echoes. Complex hydroceles may be associated with severe epididymitis and orchitis. These will have thick septations and contain low-level echoes. In severe cases, a pyocele may be present. A **pyocele** occurs when pus fills the space between the layers of the tunica vaginalis. It will usually contain internal septations, loculations, and debris. This same appearance can occur following trauma or surgery.

In severe cases of orchitis, testicular infarction may occur. The swollen testis is confined within a rigid tunica albuginea. Excessive swelling can cause obstruction to the testicular blood supply. Color Doppler will show decreased or absent flow compared with the contralateral testis. With decreased flow, spectral Doppler waveforms will have high resistance with little or no diastolic flow. A Doppler waveform demonstrating reversed diastolic flow is a serious finding indicating threatened testicular infarction (Figure 19-17). Infarction can affect the entire testis or be confined to a focal area. With focal

Figure 19-14 Complex hematoma in a patient with hemophilia following scrotal trauma. Transverse ultrasound scan of both testes shows a large heterogeneous mass adjacent to the left testis. Color Doppler (not shown) demonstrated the mass to be avascular.

Figure 19-15 **A,** Sagittal ultrasound image in a patient with severe epididymitis shows an enlarged epididymis with a heterogeneous echo texture. Focal hyperechoic areas *(arrow)* within the epididymis may represent hemorrhage. A complex hydrocele with numerous septations is shown near the epididymal head. **B,** Color Doppler shows hyperemic flow within the epididymis. A Doppler waveform obtained from the epididymal head shows increased diastolic flow associated with inflammation.

Figure 19-16 **A,** Orchitis in a patient presenting with severe scrotal pain and swelling. Transverse stitched ultrasound scan shows an enlarged left testis and normal right testis. A complex hydrocele surrounds the left testis. Marked skin thickening is present on the left side *(arrow)* compared with the normal right side. **B,** Color Doppler shows hyperemic flow.

Figure 19-17 **A,** Severe epididymo-orchitis in patient with scrotal pain, swelling, and edema. The testis is swollen against a rigid tunica albuginea. Scrotal skin thickening is evident. **B,** Power Doppler shows hyperemic perfusion surrounding the testis, but little intratesticular flow despite the use of sensitive Doppler settings. **C,** Spectral Doppler waveform of an intratesticular artery demonstrates a high-resistance waveform. Reversed flow is seen in diastole *(arrow)*. This is a serious finding, indicating threatened infarction.

infarction, color will show perfusion in only portions of the testis with an absence of color signals in the affected areas. Grayscale imaging will depict a heterogeneous pattern. The areas of infarction tend to appear hypoechoic compared with the surrounding testicular parenchyma. If the entire testis becomes infarcted, the findings cannot be differentiated from testicular torsion.

Torsion. Torsion of the spermatic cord occurs as a result of abnormal mobility of the testis within the scrotum. An anomaly termed the bell clapper deformity is the most common etiology of this condition. Normally, the testis and epididymis are surrounded by the tunica vaginalis except at the bare area where they are attached to the posterior scrotal wall. The bell clapper anomaly occurs when the tunica vaginalis completely surrounds the testis, epididymis, and distal spermatic cord, allowing them to move and rotate freely within the scrotum. This movement is similar to that of a clapper inside a bell, hence the name. Torsion results when the testis and epididymis twist within the scrotum, cutting off the vascular supply within the spermatic cord. In patients with torsion, up to 60% will have an anatomic anomaly on both sides. Undescended testes are 10 times more likely to be affected by torsion than normal testes. Torsion compromises blood flow to the testis, epididymis, and the intrascrotal portion of the spermatic cord. Venous flow is affected first with the occluded veins, causing swelling of the scrotal structures on the affected side. If torsion continues, the arterial flow is obstructed and testicular ischemia follows.

Torsion of the spermatic cord is a surgical emergency. It is important to obtain the diagnostic images as quickly as possible since the salvage rate of the testis depends on the elapsed time since torsion. If surgery is performed within 5 to 6 hours of the onset of pain, 80% to 100% of the testes can be salvaged. Between 6 and 12 hours the salvage rate is 70%, but after 12 hours only 20% will be saved. The degree of torsion (or number of twists) also affects testicular salvage.

Torsion is the most common cause of acute scrotal pain in adolescents. Although it is more common in young adults and adolescents, torsion can occur at any age, with the peak incidence at age 14. Patients with torsion most often present with a sudden onset of scrotal pain accompanied by swelling on the affected side. The severe pain causes nausea and vomiting in many patients. Patients with torsion frequently report previous episodes of scrotal pain. The clinical differentiation between torsion and epididymo-orchitis is difficult as patients have similar symptoms. Ultrasound plays a key role in helping differentiate these entities.

Sonographic Findings. Gray scale findings on ultrasound depend upon how much time has passed since the torsion occurred. In the early stages, the scrotal contents may have a normal sonographic appearance. After 4 to 6 hours, the testis becomes swollen and hypoechoic (Figure 19-18). The lobes within the testis are usually well identified during this time as a result of interstitial and septal edema. After 24 hours, the testis becomes heterogeneous as a result of hemorrhage, infarction, necrosis, and vascular congestion (Figure 19-19).

The epididymal head appears enlarged and may have decreased echogenicity or become heterogeneous. In some cases the twisted spermatic cord knot may be seen as a round or oval extratesticular mass that can be traced back to normal spermatic cord. Other findings may include scrotal skin thickening and reactive hydrocele.

Since the ultrasound grayscale findings are similar to those found with epididymo-orchitis, Doppler evaluation in testicular torsion is very important. Color Doppler imaging is used to make the diagnostic images of torsion. An absence of perfusion in the symptomatic testis with normal perfusion demonstrated in the asymptomatic side is considered to be diagnostic of torsion. The color or power Doppler parameters must be adjusted for optimal detection of slow flow. The PRF and wall filter should be set at a low level. Flow around the ischemic testis will appear normal or decreased.

Spontaneous detorsion can produce a very confusing picture both clinically and by ultrasound. Depending upon how long the testis was torsed and how long it has been since relief, the intratesticular flow may be minimal or hyperemic. Extratesticular flow is usually increased. This is very difficult to differentiate from epididymo-orchitis.

Torsion of the appendix epididymis and appendix testis also occurs and further complicates the clinical picture. The clinical presentation is similar to that of testicular torsion and epididymo-orchitis. Ultrasound may show a small, hypoechoic mass located between the head of the epididymis and superior testis. Color Doppler shows increased flow around the mass. Hemorrhage may cause the mass to appear hyperechoic.

EXTRATESTICULAR MASSES

Epididymal Cysts, Spermatoceles, and Tunica Albuginea Cysts. Cysts are benign fluid collections that may be located within the testis or in the extratesticular structures. Most scrotal cysts are extratesticular. Extratesticular cysts are found in the tunica albuginea or epididymis. These include spermatoceles, epididymal cysts, and tunica albuginea cysts. **Spermatoceles** are cystic dilatations of the efferent ductules of the epididymis. They are always located in the epididymal head. Spermatoceles contain proteinaceous fluid and spermatozoa. They may be seen more often following vasectomy.

Epididymal cysts are small, clear cysts containing serous fluid (Figure 19-20). They can be found anywhere within the epididymis. Small cysts are sometimes found between the layers of the tunica vaginalis or between the tunica vaginalis and tunica albuginea. All three entities are generally asymptomatic, although they may be palpable and cause concern to the patient.

Sonographic Findings. Spermatoceles may be seen as simple cysts or multilocular cystic collections containing internal echoes. Epididymal cysts appear as simple fluid-filled structures having thin walls and posterior acoustic enhancement. Ultrasound imaging cannot reliably differentiate epididymal cysts and spermatoceles. Tunica albuginea cysts are usually quite small and appear as anechoic, thin-walled structures with an ultrasound. They can become large and cause displacement and distortion of the testis. This helps to differentiate them from hydroceles, which do not distort the testis.

Figure 19-18   Testicular torsion in adolescent patient with sudden onset of right testicular pain, accompanied by nausea and vomiting. **A,** Color Doppler shows normal flow within the parenchyma of the left testis. **B,** The right testis and epididymis are avascular with color Doppler imaging, with the same settings used to show flow on the asymptomatic side. **C,** Transverse ultrasound image showing both testes in right testicular torsion. The right testis is swollen and hyperechoic compared with the normal left testis.

VARICOCELE

A **varicocele** is an abnormal dilation of the veins of the pampiniform plexus (located within the spermatic cord). Varicoceles are usually caused by incompetent venous valves within the spermatic vein. These are called primary varicoceles. They are more common on the left. This is probably due to the mechanics pertaining to the left spermatic vein and left renal vein. The spermatic vein empties into the left renal vein at a steep angle, which may inhibit blood flow return. The left renal vein can become compressed between the aorta and superior mesenteric artery. Secondary varicoceles are caused by increased pressure on the spermatic vein. This may be the result of renal hydronephrosis, abdominal mass, or liver cirrhosis. An abdominal malignancy invading the left renal vein may cause a varicocele with non-compressible veins. Any noncompressible varicocele in a man over 40 years of age should prompt a search for a retroperitoneal mass.

Varicoceles have a relationship with impaired fertility. They are more common in infertile men. Treatment of the varicocele has been shown to improve sperm count in up to 53% of cases, but there is controversy surrounding the treatment of varicoceles for infertility. Uncommonly, varicoceles may extend within the testis. These will be located near the mediastinum. Intratesticular varicoceles have an unknown clinical significance, but it is possible that they will affect male fertility by the same mechanism as extratesticular varicoceles.

Sonographic Findings. Ultrasound imaging of a varicocele shows numerous tortuous tubes of varying sizes within the spermatic cord near the epididymal head. The tubes may contain echoes that move with real-time imaging. This represents slow venous flow (Figure 19-21, *A, B*). Varicoceles measure more than 2 mm in diameter. They tend to increase diameter in response to the Valsalva maneuver. Scanning with the patient in an upright position will enhance the visibility of a varicocele because the veins will become more distended. Some authors advocate using a standing position routinely; however, others feel that supine scanning with the Valsalva maneuver and color Doppler imaging are adequate. With either protocol, color and spectral Doppler are used to confirm the presence of venous flow and to demonstrate retrograde filling with the Valsalva maneuver (Figure 19-21, *C*). Color Doppler settings must be sensitized for slow flow to detect the venous signal in varicoceles. Flash artifact may be a

RIGHT TESTICLE   LEFT TESTICLE

A

LEFT TESTICLE

B

RIGHT TESTICLE   LEFT TESTICLE

COMPARISON

C

Figure 19-19   Left spermatic cord torsion in adolescent with a history of scrotal pain of a duration greater than 24 hours. **A,** Transverse ultrasound image showing both testes. The left testis is enlarged and heterogeneous. **B,** Sagittal ultrasound image of the left testis. The infarcted testis has a mixed echo pattern caused by the hemorrhage, necrosis, and vascular congestion associated with spermatic cord torsion exceeding 24 hours. **C,** Transverse color Doppler image showing normal perfusion to the right testis with absence of detectable signal on the left side. Paratesticular blood flow is increased around the abnormal testis *(arrows)*.

Figure 19-20   Sagittal ultrasound image of a patient with a palpable scrotal mass. This sagittal image was obtained by scanning directly over the palpable area. It shows a fluid-filled mass with posterior acoustic enhancement located in the head of the epididymis *(arrow)*. This finding is consistent with both spermatocele and epididymal cyst.

problem with color Doppler imaging during a Valsalva maneuver. It is helpful to instruct the patient to hold as still as possible during the maneuver and to carefully adjust the color settings so that the PRF and wall filter are sensitized but not so low that flash artifact fills the screen with a small movement.

Intratesticular varicocele has the sonographic appearance of either straight or serpiginous channels coursing from the mediastinum into the testicular tissue. Color and spectral Doppler are used to identify these channels as dilated veins. On gray scale imaging, the appearance can mimic that of tubular ectasia of the rete testis. Color Doppler will differentiate between intratesticular varicocele and tubular ectasia of the rete testis, as the latter shows no flow (Figure 19-22).

SCROTAL HERNIA

Hernias occur when bowel, omentum, or other structures herniate into the scrotum. Clinical diagnosis is usually sufficient, but ultrasound imaging is helpful when there are equivocal findings. The bowel is the most commonly herniated structure, followed by the omentum.

Sonographic Findings. Peristalsis of the bowel, seen with real-time imaging, confirms the diagnosis of a scrotal hernia (Figure 19-24). This can be captured on videotape or as a cine clip for the interpreting physician to review. Unfortunately,

Figure 19-21 Varicocele in patient being evaluated for infertility. **A,** Sagittal view of the testis shows dilated tubular structures superiorly. **B,** Stitched ultrasound image showing prominent serpiginous venous channels forming a large varicocele on the left. **C,** Doppler ultrasound with Valsalva maneuver shows venous flow within the dilated vascular channels confirming the diagnosis of varicocele.

peristalsis may not always be visible. Fluid-filled bowel loops are easily recognizable by ultrasound. Air-filled loops or loops containing solid stool are more difficult to recognize. On ultrasound, air appears as bright echoes with a dirty acoustic shadow or ring artifact. Omental hernias appear brightly echogenic because of the omental fat (see Figure 19-23).

HYDROCELE, PYOCELE, AND HEMATOCELE

A potential space exists between the visceral and parietal layers of the tunica vaginalis. This space is where a hydrocele, pyocele, or hematocele will develop. Normally, a small amount of fluid is present in this cavity and should not be confused with the presence of a hydrocele. A hydrocele contains serous fluid and is the most common cause of painless scrotal swelling. Hydroceles may have an unknown cause (idiopathic), but are commonly associated with epididymo-orchitis and torsion. They may also be found in patients following trauma or having a neoplasm. Hydroceles associated with neoplasms tend to be smaller than those associated with other causes. Pyoceles and hematoceles are much less common than hydroceles.

A pyocele is a collection of pus. Pyoceles occur with untreated infection or when an abscess ruptures into the space between the layers of the tunica vaginalis. Hematoceles are

associated with trauma, surgery, neoplasms, or torsion. They are collections of blood.

Sonographic Findings. A hydrocele displays a fluid-filled collection located outside the anterolateral aspect of the testis. Hydroceles may be anechoic, but most often contain some low-level echoes as a result of cellular debris (see Figure 19-25). The display of low-level echoes is enhanced with high-frequency transducers and harmonic imaging. Hydroceles are more likely to appear anechoic with transducer frequencies below 7 MHz or when low dynamic range settings are used. Hydroceles associated with infection show more internal echoes and septations. Sonographically, pyoceles and hematoceles are indistinguishable. They both contain internal echoes, thickened septations, and loculations (Figures 19-26 and 19-27). Ultrasound depiction of air within the space indicates an abscess, although an abscess may occur without the presence of air.

SPERM GRANULOMA

Sperm granulomas occur as a chronic inflammatory reaction to extravasation of spermatozoa. They are most frequently seen in patients with a history of vasectomy. A sperm granuloma may be located anywhere within the epididymis or the vas deferens. The main role of ultrasound imaging is to determine if

Figure 19-22 Intratesticular varicocele. **A,** Sagittal ultrasound image shows prominent connecting tubes with the testis *(arrows).* **B,** Transverse ultrasound image of both testes shows both an intratesticular and extratesticular varicocele on the left side *(arrows).* **C,** Color Doppler is used to detect flow within the dilated intratesticular veins during Valsalva maneuver.

Figure 19-23 Scrotal hernia. Sagittal ultrasound image in a patient with chronic heart failure and scrotal edema. A large amount of edema is seen in the tissue surrounding the normal testis. A small hydrocele is present. A large hernia is seen protruding into the scrotum and displacing the testis inferiorly *(arrow).* The hyperechoic appearance of the hernia suggests omental fat content.

the mass is intratesticular or extratesticular. Extratesticular masses have a much lower rate of malignancy compared with intratesticular masses. Sperm granulomas cannot be reliably differentiated from epididymal tumors by ultrasound imaging. However, a clinical history of vasectomy will help to target the differential diagnosis. Additionally, sperm granulomas are often painful. This aids in their differentiation from epididymal tumors, which are usually painless.

Sonographic Findings. Sonographic imaging shows a well-defined, solid mass that may appear hypoechoic or isoechoic to the epididymis. They are often heterogeneous (Figure 19-28). Calcifications are not commonly present. They may show increased flow with color Doppler when inflammation is present.

BENIGN TESTICULAR MASSES

Tubular Ectasia of the Rete Testis. The **rete testis** is located at the hilum of the testis where the mediastinum resides. Tubular ectasia of the rete testis is an uncommon, benign condition. It is associated with the presence of a spermatocele, epididymal, or testicular cyst or other epididymal obstruction on the same side as the dilated tubules. It is more commonly seen in patients 45 years of age or older.

Sonographic Findings. The normal rete testis may not be clearly depicted with ultrasound imaging. High-resolution

Figure 19-24 Small bowel herniated into scrotum representing scrota hernia. Peristalsis was noted on real-time imaging. *B*, bowel; *F*, fluid; *T*, testicle.

Figure 19-25 Idiopathic hydrocele formation in patient with scrotal swelling. Sagittal ultrasound view shows a large, anechoic hydrocele located posterolateral to the testis.

imaging sometimes allows visualization of the normal rete testis as very tiny tubular structures near the mediastinum. Tubular ectasia appears as prominent hypoechoic channels near the echogenic **mediastinum testis** (Figure 19-29). Color Doppler can confirm the avascular nature of the tubules. Tubular ectasia has a similar sonographic appearance to intra-testicular varicocele. These conditions can be differentiated using Doppler interrogation because the varicocele will demonstrate slow venous flow. To demonstrate slow flow, the color Doppler must be sensitized by using a low PRF and wall filter setting. The Valsalva maneuver should be used to enhance flow if a varicocele is present. If these and other adjustments are not made to the color controls, flow within a varicocele may not be detected, and results may be misinterpreted.

Cyst. Intratesticular cysts were once thought to be uncommon, but are seen more often with the more frequent use of ultrasound imaging. Cysts are more common in men over 40 years of age and have an association with extratesticular spermatoceles. They are located near the mediastinum. They may be single or multiple and of variable size. Cysts are incidental findings in sonography and do not require treatment.

Sonographic Findings. The sonographic appearance of cysts is the same throughout the body. Simple cysts are anechoic with posterior acoustic enhancement and a smooth border (Figure 19-30).

Microlithiasis. This is an uncommon condition characterized by tiny calcifications within the testis. These microcalcifications are smaller than 3 mm. Microlithiasis is usually a bilateral condition. It has been reported to have an association with testicular malignancy, but the exact nature of this is unknown. Annual follow-up of patients with testicular microlithiasis is recommended by some to exclude the development of neoplasm. Microlithiasis has also been associated

A   **B**

Figure 19-26   Pyocele formation in patient with severe, untreated epididymo-orchitis. **A,** Sagittal ultrasound image shows the multiseptated fluid collection containing internal debris *(arrow).* **B,** Color Doppler image shows increased perfusion in the epididymis, testis, and the surrounding tissue.

Figure 19-27   Hematocele in patient from the emergency room with scrotal trauma. Sagittal ultrasound image shows a small fluid collection with numerous bright echoes.

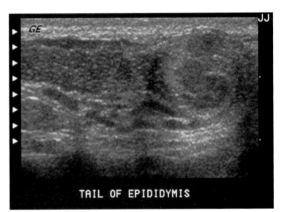

Figure 19-28   Painful epididymal mass in patient with history of vasectomy. Sagittal ultrasound image of epididymis shows a small, heterogeneous mass in the tail of the epididymis, possibly representing a sperm granuloma.

A   **B**

Figure 19-29   **A,** Mild dilation of the rete testis in patient with spermatocele. Sagittal ultrasound image shows enlarged tubular structures located near the mediastinum testis. **B,** Sagittal ultrasound image with a significant amount of dilation of the rete testis in a patient with multiple large spermatoceles.

with cryptorchidism, Klinefelter's syndrome, infertility, varicoceles, testicular atrophy, and male pseudohermaphroditism.

Sonographic Findings. The sonographic appearance of testicular microlithiasis is of multiple bright, nonshadowing foci scattered throughout the testis (Figure 19-31). The microliths may be quite numerous or few, but are not considered to be abnormal unless more than five appear on any single image (Figure 19-32).

MALIGNANT TESTICULAR MASSES

Table 19-6 lists the sonographic findings for solid malignant masses.

Germ Cell Tumors. Testicular cancer is not common, comprising only 1% of cancers in men, but it is the most common malignancy in men between the ages of 15 and 35. Fortunately, testicular cancer is one of the most curable forms of cancer. It is more common in white men than black men. Testicular cancer occurs most frequently between the ages of 20 and 34. Undescended testes are 2.5 to 8 times more likely to develop cancer.

Most patients have no other symptoms except a painless lump, testicular enlargement, or vague discomfort in the scrotum. The primary goal of the ultrasound exam in testicular tumors is to determine mass location and differentiate between cystic and solid composition. Extratesticular masses are usually benign, whereas intratesticular masses are more likely to be malignant. Intratesticular cysts are benign masses, but care must be taken to ensure a cyst is simple because some testicular cancers contain cystic components. Some benign conditions may mimic malignancy. These include hematoma, orchitis (especially when focal), abscess, infarction, and sperm granuloma. Obtaining a thorough patient history is very important because it will help to differentiate between these conditions.

In general, testicular tumors are divided into germ cell and non–germ cell tumors. Germ cell tumors are associated with an elevated level of human chorionic gonadotropin and alpha-fetoprotein. Approximately 95% of all testicular tumors are of germ cell type and are highly malignant. Non–germ cell tumors are generally benign. The most common type of germ cell tumor is seminoma, followed by mixed embryonal cell tumors and teratocarcinomas. Other less common germ cell tumors include yolk sac, choriocarcinomas, teratomas, and other combinations of these cell types. The sonographer must remember that although testicular masses can be clearly described and differentiated using ultrasound, the examination

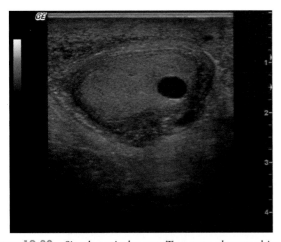

Figure 19-30   Simple testicular cyst. Transverse ultrasound image demonstrates a fluid-filled structure within the testis. Note the smooth borders and posterior acoustic enhancement.

TABLE 19-6	SOLID MALIGNANT MASSES
Tumor	Sonographic Findings
Seminoma	Hypoechoic lesion
	Smooth, well-defined borders
Embryonal cell carcinoma	Small hypoechoic mass
	Areas of increased echogenicity due to calcification
	Irregular borders
	May contain cystic areas
Teratoma	Complex mass, usually cystic and/or solid
	Well-defined borders
	Acoustic shadowing
Choriocarcinoma	Irregular borders
	Complex lesion
	Metastasis usually seen
Metastasis	Solid hypoechoic lesion (uncommonly may appear as hyperechoic or mixed echogenicity)
Lymphoma and leukemia	Enlarged testis
	Diffuse or focal areas of decreased echogenicity
Chronic lymphocytic leukemia	Well-circumscribed
	Anechoic
	Through-transmission

A   B

Figure 19-31   Testicular microlithiasis. **A,** Stitched transverse ultrasound image showing both testes with numerous brightly echogenic foci throughout. **B,** Sagittal ultrasound image showing testis with fewer microliths.

cannot confirm the histology of the neoplasm. However, the sonographic features of a mass may suggest a certain type of tumor.

Sonographic Findings. Ultrasound is nearly 100% sensitive for detecting tumors. Sonographically, most tumors appear as focal, hypoechoic masses (see Table 19-6). Seminomas tend to be homogeneous, hypoechoic masses with a smooth border (see Figure 19-27) (Figures 19-33 and 19-34). They do not often contain calcification or cystic components. In comparison, embryonal cell carcinoma is heterogeneous and less well circumscribed. It may contain areas of increased echogenicity resulting from calcification, hemorrhage, or fibrosis (see Figure 19-28). Cystic components are found in up to one third of embryonal cell carcinomas (Figure 19-35). Embryonal cell tumors are more aggressive than seminomas, often invading the tunica albuginea and distorting the testicular contour. Teratomas may show dense foci that produce acoustic shadowing. They are normally heterogeneous but have well-defined borders. Teratomas are usually benign in children but malignant in adults. Choriocarcinoma has a varied sonographic appearance because of mixed cell types. Its appearance is determined by the dominant cell type, but it typically has irregular borders (see Figure 19-29). Ultrasound imaging cannot differentiate malignant from benign masses. Neither color Doppler nor Doppler waveforms can reliably distinguish between flow patterns of benign and malignant tumors.

Metastasis. Metastasis to the testicle is rare, normally occurring later in life. The primary tumor may originate from the prostate or kidneys; less common sites include lung, pancreas, bladder, colon, thyroid, or melanoma. Metastasis to the testicle is bilateral, with multiple lesions found.

Sonographic Findings. Sonographically, metastasis appears as a solid hypoechoic mass, although it has been reported as hyperechoic or a mixture of both (see Table 19-6).

LYMPHOMA AND LEUKEMIA

Malignant lymphoma makes up 1% to 7% of all testicular tumors and is the most common bilateral secondary testicular neoplasm affecting men older than 60 years.

Leukemia involvement of the testicle is the next most common secondary testicular neoplasm, most often found in children. Of children with leukemia, 8% have been reported to have testicular involvement.

Clinically, patients may experience weight loss, anorexia, and weakness. The testicle may become enlarged, and the tumor may be bilateral or unilateral.

Sonographic Findings. Sonographically, lymphoma and leukemia appear similar. The testes may appear homogeneously hypoechoic or contain multiple focal areas of decreased echogenicity (see Table 19-6). Chronic lymphocytic leukemia may appear as a focal, well-circumscribed, anechoic mass with through-transmission. Increased vascularity is seen with color Doppler imaging.

CONGENITAL ANOMALIES

Cryptorchidism (Undescended Testicle). During fetal growth, the testes first appear in the retroperitoneum near the kidneys. They descend into the scrotum from the inguinal canal shortly before birth or early in the neonatal period. The terms *undescended testis* and **cryptorchidism** describe a condition in which the testis has not descended into the scrotum

Figure 19-32 Sagittal ultrasound image showing testis with fewer microliths. More than five microcalcifications per image is considered abnormal. Note the absence of shadowing.

A   **B**

Figure 19-33 Small seminoma. **A,** Sagittal ultrasound image shows a small, hypoechoic mass within the testis. Note the presence of a small hydrocele. **B,** Color Doppler shows increased vascularity to the mass.

A   **B**

C   **D**

Figure 19-34 Germ cell testicular tumor. **A,** Transverse ultrasound image shows heterogeneous echo texture throughout the testis. The tumor is primarily hypoechoic. **B,** Color Doppler shows distortion of the normal vessel architecture within the testis. Increased flow is seen within the mass. **C,** Power Doppler clearly shows the distorted vasculature of the testis within the mass. **D,** Spectral Doppler waveforms obtained within the mass show low resistance with prominent end diastolic velocities characteristic of tumor flow. Doppler waveforms have not been shown to reliably differentiate between benign and malignant flow patterns.

Figure 19-35 Heterogeneous testicular tumor. Sagittal ultrasound image of a testicular tumor containing calcium and cystic components. Although this pattern is not specific, it is more typical of embryonal cell tumor.

and cannot be brought into the scrotum with external manipulation. The undescended testis may be located in the abdomen, inguinal canal, or other ectopic location. In most cases (up to 80%) the testis is found in the inguinal canal and is usually palpable. Since the testes do not descend until late in pregnancy, this condition is more common in premature babies. Cryptorchidism is bilateral in 10% to 25% of cases.

Surgical treatment of an undescended testicle by freeing it from the structures and implanting it into the scrotum is known as *orchiopexy.* If orchiopexy is not performed at an early age, multiple complications can occur. The exposure of the testis to higher temperatures than when it is located in the scrotum can prohibit spermatogenesis and result in infertility. Undescended testes are much more likely to develop testicular cancer. The risk of cancer is not reduced by orchiopexy, but it does allow the testis to be more easily palpated so that a lump may be detected and treated earlier. Testicular torsion is also more common with undescended testes.

Sonographic Findings. On ultrasound, the undescended testis is smaller and less echogenic than the normal testis. It is

Figure 19-36 Undescended right testicle **(A)** with normal left testicle **(B)**. The undescended testis is smaller and hypoechoic compared with the normal left testis. The right testicle was located within the right inguinal canal.

usually oval with a homogeneous texture (Figure 19-36). Rarely, the mediastinum is seen.

Testicular Ectopia. Testicular ectopia is a very rare condition. Unlike an undescended testicle, an ectopic testicle cannot be manipulated into the correct path of descent. The most common site for the ectopic testicle to rest is the superficial inguinal pouch. Other sites include perineum, femoral canal, suprapubic area, penis, diaphragm, and the other scrotal compartment.

Anorchia. Anorchia is also rare. Unilateral anorchia, or monorchidism, is found in 4% of patients with a nonpalpable testis. It is more common on the left side, and definitive diagnosis depends on surgical diagnosis. Causes include intrauterine testicular torsion or other forms of decreased vascular supply to the testicle in utero. Bilateral anorchia is only found in 0.6% to 1.0% of patients with a nonpalpable testis. Patients have a male XY genotype. On physical examination, the **scrotum** is an empty, hypoplastic sac with a micropenis. These patients also have delayed onset of puberty, usually caused by an imbalance of hormones.

Polyorchidism (Testicular Duplication). Polyorchidism is a very rare disorder, with only 80 cases reported. It is more common on the left side (75%) and bilateral in 5% of cases. The testicular duplication is usually found in the scrotum, but has also been found in the inguinal canal or retroperitoneum. There is an increased incidence of malignancy, cryptorchidism, inguinal hernia, and torsion with polyorchidism. The duplicated testis is usually small, and its efferent spermatic system is completely absent.

SELECTED BIBLIOGRAPHY

American College of Radiology: *ACR standard for performance of scrotal ultrasound examination,* Available: http://www.acr.org, 2001.

Berman JM, Beidle TR, Kunberger LE and others: Sonographic evaluation of acute intrascrotal pathology, *AJR* 166:857-861, 1996.

Black JAR, Patel A: Sonography of the abnormal extratesticular space, *AJR* 167:507-511, 1996.

Bree RL, Hoang DT: Scrotal ultrasound, *Radiol Clin North Am* 34(6):1183, 1996.

Dambro TJ, Stewart RR, Carroll, BA: The scrotum. In Rumack CM, Wilson SR, Willi J, editors: *Diagnostic ultrasound,* vol 1, ed 2, St Louis, 1998, Mosby.

Dogra VS, Gottlieb RH, Oka M and others: Sonography of the scrotum, *Radiology* 227:18-36, 2003.

Feole JB, Lee FT Jr: Doppler sonography in testicular and scrotal imaging, *Current Opin Urol* 8(2):87, 1998.

Figler TJ, Olson MC, Kinzler GJ: Polyorchidism and rete testis adenoma: ultrasound and MR findings, *Abdom Imaging* 21(5):470, 1996.

Hall R: *The ultrasound handbook,* ed 2, Philadelphia, 1993, JB Lippincott.

Healey JE, Seybold WD: *A synopsis of clinical anatomy,* Philadelphia, 1969, WB Saunders.

Horstmann WG, Middleton WD, Melson GL: Scrotal inflammatory disease: color Doppler sonographic findings, *Radiology* 179:55, 1991.

Hricak H: *Imaging of the scrotum,* New York, 1995, Raven.

Morse MJ, Whitmere WF: Neoplasm of the testis. In Walsh P and others, editors: *Cambell's urology,* ed 5, Philadelphia, 1986, WB Saunders.

Oh C, Nisenbaum HL, Langer J and others: Sonographic demonstration, including color Doppler imaging of recurrent sperm granulomas, *JUM* 19:333-335, 2000.

Older RA, Watson LR: Tubular ectasia of the rete testis: a benign condition with a sonographic appearance that may be misinterpreted as malignant, *J Urol* 152:477-478, 1994.

Prando D: Torsion of the spermatic cord, *Ultrasound Q* 18(1):41-57, 2002.

Ragheb D, Higgins JL: Ultrasonography of the scrotum, technique, anatomy, and pathologic entities, *J Ultrasound Med* 21:171-185, 2002.

Weiss AJ, Kellman GM, Middleton WD and others: Intratesticular varicocele: sonographic findings in two patients, *AJR* 158:1061-1063, 1992.

CHAPTER 20

The Musculoskeletal System

Susan Raatz Stephenson

KEY TERMS

acromioclavicular joint (AC) – the joint found in the shoulder that connects the clavicle to the acromion process of the scapula

anisotropy – the quality of comprising varying values of a given property when measured in different directions

aponeurosis – bandlike flat tendons connecting muscle to the bone

bursa – a saclike structure containing thick fluid that surrounds areas subject to friction, such as the interface between bone and tendon

cartilage interface sign – echogenic line on the anterior surface of the cartilage surrounding the humeral head

clapper-in-the-bell sign – hypoechoic hematoma found at the end of a completely retracted muscle fragment

comet tail artifact (ring-down) – posterior linear equidistant artifact created when sound reverberates between two strong reflectors, such as air bubbles, metal, and glass

dorsiflexion – upward movement of the hand or foot

epineurium – the covering of a nerve that consists of connective tissue

fasciculi – term describing a small bundle of muscles, nerves, and tendons

Guyon's canal or tunnel – a fibrous tunnel that contains the ulnar artery and vein, ulnar nerve, and some fatty tissue

ligament – fibrous band of tissue connecting bone or cartilage to bone that aids in stabilizing a joint

muscle – a type of tissue consisting of contractile cells or fibers that affects movement of an organ or part of the body

myelin – substance forming the sheath of Schwann cells

naked tuberosity sign – the deltoid muscle is on the humeral head; seen with a full-thickness tear of the rotator cuff

pennate – featherlike pattern of muscle growth

perineurium – the surrounding connective tissue of muscle

Phalen's sign (Phalen's test, Phalen's maneuver, or Phalen's position) – an increase in wrist compression due to hyperflexion of the wrist for 60 seconds; this test is done with the patient holding the forearms upright and pressing the ventral side of the hands together

plantar flexion – pointing of the toes toward the plantar surface of the foot

refractile shadowing (edge artifact) – the bending of the sound beam at the edge of a circular structure, resulting in the absence of posterior echoes

seroma – accumulation of serous fluid within tissue

synovial sheath – membrane surrounding a joint, tendon, or bursa that secretes a viscous fluid called synovia

tendinitis (tendinopathy, tendinosis, or tenosynovitis) – inflammation of a tendon

tendon – fibrous tissue connecting muscle to bone

Thompson's test – a test used to evaluate the integrity of the Achilles' tendon that involves plantar flexion with squeezing of the calf

Tinel's sign (Hoffmann-Tinel sign, Tinel's symptom, or Tinel-Hoffmann sign) – pins-and-needles type tingling felt distally to a percussion site. Sensation can be either an abnormal or a normal occurrence (i.e., hitting the elbow creates a tingling in the distal arm).

volar – the anterior portion of the body when in the anatomical position

---

In the early 1990s a radiologist asked me to try to image a torn suprapatellar tendon. It was difficult to image the torn tendon because of technologic limitations and our inexperience in musculoskeletal (MS) ultrasound imaging. Musculoskeletal imaging is now gaining in popularity in the United States, following in the wake of the magnetic resonance imaging (MRI). However, ultrasound of the musculoskeletal system has been widely used outside of the United States.

Many things have changed in the past 10 years, both in the delivery of medical care and in the production of sonographic images. The decrease in medical reimbursements has forced development of less expensive modalities to complement or replace CT or MRI. Ultrasound equipment manufacturers have also continued to improve and refine technology, which has resulted in improved soft tissue imaging. The 5- or 7-MHz transducer commonly used in the nineties is hardly acceptable for scanning superficial structures today. Current transducers image with frequencies as high as 17 MHz.

This chapter is intended to provide a solid foundation for basic musculoskeletal ultrasound (MSUS). Imaging of the muscular system is not limited to the muscles themselves, but also includes the tendons, nerves, ligaments, and bursa. Other areas of musculoskeletal (MS) imaging include the joints, pediatric imaging, bone, skin, many disease processes, foreign bodies, and postoperative scanning. Add the joint specific scanning, shoulder, knee, ankle, elbow, and wrist, and you begin to understand that MSUS imaging is a significant area that we have just begun to explore.

ANATOMY OF THE MUSCULOSKELETAL SYSTEM

Normal Anatomy

Skeletal muscle contains long organized units called muscle fibers. The characteristic long fibers are under voluntary control, allowing us to contract a **muscle** and move a joint. The blood vessels, lymphatics, and nerves follow the fibrous partitions between the bundles of muscle.

Several different types of muscles are present in the human body. Muscles have fibers that run parallel to the bone, have a fan shape, or form a **pennate** pattern. These featherlike muscle patterns run oblique to the long axis of the muscle and are unipennate, bipennate, multipennate, or circumpennate. Think of a feather and how the fibers grow from a central section. Half of this feather is unipennate, whereas the whole feather is bipennate. A multipennate muscle is a division of several featherlike sections in one muscle, whereas the circumpennate is the convergence of fibers to a central tendon (Figure 20-1, *A*). The deltoid muscle is an example of a unipennate muscle and has featherlike fascicles with a unipennate, bipennate, or multipennate attachment (Figure 20-1, *B*). The gastrocnemius muscle in the calf is a bipennate muscle where the fibers have a central origin (Figure 20-1, *C*). The large, flat muscles of the external oblique or the trapezius attach with a large, flat aponeurosis (Figure 20-1, *D*).

Attachment of the muscle occurs at the proximal and distal portions of the bundle. This attachment, a collection of tough collagenous fibers, is a **tendon.** These attachments are either cordlike or flat sheets called **aponeuroses.** This type of attachment occurs in the flat muscles, such as the rectus abdominis in the abdomen. The elastic tendon consists of collagen fibers that enable it to stretch and flex around structures. This avascular structure heals slowly and has a whitish appearance. Due to the lack of vascularity, tendons heal slowly, which is why an injury can incapacitate a patient.

Tendons occur with or without a **synovial sheath.** This tubular sac surrounding a tendon has two layers. Fluid separates the two layers of the sheath and occurs in the shoulder, hand, wrist, and ankle. This sheath plays an important role in imaging these structures with sonography. The biceps tendon of the shoulder is one example of a tendon with a synovial sheath. Other tendons, such as the Achilles' and patellar, lack this sheath and have a surrounding fat layer or loose connective tissue. This makes this type of tendon more difficult to image with sonography.

Support and strength of a joint are due in part to the **ligaments**. These short bands of tough fibers connect bones to other bones. This type of connective tissue is especially important in the knees, ankles, and shoulders.

The saclike structure surrounding joints and tendons containing a viscous fluid is the **bursa.** This potential space provides an area for synovial fluid to aid in the reduction of friction between two musculoskeletal structures, such as tendon and bone or ligament and bone. For example, two of the knee joints that have such a bursa are the patellofemoral and femorotibial joint. The suprapatellar pouch has a continuous connection with the joint cavity, but is often referred to as a bursa. The knee joint itself has nine bursa, three located anterior and six on the popliteal side of the joint.

Nerves are the conduit for impulses to and from the muscles and central nervous system (CNS). Muscle action is under the control of the muscle system with the nerves in contact with the muscle through motor end plates. Elements of the nerves include the nerve fibers, arranged into bundles **(fasciculi)** and surrounded by dense insulating sheaths of

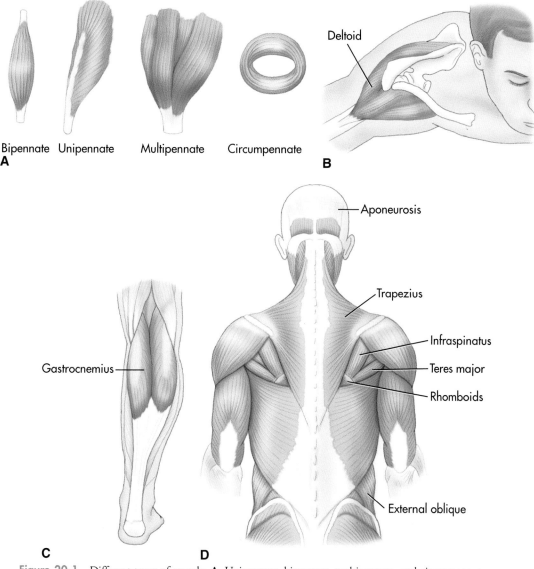

Figure 20-1   Different types of muscle. **A,** Unipennate, bipennate, multipennate, and circumpennate muscle patterns. **B,** The deltoid muscle is an example of a unipennate muscle and has featherlike fascicles with a unipennate, bipennate, or multipennate attachment. **C,** The gastrocnemius muscle in the calf is a bipennate muscle, whose fibers have a central origin. **D,** The large, flat muscles of the external oblique or the trapezius attach with a large, flat aponeurosis.

myelin (forms the sheath of Schwann cells), and connective tissue.

NORMAL SONOGRAPHIC APPEARANCE

Imaging of the musculoskeletal system can be quite overwhelming because there are so many different muscles, attachments, ligaments, and tendons. Each joint contains similar anatomic structures, with tendons and ligaments having the same sonographic imaging characteristics whether they are part of an ankle or a shoulder. Muscle attachments also have a similar sonographic appearance. The first step in sonographic imaging of any MS structure is knowledge of the normal appearance.

Tendons. Magnetic resonance imaging (MRI) has been the modality of choice for physicians in the United States when

diagnosing MS problems. The advent of high-resolution ultrasound has challenged the superiority of MRI for imaging tendons, especially when the examination is performed by a skilled sonographer using high-quality equipment. The evolution of real-time ultrasound allows demonstration of the full range of motion of the tendon. High resolution of modern transducers also allows for imaging of the fine tendon fibers and for comparison of the normal with the abnormal using dual imaging techniques. Sonography has the ability to supersede MRI in MS imaging in the hands of a skilled sonographer using high-quality equipment.

The tendon occurs in two forms, with and without a synovial sheath (Figure 20-2). Wrapped around the tendon, the smooth inner layer of this tubular sac lies in close contact with the tendon. Between this inner layer and an outer layer a small amount of thick mucinoid material helps facilitate movement. The biceps tendon is one example of a sheath-covered tendon that images well (Figure 20-3). The thickness of this sheath is only a couple of millimeters and is sonographically imaged as a hypoechoic halo surrounding the tendon. Inflammation of this sheath and tendon often aids in imaging and diagnosing problems with this tendon. Acute disease may reveal a sheath that is thicker than the contained tendon. Areas of high stress in the hand, wrist, and ankle also contain tendons with sheaths.

Paratenon, a loose areolar connective tissue, fills the fascial compartment of the tendon lacking a synovial sheath. The dense epitendineum, another layer of connective tissue, closely adjoins the tendon. The epitendineum images as an echogenic layer adjacent to the tendon. The lack of density differences in these interfaces makes the tendon somewhat difficult to image. Fortunately, many of the tendons without a synovial sheath are large and image relatively well. The accompanying bursa may also be abnormal, enhancing the tendon. Examples of this type of tendon include the Achilles', patellar, proximal gastrocnemius, and the semimembranosus tendons (Figure 20-4).

Interwoven and interconnected collagen fibers found in the tendon run in a parallel path. The numerous interfaces of the collagen fascicles provide a strong linear reflector that images well with ultrasound. The higher the frequency of the imaging transducer, the better these fibers image, underscoring the need for a transducer of 7 MHz or higher. This normal fibrillar hypoechoic pattern and imaging detail become very important when diagnosing abnormalities.

Care must be taken when imaging the tendon because even a slight rotation off axis may produce an image that incorrectly suggests tendinitis. Both the transverse and longitudinal planes help image the tendon along with a side-by-side (dual) comparison of the contralateral side.

The tendon insertion site has its own sonographic characteristics. The joining of the tendon to the bone occurs (enthesis) with a narrow band of fibrocartilage. This avascular structure is approximately 1 cm long and images longitudinally as a triangular hypoechoic area in the distal tendon. Familiarity with the normal sonographic appearance is important because injury to this area of the tendon results in thickening of the insertion site (Figure 20-5).

Ligaments. Ligaments are thin, superficial structures making them difficult to image. This superficial location requires the use of a higher frequency transducer, 10 MHz or greater, and possibly a standoff pad to aid in imaging ligaments outside the joint. Critical to ligament identification is the equipment parameter adjustment. Adding too much gain to the image with either the overall gain or time gain compensation (TGC) results in loss of detail because of the strong bone reflections. Unlike imaging in other areas of the body, longitudinal imaging of the ligament is the only method used to image injuries. Transverse planes are of little help when imaging the ligament as a result of blending with the surrounding fat. The difficulty in imaging the ligament is helped by using the dual or side-by-side technique to compare the normal and abnormal anatomy.

Many ligaments in the large joints of the body image well as hyperechoic straplike structures (Figure 20-6). One exception is the cruciate ligament within the knee joint, which appears hypoechoic. The large joints include the hip, shoulder,

Figure 20-2 Superficial and deep flexor tendons *(stars)* have a surrounding synovial sheath allowing for smooth motion of the pulley system of the hand. Tendon movement can be seen in real time with movement of the fingers.

Figure 20-3 This transverse view of the rounded biceps tendon **(A)** images the tendon as a hyperechoic structure sitting within the bicipital groove of the humerus *(arrow)*. The longitudinal view **(B)** has the characteristic pattern seen with tendons encased within a synovial sheath *(arrows)*.

Figure 20-4   A cross-section or transverse view of the distal Achilles' tendon **(A)** demonstrates the characteristic oval appearance. The tendon changes shape with decreased use, becoming round in the sedentary individual. The lack of synovial sheath is evident on the longitudinal image of the tendon **(B).** A slight increase in echogenicity *(arrows)* on each side of the tendon is the epitendineum.

Figure 20-5   The normal Achilles' tendon insertion *(arrow)* images at that insertion on the calcaneus and mimics cartilage found in other parts of the body.

Figure 20-6   The coracohumeral ligament *(between arrows)* helps maintain the proper location of the long biceps tendon within the bicipital groove. This biceps tendon demonstrates tenosynovitis, inflammation of the tendon and sheath, which results in a hypoechoic appearance.

ankle, wrist, and knee. Part of the difficulty in imaging the ligament is the lack of a contiguous structure, such as muscle, to aid in location. The dense fibers have a slightly less regular appearance and may help hold a tendon in place. Usually the ligament measures 2 to 3 mm thick and images as a hypoechoic band with a homogeneous appearance. These ligament structures are found close to both ends attaching to the bony cortex.

One ligament—the median collateral ligament (MCL) or tibial collateral ligament, which connects the medial femoral condyle to the medial proximal tibia—deviates from the usual ligament appearance. This wide, smooth ligament is about 9 cm long and has deep and superficial portions. The external superficial portion is connective tissue appearing as a dense band that connects the medial femoral condyle to the proximal tibia. The deep layer connects the medial meniscus to the femur and tibia.

Sonographic imaging of the MCL reveals a three-layer structure. The superficial and deep layers have a hypoechoic-separating layer. Loose connective tissue forms this middle layer and is a potential space for bursa in some individuals (Figure 20-7).

Muscle.   Discussions of muscle quite often contain references to the origin and insertion of the muscle. The proximal portion of the muscle is considered the origin, whereas the

insertion is the distal end. A muscle with two or more heads has an origin in more than one place on the bone. Most of us do not think in terms of origins and insertions, so for the purpose of this discussion, we will talk in terms of the location or attachment of the muscle will be used.

To begin learning the normal appearance of the muscle, it is easy to use the large quadriceps muscle located in the anterior thigh or the posterior calf muscles. Skeletal muscle imaged on a longitudinal plane appears homogeneous with multiple, fine, parallel echoes (Figure 20-8). Connective tissue surrounding the fiber bundles produces these echogenic bands. The main portions of the muscle fibers are hypoechoic and radiate toward a central tendon or aponeurosis (Figure 20-9). The transverse plane discloses a less organized pattern of fine punctuate echoes scattered through the muscle bundle. Encasing the muscle is a connective tissue fascia that has a bright echogenic appearance (Figures 20-10 and 20-11). This fascia layer, though brighter than the sheathed muscle fibers, has less echogenicity than subcutaneous fat or tendons.

The muscle bundle contains nerves, fascia, tendons, fat, and the fibrous connective tissue surrounding the muscle. The

Figure 20-7 The fibular collateral ligament connects the fibula to the lateral side of the femur. This hypoechoic linear structure *(arrows)* passes over the lateral meniscus and has a slightly oblique course.

Figure 20-9 The dense aponeurosis tissue that connects the muscle to bone images as an echogenic linear structure *(arrows).*

Figure 20-8 The bipennate gastrocnemius muscle has echogenic obliquely oriented connective tissue *(solid arrow)* between the muscle bundles. A small central tendon *(open arrow)* serves as the anchor for these bundles.

Figure 20-10 Panoramic imaging allows for a global study of this normal gastrocnemius muscle.

epimysium continues into the muscle developing into the perimysium, which separates the bundles into muscle fibers. These hypoechoic structures, when compared with the muscle fibers, help differentiate muscles. The sonographic appearance of muscle can be deceiving in some areas, such as the hand, because of the similarity of echo texture to a mass or tenosynovitis. Careful scanning and transducer rotation help image the pinnate structure of the muscle, aiding in identification of a possible normal muscle variant.

Normal dynamics of the muscle image easily in real time since contraction of the muscle increases the muscle thickness and hypoechogenicity. In addition, the echogenic connective tissue bands increase in obliquity. Sustained contraction of the muscle has the same sonographic appearance as the muscle bundles found in the athletic patient. This decreased echogenic muscle, as a result of hypertrophy, is normal for this patient population. Compression of the muscle with the transducer condenses the tissue, resulting in an increase in the echogenicity of the muscle.

Transducer orientation is another factor that influences the muscle echogenicity. Ensuring a longitudinal and transverse

Figure 20-11 Small punctuate echogenicities *(arrows)* image on the transverse muscle.

plane with good contact helps negate the possibility of introducing artifactual information. It is helpful to scan the contralateral normal side to ensure technique or to ensure that normal variants do not result in a misdiagnosis.

Nerves. The normal nerve has a hyperechoic appearance when compared with muscle but is hypoechoic compared with tendons. The echogenicity depends on the surrounding structures and is not constant within the body. The longitudinal plane reveals a fibrillar pattern with parallel inner linear echoes similar to the tendon. In transverse imaging the nerve fibers appear hypoechoic, with a hyperechoic **perineurium** surrounding each fiber. The collagenous **epineurium**, the outer layer of the nerve, appears as a hyperechoic layer (Figures 20-12 and 20-13).

Differentiating the nerves from tendons is a simple task when you contrast the two structures. Real-time imaging shows tendons that move when the corresponding joint or muscle contracts. The nerve will remain stable within the muscle tissue. Sonographic artifacts (anisotropy) are not as evident on the nerve as they are on the tendon, and the nerves are imaged best with a transducer of 10 MHz or higher. Power Doppler is especially helpful because vessels accompany the nerves. Table 20-1 lists the nerves that are identifiable with sonography.

Bursa. The small sac between two moving surfaces, usually tendon and bone, is the bursa. These fluid-filled cavities facilitate the movement of tendons or muscles over bony projections. The minute amount of viscous fluid contained within the bursa helps reduce friction between the moving parts of the joint (Figures 20-14 and 20-15). The major bursa of the body is the subacromial-subdeltoid bursa found in the shoulder covering the deep surface of the deltoid muscle.

Two types of bursa are found in the body: communicating and noncommunicating. This categorization helps explain the relationship of the bursa to the joint space. One communicating bursa sonographers often see is the Baker cyst, which is located in the medial popliteal fossa. This bursa, located between the semimembranosus and medial gastrocnemius tendons, has a connecting neck to the bursa contained within the knee joint. Usually, sonographers image bursa that do not communicate with the joint space. An example of a superficial noncommunicating type of bursa is the prepatellar bursa.

In the normal patient, the bursas are difficult to image because they often blend in with the surrounding tissue and fat. The thin film of viscous fluid found within the bursa contributes to the hypoechoic appearance of the structure since the walls are too thin to image. These potential spaces will

Figure 20-12   The median nerve runs on the ventral side of the forearm and wrist supplying the muscles of the superficial layers of the forearm and hand. The hypoechoic nerve *(arrows)* sits just anterior to the echogenic deep flexor tendon of the index finger *(T)*.

TABLE 20-1	NERVES IDENTIFIABLE WITH SONOGRAPHY
Lower Limb	Location
Sciatic	Posterior thigh lateral to the hamstring muscle
Popliteal	Popliteal fossa superficial to the popliteal artery and vein
Upper Limb	Location
Suprascapular	Deep to the trapezius to the infraspinatus fossa
Median	Medial to the biceps tendon and brachial artery, elbow, right side of the carpal tunnel
Radial	Between the brachioradialis and brachialis muscles
Ulnar	Median epicondyle of the elbow, medial to the ulnar artery in the Guyon's canal

Figure 20-13   The transverse scan of the median nerve reveals the hyperechoic nerves with hypoechoic nerve fiber fascicles.

Figure 20-14   This normal infrapatellar tendon has multiple bursas, which usually blend in with the surrounding tissue. One lies between the skin and fascia anterior to the tibial tuberosity *(arrow)* and a deep bursa lies between the patellar ligament and the tibial tuberosity *(open arrow)*. The knee itself has a total of nine bursa located in and around the joint.

appear on ultrasound in the presence of an inflammatory process caused by fluid accumulation. Any bursa measuring greater than 2 mm is enlarged and needs to be compared with the normal contralateral side.

Table 20-2 summarizes the normal sonographic appearance of tendons, ligaments, nerves, muscle, and bursa.

ARTIFACTS

Sonographers and sonologists have the daily challenge of separating artifacts from useful image information. All equipment manufacturers program in some basic assumptions about the interaction between tissue and sound: that the speed of sound is 1540 m/sec, that the area imaged is within the central beam, and that sound travels out and back in a straight line. Artifacts occur when these basic assumptions are not met and create something that is not real, is erroneously positioned, has improper brightness, or is absent from the image. Many manufacturers have developed technology to reduce and often

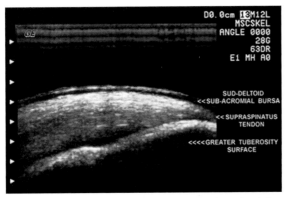

Figure 20-15 New technologies, such as 3-D, have the ability to remove surrounding tissue signals from the data set. This capability makes this modality ideal for imaging of the bursa. This subdeltoid-subacromial bursa image clearly demonstrates the external synovial layer with the hypoechoic lubricating fluid.

eliminate some types of artifacts caused by compound and harmonic imaging.

Musculoskeletal imaging displays the same gamut of artifacts seen in other areas of the body. The superficial nature of the MS structures, often anterior to the highly reflective bone, results in artifacts becoming more of a problem. Some artifacts aid in identifying pathologic conditions and structures; however, others hinder and even mimic disease.

Several artifact types—anisotropy, reverberation, time of flight artifact, and refractile shadowing—are important in MSUS. Understanding how artifacts occur and how to correct images increases both diagnostic confidence and image accuracy.

ANISOTROPY

The anisotropic phenomenon is one that occurs not only in sonography but also in other professions, such as astronomy, geology, and chemistry. **Anisotropy** occurs when the sound beam misses the transducer on the return because of the curve of the structure (Figure 20-16). The angle and direction of the reflected beam depend upon the angle of incidence.

The reflection coefficient is a function of angle and becomes a problem when the reflected beam misses the receiver. The nonperpendicular tissue interfaces return echoes at an angle that does not return to the transmitting transducer, creating an imaging challenge. This results in differing image properties depending on the angle of incidence.

The loss of definition of the curved upper pole of the right kidney is one example of this artifact. The muscle, ligaments, and nerves also image as an anisotropic reflector because of the plane they occupy, with tendons having the most pronounced anisotropy in MS imaging. This loss of image requires a heel-to-toe rocking of the transducer to create the optimal 90-degree angle (Figures 20-17 and 20-18).

REVERBERATION

A reflective surface reverberates sound and is either beneficial or detrimental. We often experience this phenomenon without

TABLE 20-2	NORMAL SONOGRAPHIC APPEARANCE		
Anatomy	General Sonographic Appearance	Longitudinal Appearance	Transverse Appearance
Tendon	Hyperechoic linear structure Dynamic with movement of corresponding joint/muscle	Cordlike	Oval, round, or cuboid

Ligament	Isoechoic, weakly hyperechoic	Striated structures connecting bone
		  to bone
			Difficult to image on the transverse
			  plane

Nerve	Hypoechoic to tendons Hyperechoic to muscle Cannot be mobilized with movement Posterior enhancement lacking	Cordlike tubular structure	Hypoechoic with fascicles

Muscle	Muscular bundles—hypoechoic
	Perimysium, epimysium, fascia, fat
	  plane—hyperechoic
		Parallel echogenic linear appearance
		  within hypoechoic muscle tissue;
		  may appear featherlike depending
		  on the type of muscle imaged
			Punctate echogenic areas within
			  the hypoechoic muscle

Bursa	Thin, hypoechoic structure that merges
	  with the surrounding fat
		Thin linear hypoechoic structure
		  adjacent to a tendon
			Normal bursa are difficult to
			  image on the transverse plane

realizing its impact. Our senses use reverberation as a clue to the location of structures in a room through reflection of sound back to our ears. Any acoustic environment, such as an auditorium, relies on reverberation to transmit sound.

The same is true of sound transmitted into the body. The initial sound beam transmits and returns. Multiple delayed reflections from strong tissue boundaries, such as bone, result in a linear artifact that *decreases* in intensity with depth. This collection of reflected sound is superimposed over the primary signal, often adding distracting information to the image (Figure 20-19).

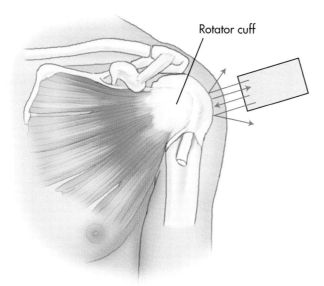

Figure 20-16   A perpendicular or 90-degree angle of the sound beam to the reflecting tissue surface results in the greatest amount of reflection occurring providing optimal images. At nonperpendicular incidence, part of the incident sound beam misses the transducer resulting in the display of decreased brightness of the returning echoes.

Reverberation is not always a detrimental process. One type of artifact, comet tail, results from reverberation from metal, such as clips, sutures, staples, or a foreign object like a BB. This type varies slightly from the traditional reverberation, which bounces between the transducer face and the strong reflector. The **comet tail artifact** is a function of the sound bouncing between two closely placed reflectors within the imaged structure. In the case of a pin surgically placed within a bone, the reflecting surfaces are the anterior and posterior borders of the hardware. The ringing occurs within the metal object, and each time the sound returns to the anterior border some of the sound escapes. The resultant artifact resembles a comet tail, hence its name (Figure 20-20).

REFRACTILE SHADOWING

The bending of the transmitted sound beam to an oblique path occurs often and is seen as an edge artifact (**refractile shadowing**) on the sonographic image. This change in direction of the sound beam results in a hypoechoic band posterior to the structure. Another cause of refractile shadowing is a tissue impedance mismatch different than the average speed of sound within soft tissue (1540 m/sec). This is seen at the edge of a round or oval ligament or as the result of a traumatic tear of an MS structure (Figures 20-21 and 20-22). Most commonly seen with a complete tendon tear, the angles formed from the retracted tendon cause refractile shadowing. This shadowing is often used to determine the distance between the ligaments by measuring from one artifact edge to the other.

TIME OF FLIGHT ARTIFACT

Time of flight or speed of sound artifacts occur when the returning sound wave has passed between two tissues with markedly different speeds. This misrepresentation of the return time results from the assumption that the speed of sound is a constant 1540 m/sec. If the speed of sound is less than the average in tissue, the artifact appears to be further away from the transducer. Faster speed results in the artifact being closer

A   **B**

Figure 20-17   These images of the median nerve and the deep flexor tendon illustrate the effects of anisotropy. **A,** A large artifact occurred because the angle of incidence is not 90 degrees, resulting in a hypoechoic appearance of the tendon and nerve *(arrow).* **B,** Rocking the transducer or repositioning the structure allows for the angle of incidence to be closer to 90 degrees, thus reducing or eliminating the artifact.

Figure 20-18   Change in direction of the imaged structure (digital flexor tendon) causes multiple areas of anisotropy (yellow arrows) because of the changes in the angle of incidence.

Figure 20-19   Reverberation artifact resultant from sound bouncing between the strongly reflecting bone and the transducer face.

Figure 20-20   Comet tail artifact *(arrows)* seen posterior to tibial pins placed to stabilize a tibial fracture. Note the widening of the posterior reverberation, which is due to the reverberation within the metal pins. This widening is common with metal placed within MS structures and is still a comet tail artifact even though it does not narrow in the distal area.

Figure 20-21   This ganglion located in the ankle demonstrates retractile shadowing.

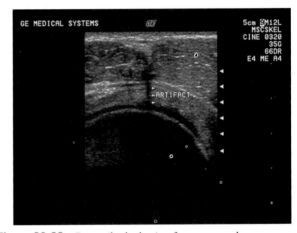

Figure 20-22   Retractile shadowing from a normal structure anterior to the area of interest (supraspinatus tendon) makes it difficult to diagnose abnormalities.

Figure 20-23   This panoramic rotator cuff tear demonstrates the very subtle time of flight artifact.

to the transducer on the image. Creation of this type of false information occurs most commonly with MSUS when imaging obese patients at a muscle-fat interface (Figure 20-23).

The speed of sound artifact displaces the image in the anteroposterior (axial) plane. When this speed artifact is coupled with refraction, a structure displays with an incorrect shape. For example, think of a wall of bricks. If one section

fails and drops down, the result is that one section is asymmetric from the surrounding areas. Do not mistake this very subtle artifact with a transducer crystal malfunction. A mechanical failure produces a decrease in image information

TABLE 20-3	CORRECTION TECHNIQUES FOR ARTIFACTS
Artifact	Correction Technique
Anisotropy	Heel-to-toe rocking of the transducer creates a perpendicular angle of incidence removing the anisotropy.
Reverberation	Anterior reverberation can be minimized with the use of a standoff pad or changing the angle of incidence.
Refractile shadowing	Use of newer technologies, such as compound imaging or tissue harmonics, helps reduce or eliminate this artifact. Changing the angle of incidence may move the artifact out of the region of interest.
Time of flight artifact	May not be able to eliminate as a result of tissue sound properties. Change the angle of incidence to demonstrate surrounding tissue.

Figure 20-24 The subscapularis, biceps tendon, and the acromioclavicular joint image easily from the anterior approach. This is considered a neutral position for the shoulder.

that begins at the transducer face, while the time of flight artifact affects only the image.

Table 20-3 lists the techniques for correcting the artifacts discussed previously.

SONOGRAPHIC EVALUATION OF THE MUSCULOSKELETAL SYSTEM

Sonographic imaging of the joints begins with the proper choice of transducers. Superficially located joints and structures image well with high-frequency transducers of 5 MHz or higher. The more superficial the imaged structure is, the higher the transducer frequency must be to ensure maximal detail; however, larger joints, such as the shoulder, may require a lower frequency to penetrate the MS structures.

Positioning of the joint of interest is an important part of the examination. The patient should be placed in a comfortable position that allows the sonographer to maintain correct scanning ergonomics to prevent development of MS problems. A final consideration is the dynamic portion of the examination. It is often helpful to be able to move the joint to confirm the imaged structure. Space must be allowed for a full range of motion for the imaged joint.

ROTATOR CUFF

The American Institute for Ultrasound Medicine (AIUM) recommends middle frequencies of 7 and 10 MHz for imaging the shoulder structures; however, the deeper rotator cuff structures may require a frequency of 5 MHz. Shoulder anatomy is quite complex with the numerous bursas, muscles, and tendons that surround the joint. A basic sonographic examination of the structures found in the rotator cuff includes 11 images. Comparison with the contralateral normal shoulder is always helpful in determining the absence or presence of a pathologic condition.

The biceps tendon is one of the easiest structures to image in the adult shoulder. Similar to any examination, documen-

tation includes both longitudinal and transverse views. Begin by having the patient sit erect on a rotating chair with a back. The rotation of the chair allows for quick and easy readjustments to the shoulder. To begin the examination of the biceps tendons, place the patient with a slight internal rotation of the shoulder. To obtain this position, have the patient place the arm on the lap with the fingers of the hand facing the opposite shoulder (Figure 20-24).

Begin the examination by facing the patient and checking the transducer orientation to prevent confusion during scanning. The structures will change with the particular shoulder being imaged. When facing the patient and imaging the right shoulder, the lateral anatomy displays on the left side of the image and the medial anatomy on the right side of the screen. When scanning posterior shoulder structures, the image corresponds to the patient position.

Begin the examination with the 3 to 5 mm thick biceps tendon. This tendon is easily located in the transverse plane and images as an echogenic oval structure within the bicipital groove of the humerus. This groove, located between the greater and lesser tuberosities, coupled with the overlying transverse ligament, maintains the biceps tendon location. Once identified, images at several different levels help determine normalcy. A small amount of fluid, less than 1.5 mm, is a normal finding. Care must be taken to use minimal transducer pressure because small amounts of fluid may be compressed out of the imaging plane (Figure 20-25). A longitudinal image of the tendon requires some rocking of the transducer to obtain images with minimal anisotropic artifacts. When scanning the biceps tendon, take note of the fibrillar pattern of the normal tendon because disruptions indicate a possible pathologic condition (Figure 20-26).

Finding the subscapularis tendon begins by imaging the biceps tendon on the transverse plane at the level of the

Figure 20-25   A, The transverse view of the normal biceps tendon has the echogenic tendon *(T)* within the bicipital groove. The anechoic effusion of tenosynovitis surrounding the tendon aids in visualization. **B,** Diagram of the anatomy.

Figure 20-26   A, The longitudinal image of the biceps tendon *(arrows)* images the fibrillar pattern seen with tendons. The small amount of effusion *(open arrow)* seen posterior to the tendon indicates mild tenosynovitis. **B,** Diagram of the anatomy.

humeral head. Using the biceps tendon as a landmark, angle the transducer anteromedially, locating the subscapularis. The transverse view images the tendon as an oval soft tissue structure. Note that the transverse view of the tendon requires a longitudinal transducer orientation (Figure 20-27). Externally rotating the arm while scanning aids in visualization of the tendon and determination of normal movement. This tendon inserts into the lesser tuberosity at an angle requiring slight rotation to obtain the longitudinal view (transverse transducer position).

The next structure to locate is the 3- to 7-mm supraspinatus tendon located laterally and posteriorly from the biceps tendon. This bandlike tendon has a medium-level echo texture and originates from the greater tuberosity of the humerus. The acromion limits the field of view, necessitating careful transducer and patient positioning. A portion of the tendon, called the critical zone and located 1 cm posterolateral to the biceps tendon, is the most likely location for injury. Care must be taken here because improper scanning results in a false-

**Figure 20-27   The biceps tendon *(B)* is a good landmark to locate the subscapularis and supraspinatus tendons. This image shows the transverse tendon between the anteromedially located subscapularis tendon and the posterolateral supraspinatus. Note the anisotropy artifact *(arrows)* seen as the tendons curve with the humeral head.

positive or false-negative finding. The dual or split screen function allows for normal versus injured-shoulder comparisons, which helps to pinpoint tears.

Initial transverse and longitudinal views begin with the patient's arm in a neutral position; however, after localization of the tendon, the arm is repositioned into the Bouffard or Crass position (Figure 20-28). Externally rotating the shoulder into these positions depends on the patient's ability to place the arm behind the back or on the hip. This stresses the tendons of the rotator cuff, helping to emphasize any abnormalities. Another benefit is that the supraspinatus moves anterior and out from under the acromion, allowing for better visualization of the tendon (Figures 20-29 through 20-32).

The infraspinatus tendon is the next structure to image, and there are two methods of localizing the tendon. The first involves rotating the patient to gain access to the posterior shoulder and positioning the hand on the patient's opposite shoulder. The posterior glenoid labrum is a good landmark to help find the anteriorly located infraspinatus tendon (Figure 20-33). A second method has the patient's arm in the same position used in imaging the biceps tendon, locating the supraspinatus tendon, moving posterior and parallel to the scapular spine, and locating the infraspinatus tendon at its attachment to the posterior greater tuberosity of the humerus. Fluid imaged superficial to the infraspinatus tendon indicates bursal fluid, whereas posterior fluid indicates joint effusion. Take note of the humeral head contours because irregularities indicate a pathologic condition.

Although injury to the teres minor tendons is uncommon, imaging ensures complete visualization of the infraspinatus tendon because of their close proximity. This tendon lies

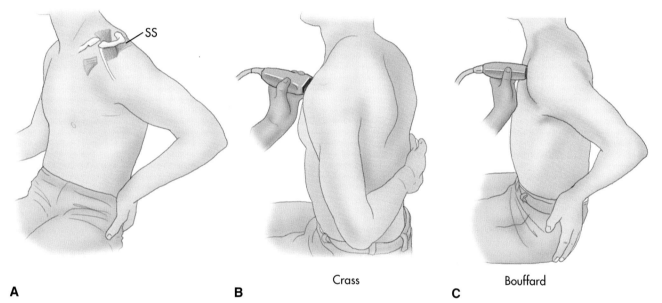

A   Crass **B**   Bouffard **C**

Figure 20-28   Once the supraspinatus *(SS)* has been located in the neutral position **(A),** move the hand to position the patient in the Crass **(B)** or Bouffard **(C)** position.

Figure 20-29   **A,** The medially located biceps tendon *(arrow)* helps locate the supraspinatus *(SS)*. Scan this tendon from the acromion to the greater tuberosity to locate any echogenicity changes or the presence of fluid. **B,** Diagram of the anatomy.

Figure 20-30   The transverse scan of the supraspinatus shows the tendon *(arrow)* to be mildly hyperechoic.

Figure 20-31   This image has the arm in a neutral position. To locate the supraspinatus use the biceps tendon (star) as a landmark and then rotate the transducer until the acromion *(A)* comes into view. The supraspinatus tendon *(arrow)* appears between these two structures. Note the anisotropy artifact that hinders visualization of part of the tendon.

Figure 20-32   This image shows the supraspinatus tendon *(arrow)* seen extending to the acromion *(A)* with the shoulder internally rotated into the Bouffard position. Most of the anisotropic artifact disappears since the tendon is closer to parallel to the transducer.

Figure 20-33   The infraspinatus tendon *(black arrow)* lies lateral and inferior to the scapular spine *(green arrow)*.

parallel to the scapular spine and inferior to the infraspinatus tendon. To differentiate the infraspinatus tendon from the teres minor, pay close attention to the plane of the tendon fibers. Horizontal fibers indicate the infraspinatus, whereas the teres minor is on an oblique plane. The teres minor appears as a trapezoidal structure inferior to the infraspinatus tendon.

During the examination of the rotator cuff structures it is important to note any bursal thickening, tendon calcifications, bony irregularities, loose bodies, or fluid collections. Many other nonrotator cuff structures can also be imaged, such as the **acromioclavicular joint (AC)**. Due to the superficial location of the AC, joint separations are easily imaged, especially when compared with a normal contralateral joint. As with any other portion of the body, soft tissue masses and injury, foreign body localization, and fluid collections are easily identified (Figures 20-34 and 20-35).

Box 20-1 lists the main indications for shoulder sonography. Box 20-2 lists the minimum shoulder views of the rotator cuff.

CARPAL TUNNEL

The wrist joint is easily examined because of its accessibility, size, and lack of overlying bony structures. This ease of imaging implies the wrist is an uncomplicated joint to image; however, familiarity with the wrist anatomy reveals a very complex set of structures. The complexity of the wrist is underscored by the fact that some orthopedic surgeons specialize in just this one joint.

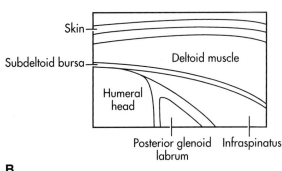

A   **B**

Figure 20-34 **A,** The posterior glenoid labrum *(star)* is a triangular hyperechoic structure deep to the infraspinatus tendon. The humeral head cartilage *(arrow)* images as a thin, hypoechoic layer superficial to the bony surface. **B,** Diagram of the anatomy.

Figure 20-35 The infraspinatus tendon *(IT)* has a triangular appearance at the attachment to the posterior greater tuberosity. This image helps determine the echogenic consistency of the tendon when coupled with external and internal rotation maneuvers.

BOX 20-2

MINIMUM SHOULDER VIEWS OF THE ROTATOR CUFF

View: 1/2: Biceps longitudinal and transverse
View: 3/4: Subscapularis longitudinal and transverse
View: 5/6/7/8: Supraspinatus in neutral and internal rotation
View: 9/10: Infraspinatus/posterior glenoid labrum
View: 11: Teres minor

BOX 20-1

INDICATIONS FOR SHOULDER SONOGRAPHY

• Shoulder pain or swelling
• Pain with joint rotation
• Weakness with arm elevation
• Trauma
• Decreased range of motion
• Evaluation of soft tissue masses

Positioning of the wrist entails placing the arm at a 90-degree angle with the palm pronated or supinated on the lap of the patient (Figure 20-36). Placing a small rolled up towel under the wrist when examining the palmar (**volar**) portion of the wrist places the joint in a neutral position. The towel also helps dorsal imaging of the wrist when the hand is palm down. These positions allow for imaging of carpal tunnel

structures, ganglion and synovial cysts, tears of the triangular fibrocartilage, tenosynovitis, and any other tumors. Another benefit of sonographic imaging of the wrist is the ability to demonstrate the dynamics of the wrist and associated masses with finger movement. The smaller wrist joint requires a higher frequency transducer in the 10- to 20-MHz range. Manufacturers also offer transducers with smaller footprints, which allow for easier scanning than some of the larger linear transducers.

The carpal tunnel is located between the carpal bones and the flexor retinaculum on the palmar side of the wrist. This fibro-osseous space contains the median nerve, the flexor pollicis longus, and the eight tendons that connect digital muscles to the wrist (flexor digitorum tendons). The ulnar artery and veins indicate the medial border of the carpal tunnel, whereas the most lateral structures are the radial artery and veins. The flexor retinaculum forms the anterior border by attaching to the scaphoid tubercle, trapezium ridge, pisiform bone, and the hook of the hamate. The median nerve, of particular interest in diagnosing carpal tunnel syndrome, lies superficial and towards the radial side of the tunnel. **Guyon's canal** is a tunnel on the ulnar side of the wrist formed by the hook of the hamate and pisiform bones. The ulnar nerve may be compressed at this site in long-distance cyclists, by falling on the wrist, or by repetitive wrist actions.

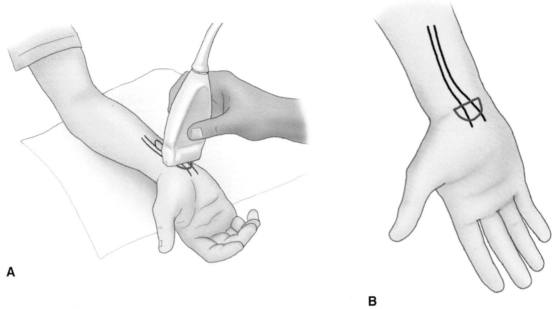

A

B

Figure 20-36   **A,** The wrist can be positioned on a pillow on the patient's lap to aid in imaging the volar structures. **B,** The retinaculum *(red structure),* a strong fibrous structure, attaches to the pisiform on the lateral side and the hook of the hamate.

The transverse imaging plane is the easiest approach to use to begin an examination of the carpal tunnel. Locating the ulnar artery at the wrist crease helps orientation and subsequent identification of the wrist structures. Care must be taken to maintain a perpendicular scan plane to reduce anisotropic effects. Use of large amounts of gel or a standoff pad may help in imaging the anterior structures of the wrist. The flexor digitorum tendons are a hypoechoic structure just posterior to the median nerve. Fibrillary hyperechoic tendon patterns help differentiate the median nerve because the nerve is hypoechoic with a hyperechoic border. The rounded or oval median nerve flattens as it continues through the carpal tunnel (Figure 20-37).

The longitudinal nerve images as a parallel structure superficial to the flexor digitorum tendons. The nerve sheath appears as a continuous hyperechoic structure on the anterior and posterior borders of the nerve. Tendons located posterior to the median nerve have the characteristic hyperechoic fibrillar pattern seen with tendons in other areas of the body (Figure 20-38).

Box 20-3 lists the main indications for wrist sonography.

Figure 20-37   This image taken from the volar side of the wrist at the crease demonstrates the complicated anatomy from this view. Large amounts of gel allow for imaging with minimal artifact on the lateral curved edges. Guyon's canal *(circle)* contains the ulnar vein and vessels demarcating the medial carpal tunnel border. The lunate *(L)* and scaphoid bone *(S)* mark the posterior boundaries of the carpal tunnel. Laterally the radial artery and vein mark this border. The median nerve is slightly flattened at this level, which is a normal finding.

ACHILLES' TENDON

The Achilles' tendon is named after a figure in Greek mythology. Achilles' mother wished to have her son invulnerable to all weapons, so she dipped him in the waters of the river Styx. The only portion that was not bathed in the water was his heel, resulting in a vulnerable spot. A poison arrow would later pierce the unprotected heel during the Trojan wars, resulting in Achilles' death.

This large, strong fibrous tendon connects the gastrocnemius and soleus muscles to the calcaneus. Though there are many variations of this tendon (as with any tendon), approximately two thirds of the tendon originates from the gastrocnemius muscle and one third from the soleus muscle. This tendon helps move your foot downward, push off when walking, and rise up on your toes. Injury to this tendon can make it impossible to walk without pain.

A limited blood supply increases the Achilles' tendon risk of injury and slows the healing process. The longitudinal arteries that run the length of the gastrocnemius and soleus muscle provide the blood supply. The poorest blood supply is above

Figure 20-38   This image taken proximal to Figure 20-37 demonstrates a rounder median nerve *(solid arrow)*. The flexor pollicis longus tendon and the beginning of the muscle *(open arrow)* appear as a hypoechoic structure.

> **BOX 20-3   INDICATIONS FOR WRIST SONOGRAPHY**
>
> - Masses
> - Loss or decrease of digital mobility
> - Pain and swelling
> - Trauma
> - Foreign body location
> - Numbness of the middle and index fingers
> - Weakness or clumsiness of the hand
> - Tingling with nerve percussion (Tinel's sign)
> - Pain with wrist flexion when sustained for a minute or longer (Phalen's sign)

the insertion of the tendon into the calcaneus, which is also the most frequent site of tendon tears. Chances of rupture and inflammation increase with age as a result of a diminishing blood supply.

A connective tissue sheath called the paratenon surrounds the Achilles' tendon. This allows for a gliding action of 2 to 3 cm with movement, and the tendon may thicken with increased activity. The lack of a true synovial sheath results in a less echogenic border between the tendon and the surrounding tissue.

The largest tendon of the body, the Achilles' tendon may develop tendinitis in the athletic patient. Any activity that involves jumping and sudden stops and starts will stress the tendon. Female athletes who wear high-heeled shoes and then change into sneakers to exercise also increase their risk of tendinitis. Overstretching the tendon can result in a partial or complete tear, with the most common site being the distal tendon at the area of decreased blood flow (2 to 6 cm from the calcaneus).

Fortunately the Achilles' tendon is relatively easy to scan because of the echo characteristics and location. To begin the examination, position the patient prone with the foot hanging over the edge of the cart or bed. The foot may also be supported on a pillow or sponge for easier scanning and patient

> **BOX 20-4   INDICATIONS FOR ACHILLES' TENDON SONOGRAPHY**
>
> - Abnormal Thompson's test (Toes point toward the plantar surface of the foot when the calf is squeezed.)
> - Trauma
> - Displacement of Kager's fat pad on a radiograph
> - Knot or bulge over the proximal tendon
> - Audible pop or snap followed by a sharp pain
> - Inability to stand on toes
> - Swelling
> - Heel pain for more than 4 weeks
> - Decreased strength or mobility
> - Postoperative monitoring

comfort. Patients who are unable to lie prone may also be scanned while on their side if the injured Achilles' tendon is on the upside.

The size of this tendon allows for imaging with a 5-MHz linear transducer. Scan the tendon from the origin at the gastrocnemius and soleus muscles to the insertion on the calcaneus. A complete scan includes transverse and sagittal views and measurements of the transverse tendon. The anteroposterior (AP) diameter of the normal tendon is approximately 5 to 6 mm, varying with patient gender and body habitus. Measurement of the AP tendon diameter on the longitudinal plane tends to overestimate the distance because of the oblique course of the tendon. **Dorsiflexion** and **plantar flexion** of the foot, best imaged on the sagittal plane, increase the chances of imaging an Achilles' tendon tear. The **Thompson's test** (plantar flexion with squeezing of the calf) may be used to evaluate the integrity of the Achilles' tendon. The patient kneels on the examination table with the feet hanging off; the examiner then squeezes the calf while observing for plantar flexion. The result is positive if there is no movement of the foot; this indicates an Achilles' tendon rupture.

Special attention must be given to the hypoechoic Kager's fat pad or pre-Achilles' fat pad located deep in the Achilles' tendon when scanning the patient in the prone position. Displacement of this triangular fat pad is one radiographic marker for the Achilles' tendon and can serve as a landmark during the sonographic examination. Scanning the contralateral side also aids in determining normalcy of the tendon (Figures 20-39 and 20-40).

Box 20-4 lists the indications for Achilles' tendon sonography.

PATHOLOGY OF THE MUSCULOSKELETAL SYSTEM

Familiarity with the sonographic appearance of injury, inflammation, and chronic problems allows for a confident diagnosis of MS problems. Some pathology occurs with an increased frequency in a specific joint, but the same problem images similarly in the tendons, ligaments, and muscles, regardless of location.

A   **B**

Figure 20-39   **A,** The Achilles' tendon imaging extends from the origin at the gastrocnemius and soleus muscle to the insertion on the calcaneus. **B,** Placing the patient prone with the foot over the cart edge allows for easy access to the tendon and dorsal and plantar flexion of the foot.

Figure 20-40   Panoramic or extended field of view (EFOV) imaging allows for imaging of a greater length of the Achilles' tendon. This ensures comparison of the echo texture in different areas of the tendon. Kager's fat pad *(star)* images as a hypoechoic structure.

Figure 20-41   Subluxation and complete or incomplete dislocation of the biceps tendon *(star)* out of the bicipital groove *(arrow)* of the humerus.

SHOULDER BICEPS TENDON SUBLUXATION/DISLOCATION

The dislocation (also called *subluxation*) of the biceps tendon from the bicipital groove may be due to a problem with the transverse humeral ligament, abnormal development of the bicipital groove or supraspinatus, and/or subscapularis tears. The most common dislocation is deep to the subscapularis anterior to the glenohumeral joint capsule. This medial dislocation results in an empty groove that may fill with granulation and fibrous tissue. Rotating the arm from a neutral to external position allows for real-time imaging of the tendon dislocation or subluxation (Figures 20-41 and 20-42).

ROTATOR CUFF TEARS

Tears of the rotator cuff are classified as either partial-thickness or full-thickness tears (Figure 20-43). Differentiation between the two types is done through determination of the abnormal communication between the glenohumeral joint and the subacromial bursa. The full-thickness tear has this communication, although the partial thickness does not.

Rotator cuff problems occur as either an acute or chronic process. Biceps tendon ruptures, falls, and shoulder dislocations are a few causes of an acute rotator cuff tear. A chronic process occurs as a cumulative progression of injury from activities involving placing the arms over the head. This may be due to actions such as placing items on high shelves, playing tennis, swimming, or rock climbing. This microtrauma, due to impingement of the tendon between the humeral head and acromion, results in cuff degeneration and an eventual tear. Rotator cuff tears are divided into three stages—Stage I: swelling and mild pain; Stage II: inflammation and scarring; Stage III: partial or complete tears of the rotator cuff.

The supraspinatus, like all tendons of the shoulder, is a strap-like tendon with three dimensions. Tears occur on tendons in the width, length, and thickness, and a complete examination includes a description of the tear in all the planes. A tear located on the sagittal plane of the tendon images as a disruption on the thickness or anteroposterior (AP) dimension of the tendon. This is only part of the picture and an orthogonal image will identify the location and extent of the tear on the width of the tendon.

Another consideration is that the curved tendons will have an increased chance of producing an anisotropic artifact, which will appear similar to a tear. Moving the patient's arm to an internal rotation or an extended position changes the imaging plane and helps not only to reduce the artifact, but to accentuate the defect.

Partial-Thickness Tear. The partial-thickness tear involves either the bursal or articular cuff surface or the intrasubstance material. An intrasubstance tear is very rare. Tears begin in the critical zone of the anterolateral supraspinatus tendon and image as focal disruptions of the tendon fibers. This zone is located 1 cm from its insertion into the greater tuberosity. When injured, the acute tendon tear images as an anechoic defect in the rotator cuff. A chronic tear may image as an area of hyperechogenicity because of the mixing of blood and bursal granulation tissue in the frayed tendon area. Diffuse thinning of the tendon is another indication of a chronic partial-thickness tear.

The most common type of tear is the articular cuff surface defect. The following criteria help in establishing the presence of a partial-thickness tear:

1. A critical zone focus of mixed hyperechoic and hypoechoic echo texture (focal discontinuity).
2. Bursal or articular extension of any hypoechoic areas imaged in two orthogonal planes.
3. An irregularity of the anterior greater tuberosity is seen in up to three fourths of partial-thickness tears. These may

Figure 20-42 Complete dislocation of the biceps tendon *(star)* outside of the biceps groove of the humerus.

A

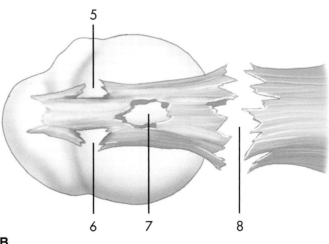

B

Figure 20-43 Coronal view **(A)** and view from above **(B)** showing tears of the supraspinatus tendon. These tears can occur anywhere along the tendon and range from an intrasubstance tear (1) to a complete full-thickness, full-width tear (8). The range includes partial-thickness humeral surface tear (2), partial-thickness bursal surface tear (3), full-thickness tear (4), full-thickness tear posteriorly (partial width) (5), full-thickness tear posteriorly (partial width) (6), and full-thickness tear centrally (partial width) (7).

appear as bone cortex defects, fragmentation, and/or spurring.

4. Decreased thickness of the tendon with chronic partial-thickness tears.

Fluid seen within the biceps tendon indicates the possibility of an articular surface tear. The presence of large amounts of fluid in the subacromial-subdeltoid bursa raises the chance of a nonvisualized full-thickness tear.

The hypoechoic concave bursal surface tears are the next most common type of partial rotator cuff tears (Figure 20-44). These defects, close to the joints and bursa, are tender to palpation.

Box 20-5 lists the sonographic criteria for partial-thickness tears.

Full-Thickness Tear. A tear of the rotator cuff that involves the full thickness and full width of the tendons is considered a full-thickness tear. Retraction of multiple tendons occurs with a separation of 2 to 4 cm between the torn tendon ends. The frequency of tendon tearing in descending order is the supraspinatus, infraspinatus, subscapularis, and very rarely the teres minor.

Images of the tear on both the sagittal and transverse planes not only confirm the full-thickness tear, but also provide for measurement between the torn tendon edges (Figures 20-45 through 20-47). The largest distance measurement is used to classify the tear. The four classifications of rotator cuff vary with author, but the criteria listed are a composite of published cate-

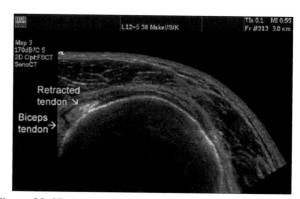

Figure 20-45   This complete full-thickness tear (complete rupture) panoramic image shows the biceps tendon retraction in the far left of the image. The deltoid muscle is located anterior to the greater tuberosity.

Figure 20-46   This magnification and panoramic image shows a complex subdeltoid bursa representing hemorrhage after a rotator cuff tear. The retracted supraspinatus (SS) leaves a space for fluid and blood to collect. Note the irregularity of the biceps groove.

> **BOX 20-5   SONOGRAPHIC CRITERIA FOR PARTIAL-THICKNESS TEARS**
>
> - Critical zone of the supraspinatus imaging with a hypoechoic or hyperechoic focus
> - Articular or bursal extension of a hypoechoic lesion on two orthogonal planes
> - Hypoechoic or echogenic line within the cuff substance
> - Anterior greater tuberosity regional irregularities
> - Effusions of the biceps tendon sheath
> - Concave subdeltoid bursal surface

Figure 20-44   This bursal side partial-thickness tear (solid arrow) has a hypoechoic appearance when compared with the surrounding rotator cuff. Fluid, blood, and debris collect in the bursa, producing an anechoic structure (open arrow).

Figure 20-47   The cartilage interface sign (arrow) is the echogenic anterior linelike border of the cartilage surrounding the humeral head. This is seen through the anechoic or hypoechoic complete rotator cuff tear.

gorizations. The **cartilage interface sign** is the echogenic line on the anterior surface of the cartilage surrounding the humeral head.

1. Partial-thickness tear
2. Small full-thickness tear 1 to 2 cm in AP dimension over the greater tuberosity
3. Large full-thickness tear of 2 to 4 cm
4. Complete tears of more than 4 cm

During the real-time examination, perform a simple compression test over the area of concern. The normal tendon cannot be compressed; however, the injured tendon flattens as the torn edges move apart. Long-standing cuff injury may also result in atrophy or nonvisualization of a muscle. Rupture of the subscapularis tendon results in the muscle retracting between the scapula and chest wall. Fatty infiltration of the supraspinatus and infraspinatus fossa changes the echo appearance of this area giving a false appearance of normalcy and underscoring the importance of scanning the normal contralateral side. The naked tuberosity sign is defined as the deltoid muscle on the humeral head; it is seen with a full-thickness tear of the rotator cuff.

Joint effusion around the biceps tendon combined with subacromial-subdeltoid (SASD) bursitis results in the double effusion sign. This is a specific sign of a rotator cuff tear and has been quoted as having a positive predictive value of as high as 95%. Arm extension and internal rotation help image lateral greater tuberosity bursal fluid. Light transducer pressure is important because a heavy scan technique may compress the fluid into other nonimaged areas of the joint. This indirect sign is important enough to warrant complementary imaging of arthroscopy or MRI.

Box 20-6 lists the primary and secondary sonographic signs of a full-thickness tear.

BOX 20-6

PRIMARY AND SECONDARY SONOGRAPHIC SIGNS OF A FULL-THICKNESS TEAR

PRIMARY SIGNS
- Naked tuberosity sign
- Tendon edge atrophy in a chronic tear
- Retracted tendons
- Fiber discontinuity with interposed fluid
- A cleft in the cuff of either hypoechoic or anechoic echo texture
- Distended SASD bursa in direct communication with the joint
- Compressed tendon
- Absence of the rotator cuff
- Deltoid muscle or SASD bursa herniation into the rotator cuff

SECONDARY SIGNS
- Long head biceps tendon effusion
- Double effusion sign
- Erosions of the greater tuberosity of the humerus
- Cartilage interface sign
- Double effusion sign
- Glenohumeral joint effusion

TENDINITIS

One of the most common tendon abnormalities is inflammation due to age-related elasticity loss, disease such as rheumatoid arthritis, overuse, or acute trauma. **Tendinitis** occurs in any tendon, but is seen more often in the shoulder, wrist, heel, and elbow. This inflammatory condition has a characteristic clinical symptom of pain at the tendinous insertion into the bone, palpable mass in the area of pain, and a decreased range of movement. Treatment is important since chronic tendinitis may lead to weakening of the tendon, resulting in rupture (Figure 20-48).

Sonography images tendinitis well because of the changes in the inflamed area in the surrounding tissue (Figure 20-49). Acute tendinitis (also called *tenosynovitis*) involves not only the tendon but also the surrounding synovial sheath as well. Imaging demonstrates an increase in fluid within the synovial sheath, appearing as a halo effect on the transverse image (Figure 20-50). The normal synovial sheath appears as a hypoechoic halo around the tendon. Fluid surrounding the tendon may be anechoic or complex due to debris. To differentiate complex fluid from edema, tap the area or increase the output power to encourage movement of the debris.

A focal or diffuse decrease in echogenicity within the tendon fibers is one sonographic sign of tendinitis. This hypoechoic area also demonstrates increased Doppler flow in the periphery, caused by hyperemia. These areas of injury may be very subtle; comparing the normal to the abnormal side helps confirm the diagnosis (see Figure 20-49). Any discrepancy in thickness measurements of more than 1.5 mm is highly suspicious of a focal lesion.

de Quervain's tendinitis is one form of tendinitis with which many sonographers and sonologists may be inherently familiar. This type of tendon inflammation results in symptoms of pain over the thumb side of the wrist and may even result in an audible creaking called *crepitus*. Continuous use of the hand and thumb in a twisting, pinching, or grasping fashion increases the chances of developing swelling on the thumb side of the wrist. During the acute phase of this disease, sonographic imaging of the large abductor pollicis longus and small extensor pollicis brevis tendon reveal hypoechoic tendons and synovium. As the process becomes chronic, fibrosis forms,

Figure 20-48   Intratendinous calcifications *(arrow)*, as seen in this rotator cuff, are a common finding with chronic tendinitis.

increasing the echogenicity. Fibrosis results in restriction of the tendons through the dorsal compartment of the hand, leading to the inability to move the thumb away from the rest of the hand or straighten the thumb after grasping.

Box 20-7 lists the sonographic features of tendinitis.

BOX 20-7   SONOGRAPHIC FEATURES OF TENDINITIS

- Focal or diffuse hypoechogenicity
- Enlargement of the tendon in either a focal or diffuse pattern
- Echogenic tendon fibrils within the area of inflammation
- Calcifications with chronic tendinitis
- Increased color or power Doppler signal in the periphery
- Coexisting bursitis
- Synovial sheath fluid

Figure 20-49   Comparison of the normal with the injured tendon identifies a focal area of inflammation *(arrow)*.

MUSCLE TEARS

Ultrasound demonstrates traumatic muscle injury because of its ability to reveal subtle changes in the internal structure of the muscle. A tear is the most common pathologic condition of the muscles of the limbs, though other sites are also affected. A muscle strain related to exertion does not image with ultrasound because of the lack of a lesion; however, imaging of this type of pain-related problem helps differentiate a tear from a strain. Two types of tears occur in the muscle: a distraction (indirect) or compression (direct) tear. The abrupt stretching of the muscle beyond the maximum length results in distraction tears. These are usually due to the sudden interruption of a movement, such as kicking, or improper body alignment. External force resulting in a crush injury is considered a compression tear. This type of trauma, resultant from muscle crushing against the underlying bone, ranges from a bruise to a large hematoma. Hematomas also occur with muscle injury and have a variable sonographic appearance. This characteristic of a muscle injury helps determine the extent of the underlying damage. The new hematoma is a hyperechoic mass structure pushing the muscle fibers apart. Often diffuse and ill-defined, the acute hematoma images as an area of enlargement with increased echogenicity within the muscle fibers. Within a few days, the hematoma becomes organized, which often increases detection (Figure 20-51). As the hematoma ages, it liquefies into a hypoechoic to anechoic mass, and a **seroma**, an accumulation of serous fluid within tissue, forms within the defect in a few weeks. Healing of this type of injury results in a hyperechoic fibrous scar or calcifications within the muscle after reabsorption of the serous material. The hematoma that conforms to the fibrous layers may also mimic deep vein thrombosis (DVT) within the calf or arm muscles.

The sonographic appearance of a muscle tear varies with the type of injury. A tear of the full thickness of the muscle images with the torn muscle end outlined by fluid. The muscle belly

Figure 20-50   **A,** Tenosynovitis of the extensor tendons of the hand displays the characteristic anechoic fluid *(star)* surrounding the tendon *(T)*. **B,** The fluid within the tendon sheath creates a halo effect *(arrows)* around the tendon on the transverse image.

Figure 20-51 This intramuscular hematoma images an organized clot with a heterogeneous appearance.

Figure 20-53 The right median nerve is notably flattened in this symptomatic patient. The left median nerve is also mildly flattened.

Figure 20-52 A tear of the gastrocnemius muscle *(M)* results in a hematoma *(star)* at the area of the injury. Comparison of the normal and injured side confirms the muscle tear and may be seen in athletes participating in jumping activities.

TABLE 20-4	SONOGRAPHIC APPEARANCE OF MUSCLE TEAR GRADES
Muscle Tear Grade	Sonographic Appearance
I (elongation injury)	Normal, flame-shaped focal fiber discontinuity, small hematoma (<1 cm)
II (partial rupture)	<1/3 of muscle fibers disrupted, hematoma <3 cm, interfascial hematoma, hypoechoic gap within the muscle that changes position with transducer pressure
III (complete rupture)	>1/3 rupture of muscle resembling a soft tissue mass, hematoma >3 cm, large interfascial hematoma

will appear thicker with a whorled circular pattern when compared with the contralateral side (Figure 20-52). As the hematoma resolves, it becomes smaller and the echogenicity increases.

A complete tear of a muscle has a straightforward appearance of a retracted hyperechoic muscle surrounded by a hematoma (**clapper-in-the-bell sign**). The partial tear may be as subtle as a discontinuity of the muscle fibers and septa or as obvious as a hematoma with echoic debris. This type of tear may be difficult to separate from the earlier mentioned edge artifact because of the similar appearance. The true torn muscle with the irregular margins will maintain the same sonographic appearance at different angles of incidence, whereas the edge artifact will only appear with the 90-degree angle. The examination of the injured muscle includes images with the muscle contracted and at rest in both the longitudi-

nal and transverse planes. An area of rupture may also image with a hyperechoic halo surrounding the jagged rupture margins. As the muscle heals, the edges of the tear increase in echogenicity and thickness. The normal muscle architecture becomes evident with healing. The hyperechoic linear, stellate, or nodular scar or an intramuscular cyst is evidence of an abnormal healing process.

Table 20-4 lists the sonographic appearance of muscle tear grades.

CARPAL TUNNEL SYNDROME

Carpal tunnel syndrome (CTS) is primarily entrapment or compression neuropathy of the median nerve. Occupations requiring repetitive motion produce the repetitive stress on the nerve, resulting in the pain and paresthesias characteristic of this syndrome. The continued use of the same muscle group results in hypertrophied muscles, and repeated trauma to the tendon sheath may cause enlargement (traumatic synovitis). This increase in size of the muscle and tendon sheath results in tunnel narrowing (Figure 20-53). We are most familiar with the repetitive causes of CTS, but there are other causes for this group of problems, which include pregnancy, chronic renal failure, diabetes mellitus, rheumatoid arthritis, amyloidosis, and tenosynovitis. Extrinsic causes include accessory muscles, soft tissue masses, and ganglions.

> **BOX 20-8   SONOGRAPHIC APPEARANCE OF MEDIAN NERVE COMPRESSION**
>
> - Focal or diffuse proximal enlargement
> - Increased cross-sectional area (>15 mm^2)
> - >3 flattening ratio of the median nerve in distal carpal tunnel
> - Tenosynovitis with >4 mm dorsal bowing of the flexor retinaculum

The patient suffering from CTS typically presents with numbness of the middle and index fingers, weakness or clumsiness of the hand, and pain. The clinical examination is positive for **Tinel's sign** or **Phalen's sign,** and weakness in the affected hand.

Normal median nerves are elliptical and flatten with distal progression. The transverse scan on a patient with CTS reveals a nerve that flattens in the distal tunnel and nerve swelling in the distal tunnels; at the level of the distal radius and palmar, bowing is seen in the flexor retinaculum. Due to the varied cross-sectional area, calculation of the area is helpful in determining the presence of an increase in the median nerve. This area estimate uses the formula for the ellipse (area $= \pi(\text{D1} \times \text{D2})/4$). Any cross-sectional area greater than 15 mm^2 at the level of the proximal tunnel is considered diagnostic for an increased median nerve.

Box 20-8 lists the sonographic appearance of median nerve compression.

SELECTED BIBLIOGRAPHY

American Institute of Ultrasound in Medicine: AIUM practice guidelines for the performance of a shoulder ultrasound examination, *J Ultrasound Med* 22(10):1137-1141, 2003.

Chhem R, Cardinal E, editors: *Guidelines and gamuts in musculoskeletal ultrasound*, New York, 1999, Wiley-Liss.

Disler D, Raymond E, May D and others: Articular cartilage defects: in vitro evaluation of accuracy and interobserver reliability for detection and grading with US, *Radiology* 215:(3):846, 2000.

Dondelinger R, editor: *Peripheral musculoskeletal ultrasound atlas*, New York, 1996, Thieme.

Formnage B, editor: *Musculoskeletal ultrasound*, New York, 1995, Churchill Livingston.

Kremkau F: *Diagnostic ultrasound: principles and instruments*, ed 7, Philadelphia, 2006, WB Saunders Co.

Lin J, Fessell D, Jacobson J and others: An illustrated tutorial of musculoskeletal sonography: part 3, lower extremity, *Am J Roentgenol* 175:1313-1321, 2000.

Ly J, Bui-Mansfield L: Anatomy of and abnormalities associated with Kager's fat pad, *Am J Roentgenol* 182(1):147-154, 2004.

Moore K, Dalley A: *Clinically oriented anatomy*, ed 4, Philadelphia, 1999, Lippincott Williams & Wilkins.

Peetrons P: Ultrasound of muscles, *Eur Radiol* 12(1):35-43, 2002.

Teefy S, Middleton W, Boyer M: Sonography of the hand and wrist, *Seminars in Ultrasound, CT & MR* 21(3):192-204, 2000.

Torriani M, Kattapuram S: Dynamic sonography of the forefoot: the sonographic Mulder sign, *AJR* 180:1121, 2002.

van Holsbeeck M, Introcaso J: *Musculoskeletal ultrasound*, ed 2, St Louis, 2001, Mosby.

Walker F, Cartwright M, Wiesler E and others: Ultrasound of nerve and muscle, *Clin Neurophysiol* 115(3):495-507, 2004.

Winter T, Teefey S, Middleton W: Musculoskeletal ultrasound: an update, *Radiol Clin North Am* 39(3):465-483, 2004.

Zagzebski J: *Essentials of ultrasound physics*, St Louis, 1996, Mosby.

PART IV

Pediatric Applications

• • •

CHAPTER 21

Neonatal Echoencephalography

Sandra L. Hagen-Ansert

KEY TERMS

aqueductal stenosis – congenital blockage of the aqueduct connecting the third and fourth ventricles, which causes dilatation of the third and fourth ventricles

asphyxia – severe hypoxia, or inadequate oxygenation

atrium (trigone) of the lateral ventricles – the ventricle is measured at this site (anterior, occipital, and temporal horn junction) on the axial view

axial plane – transducer is placed above the ear (above the canthomeatal line)

brain stem – composed of the midbrain, pons, and medulla oblongata

caudate nucleus – forms the lateral borders of the anterior horns, anterior to the thalamus

cavum septum pellucidum – prominent structure best seen in the midline filled with cerebrospinal fluid in the premature infant

cerebellum – lies posterior to the brain stem below the tentorium

cerebrum – two equal hemispheres; largest part of the brain

Chiari malformation – congenital defect in which the cerebellum and brainstem are pulled toward the spinal cord (banana sign); frontal bossing or "lemon head" is also evident on ultrasound

choroid plexus – echogenic cluster of cells important in the production of cerebrospinal fluid that lies along the atrium of the lateral ventricles

cistern – reservoir for cerebrospinal fluid

coronal plane – transducer is perpendicular to the anterior fontanelle in the coronal axis of the head

corpus callosum – prominent group of nerve fibers that connect the right and left sides of the brain; found superior to the third ventricle

Dandy-Walker malformation – abnormal development of the fourth ventricle, often accompanied by hydrocephalus

extracorporeal membrane oxygenation (ECMO) – term used for the treatment of infants with severe respiratory failure who have not responded to maximal conventional ventilatory support

falx cerebri (interhemispheric fissure) – echogenic fibrous structure (portion of the dura matter) that separates the cerebral hemispheres

fontanelle – soft space between the bones; the space is usually large enough to accommodate the ultrasound transducer until the age of 12 months

germinal matrix – periventricular tissue within the caudate nucleus, which before 32 weeks' gestation is fragile and bleeds easily

holoprosencephaly – abnormal single ventricular cavity with some form of thalami fusion

hydrocephalus – dilation of the ventricular system; may be partial or complete

hypoxia – decreased oxygen in the body

meninges – three membranes enclosing the brain and spinal cord

neonatal – early newborn period

periventricular leukomalacia (PVL) – echogenic white matter necrosis (WMN) best seen in the posterior aspect of the brain or adjacent to the ventricular structures

sagittal plane – perpendicular to the coronal plane with the transducer in the anterior fontanelle

subependyma – area beneath the ependyma. In the caudate nucleus, this area is the site of hemorrhage for the germinal matrix. This area is subject to bleeding in the premature neonate.

subependymal cyst – cyst that occurs at the site of a previous bleed in the germinal matrix.

sulcus – groove on the surface of the brain that separates the gyri

tentorium cerebelli – echogenic "V-shaped/tent" structure in the posterior fossa that separates the cerebellum from the cerebrum

thalamic-caudate groove or notch – the region at which the thalamus and caudate nucleus join; the most common location of germinal matrix hemorrhage

thalamus – two ovoid brain structures located midbrain, situated on either side of the third ventricle superior to the brain stem

trigone – see *atrium (trigone) of the lateral ventricles*

ventriculitis – inflammation/infection of the ventricles, which appears as echogenic linear structures along the gyri; may also appear as focal echogenic structures within the white matter

ventriculomegaly – enlargement of the ventricles in the brain

---

With advancements in ultrasound, computed tomography, and magnetic resonance imaging, the last two decades have brought increased understanding of the intracranial lesions of premature babies. Ultrasound has been the primary imaging modality for the neonatal head because it is portable and readily available at the neonatal bedside, nonionizing and noninvasive, and tolerated by even the sickest infants. Ultrasound of the neonatal brain may be performed if there are abnormal findings in the prenatal ultrasound examination or in the premature infant (to evaluate for intracranial bleeds) or if the postnatal examination is abnormal. Neonates who suffered a difficult delivery associated with **hypoxia** or **asphyxia** may be examined with ultrasound. Brain damage is one of the primary concerns about the health of premature infants. Intraventricular and subependymal hemorrhages occur in 40% to 70% of premature neonates under 34 weeks gestation. Multifocal necrosis of the white matter or periventricular leukomalacia may develop in 12% to 20% of infants weighing less than 2000 g. These lesions are associated with increased mortality and an abnormal neurologic outcome.

This chapter will focus on embryology, normal cranial anatomy, sonographic protocols for the neonatal head examination, common developmental problems of the brain, and ultrasound evaluation of neonatal brain lesions. The primary focus of this chapter is on neural tube defects, hydrocephalus, infections, and hemorrhagic pathologic conditions of the premature infant. For further detail on lesions of the brain, the reader is referred to Chapter 55.

EMBRYOLOGY OF THE BRAIN

The central nervous system develops from the neural plate. Before the neural tube forms, the neural plate is expanded rostrally where the brain will develop (Figure 21-1). The neural plate develops at 18 to 20 days after conception. The neural plate forms the neural tube and the neural crest. The neural tube differentiates into the central nervous system, consisting of both the brain and the spinal cord. The neural crest gives rise to most of the structures in the peripheral nervous system.

Temporarily the neural tube is open at both the cranial and the caudal ends (Figure 21-2). The cranial opening closes first at around 24 days after conception. The caudal opening closes two days later. The walls of the tube thicken to form the various portions of the brain and the spinal cord. The lumen of the neural tube becomes the ventricular system of the brain cranially and the central canal of the spinal cord caudally.

The greatest growth and differentiation of the neural tube are at the cranial end. At the end of the fourth week after conception, the cranial end of the neural tube differentiates into

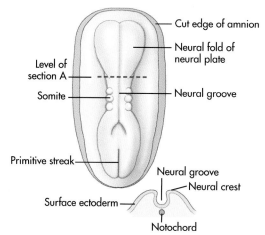

Level of section A — - - -
Somite
Primitive streak —
Surface ectoderm —
Cut edge of amnion
Neural fold of neural plate
Neural groove
Neural groove
Neural crest
Notochord

Figure 21-1 Dorsal view of the nervous system at 22 days. The neural folds have fused near the middle of the embryo to form the neural tube.

three primary brain vesicles. These vesicles consist of the prosencephalon (forebrain), mesencephalon (midbrain), and rhombencephalon (hindbrain) (Figure 21-3). The following week the forebrain differentiates into the telencephalon (end brain), which is the rostral portion of the brain, and the diencephalon (immediate brain). The hindbrain divides into the metencephalon and the myelencephalon (Table 21-1).

THE FOREBRAIN

As the brain flexures form, the forebrain develops rapidly. During the fifth week it develops diverticula called optic vesicles (Figure 21-3, *B*) that will develop into the eyes, and cerebral vesicles that will become cerebral hemispheres (Figure 21-3, *C*). The diencephalon is positioned centrally, whereas the telencephalon consists of lateral expansions. The diencephalon (Figure 21-3, *D*) develops from the tissues of the walls of the third ventricle that form three discrete swellings: the epithalamus, the **thalamus**, and the hypothalamus.

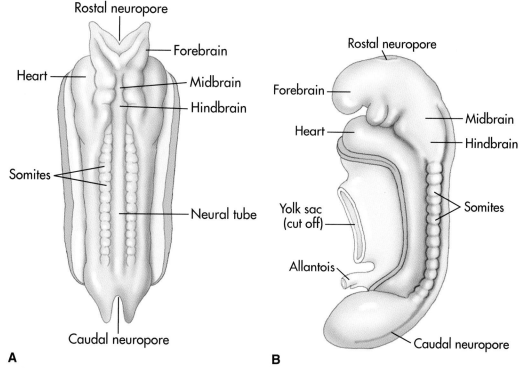

Figure 21-2 **A,** Dorsal view of an embryo at 23 days. Note that the hindbrain and midbrain vesicles have formed and that the neural tube is much longer. **B,** Lateral view. The rostral and caudal neuropores are still open. The rostral neuropore closes on day 25 or 26 and the caudal neuropore closes about 2 days later. Failure of these openings to close results in severe neural tube defects.

TABLE 21-1	PROGRESSION OF DEVELOPING REGIONS OF THE BRAIN	
Primary Brain Vesicles	Secondary Brain Vesicles	Regions of the Mature Brain
Forebrain (Prosencephalon)	Diencephalon	Thalamus, epithalamus, hypothalamus, subthalamus
	Telencephalon	Cerebral hemispheres (consisting of the cortex and medullary center, the corpus striatum, and the olfactory system)
Midbrain (Mesencephalon)	Mesencephalon	Midbrain
Hindbrain (Rhombencephalon)	Myelencephalon	Medulla
	Metencephalon	Pons and cerebellum

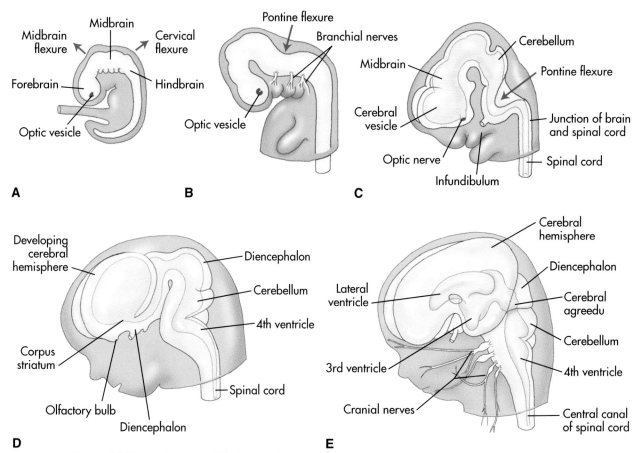

Figure 21-3   Development of the brain and the ventricular system. Note how the brain flexures affect the shape of the brain, enabling it to be accommodated in the head. The cerebral hemispheres expand and gradually cover the diencephalon and midbrain. The nerves of the branchial arches become the cranial nerves. **A,** 28 days. **B,** 35 days. **C,** 56 days. **D,** 10 weeks. **E,** 14 weeks.

The cerebral vesicles enlarge rapidly, expanding in all directions until they cover the diencephalon and part of the brain stem (Figure 21-3, *E*). In the floor and lateral wall of each vesicle, a thickening of nerve cells develops that will become the corpus striatum (see Figure 21-3, *D*) from which the basal ganglia will develop. Fibers from the developing cerebral hemispheres pass through the corpus striatum on their way to the brain stem and spinal cord, dividing the corpus striatum into two parts, the caudate nucleus and the lentiform nucleus. These fibers form the internal capsule.

Thickenings appear in the lateral walls of the diencephalon, which will become the thalamus. The thalamus is the dominant portion of the diencephalon and enlarges rapidly. At the same time, the thalami bulge into the third ventricle to reduce the ventricular lumen to a narrow cleft. The thalami fuse in the midline and form a fusion called the *massa intermedia.*

The diencephalon also participates in the formation of the pituitary gland. The posterior lobe of the pituitary gland develops from a down growth from the diencephalons known as the infundibulum (see Figure 21-3, *C*). The anterior lobe of the pituitary gland develops from an evagination of the primitive mouth cavity.

The telencephalic or cerebral vesicles communicate with the cavity of the third ventricle. Along the choroidal fissure, the medial wall of the developing cerebral hemisphere becomes thin. Invaginations of vascular pia form the choroid plexus of the lateral ventricles at this site. The hemispheres cover the surfaces of the diencephalon, the midbrain, and eventually, the hindbrain. The falx cerebri, or interhemispheric fissure, is formed as the mesenchyme is trapped in the midline with the growth of the hemispheres. This development separates the lateral ventricles from the third ventricle. At this point in development, only the frontal horns, bodies, and atria of the lateral ventricles are developed.

THE MIDBRAIN

The midbrain does not change as much as the other parts of the brain, except for considerable thickening of its walls. It is the growth of large nerve fiber tracts through it that thickens its walls and reduces its lumen, which become the cerebral aqueduct (see Figure 21-3, *E*). Four large groups of neurons form in the roof of the midbrain known as the superior and inferior colliculi (quadrigeminal body). In the basal portion of the midbrain, fibers passing from the cerebrum form the cerebral peduncles. A broad layer of gray matter adjacent to these large fiber tracts is known as the substantia nigra.

THE HINDBRAIN

The hindbrain undergoes flexion, which divides the hindbrain into the metencephalon and myelencephalon. The pontine flexure demarcates the division between these two parts (see Figure 21-3, *B*). The myelencephalon becomes the closed part of the medulla oblongata. It resembles the spinal cord both developmentally and structurally.

The metencephalon becomes the pons and the **cerebellum.** The fourth ventricle forms from the cavity of the hindbrain and also contains choroid plexus, as do the lateral and third ventricles. At 12 weeks, the vermis and cerebellar hemispheres are recognizable.

ANATOMY OF THE NEONATAL BRAIN

The sonographer must be familiar with specific anatomic structures within the brain to perform a complete ultrasound examination of the neonatal head. The anatomy presented in this chapter will focus on cranial anatomy the sonographer needs to understand in order to perform a neonatal cranial ultrasound. The cranial cavity contains the brain and its surrounding meninges and portions of the cranial nerves, arteries, veins, and venous sinuses.

FONTANELLE

Fontanelles are the spaces between the bones of the skull (Figure 21-4). In the neonate, the fontanelles have not closed completely. The anterior fontanelle is located at the top of the neonatal head and may be easily felt as the "soft spot." If hydrocephalus is present, this fontanelle is felt to be bulging. If there is overlapping of the cranial bones, the fontanelle may be difficult to palpate and provides a limited window for the transducer to image the cranial structures. The transducer is placed carefully on the anterior fontanelle to record multiple images of the brain in the coronal, axial, and sagittal planes.

MENINGES

There are three membranes called **meninges** that surround and form a protective covering for the brain: the dura mater, arachnoid, and pia mater membranes. The dura mater is a double layered outer membrane that forms the toughest barrier. The **falx cerebri** is a fibrous structure separating the two cerebral hemispheres. The **tentorium cerebelli** is a V-shaped echogenic structure separating the cerebrum and the cerebellum; it is an extension of the falx cerebri.

VENTRICULAR SYSTEM

The lateral ventricles are the largest of the cerebral spinal fluid cavities located within the cerebral hemispheres. They communicate with the third ventricle through the interventricular foramen. There are two lateral ventricles located on either side of the brain. The lateral ventricles are divided into the following four segments: frontal horn, body, and occipital and temporal horns (Figures 21-5 and 21-6). The **atrium** or **trigone** is the site where the anterior, occipital, and temporal horns join together.

The body of the lateral ventricle extends from the foramen of Monro to the trigone. The corpus callosum forms the roof, and the cavum septum pellucidum forms the medial wall. The thalamus touches the inferior lateral ventricular wall, and the body of the caudate nucleus borders the superior wall.

The temporal horn extends anteriorly from the trigone through the temporal lobe. The roof is formed by the white matter of the temporal lobe and by the tail of the caudate nucleus. The hippocampus forms the medial wall.

The occipital horn extends posteriorly from the trigone. The occipital cortex and white matter form the medial wall. The corpus callosum forms the proximal roof and lateral wall.

The frontal horn is divided posteriorly by the foramen of Monro near the body of the ventricle. The roof is formed by the corpus callosum. The septum pellucidum forms the medial wall and the head of the caudate nucleus forms the lateral wall.

The third ventricle is connected by the foramen of Monro to the lateral ventricles. The aqueduct of Sylvius connects the third and fourth ventricles. The medulla oblongata forms the floor of the fourth ventricle. The roof is formed by the cerebellar vermis and posterior medullary velum. The lateral angles of the fourth ventricle form the foramen of Luschka. The inferior angle, foramen of Magendie, is continuous with the central canal of the spinal cord.

Cerebrospinal Fluid. The cerebrospinal fluid (CSF) surrounds and protects the brain and spinal cord from physical impact. Approximately 40% of the CSF is formed by the choroid plexuses of the lateral, third, and fourth ventricles. The remainder is produced by the extracellular fluid movement from blood through the brain and into the ventricles. The fluid from the lateral ventricles passes through the foramen of Monro to the third ventricle. The fluid then passes through the aqueduct of Sylvius to the fourth ventricle. From that

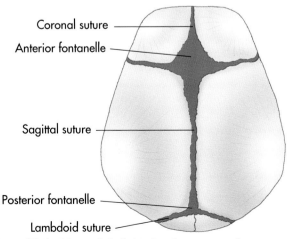

Figure 21-4   Neonatal skull showing the sutures and open anterior fontanelle.

Coronal suture

Anterior fontanelle

Sagittal suture

Posterior fontanelle

Lambdoid suture

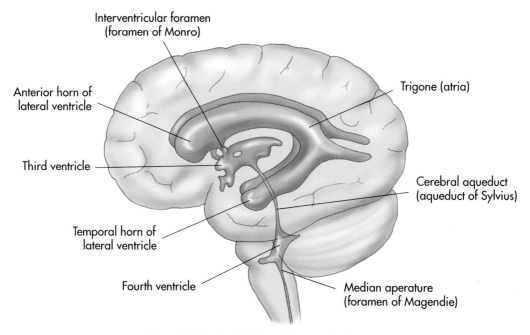

Figure 21-5   Sagittal view of the ventricular system.

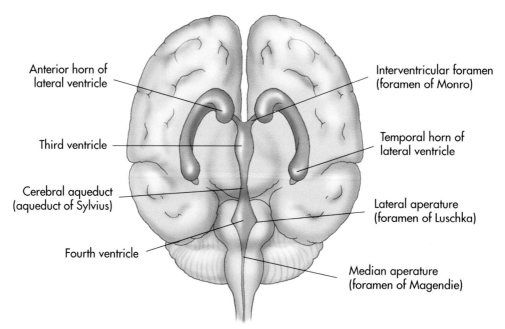

Figure 21-6   Anterior view of the ventricles.

point, the fluid may leave through the central foramen of Magendie or the lateral foramen of Luschka into the cisterna magna and the basal subarachnoid cisterns. The anterior flow continues upward through the chiasmatic cisterns, sylvian fissure, and the pericallosal cisterns up over the hemispheres, where it is reabsorbed by the arachnoid granulations in the sagittal sinus. Posteriorly the cerebrospinal fluid flow moves around the cerebelli, through the tentorial incisure, the quadrigeminal cistern, the posterior callosal cistern, and up over the hemispheres. A small amount flows down the spinal subarachnoid space.

The cerebrospinal fluid results from the production of fluid by the choroid plexus and from the respiratory and vascular pulsations, ciliary action in the ependyma, and a downhill pressure gradient between the subarachnoid spaces and the venous sinuses. The CSF fluid production does not change appreciably with increased intracranial pressure; however, when the pressure is significantly increased, there will be a change in intracranial pressure.

Cavum Septum Pellucidum. The cavum septum pellucidum is a thin triangular space filled with cerebrospinal fluid, which lies between the anterior horn of the lateral ventricles and forms the floor of the corpus callosum. Thus the cavum septum pellucidum is anterior to the corpus callosum. The cavum vergae is found at the posterior extension of the cavum septum pellucidum. The cavum septum pellucidum is present at birth and closes within 3 to 6 months of life.

Choroid Plexus. The **choroid plexus** is a mass of special cells located in the atrium of the lateral ventricles. These cells regulate the intraventricular pressure by secretion or absorption of cerebral spinal fluid. The glomus is the tail of the choroid plexus and is a major site for bleeding (Figure 21-7).

CISTERNS

The narrow subarachnoid space surrounding the brain and spinal cord contains a small amount of fluid. The subarachnoidal cisterns are the spaces at the base of the brain where the arachnoid becomes widely separated from the pia, giving rise to large cavities. The cisterna magna is one of the largest of these subarachnoidal **cisterns;** it is located in the posterior fossa between the medulla oblongata, cerebellar hemispheres, and occipital bone (Figure 21-8).

CEREBRUM

Cerebral Hemispheres. There are two cerebral hemispheres connected by the corpus callosum. They extend from the frontal to the occipital bones above the anterior and middle cranial fossae. Posteriorly, they extend above the tentorium cerebelli. They are separated by a longitudinal fissure into which projects the falx cerebri. The **cerebrum** consists of the gray and white matter. The outermost portion of the cerebrum is the cerebral cortex (composed of gray matter). The white matter is located within the cerebrum. The largest and densest bundle of white matter is the corpus callosum.

Figure 21-7   Sagittal view of choroid plexus and cisterns of the ventricular system.

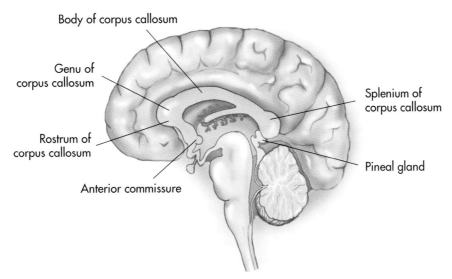

Figure 21-8   Sagittal view of cerebral cortex.

Lobes of the Brain. The cortex is divided into four lobes: frontal, parietal, occipital, and temporal, which correspond to the cranial bones with the same names (Figure 21-9).

Gyrus and Sulcus. The gyri are convolutions on the surface of the brain caused by infolding of the cortex. The **sulcus** is a groove or depression on the surface of the brain separating the gyri. The sulci further divide the hemispheres into frontal, parietal, occipital, and temporal lobes.

Fissures. The interhemispheric fissure is the area in which the falx cerebri sits and separates the two cerebral hemispheres. The sylvian fissure is located along the lateral most aspect of the brain and is the area where the middle cerebral artery is located (Figure 21-10). The quadrigeminal fissure is located posterior and inferior from the cavum vergae. The vein of Galen is posterior, so the sonographer must be aware that Doppler should be performed to make sure it is a fissure and not an enlarged vein of Galen.

Corpus Callosum. The corpus callosum forms broad bands of connecting fibers between the cerebral hemispheres. This structure forms the roof of the lateral ventricles. The corpus callosum sits superior to the cavum septum pellucidum (see Figure 21-7). The development of the corpus callosum occurs between the 8th and 18th week of gestation, beginning ventrally and extending dorsal. The anterior body of the corpus callosum develops earlier than the *genu* (the dorsal element).

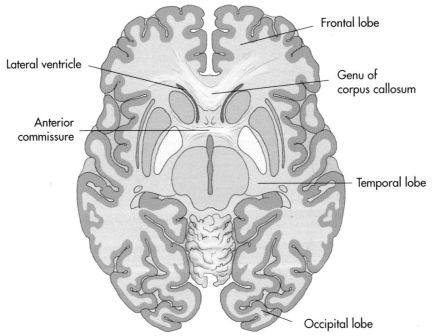

Figure 21-9   Axial view of cerebral cortex and corpus callosum.

Figure 21-10   Coronal view of cerebral lobes, corpus callosum, and sylvian fissure.

If a uterine insult occurs, development may be partially arrested or complete agenesis may occur. If partial, then the genu, the splenium (posterior element), and the rostrum are absent. This is known as agenesis of the corpus callosum.

BASAL GANGLIA

The basal ganglia are a collection of gray matter that include the caudate nucleus, lentiform nucleus, claustrum, and thalamus. The caudate nucleus is the portion of the brain that forms the lateral borders of the frontal horns of the lateral ventricles and lies anterior to the thalamus (Figure 21-11). It is further divided into the head, body, and tail. The head of the caudate nucleus is a common site for hemorrhage. The caudate nucleus and lentiform nucleus are the largest basal ganglia. They serve as relay stations between the thalamus and the cerebral cortex. The claustrum is a thin layer between the insula and the lentiform nucleus.

The thalamus consists of two ovoid, egg-shaped brain structures situated on either side of the third ventricle superior to the brain stem. The thalamus borders the third ventricle and connects through the middle of the third ventricle by the massa intermedia.

The hypothalamus forms the floor of the third ventricle. The pituitary gland is connected to the hypothalamus by the infundibulum.

The germinal matrix includes periventricular tissue and the caudate nucleus. It is located 1 cm above the caudate nucleus in the floor of the lateral ventricle. It sweeps from the frontal horn posteriorly into the temporal horn.

BRAIN STEM

The **brain stem** is the part of the brain connecting the forebrain and the spinal cord. It consists of the midbrain, pons, and medulla oblongata.

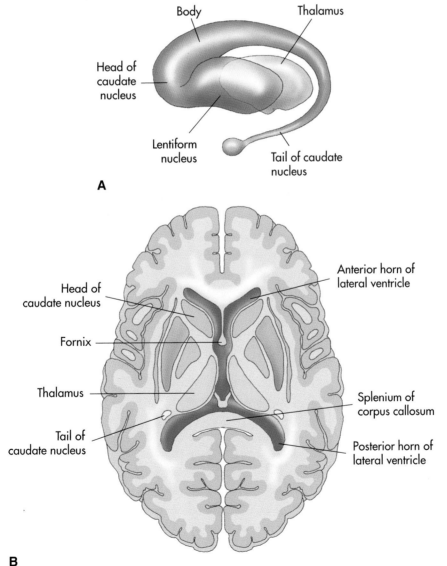

Figure 21-11 **A,** Lateral view of the basal ganglia with the caudate nucleus. **B,** Axial view of the basal ganglia with the thalamus, corpus callosum, and caudate nucleus.

Midbrain. The midbrain portion of the brain is narrow and connects the forebrain to the hindbrain. It consists of two halves called the cerebral peduncles (Figure 21-12). The cerebral aqueduct is a narrow cavity of the midbrain that connects the third and fourth ventricles. The tectum is part of the tegmentum located behind the cerebral aqueduct. It has four small surface swellings called the superior and inferior colliculi.

Pons. The pons is found on the anterior surface of the cerebellum below the midbrain and above the medulla oblongata.

Medulla Oblongata. The medulla oblongata extends from the pons to the foramen magnum where it continues as the spinal cord (see Figure 21-9). This structure contains the fiber tracts between the brain and the spinal cord, and the vital centers that regulate important internal activities of the body (heart rate, respiration, and blood pressure).

CEREBELLUM

The **cerebellum** is composed of two hemispheres that have the appearance of cauliflower. The cerebellum lies in the posterior cranial fossa under the tentorium cerebelli. The two hemispheres are connected by the vermis (Figure 21-13). Three pairs of nerve tracts, the cerebellar peduncles, connect the cerebellum to the brain stem. The superior cerebellar peduncles connect the cerebellum to the midbrain. The middle cerebellar peduncles connect the cerebellum to the pons and the inferior cerebellar peduncles connect the cerebellum to the medulla oblongata.

CEREBROVASCULAR SYSTEM

The cerebrovascular system consists of the internal cerebral arteries, vertebral arteries, and circle of Willis (Figure 21-14). The middle cerebral artery (branch of the internal carotid artery) and the circle of Willis are often evaluated with Doppler ultrasound in determining cerebral blood flow patterns. The cerebrovascular system will be discussed in more detail in Chapter 32.

SONOGRAPHIC EVALUATION OF THE NEONATAL BRAIN

Most **neonatal** examinations are performed in the nursery at the bedside. The sonographer must be aware of the infant's condition before the examination. Contact the infant's neona-

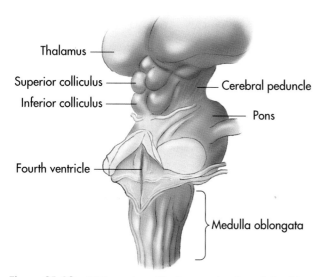

Figure 21-12   Oblique view of brain stem showing relationship of thalamus to cerebral peduncles, fourth ventricle, and medulla oblongata.

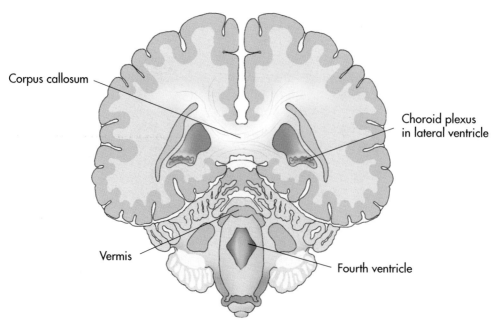

Figure 21-13   Coronal view of the medulla oblongata with the vermis and fourth ventricle.

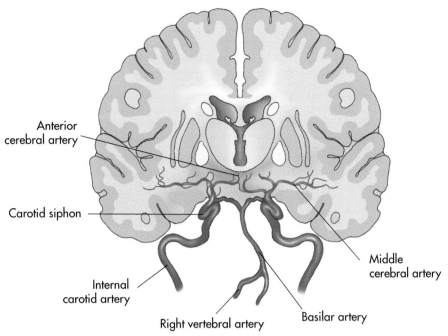

Figure 21-14 Coronal view of the cerebral arterial system.

tal nurse to find out the status of the neonate before the examination. A small amount of warm gel should be used; keep in mind the infant's temperature may be reduced if the Isolette is open for extended time during the examination, or if a large amount of cold gel is applied to the fontanelle.

If the patient is stable enough to travel to the ultrasound department, the sonographer should take the following considerations into account: First, even though the neonate may be well enough to come to the laboratory, he or she is still fragile and susceptible to any environmental changes. Consequently, blankets, radiant heaters, oxygen hookups, and heating pads are all essential to making the environment in the laboratory suitable. Second, if there are any problems with the child, a crash cart and life support systems must be immediately available. A neonatal nurse specialist will probably accompany the neonate to the laboratory. After all these considerations, you may decide to transport the ultrasound equipment to the neonatal intensive care unit for initial evaluation and follow-up.

NEONATAL HEAD EXAMINATION PROTOCOL

Phased array or small linear sector transducers are the equipment of choice to perform echoencephalography studies. The small diameter transducer makes it possible to obtain excellent contact with the skull through the fontanelles and sutures and to avoid the curvature of the calvarium. Consequently, the brain is visualized well even in infants with small fontanelles. The broadband with transducer frequencies ranging from 7 to 4 MHz or 10 to 5 MHz are most commonly used with the premature infant. In larger babies the studies can be obtained with the higher frequency transducer for structures located

> **BOX 21-1** **TRANSDUCER SELECTION**
>
> 5.0 MHz for over 34 weeks or macrocephaly
> 7.0 MHz for under 34 weeks
> <12 MHz for 24 to 26 weeks

close to the fontanelles and a slightly lower frequency transducer for visualization of the anatomy in areas situated farther away from the transducer (Box 21-1). The use of multiple focal zones throughout the depth of the image is used for the best lateral resolution.

Multiple planes and views are used to study the supratentorial and infratentorial compartments. Supratentorial studies show both cerebral hemispheres, the basal ganglia, the lateral and third ventricles, the interhemispheric fissure, and the subarachnoid space surrounding the hemispheres. Infratentorial studies visualize the cerebellum, the brain stem, the fourth ventricle, and the basal cisterns.

Both compartments are studied in the coronal, modified coronal, sagittal, and parasagittal planes. The sagittal, parasagittal, and modified coronal planes are imaged from the anterior fontanelle. Since the structures in the infratentorial compartment are located relatively far from the transducer, the alteration of a deep focal placement or lowering the transducer frequency is recommended, particularly in older infants. The coronal views for the infratentorial compartment are obtained from the mastoid fontanelle and the occipitotemporal area.

At this point, we examine the cross-sectional relationship of structures within the brain so correlation can be made with ultrasound. There are many ways to divide the brain in a cross section. We will deal only with the three planes that are commonly used in ultrasound: axial, coronal, and sagittal.

CORONAL AND MODIFIED CORONAL PLANES

Technically a **coronal** view is 90 degrees to Reid's baseline, but a number of different angles to Reid's baseline are actually used in performing the examination. Reid's baseline is the line extending from the lower edge of the orbit to the center of the aperture of the external auditory canal and backward to the center of the occipital bone. When looking at the coronal sections, the vertex of the skull is at the top and the left side of the brain is to the right of the image.

To perform these studies, the transducer is placed on the anterior fontanelle with the scanning plane following the coronal suture (Figure 21-15). The middle of the transducer must be centered in the coronal suture to reduce bone interference and to procure the most extensive image of the brain. It is critical that symmetric images be obtained; this is accomplished by using the skull bones and the middle cerebral arteries at the sylvian fissure as landmarks (Figure 21-16). The skull bones and the arteries should be the same size bilaterally. In the coronal plane, the transducer is angled from the anterior to the posterior of the skull to completely visualize the lateral and third ventricles, the deep subcortical white matter, and the basal ganglia (Box 21-2).

When the transducer is angled anteriorly, the frontal horns of the lateral ventricles appear as slitlike hypoechoic to cystic formations. As the transducer is angled posteriorly, the ventricles acquire a commalike shape; the ventricular width increases from 2 mm at the frontal lobes to a maximum of 3 to 6 mm at the region of the choroid plexus (bodies of the lateral ventricles) (Figure 21-17).

The sonographer should be aware that ventricular size varies with gestational age and that the premature infant will normally have larger ventricles than the term infant. The term infant has small ventricles, which are "slitlike" in shape. It is important to note the approximate "gestational age" of the premature infant when performing a neonatal sonogram of the head.

The choroid plexus is an intraventricular structure lying along the floor of the lateral ventricles, extending from the temporal horn into the atrium and body of the lateral ventricles (see Figure 21-17). At the foramen of Monro, the choroid plexus enters into the third ventricle. Consequently the frontal (anterior) and the occipital (posterior) horns are devoid of choroid plexus. The choroid plexus becomes enlarged at the level of the atria (glomus of the choroid plexus). At the atria, the plexus can almost entirely fill the ventricular cavity.

Ultrasound depicts the choroid plexus as a very echogenic structure inside the ventricular cavities surrounding the thalamic nuclei. The size of the choroid plexus depends on the gestational age of the infants. The plexus is very large in very immature infants (less than 25 weeks), and it should not be mistaken for intraventricular hemorrhages. The plexus becomes smaller with increasing gestational age. Between 30

BOX 21-2   CORONAL PROTOCOL

- Anterior: orbits
- Anterior: anterior horns and lateral ventricles
- Middle: lateral ventricles, cavum septum pellucidum, third ventricle, and corpus callosum
- Posterior: ambient wings and cisterna magnum
- Posterior: tentorium and cisterna magnum
- Posterior: choroid
- Posterior: glomus of choroids
- Posterior: far posterior brain (occipital)

Coronal plane

A

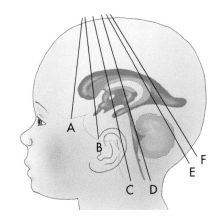

B

Figure 21-15   A, The transducer is placed on the anterior fontanelle, perpendicular to the neonatal head. **B,** Coronal scan planes as the transducer is angled from the anterior to posterior skull as described in the text. *A* through *F* indicate the different scanning planes. *A* is the most anterior, and *F* is the most posterior.

Figure 21-16 Normal protocol for coronal images beginning with the transducer angled toward the anterior skull (**A** and **B**); then angled to the midcoronal section (**C, D, E,** and **F**); and finally angled toward the posterior occipital area of the skull (**G** and **H**).

Figure 21-17 A, First anterior coronal image. *CN,* Caudate nucleus; *F,* falx; *SP,* septum pellucidum.
B, Second anterior coronal image. *CN,* Caudate nucleus; *SP,* septum pellucidum. **C,** Midcoronal image. *AH,*
Anterior horn; *CC,* corpus callosum; *CN,* caudate nucleus; *SF,* sylvian fissure; *SP,* septum pellucidum; *Tent,*
tentorium. **D,** Midcoronal image. *AH,* Anterior horn; *CP,* choroid plexus. **E,** Posterior coronal image. *CP,*
Choroid plexus. **F,** Posterior coronal image beyond the level of the ventricles.

weeks of gestation and term, the size is approximately 2 to 3 mm at the body of the lateral ventricles and 4 to 5 mm at the atria (glomus of the choroid plexus).

The third ventricle is not visualized in normal conditions in the coronal or modified coronal studies in the full-term fetus. Occasionally a thin and very echogenic formation can be seen in the midline immediately below the septum pellucidum. This echogenic image corresponds to the choroid plexus extending into the third ventricle. The septum pellucidum appears as a midline hypoechoic to cystic structure separating the bodies and frontal horns of the lateral ventricles. The septum constitutes the internal wall of the bodies and posterior part of the frontal horns. The cavum septum pellucidum is anterior to the corpus callosum. In the premature fetus, less than 32 weeks, the third ventricle is prominent and easily seen on sonography.

Coronal and modified coronal views also visualize the basal ganglia and the white matter. The caudate nuclei constitute the inferior and lateral walls of the ventricles at the bodies and posterior part of the frontal horns (see Figure 21-17). In premature infants the caudate nuclei may have higher echogenicity than the rest of the brain parenchyma. In these infants, the nuclei should not be mistaken for **subependymal** hemorrhages. The thalamic ganglia are located laterally to the third ventricle, and they are visualized as areas of low echogenicity. The white matter is situated between the lateral ventricles and the cortex. The white matter has low echogenicity with thin echogenic streaks that correspond to small vessels. This area is known as "watershed zones," which are the terminal ends of the vessel bed and may be used to describe the periventricular white matter.

MODIFIED CORONAL STUDIES OF THE VENTRICLES AND POSTERIOR FOSSA

The modified coronal plane demonstrates the body of the lateral ventricles, the third ventricle, and the posterior fossa. To obtain this view, the transducer is positioned over the anterior fontanelle with an angle of approximately 30 to 40 degrees between the scanning plane and the surface of the fontanelle. In this view the tentorium, the cerebellar vermis, the fourth ventricle, the cerebellar hemispheres, and the cisterna magna can be seen in the infratentorial compartment.

The vermis is a very echogenic structure in the midline (Figure 21-18). The fourth ventricle appears in the midline as a small anechoic space approximately 2 to 3 mm wide, located anteriorly to the vermis. The cerebellar hemispheres have low echogenicity and are contiguous with the echogenic vermis. The cisterna magna corresponds to a nonechogenic space between the vermis, the cerebellar hemispheres, and the occipital bone.

CORONAL STUDIES THROUGH THE POSTERIOR FONTANELLE

If the anatomical structures are difficult to image because of overlapping bones in the area of the fontanelle, the posterior fontanelle is used as an alternative window to image the choroid plexus and lateral ventricles.

Figure 21-18 Midcoronal image of the septum pellucidum *(SP)*, third ventricle *(3V)*, vermis *(V)*, and fourth ventricle *(4V)*.

BOX 21-3 **SAGITTAL AND PARASAGITTAL PROTOCOL**

These steps should be done separately for each side of the brain:

- Midline: cavum septum pellucidum, corpus callosum, third ventricle, and foramen of Monroe, aqueduct of Sylvius, fourth ventricle, cerebellum (tentorium), cisterna magna
- Thalamus
- Caudothalamic groove (notch)
- Lateral ventricle: anterior, body, and occipital (temporal if hydrocephalic)
- Angle slightly lateral from the lateral ventricle to show the white matter
- Very lateral—sylvian fissure (middle cerebral artery)

SAGITTAL AND PARASAGITTAL PLANE

Sagittal plane sections are made by rotating the coronal plane approximately 90 degrees. These sections are viewed with the anterior brain to the left and the occipital portion of the brain to the right. To obtain these studies, the transducer is positioned over the anterior fontanelle with the scanning plane following the sagittal suture (Figures 21-19 and 21-20). Sagittal studies provide the most extensive visualization of the brain (Box 21-3).

The straight sagittal study (the only view strictly in the sagittal plane) shows the midline structures in the supratentorial and infratentorial compartments. The straight midline view should be obtained before performing the right and left parasagittal studies. This view is a guide to determine if a parasagittal study corresponds to the right or left side (Figure 21-21).

The supratentorial structures shown by the sagittal studies are the corpus callosum, septum pellucidum, and third ventricle (Figure 21-22). The corpus callosum appears as two thin parallel lines separated by a thin echogenic space. The genu and splenium of the corpus callosum may be identified as the anterior-dorsal and posterior portions, respectively. The

Figure 21-19   The transducer is placed in the anterior fontanelle, perpendicular to the skull, and rotated 90 degrees from the coronal plane to the sagittal plane. The transducer uses the midsagittal plane as the primary landmark; slight angulation of the transducer away from the midline will show the parasagittal and midsagittal planes. *A* and *C* indicate the lateral sagittal planes through the ventricles. *B* indicates the midline sagittal plane.

cingulate sulcus is found anterior and parallel to the corpus callosum. This is a helpful landmark to identify; as with agenesis of the corpus callosum, it is randomized or spiraled because of the midline defect. The septum pellucidum appears as an anechoic (cystic) structure immediately below the corpus callosum. The third ventricle is normally anechoic and is located inferiorly to the septum. The echogenic choroid plexus appears to enter the top of the third ventricle through the foramen of Monro. The supraoptic recess of the third ventricle is shown as a triangular nonechogenic structure extending inferiorly and anteriorly toward the suprasellar region.

In the straight sagittal plane, the infratentorial structures visualized are the cerebellar vermis, the fourth ventricle, the cisterna magna, the supracerebellar and quadrigeminal cisterns, and the brain stem. The vermis of the cerebellum appears as a very echo-dense formation, separated from the occipital bone by an anechoic space that corresponds to the cisterna magna.

The other cisterns also are anechoic spaces located above and behind the cerebellar vermis. The fourth ventricle appears as a small v with the vertex oriented posteriorly inside the echogenic vermis. The fourth ventricle is limited anteriorly by the brain stem. The brain stem has low echogenicity, with an echo-dense anterior border demarcated by the basilar artery.

PARASAGITTAL STUDIES

After having studied the midline, the transducer is moved/angled slightly to the left and right sides to visualize the cerebellar hemispheres in the parasagittal plane (see Box 21-3). The cerebellar hemispheres appear as round, low echogenic formations with moderately hyperechoic surfaces.

The parasagittal views are obtained by angling the transducer to the right or left side of the skull. Three parasagittal studies should be performed. The first parasagittal image should be close to the midline to visualize the caudate nuclei in detail since subependymal hemorrhages begin in the germinal matrix that is located at the level of these ganglia. These views image the frontal horn and body of the lateral ventricles, the thalamus, the head of the caudate nucleus, and the choroid plexus.

The frontal horns and bodies of the lateral ventricles appear as narrow sonolucent cavities (Figure 21-23). The height of the bodies of the ventricles normally is less than 7 mm at the level of the midthalamus. The floor of lateral ventricles is determined by the boundary between the very echogenic choroid plexus and the less echogenic thalamus. The choroid plexus appears as a small (2 to 3 mm height), very echogenic structure lying against the thalamus. The plexus appears to end at the thalamic-caudate groove, which is the most common location of subependymal hemorrhages. The floor of the ventricles ventral to the groove is formed by the head of the caudate nucleus, which in very small infants has higher echogenicity than the surrounding tissue.

The second parasagittal image is made slightly lateral to the first image and includes the entire ventricular cavity. Since the ventricular cavity is not entirely parallel to the midline (i.e., the posterior horns are more lateral or external than the anterior horns), the transducer must be rotated slightly counterclockwise to form an acute angle with the sagittal suture anteriorly. These views show the entire ventricular horns; the choroid plexus, including the glomus; the thalami; the caudate nuclei; and the white matter superior and anterior to the lateral ventricles.

Figure 21-20 Normal protocol for sagittal images beginning with the transducer perpendicular to the skull (**A**), then to the right (**B, C, D,** and **E**), back to the midline (**F**), and then to the left (**G** and **H**).

The third parasagittal view images the white matter located lateral (externally) to the lateral ventricles (Figure 21-24). This view is useful in studying intraparenchymal hemorrhages, porencephaly, and periventricular leukomalacia.

A fourth parasagittal view should demonstrate the lateral most aspect, the sylvian figure, middle cerebral artery, and insula.

DEVELOPMENTAL PROBLEMS OF THE BRAIN

NEURAL TUBE DEFECTS

A number of different anomalies may occur in fetal brain development. These anomalies, such as anencephaly, meningomyelocele, meningocele, and encephalocele, are discussed in more detail in Chapter 55.

Chiari Malformations. A Chiari malformation is a congenital anomaly associated with spina bifida in which the cerebellum and brain stem are pulled toward the spinal cord and secondary hydrocephalus develops. Chiari malformations have been characterized by variations of the following findings: (1) displacement of the fourth ventricle and upper medulla into the cervical canal; (2) displacement of the inferior part of the cerebellum through the foramen magnum; and (3) defects in the calvarium and spinal column.

Chiari malformations have been classified into four groups:

Chiari I—downward displacement of the cerebellar tonsils, without displacement of the fourth ventricle or medulla

Chiari II—most common (and of greatest clinical importance) because of its association with meningomyelocele

Chiari III—high cervical encephalomeningocele in which the medulla, fourth ventricle, and cerebellum reside

Chiari IV—severe hypoplasia of the cerebellum without displacement

Figure 21-22   "Straight" sagittal view of the midline structures. Supratentorial structures: choroid plexus *(CP)*, corpus callosum *(CC)*, septum pellucidum *(SP)*, and third ventricle *(3V)*. Infratentorial structures: brain stem *(BS)*, cerebellar vermis *(V)*, cisterna magna *(CM)*, and fourth ventricle *(4V)*.

Figure 21-21   Slight parasagittal view of the third ventricle *(3V)*, fourth ventricle *(4V)*, vermis *(V)*, foramen magnum *(FM)*, and cisterna magna *(CM)*.

A   B

Figure 21-23   Parasagittal images of the right **(A)** and left **(B)** ventricles *(LV)* with choroid plexus (CP).

A   **B**

Figure 21-24   Parasagittal images of the brain are made as the transducer is angled toward the sylvian fissure to show the white matter of the brain. **A,** Right brain; **B,** left brain.

Chiari malformation is frequently associated with myelomeningocele, hydrocephalus, dilation of the third ventricle, and absence of the septum pellucidum. About 80% to 90% of infants with myelomeningocele have Chiari malformations. Hydrocephalus is usually caused by obstruction of the CSF pathway at the fourth ventricle or in the posterior fossa, or secondary to aqueductal stenosis, which is present in 40% to 75% of infants with Chiari malformations.

Sonographic Findings. Chiari malformations can be diagnosed with ultrasound. A failure in the neural tube closure results in a small posterior fossa. In addition, the formation of a myelomeningocele may develop as a result of the open neural tube defect. The myelomeningocele in turn decompresses the ventricles, causing underdevelopment of the posterior fossa. Sagittal studies from the anterior fontanelle show a small cerebellum, absence of the cisterna magna, low position of the fourth ventricle, and displacement of the cerebellum through the foramen magnum associated with hydrocephalus, absence of the septum pellucidum, and widening of the third ventricle (Figures 21-25 and 21-26). With compression of the cerebellum, the cerebellar tonsils and vermis herniated into the spinal canal through an enlarged foramen magnum. The pons and medulla are inferiorly displaced and the fourth ventricle becomes elongated (Figure 21-27). In addition, enlargement of the massa intermedia may be noted on the coronal and midline sagittal images. This enlargement of the massa intermedia may cause the third ventricle to appear slightly larger than normal. The frontal horns are often small ("bat wing" sign of the anterior and inferior pointing of the frontal horns), whereas the posterior horns of the ventricles are quite enlarged. The septum pellucidum may be partially or completely absent. The interhemispheric fissure may appear widened on the coronal scans. The posterior fossa is small and the tentorium is low and hypoplastic. Hydrocephalus is usually present.

Holoprosencephaly. Holoprosencephaly is characterized by a grossly abnormal brain in which there is a common large

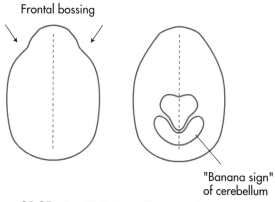

Figure 21-25   Arnold-Chiari malformation shows a small displaced cerebellum, absence of the cisterna magna, malposition of the fourth ventricle, absence of the septum pellucidum, and widening of the third ventricle.

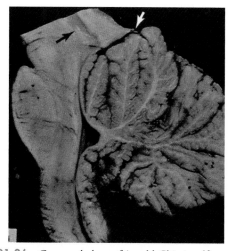

Figure 21-26   Gross pathology of Arnold-Chiari malformation shows breaking of the tectum *(arrow)* and dilatation of the aqueduct *(open arrow)* caused by compression of the fourth ventricle. (From Damjanov I, Linder J: *Pathology: a color atlas,* St Louis, 2000, Mosby.)

central ventricle (Figure 21-28). **Holoprosencephaly** is caused by disturbances in the process of ventral induction very early in life. Holoprosencephaly represents a spectrum of malformations that form a continuum from most severe, with no separation of the telencephalon (alobar), to least severe, with partial separation of the dorsal aspects of the brain (lobar). A third classification of intermediate severity between alobar and lobar is semilobar holoprosencephaly. The neuropathologic features include a single cerebrum with a single ventricular cavity, absence of the corpus callosum and frontal horns, and a thin membrane arising from the roof of the third ventricle, which may extend posteriorly forming a supratentorial cyst (Figure 21-29). In addition, anomalies of the face also accompany this condition.

Alobar holoprosencephaly. This is the most severe form of holoprosencephaly. Multiple facial anomalies (i.e., cebocephaly, cyclopia, and ethmocephaly) are present. The brain surrounds a single midline crescent-shaped ventricle with the thin, primitive cerebral cortex surrounding the large ventricle. The thalami and hemispheres are fused; no falx, corpus callosum, or interhemispheric fissure is present. The fused thalami are seen anterior to the fused hyperechogenic choroid plexus (Figure 21-30). The third ventricle is absent, causing the dilated single ventricle to communicate directly with the aqueduct of Sylvius.

Figure 21-27   Infant was delivered by cesarean section at 39 weeks' gestation for thoracic spina bifida. Chiari's malformation, type II, was identified. Enlarged ventricles can be seen in **(A)** anterior and **(B)** posterior coronal views. **C,** Lateral sagittal view of head. **D,** Magnetic resonance imaging shows spinal defect. (From Henningsen C: *Clinical guide to ultrasonography,* St Louis, 2004, Mosby.)

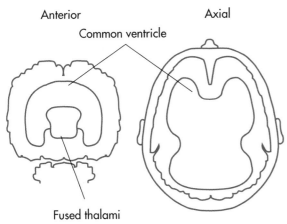

Figure 21-28   Holoprosencephaly features a single ventricular cavity with abnormalities of the cerebrum.

A

B

Figure 21-30   **A**, Alobar holoprosencephaly is identified in image demonstrating single ventricle. **B**, Variable fusion identified in semilobar holoprosencephaly is seen in image. (From Henningsen C: *Clinical guide to ultrasonography,* St Louis, 2004, Mosby.)

Figure 21-29   This posterior view shows the reflected cyst wall communicating with a univentricle. (From Damjanov I, Linder J: *Pathology: a color atlas,* St Louis, 2000, Mosby.)

Semilobar holoprosencephaly. A single ventricle is evident; however, more brain parenchyma is present with pieces of the falx and interhemispheric fissure developed in the posterior segment. There may be separate occipital and temporal horns. The splenium of the corpus callosum is often formed and may be seen on midline sagittal images. The thalami are partially separated and the third ventricle is rudimentary. Mild facial anomalies (i.e., hypotelorism and cleft lip) may be present.

Lobar holoprosencephaly. This is the least severe form of holoprosencephaly. There is nearly complete separation of hemispheres with development of a falx and interhemispheric fissure. There may be fusion of the frontal lobes. The septum pellucidum is absent. The anterior horns of the lateral ventricles are fused; however, the occipital horns are separated. The third ventricle is present and separates the thalami. The splenium and body of the corpus callosum are present with the absence of the genu and rostrum. Facial anomalies are mild.

Ischemic lesions. After the ventral induction has occurred, ischemic lesions in the midline may induce malformations of

the telencephalon similar to holoprosencephaly. As in holoprosencephaly, there is a single ventricular cavity and absence of the corpus callosum. However, the presence of two frontal horns helps differentiate these malformations caused by ischemic lesions from true holoprosencephaly.

Sonographic Findings. When holoprosencephaly is suspected, it is important to obtain modified coronal studies of the whole frontal lobes to determine whether two frontal horns are present.

Dandy-Walker Malformation. Dandy-Walker syndrome is a congenital anomaly in which a huge fourth ventricle cyst occupies the area where the cerebellum usually lies, with secondary dilation of the third and lateral ventricles. The **Dandy-Walker malformation** of the cerebellum is the result of a disturbance of the growth of the roof of the fourth ventricle. The vermis is absent in 25% of the population. The fourth ventricle is enlarged. The posterior fossa is enlarged with the sinuses displaced upward. It may be associated with the following malformations: hydrocephalus, agenesis of the corpus callosum, infundibular hamartomas, or brain-stem lipomas.

Sonographic Findings. The typical Dandy-Walker malformation is characterized by absence of the cerebellar vermis, cystic changes in the fourth ventricle with the development of a large cyst in the posterior fossa (Dandy-Walker cyst), and hydrocephalus (Figure 21-31). The hydrocephalus is caused by the atresia of the foramina of Luschka and Magendie (congenital obstructive hydrocephalus) (Figure 21-32). When the vermis is absent, the fourth ventricle communicates directly with the cyst. A Dandy-Walker variant is present when there is an enlarged cisterna magna communicating with the fourth ventricle in the presence of a normal or hypoplastic cerebellar vermis (Figure 21-33).

Agenesis of the Corpus Callosum. Agenesis of the corpus callosum is a condition in which the fibers of the corpus callosum cross from side to side on a glial sling; agenesis may occur as an isolated anomaly without any clinical effect. The corpus callosum is the great commissure connecting the brain hemispheres. Hypoplasia or agenesis of the corpus callosum may occur during the processes of ventral induction or cellular migration. Agenesis of the corpus callosum is often combined with migrational disorders, such as heterotopias and polymicrogyria. Absence of the corpus callosum may also be induced by ischemic lesions in the midline or by intrauterine encephalomalacia. Other defects associated with this defect are porencephaly, hydrocephalus, microgyria, and fusion of the hemispheres.

The corpus callosum is absent in severe holoprosencephaly. Agenesis of the corpus callosum may be associated with Arnold-Chiari malformation and hydrocephalus. In neonates with this anomaly, the cerebral hemispheres have ventricles with pointed upper corners (bat-wing appearance).

Sonographic Findings. Complete absence of the corpus callosum is distinguished by narrow frontal horns and marked separation of the anterior horns and bodies of the lateral ventricles associated with widening of the occipital horns and the third ventricle (Figure 21-34). The ventricular cavities acquire the distinctive appearance of "vampire wings." These characteristics are easily identified by ultrasound (Figure 21-35). Partial agenesis of the corpus callosum occurs when the genu, the splenium, and the rostrum are absent.

HYDROCEPHALUS

Congenital Hydrocephalus. Hydrocephalus refers to any condition in which enlargement of the ventricular system is caused by an imbalance between production and reabsorption of cerebrospinal fluid (CSF). Hydrocephalus is caused by a variety of conditions that cause the ventricles to dilate when there is obstruction of cerebral spinal fluid. Congenital structural malformations, such as myelomeningocele, agenesis of the corpus callosum, and aqueductal stenosis, are all associated with ventricular dilatation. Acquired hydrocephalus occurs after the loss of deep white matter in periventricular leukomalacia (PVL), and after intraventricular hemorrhage caused by either acquired aqueductal stenosis or occlusion of resorptive arachnoid granulations. Posthemorrhagic hydrocephalus (PHH) should not be confused with grade III intraventricular hemorrhage. Hydrocephalus is divided into communicating and noncommunicating forms; the former is produced by occluded granulations and the latter by some anatomic obstruction to CSF flow.

The earlier the hydrocephalus occurs, the greater the enlargement of the neonatal head. This dilation results in widely separated sutures and huge, bulging fontanelles.

Sonographic Findings. The sonographer should look for the blunting of the lateral angles of the lateral ventricles (Figure 21-36).

When this instability of hydrocephalus ensues in the fetus, the widening of the ventricular system is present at birth. Infants born with ventricular enlargement are considered to have congenital hydrocephalus. Hydrocephalus is infrequently caused by overproduction of fluid. Excessive fluid production may occur in infants with papilloma of the choroid plexus, a tumor that actively secretes CSF. Two anatomic

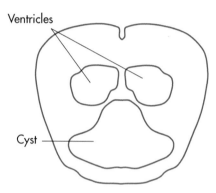

Ventricles

Cyst

Posterior fossa

Figure 21-31 Dandy-Walker malformation is characterized by the absence of the cerebellar vermis and cystic changes in the fourth ventricle. Hydrocephalus may also be present.

Figure 21-32 Dandy-Walker malformation. Hypoplastic vermis and cyst are reflected to expose a dilated fourth ventricle. (From Damjanov I, Linder J: *Pathology: a color atlas,* St Louis, 2000, Mosby.)

Figure 21-33 Dandy-Walker malformation. **A** and **B,** Female infant was born at 37 weeks' gestation, and neonatal head ultrasound was ordered. Mother of the infant had no prenatal care. Sonographic evaluation showed posterior fossa cyst and splaying in cerebellar hemispheres as noted in the coronal images. No hydrocephalus was identified. **C** and **D,** Hydrocephalus was identified in infant with DWM. **C,** Lateral sagittal and **D,** coronal views show large posterior fossa cyst and accompanying ventricular enlargement. (From Henningsen C: *Clinical guide to ultrasonography,* St Louis, 2004, Mosby.)

types of hydrocephalus are distinguished: obstructive and communicating.

Obstructive hydrocephalus. Obstructive hydrocephalus is characterized by interference in the circulation of CSF within the ventricular system itself, causing subsequent enlargement of the ventricular cavities proximal to the obstruction.

Communicating hydrocephalus. In communicating hydrocephalus, the CSF pathways are open within the ventricular system, but there is decreased absorption of CSF. Absorption of CSF can be impeded by occlusion of the subarachnoid cisterns in the posterior fossa or the obliteration of the subarachnoid spaces over the convexities of the brain. The entire ventricular system becomes uniformly distended.

The most common cause of congenital hydrocephalus is **aqueductal stenosis**. The aqueduct of Sylvius is narrowed or replaced by multiple small channels with blind ends. Occasionally, aqueductal stenosis may be caused by extrinsic lesions posterior to the brain stem, such as congenital aneurysm of the vein of Galen.

Sonographic Findings. Aqueductal stenosis can be diagnosed with ultrasound when an infant is born with widening of the lateral and third ventricles and a normal-size fourth ventricle. If the hydrocephalus is very large, the posterior fossa is smaller than usual, and the cerebellum is displaced toward the occipital bone with the disappearance of the cisterna magna. However, the cerebellum is not dislodged into the foramen

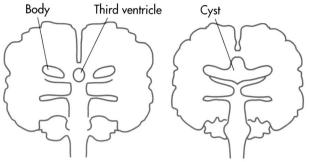

Body   Third ventricle   Cyst

Figure 21-34 Complete agenesis of the corpus callosum is characterized by narrow frontal horns with marked separation of the anterior horns and bodies of the lateral ventricles.

magnum, thus differentiating aqueductal stenosis from the Arnold-Chiari malformation. Arnold-Chiari and Dandy-Walker malformations, other important causes of congenital hydrocephalus, already have been described.

SUBARACHNOID CYSTS

Subarachnoid cysts are lined by arachnoid tissue and contain cerebrospinal fluid. There are three major causes postulated to explain the formation of these cysts: (1) localized entrapment of fluid during embryogenesis, (2) residual subdural hematoma, and (3) fluid extravasation secondary to leptomeningeal tear or ventricular rupture.

The cysts may be located in the infratentorial or supratentorial compartments. Subarachnoid cysts in the posterior fossa

A   B

C

Figure 21-35 **A,** Agenesis of the corpus callosum (ACC) is noted in midline sagittal image of preterm infant. Cingulated gyri also display abnormal configuration. **B,** Rounded occipital horns are also evidence of ACC. **C,** Coronal view shows monoventricle present. Infant was diagnosed with semilobar holoprosencephaly. Bilateral cleft lip was also present. Infant died shortly after birth. (From Henningsen C: *Clinical guide to ultrasonography,* St Louis, 2004, Mosby.)

Figure 21-36   **A through D,** A 4-month-old infant with hydrocephalus shows dilation of the lateral ventricles. **E and F,** Follow-up study of the infant shows the shunt tubing in place for drainage of the hydrocephalus. Ultrasound is very useful in following the shunt placement and monitoring the drainage of the dilated ventricle.

are associated with a normal vermis and a normal fourth ventricle, which differentiates subarachnoid cysts from the Dandy-Walker malformation. In a supratentorial compartment, these cysts usually arise from the suprasellar or quadrigeminal plate cisterns. The most frequent locations are the interhemispheric fissure, the suprasellar region, and the cerebral convexities. These cysts may be symptomatic secondary to cerebral compression or hydrocephalus, or they may be totally asymptomatic.

Sonographic Findings. Subarachnoid cysts usually appear on ultrasound studies as a sonolucent structure arising from the quadrigeminal plate cistern or the suprasellar region. Sagittal studies are useful to determine the location and size of these cysts. Sequential studies should be obtained in infants with this complication since the cysts may have progressive growth and may need to be drained by ventriculoperitoneal shunts. Color Doppler may be used to verify that these are not venous malformations, especially when the cysts occur within the quadrigeminal plate cistern or the suprasellar region.

SONOGRAPHIC EVALUATION OF NEONATAL BRAIN LESIONS

Sonography is ideal for timing the onset and sequentially following the evolution of brain lesions that may develop in the premature infant.

HEMORRHAGIC PATHOLOGY

Subependymal-Intraventricular Hemorrhages. Subependymal-intraventricular hemorrhages (SEHs-IVHs) are the most common hemorrhagic lesions in preterm newborn infants. There is an increased risk of subependymal-intraventricular hemorrhage in infants less than 32 weeks gestational age and/or less than 1500 grams birth weight. These lesions affect 30% to 50% of infants less than 34 weeks of gestation. SEHs-IVHs are a developmental disease since they originate in the subependymal germinal matrix (Figure 21-37).

The germinal matrix is the tissue where neurons and glial cells develop before migrating from the subventricular (subependymal) region to the cortex. The germinal matrix is highly cellular, has poor connective supporting tissue, and is richly vascularized with very thin capillaries. This increased capillary fragility may explain the high frequency of these hemorrhages in tiny infants. Furthermore, the germinal matrix has a high fibrinolytic activity that may be important for the extension of the capillary hemorrhages that originate in this tissue. By 24 weeks of gestation, most of the neuronal and glial migration has occurred. However, pockets of germinal matrix remain until 40 weeks of gestation in the subependymal area at the head of the caudate nuclei. This may explain why subependymal hemorrhages occur less frequently in term infants and why the majority of the intraventricular hemorrhages in these infants originate in the choroid plexus.

Subependymal hemorrhages (SEHs) are caused by capillary bleeding in the germinal matrix. The most frequent location is at the thalamic-caudate groove (Figure 21-38). If bleeding continues, the hemorrhage enlarges, pushing the ependyma into the ventricular cavity, which can then become completely occluded by the subependymal hemorrhage. Eventually, large SEHs rupture through the ependyma into the ventricular cavity, forming an intraventricular hemorrhage (IVH).

Sonographic Findings. IVHs and SEHs are easily detected with ultrasound as echogenic structures since fluid and clotted blood have higher acoustic impedance than the brain parenchyma and the CSF. The degree of echogenicity will depend upon the acute-chronic process of the hemorrhage. The acute hemorrhage will appear more echogenic than the chronic hemorrhage. SEHs-IVHs can be studied in the coronal, modified coronal, sagittal, parasagittal, and axial planes. A subependymal hemorrhage is usually seen at the thalamic-caudate notch as a very echogenic lesion pushing up the floor and external wall of the lateral ventricle with partial obliteration of the ventricular cavity. The SEH can extend by continuous bleeding and perforate the ventricular wall with partial or total flooding of the ventricular system (intraventricular hemorrhage, IVH) (Figure 21-39).

IVHs appear as echogenic structures inside the anechoic ventricular cavities. Depending on the amount of blood, the ventricle can become full and dilated. Subsequently the SEH may obstruct the circulation and absorption of the cerebrospinal fluid, causing the ventricles to dilate further with CSF and ultimately resulting in posthemorrhagic hydrocephalus.

Studies from the anterior fontanelle may not detect small IVHs, since intraventricular blood tends to "settle out" in the posterior horns. These small IVHs can be diagnosed when the occipital horns are visualized in the axial plane from the mastoid or from the posterior fontanelles. Since these fontanelles are closer to the occipital horns than the anterior fontanelle, the occipital horns are within the focal range of the

Figure 21-37 Subependymal hemorrhage extending into the ventricles. The ventricles contain coagulated blood. (From Damjanov I, Linder J: *Pathology: a color atlas,* St Louis, 2000, Mosby.)

Figure 21-38 Sagittal image of a premature neonate with a small subependymal bleed *(arrow).*

Figure 21-39   **A** and **B,** Coronal and sagittal images of a premature twin with a grade II bleed shortly after birth that progressed to a grade III bleed in 1 day (**C** and **D**).

transducer, and a greater amount of ultrasonic energy can reach the sedimented red blood cells.

IVHs-SEHs are not a sudden event; they usually expand slowly. This phenomenon is probably secondary to the high fibrinolytic activity of the germinal matrix. However, in some infants the IVHs-SEHs extend very fast; sudden flooding and distension of the ventricles by hemorrhage is associated with the clinical symptoms of shock, seizures, hypoxemia, and a sudden decrease in the hematocrit. Typically, when a small IVH-SEH progresses to a large IVH-SEH (usually during the first 4 postpartum days), the IVHs-SEHs are asymptomatic. Since approximately 70% of hemorrhages are asymptomatic, it is necessary to have a technique, such as ultrasound, to routinely scan all the infants at risk for these lesions.

Classification of subependymal intraventricular hemorrhages (SEH-IVH) is based on the extension of the hemorrhage and the resultant changes in the ventricular size (Box 21-4). Only ventricular enlargement produced by the intraventricular hemorrhage should be considered. Small SEHs-IVHs may occlude the foramen of Monro or the aqueduct of Sylvius and thereby produce moderate to large dilation of the lateral ventricles by CSF.

The ventricular size is measured in the sagittal plane (height of the body of the ventricles at the midthalamus) and in the

---

BOX 21-4   CLASSIFICATION OF SUBEPENDYMAL INTRAVENTRICULAR HEMORRHAGES

Grade I: SEH or IVH without ventricular enlargement
Grade II: SEH or IVH with minimal ventricular enlargement
Grade III: SEH or IVH with moderate or large ventricular enlargement
Grade IV: SEH or IVH with intraparenchymal hemorrhage

---

axial plane (width of the atrium at the level of the choroid plexus). Based on these measurements, ventricular dilation may be classified as follows:

- **Mild dilation:** Ventricular size measuring 8 to 10 mm
- **Moderate dilation:** Ventricular size measuring 11 to 14 mm
- **Large dilation:** Ventricular size greater than 14 mm

After the hemorrhage has occurred, the blood spreads following the CSF pathways, reaching the fourth ventricle and eventually the cisterns in the posterior fossa, with the development of subarachnoid hemorrhages (SAH) (Figure 21-40). Subsequently, obstruction of the CSF pathways and obliterans arachnoiditis occurs, causing imbalance between production

Figure 21-40   Multiple coronal and sagittal images in a premature infant born after 27 weeks of gestation with a large cerebellar bleed *(arrows)*. In 5 days the bleed had progressed throughout the cerebellar compartment.

and reabsorption of CSF. Posthemorrhagic ventricular dilation develops as a consequence of this imbalance. If the ventricular dilation is progressive, the patient is considered to have posthemorrhagic hydrocephalus. This complication occurs in approximately 35% of infants with large hemorrhages. Usually mild to moderate ventricular dilation resolves spontaneously. However, placement of a ventriculoperitoneal shunt may be necessary for severely dilated ventricles.

Posthemorrhagic hydrocephalus may be silent since the white matter of newborn infants is very compliant and easily compressed as the ventricles widen. This factor explains why initial ventricular dilation occurs without changes in the head circumference. The head circumference starts to enlarge only after significant compression of the white matter has developed. Sequential studies are required in infants with SEHs-

IVHs to diagnose posthemorrhagic ventricular dilation in the silent phase.

Ultrasound is the most reliable technique to diagnose and follow changes in the ventricular size and in the intraventricular clots. IVHs-SEHs resolve in several days or weeks, depending on the size of the bleed and on the individual patient. Although intraventricular clots are easily detected by CT, they resolve as the concentration of hemoglobin decreases, and they are not seen after 10 to 14 days in CT studies.

Intraventricular clots undergo characteristic changes with time. Initially, they are very echogenic, but then low echogenic areas appear. Eventually they become completely cystic with visualization of the choroid plexus inside the cystic ventricular cast. Large cystic intraventricular clots may cause persistent ventricular dilation despite drainage of the CSF by a ventriculoperitoneal shunt. If the bleed completely fills the ventricular cavity, the ventricle becomes isoechoic with the other structures in the brain and is more difficult to define the borders of the ventricular wall.

Intraparenchymal Hemorrhages. Intraparenchymal hemorrhages (IPHs) complicate SEHs-IVHs in approximately 15% to 25% of the infants. IPHs are a severe complication since they indicate that the brain parenchyma has been destroyed. Although IPHs originally were considered an extension of SEHs-IVHs, evidence suggests that this lesion may actually be a primary infarction of the periventricular and subcortical white matter with destruction of the lateral wall of the ventricle. When the necrotic tissue liquefies, the IVH extends into the necrotic areas.

Sonographic Findings. Intraparenchymal hemorrhages appear as very echogenic zones in the white matter adjacent to the lateral ventricles. Echogenic areas in the white matter may correspond to IPHs or to hemorrhagic infarctions or extensive periventricular leukomalacia. In the classic grade IV IPH, there is a clot extending from the white matter into the ventricular cavity (Figure 21-41).

Intraparenchymal clots follow the same evolution as intraventricular clots. A few days after the acute bleeding, the clots become cystic and are reabsorbed completely in 3 or 4 weeks, leaving a cavity communicating with the lateral ventricle (porencephalic cyst).

When SEHs-IVHs associated with IPH evolve to posthemorrhagic hydrocephalus, the increased intraventricular pressure is transmitted to the porencephalic cyst. Hydrocephalus after hemorrhage associated with porencephaly is an indication for early ventriculoperitoneal shunt placement to minimize the deleterious effects of progressive compression and ischemia of the brain parenchyma.

Intracerebellar Hemorrhages. Four categories of intracerebellar hemorrhage are described as follows:

1. Primary intracerebellar hemorrhage
2. Venous infarction
3. Traumatic laceration resulting from occipital diastasis
4. Extension to the cerebellum of a large SEH-IVH

In premature neonates, there are areas of germinal matrix located around the fourth ventricle in the cerebellar

Figure 21-41 A 3-day-old premature infant has a grade III bleed on the right and grade IV bleed on the left with extension into the brain parenchyma.

hemispheres. The cerebellar germinal matrix has the same vulnerability to hemorrhage as the telencephalic germinal matrix. Intracerebellar hemorrhages have been reported in approximately 5% to 10% of postmortem studies of neonatal populations. The incidence in live infants is significantly lower. This discrepancy is probably a result of the difficulties in diagnosing these hemorrhages.

Sonographic Findings. Using modified coronal, sagittal, and parasagittal views of the posterior fossa (infratentorial compartment), it is possible to diagnose unequivocally intracerebellar hemorrhages. These hemorrhages appear as very echogenic structures inside the less echogenic cerebellar parenchyma. Coronal views through the mastoid fontanelle may be essential to differentiate intracerebellar hemorrhages from large SAHs in the cisterna magna, the supracerebellar cistern, or both. Intracerebellar hemorrhages become cystic with time, leaving cavitary lesions in the cerebellar hemispheres. These characteristic sequential changes are useful in making a positive diagnosis of intracerebellar hemorrhages.

Epidural Hemorrhages and Subdural Collections. Epidural hemorrhages and subdural fluid collections are better diagnosed by CT. Since these lesions are located peripherally along the surface of the brain, they are often not adequately visualized by ultrasound.

Sonographic Findings. Subdural collections appear as nonechogenic spaces between the echogenic calvarium and the cortex. Epidural hemorrhages are seen as echogenic formations located immediately underneath the calvarium.

ISCHEMIC-HYPOXIC LESIONS

Ischemic-hypoxic cerebral injury is a frequent complication of sick newborn infants. The premature neonate is physiologically delicate at birth and as a result is subject to many stresses that in turn can cause hemorrhage and brain injury. Hypoxia is the lack of adequate oxygen to the brain, whereas ischemia is the lack of adequate blood flow to the brain. These occurrences can result from a variety of insults, including respiratory failure, congenital heart disease, and sepsis.

In the term neonate, hypoxic-ischemic injury tends to occur in watershed regions between the vascular territories of the major cerebral vessels. With severe insults, the basal ganglia and thalami may also be involved. The cortex is usually preserved in the preterm infant as a result of anastomotic communicating vessels from the meningeal circulation that serve to preserve cortical blood flow. The preterm infant suffers injury primarily to the periventricular white matter, occurring most commonly near the atria of the lateral ventricles posteriorly and near the foramen of Monro, but can occur anywhere within the corona radiata and even the corpus callosum. White matter ischemia leads to white matter volume loss or periventricular leukomalacia (PVL). These lesions in the brain are usually associated with abnormal neurologic outcome. Five major types of neonatal hypoxic-ischemic brain injury have been described:

1. Selective neuronal necrosis
2. Status marmoratus
3. Parasagittal cerebral injury
4. Periventricular leukomalacia or white-matter necrosis
5. Focal brain necrosis

Sonographic Findings. Ultrasound is not a very precise technique to diagnose necrotic ischemic lesions. In ischemic-hypoxic encephalopathy, ultrasound may show areas of increased echogenicity in the subcortical and deep white matter and in the basal ganglia (Figure 21-42). The increased echogenicity is caused by congestion and microhemorrhages, which are characteristically present in the acute stage of ischemic injuries (Figure 21-43). However, echodensities are not pathognomonic of ischemic necrosis, inasmuch as they have been observed in infants having only congestion and microhemorrhages without necrosis. If necrosis is present in the echogenic areas, cavitary lesions appear 2 or more weeks after the ischemic insult. Echolucencies or cysts are the landmark for the diagnosis of ischemic brain injury in newborn infants. Ultrasound is useful in diagnosing multifocal white matter necrosis (periventricular leukomalacia) and focal ischemic lesions.

Periventricular Leukomalacia or Multifocal White Matter Necrosis. Multifocal white matter necrosis (WMN) or **periventricular leukomalacia (PVL)** is the most frequent ischemic lesion in the immature brain. This lesion is associated with anomalous myelination of the immature brain and abnormal neurologic development, including cerebral palsy. WMN is probably the most important cause of abnormal neurodevelopmental sequelae in preterm infants.

WMN is found in 20% to 80% of neonatal autopsies. Pathologists describe an acute phase characterized by multiple foci or coagulation necrosis in deep and periventricular white matter, and a chronic phase depicted by cavitation and scarring appearing 1 or more weeks after the cerebral insult. Early in the chronic stage, multiple cavities develop in the necrotic white matter adjacent to the lateral walls of the frontal horns, body, atria, and occipital horns of the lateral ventricles. These lesions are frequently located in the lateral wall of the atria and occipital horns, causing damage to the optic radiations. Eventually the cavities resolve, leaving gliotic scars and diffuse cerebral atrophy. Necrotic lesions with only microscopic cavities may also lead to cerebral atrophy.

Currently, WMN may be diagnosed in infants with echoencephalography. The acute stage of WMN is characterized by highly echogenic areas in the cerebral white matter superior and lateral to the frontal horns, bodies, atria, and occipital horns of the lateral ventricles (Figure 21-44). Echogenic areas are present during the first week after delivery and usually resolve in the following weeks. Microscopically, the echogenicity consists of congestion, microhemorrhages, and foci of necrosis. However, echogenicities may be associated only with congestion and microhemorrhages without necrosis.

Sonographic Findings. The chronic stage of WMN is identified with ultrasound when echolucencies develop in the echogenic white matter (Figure 21-45). Pathologic studies have confirmed that echolucent lesions correspond to cavitary lesions in the white matter. The presence of echolucencies is

Figure 21-42   Progression of periventricular leukomalacia (PVL) in a premature infant. **A,** Posterior coronal image. **B,** Left sagittal image shows white matter congestion and cavitation on day 1. **C,** Day 3 shows progression of the PVL. **D,** Day 14 shows further progression of white matter congestion and cavitation on this sagittal image. **E,** Day 42 demonstrates extensive cavitation throughout both right and left cerebral areas. **F,** Sagittal image shows multiple cavities.

Figure 21-43   Periventricular leukomalacia. Chalky white lesions are indicated by arrows. (From Damjanov I, Linder J: *Pathology: a color atlas,* St Louis, 2000, Mosby.)

prima facie evidence that necrotic injury exists in the cerebral white matter. Echogenicity alone suggests, but does not prove, that the echogenic white matter is necrotic. The absence of cystic lesions in the echoencephalogram precludes definitive diagnosis of WMN. Since very echogenic white matter can be simply congestion without coagulation, and in fact not necessarily white matter necrosis at all, careful sequential observations must be made to identify cavitary lesions developing in the echo-dense white matter. Cystic lesions in WMN may be microscopic or smaller than the resolution of the ultrasound scanners. Consequently WMN may exist in the absence of cavitary lesions in the sonograms.

Both neuropathologic and echoencephalographic studies have shown that a period of 1 to 6 weeks ensues between the acute stage of WMN and the development of cystic lesions. Echogenic areas and cysts decrease in size and eventually disappear 2 to 5 months after the diagnosis of acute necrosis. If

A

B

C

Figure 21-44   **A,** Coronal posterior. **B** and **C,** Sagittal scans of a 33-week premature infant with white matter necrosis along the lateral ventricular borders. Follow-up studies will show if this congestion develops into a hemorrhage or clears up completely.

Figure 21-45   A and **B,** Follow-up study of the patient in Figure 21-44 shows a septal vein in the cavum septum pellucidum and increased ventricular size.

the necrosis was extensive, brain atrophy may be the only indication that WMN occurred during the perinatal period. Ultrasound is also useful to diagnose the atrophic phase of the chronic stage. This phase is identified by an enlarged subarachnoid space, widened interhemispheric fissure, and persistent ventricular dilation in an infant with a normal or small head circumference.

Focal Brain Necrosis. These necrotic lesions occur within the distribution of large arteries. This complication is present in term and preterm infants, but it is infrequent under 30 weeks' gestational age. Vascular maldevelopment, asphyxia or hypoxia, embolism from the placenta, infectious diseases, thromboembolism secondary to disseminated intravascular coagulation, and polycythemia have been implicated as causal factors in this condition. These insults may occur prenatally or early in postnatal life, leading subsequently to the dissolution of the cerebral tissues and formation of cavitary lesions. The term *porencephaly* is used to describe a single cavity; *multicystic encephalomalacia* for multiple cavities; and *hydranencephaly* for a large single cavity with the entire disappearance of the cerebral hemispheres.

Sonographic Findings. Ultrasound images of these injuries show very echogenic localized lesions within the distribution of the major vessel. The echo-dense lesions are considered to correspond to cerebral infarctions. After several days, sonolucencies appear within the echogenic areas. Subsequently the infarcted regions are replaced by cavities that may or may not communicate with the ventricle.

Extracorporeal Membrane Oxygenation. Extracorporeal membrane oxygenation (ECMO) is used for pulmonary and circulatory support in many neonatal conditions to allow additional time for the lungs to develop. Infants born with diaphragmatic hernia, persistent pulmonary hypertension, meconium aspiration, and congenital heart disease may be recommended for ECMO to give the infant's lungs a chance to mature. The ECMO cannula is inserted into the right internal jugular vein and carotid artery (the vessels are ligated above their insertion site). Therefore the ECMO pump procedure can cause a notable change in cerebral circulation, and neonatal ultrasound is used to monitor hemorrhage in the brain tissue.

After the vessel ligation, there is a 50% abrupt decrease in intracranial blood flow with a return of peak systolic velocities to nearly pre-ECMO levels within 3 to 5 minutes. The end-diastolic velocity is increased, and the Doppler used to monitor for hypoxic-ischemic encephalopathy.

Hemorrhage and ischemia are common in children on ECMO, both from the effects of ECMO itself and from the conditions leading to the use of ECMO. Preexisting hypoxic-ischemic encephalopathy with an abnormal resistive index has been shown to lead to intracranial hemorrhage in a high percentage of infants. Bleeding may occur in the parenchyma, ventricle, or posterior fossa, but the cerebellum also is a common site. Increased extraaxial fluid is a common finding in children on ECMO, usually in the subarachnoid space, and is of little consequence.

BRAIN INFECTIONS

Congenital infections of the brain can have serious consequences for the neonate including mortality, mental retardation, or developmental delay. The most frequent congenital infections are commonly referred to by the acronym TORCH. This refers to the infections Toxoplasma gondii, rubella virus, cytomegalovirus (CMV), and herpes simplex type 2. The "O" stands for *other,* such as syphilis, which may cause acute meningitis.

VENTRICULITIS

Ventriculitis is a common complication of purulent meningitis in newborn infants. Ventriculitis probably is caused by hematogenous spread of the infection to the choroid plexus. The presence of a foreign body in the ventricular cavity, such

Figure 21-46　A 1-month-old infant with bright calcifications bilaterally secondary to cytomegalovirus.

as a catheter from a ventriculoperitoneal shunt, may provide a nidus for persistent infection of the ventricular cavities.

Sonographic Findings. Ventriculitis leads to compartmentalization of the ventricular cavities by inflammatory adhesions extending from wall to wall. The first stage of ventriculitis is seen in ultrasound as very thin septations extending from the walls of the lateral ventricles (Figure 21-46). The septa become thicker and lead to multilocular hydrocephalus and extensive disorganization of the brain anatomy. Sequential studies in patients with meningitis or with ventriculoperitoneal shunts can provide early diagnosis of this severe complication.

EPENDYMITIS

Ependymitis occurs when the ependyma become thickened and hyperechoic as a result of irritation from hemorrhage within the ventricle. This is more common and occurs earlier than ventriculitis developing from interventricular hemorrhage.

SELECTED BIBLIOGRAPHY

Babcock D: *Cranial ultrasonography of infants,* Baltimore, 1981, Williams & Wilkins.

Bejar R, Coen R, Merritt TA and others: Focal necrosis of the white matter (periventricular leukomalacia): sonographic, pathologic, and electroencephalographic features, *AJNR* 7:1073, 1986.

Bowerman RA, Donn SM, Silver TM and others: Natural history of neonatal periventricular/intraventricular hemorrhage and its complications: sonographic observations, *AJNR* 5:527, 1985.

Bozynski MEA, Nelson MN, Matalon TAS and others: Cavitary periventricular leukomalacia: incidence and short term outcome in infants weighing <1200 grams at birth, *Dev Med Child Neurol* 27:572, 1985.

Calame A, Fawer CL, Anderegg A and others: Interaction between perinatal brain damage and processes of normal brain development, *Dev Neurosci* 7:1, 1985.

Calvert SA, Hoskins EM, Fong KW and others: Periventricular leukomalacia: ultrasonic diagnosis and neurological outcome, *Acta Paediatr Scan* 75:489, 1986.

Chow PP, Horgan JG, Taylor KJW: Neonatal periventricular leukomalacia: real-time sonographic diagnosis with CT correlation, *Am J Roentgenol* 145:155, 1985.

Donn S, Bowerman R, Dipietro M and others: Sonographic appearance of neonatal thalamic-striatal hemorrhage, *J Ultrasound Med* 3:231, 1984.

Dubowitz LMS, Bydder GM, Mushin J: Developmental sequence of periventricular leukomalacia, *Arch Dis Child* 60:349, 1985.

Ecker JL, Shipp TD, Bromley B and others: The sonographic diagnosis of Dandy-Walker and Dandy-Walker variant: associated findings and outcomes, *Prental Diagn* 20:328-332, 2000.

Evans DH: Doppler ultrasound and the neonatal cerebral circulation: methodology and pitfalls, *Biol Neonate* 62:271, 1992.

Fenton AC, Papathoma E, Evans DH and others: Neonatal cerebral venous flow velocity measurement using a color flow Doppler system, *J Clin Ultrasound* 19:69, 1991.

Fenton AC, Shortland DB, Papathoma E, and others: Normal range for blood flow velocity in cerebral arteries of newly born term infants, *Early Hum Dev* 22:73, 1990.

Hamrick SE, Miller SP, Leonard C, and others: Trends in severe brain injury and neurodevelopmental outcome in premature newborn infants: the role of cystic periventricular leukomalacia, *J Pediatri* 145(5):593-599, 2004.

Horgan JG, Rumack CM, Hay T and others: Absolute intracranial blood-flow velocities evaluated by duplex Doppler sonography in asymptomatic preterm and term neonates, *Am J Roentgenol* 152:1059, 1989.

Jelliger K, Gross H, Kaltenback E and others: Holoprosencephaly and agenesis of the corpus callosum: frequency of associated malformation, *Acta Neuropathol* 55:1, 1981.

Kreusser K, Schmidt R, Shackelford G and others: Value of ultrasound for identification of acute hemorrhagic necrosis of thalamus and basal ganglia in an asphyxiated term infant, *Ann Neurol* 16:361, 1984.

Levene M, Wigglesworth J, Dubovitz V: Hemorrhagic periventricular leukomalacia in the neonate: a real time ultrasound study, *Pediatrics* 71:794, 1983.

McMenamin J, Shackelford G, Volpe J: Outcome of neonatal intraventricular hemorrhage with periventricular echo-dense lesions, *Ann Neurol* 15:285, 1984.

Monteagudo A: Fetal neurosonography: should it be routine? Should it be detailed? *Ultrasound Obstet Gynceol* 12(1):1-5, 1998.

Perlman JM: White matter injury in the preterm infant: an important determination of abnormal neuro development outcome, *Early Hum Dev* 53:99-120, 1998.

Rumack C, Johnson M: *Perinatal and infant brain imaging role of ultrasound and computed tomography*, Chicago, 1984, Mosby Year Book.

Rumack CM: *Diagnostic ultrasound*, ed 3, St Louis, 2005, Mosby.

Schelliner D, Grant EG, Richardson JD: Neonatal leukoencephalopathy: a common form of cerebral ischemia, *Radiographics* 5:221, 1985.

Schmitt H: Multicystic encephalopathy, a pathological condition in early infancy: morphologic, pathogenic and clinical aspects, *Brain Dev* 1:1, 1984.

Seibert JJ, Avva R, Hronas TN and others: Use of power Doppler in pediatric neurosonography: a pictorial essay, *Radiographics* 8(4):879-890, 1998.

van de Bor M, Walther FJ, Sims ME: Acceleration time in cerebral arteries of preterm and term infants, *J Clin Ultrasound* 18:167, 1990.

Volpe JJ: Brain injury in the premature infant: overview of clinical aspects, neuropathology, and pathogenesis, *Semin Pediatr Neurol* 5:135-151, 1998.

Whitelaw A: Intraventricular hemorrhage and post-hemorrhagic hydrocephalus: pathogenesis, prevention and future interventions, *Semin Neonatol* 6:135-146, 2001.

Young RSK, Hernandez MJ, Yagel SK: Selective reduction of blood flow to white matter during hypotension in newborn dogs: a possible mechanism of periventricular leukomalacia, *Ann Neurol* 12:445, 1985.

CHAPTER 22

The Pediatric Abdomen: Jaundice and Common Surgical Conditions

Sandra L. Hagen-Ansert

EXAMINATION PREPARATION

SONOGRAPHIC EVALUATION OF NEONATAL/PEDIATRIC ABDOMEN

PATHOLOGY

JAUNDICE
COMMON SURGICAL CONDITIONS

KEY TERMS

acholic – absence or deficiency of bile secretion or failure of the bile to enter the alimentary tract (i.e., secondary to obstruction). The stool is claylike and colorless.

appendicitis – inflammation of the appendix

appendicolith – echogenic structure within the appendix

atretic – congenital absence or closure of a normal body opening or tubular structure

Beckwith-Widemann syndrome – an autosomal recessive condition characterized by macroglossia, gigantism, hemihypertrophy, and exophthalmus; individuals may also manifest with organomegaly and are at increased risk for development of certain abdominal neoplasms

biliary atresia – closure or absence of some or all of the major bile ducts

choledochal cyst – congenital cystic malformation of the common bile duct

hemihypertrophy – the excessive development of one side or one half of the body or an organ

hypertrophic pyloric stenosis – thickened muscle in the pylorus that prevents food from entering the duodenum; occurs more frequently in males

inspissated – thickened by absorption, evaporation, or dehydration

intussusception – occurs when bowel prolapses into distal bowel and is propelled in an antegrade fashion

neonate – infant in the first 28 days of life

neuroblastoma – a malignant hemorrhagic tumor principally consisting of cells resembling neuroblasts that give rise to cells of the sympathetic system (especially the adrenal medulla)

projectile vomiting – condition in pyloric stenosis in the neonatal period; after drinking, the infant experiences projectile vomiting secondary to the obstruction in the pylorus

pyloric canal – located between the stomach and duodenum

scintigraphy – photographing the scintillations emitted by radioactive substances injected into the body; this test is used to determine the outline and function of organs and tissues in which the radioactive substance collects or is secreted

target (donut) sign – frequently associated with sectional areas of the gastrointestinal tract; the muscle is hyperechoic, and the inner core is hypoechoic

Wilms' tumor – (nephroblastoma) a rapidly developing tumor of the kidney that usually occurs in children

In many medical institutions, sonography is the first imaging procedure used to evaluate infants and children with acute abdominal problems. This chapter focuses on the cause and sonographic appearance of jaundice in the neonate and pediatric patient. The chapter also focuses on sonographic examination techniques for detecting the more common surgical conditions that may cause pain or vomiting and the ultrasound appearance of these conditions. Hypertrophic pyloric stenosis, appendicitis, and intussusception are discussed.

EXAMINATION PREPARATION

Gaining the trust of the patient and the patient's family can do much to facilitate the examination. Therefore, the sonographer should first allow sufficient time to explain the examination to the parents and to the child who is old enough to comprehend the proceedings. Sedation and immobilization techniques are generally not required. Toys, books, keys, mobiles, and a variety of other distracting devices can be very helpful in quieting the frightened young child. A pacifier may likewise serve well when examining infants. Formula feeding is not recommended if the child is a surgical candidate. Some laboratories offer glucose water or Pedialyte feedings when examining a neonate for pyloric stenosis. Parents are encouraged to be present during the examination and can help reassure and quiet the patient. Box 22-1 outlines scanning considerations for the pediatric patient.

Virtually no routine patient preparation is required. However, to image the biliary system completely, it is recommended that feeding be withheld for a short time according to the age of the patient (Box 22-2). Adequate distention of the urinary bladder is desirable in many   situations. This not only allows assessment of the bladder itself, but also facilitates identification of dilated distal ureters, free peritoneal fluid, the pelvic genitalia, and a pelvic mass. A urine-filled bladder may also help localize gastrointestinal abnormalities, such as appendicitis and intussusception. In females, pelvic structures are examined with a full bladder and then emptied for the graded compression portion of the examination.

SONOGRAPHIC EVALUATION OF NEONATAL/PEDIATRIC ABDOMEN

The neonatal/pediatric sonographic examination should evaluate the abdomen and pelvis, with particular concentration on the right upper quadrant: liver, bile ducts and gallbladder, pancreas, spleen, and portal system (Box 22-3).

The size and texture of the liver should be evaluated (Figure 22-1). The right hepatic lobe should not extend more than 1 cm below the costal margin in a young infant without pulmonary hyperaeration and should not extend below the right costal margin in older infants and children. The echogenicity is normally low to medium homogenicity with clear definition of the portal venous vasculature.

Careful evaluation of the biliary system should be made to exclude ductal dilatation (Figure 22-2). The common bile duct should measure less than 1 mm in neonates, less than 2 mm in infants up to 1 year old, less than 4 mm in older children, and less than 7 mm in adolescents and adults. The gallbladder size and wall thickness should be assessed. In infants under 1 year of age, the gallbladder length is 1.5 to 3 cm and in older children it is 3 to 7 cm. The length of the gallbladder should not exceed the length of the kidney. Careful evaluation of the normal gallbladder should show a smooth-walled anechoic structure without internal echoes. Pericholecystic fluid should not be present.

The pancreas should be examined for size, echotexture, and evidence of dilatation of the pancreatic duct (Figure 22-3). The

---

BOX 22-1   GENERAL PEDIATRIC SCANNING CONSIDERATIONS

- Always use warm gel
- Keep infant warm and secure
  - Wrap blankets around infant
  - Use as little gel as possible
  - Remove gel as soon as possible; it gets cold quickly
- "Bottle, binky, and diaper"
  - Glycogen and water bottles should be handy (Dip binky into sugar solution; may repeat while scanning until able to give milk/formula)
  - Examine gallbladder and pancreas quickly, then give infant bottle for remainder of examination
  - Always keep dry diaper on infant
  - Have plenty of distractions ready (e.g., noisy bright colored toys, stickers, keys, etc.)
  - Two sonographers to one child is preferred (one to scan, one to occupy child); if not possible, use the parent or nurse
- Transducers
  - Use highest frequency transducer for area imaged
  - Linear, curved array, or sector:
    - 0-1 yr: use 7.5 MHz linear
    - 1-2 yr: use 5-7.5 MHz linear, curved array, or sector
    - 2+ yr: use 5 MHz sector or linear
    - Use sequential focusing and zoom instead of decreasing depth for better resolution
- Take breaks
  - If child becomes too stressed, give the child a rest
  - Let mother hold child until calm
  - Feasible to allow child to lie next to mother on stretcher to continue exam
- Older child
  - Explain procedure before child undresses
  - Have mother and child touch the transducer and gel and be ready to "watch the movies"

BOX 22-2   PEDIATRIC ULTRASOUND EXAMINATION PREP

ABDOMINAL ULTRASOUND
0-2 yr: NPO × 4 hr
3-5 yr: NPO × 5 hr
6+ yr: NPO × 6 hr

PELVIC ULTRASOUND
0-9 yr: Plenty of juice or water 30 min before examination. No voiding 30 min before examination time.
10+ yr: 32 oz water 1 hr before examination. No voiding.

pancreatic head should measure 1.0 to 2.2 cm; the body, 0.4 to 1.0 cm; and the tail, 0.8 to 1.8 cm. The pancreatic duct should not exceed 1 to 2 mm. The size of the pancreas should increase with the child's age (Table 22-1). The normal texture is hypoechoic compared with the normal liver texture as little fatty tissue has invaded the islets of Langerhans.

The splenic size and texture should be evaluated (Figure 22-4). The upper limits of normal splenic length ranges from 6.0 cm in infants less than 3 months old to 12 cm in children over 12 years of age.

The diameter of the portal vein may be helpful in determining the presence of portal hypertension (Figure 22-5). The mean portal vein measurement is 8.5 mm in children less than

10 years of age and 10 mm in patients 10 to 20 years old. Color Doppler should be used to determine flow direction and patency.

PATHOLOGY

JAUNDICE

During the first few weeks of life many neonates experience transient jaundice. The benign causes lead to increased unconjugated (indirect) bilirubin and follow a self-limiting course. Possible causes for this condition include breast-feeding or the mobilization of sequestered blood from a large cephalohematoma. An increased conjugated (direct) bilirubin level is never benign.

The cause of persistent jaundice in the neonate may be difficult to define because clinical and laboratory features may be similar in hepatocellular and obstructive jaundice. If bile obstruction, **biliary atresia**, or metabolic diseases are to be treated early before cirrhosis occurs, then diagnosis must be made soon after delivery. Jaundice may be either an extrahepatic or intrahepatic obstruction to bile flow. The extrahepatic obstruction in the neonate includes conditions such as **choledochal cyst**, biliary atresia, or spontaneous perforation of the bile ducts. The intrahepatic causes of neonatal jaundice include hepatitis and metabolic disease. Systemic diseases that cause cholestasis include heart failure, shock, sepsis, neonatal lupus, histiocytosis, and severe hemolytic disease.

Obstructive and nonobstructive jaundice may be differentiated with sonographic evaluation. The occurrence of unconjugated hyperbilirubinemia occurs in approximately 60% of normal term infants and in 80% of preterm infants. If the neonate has jaundice that persists beyond 2 weeks after delivery, an ultrasound may be ordered to differentiate among the three most common causes for jaundice: hepatitis, biliary atresia, and choledochal cyst. With each of these conditions, the liver appears coarse and echogenic on ultrasound; a variety of other conditions (e.g., hepatic inflammatory, obstructive, and metabolic processes) have a similar sonographic appearance. Other studies, such as hepatic **scintigraphy** or liver biopsy, may be necessary to narrow the differential considerations further. Ultrasound is very useful in demonstrating the gallbladder with **inspissated** bile and biliary duct stones. Jaundice in infants and children may be due to cirrhosis, benign strictures, and neoplastic processes.

BOX 22-3	NORMAL SONOGRAPHIC MEASUREMENTS

LIVER
- Infant: right lobe not extend >1 cm below costal margin
- Older infants and children: right lobe not extend below right costal margin

BILIARY DUCTS
- Neonates: CBD <1 mm
- Infants (up to 1 yr old): CBD <2 mm
- Older children: CBD <4 mm
- Adolescents: CBD <7 mm

GALLBLADDER LENGTH
- Infants (under 1 yr old): 1.5-3 cm
- Older children: 3-7 cm

PANCREAS (SIZE INCREASES WITH AGE)
- Head: 1.0-2.2 cm
- Body: 0.4-1.0 cm
- Tail: 0.8-1.8 cm
- Duct: 1-2 mm

SPLEEN LENGTH
- Infants (0-3 mo): 6.0 cm
- Children (>12 yr): 12.0 cm

PORTAL VEIN DIAMETER
- Children <10 yr: 8.5 mm
- Children >10 yr: 10 mm

TABLE 22-1 NORMAL DIMENSIONS OF THE PANCREAS AS A FUNCTION OF AGE

Patient Age	Patients (N)	Maximum Anteroposterior Dimensions of Pancreas (cm ±1 Standard Deviation)		
		Head	Body	Tail
<1 mo	15	1.0 ± 0.4	0.6 ± 0.2	1.0 ± 0.4
1 mo-1 yr	23	1.5 ± 0.5	0.8 ± 0.3	1.2 ± 0.4
1-5 yr	49	1.7 ± 0.3	1.0 ± 0.2	1.8 ± 0.4
5-10 yr	69	1.6 ± 0.4	1.0 ± 0.3	1.8 ± 0.4
10-19 yr	117	2.0 ± 0.5	1.1 ± 0.3	2.0 ± 0.4

Data from Siegel MJ, Martin KW, Worthington JL: Normal and abnormal pancreas in children: US studies, *Radiology* 165:15-18, 1987.

Figure 22-1   Normal pediatric liver. The liver is normal in size and contour without focal mass or marginal irregularity. **A,** Sagittal left lobe liver with aorta. **B,** Sagittal left lobe liver with inferior vena cava. **C,** Sagittal right lobe liver. **D,** Sagittal right lobe liver/gallbladder. **E,** Transverse liver with hepatic veins. **F,** Transverse liver with portal veins. **G,** Transverse liver with diaphragm. **H,** Transverse liver, gallbladder, and right kidney.

Figure 22-2 Normal pediatric gallbladder and common bile duct. Gallbladder is unremarkable without wall thickening, pericholecystic fluid, or cholelithiasis. No ductal dilatation is seen. **A-C,** Sagittal gallbladder. **D,** Transverse gallbladder. **E,** Transverse common bile duct, hepatic artery, and portal vein.

In an infant who has jaundice beyond the 2-week postdelivery date, a number of differentials is possible. In these patients, clinical and laboratory work-up is necessary to identify the underlying infectious, metabolic, or structural causes of jaundice. Laboratory work-up may include liver function tests, evaluation for hepatitis B antigen, TORCH (to rule out maternal infections), work-up for sepsis, metabolic screening, and sweat test. See Table 22-2 for clinical findings, sonographic findings, and differential considerations for the diseases and conditions discussed here.

Causes and Diagnosis of Neonatal Jaundice. The three most common causes of jaundice in the neonatal period are hepatitis, biliary atresia, and choledochal cyst.

Neonatal hepatitis. Neonatal hepatitis is an infection of the liver that occurs within the first 3 months. There are a number of causes of neonatal hepatitis, including infections, metabolic disorders, familial recurrent cholestasis, metabolism errors, or idiopathic causes. The infection reaches the liver through the placenta, via the vagina from infected maternal secretions, or through catheters or blood transfusions. Transplacental infection occurs most readily during the third trimester of pregnancy; the most common agents include syphilis, toxoplasma, rubella, and cytomegalovirus (CMV). Bacterial hepatitis is most commonly secondary to an upward spread of organisms from the vagina, infecting endometrium, placenta, and amniotic fluid. During delivery, direct contact with the viruses of herpes, CMV, human immunodeficiency (HIV) virus, and Listeria may lead to hepatitis. Blood transfusions may contain the hepatitis virus, Epstein-Barr virus, or HIV. In addition, bacterial hepatitis or abscess formation may be obtained from an umbilical vein catheter after delivery.

Figure 22-3   A-D, Normal pediatric pancreas seen in transverse plane. Evaluation of the pancreas is unremarkable without evidence of focal mass.

Figure 22-4   Normal pediatric spleen. The spleen is normal in size, contour with echogenicity measuring 109 cm in greatest pole-to-pole diameter. No focal masses are seen. **A,** Sagittal spleen and left kidney. **B,** Sagittal spleen with hilum. **C,** Sagittal spleen with measurement of the long axis.

Figure 22-5   Normal pediatric portal vein. The portal vein is normal in size with normal flow patterns. **A,** Transverse main portal vein/right portal vein. **B,** Transverse main portal vein. **C,** Transverse left portal vein.

Sonographic findings reveal a liver size that may be normal or enlarged (Figure 22-6). The parenchyma pattern is echogenic with decreased visualization of the peripheral portal venous structures. The biliary ducts and gallbladder are not enlarged. If the hepatocellular dysfunction is severe, the gallbladder may be small in size because of the decreased volume of bile. The differential of neonatal hepatitis and biliary atresia may be difficult when the gallbladder is small; therefore, nuclear scintigraphy will allow visualization of the biliary function.

Biliary atresia.   Biliary atresia is the narrowing or underdevelopment of the biliary ductal system. This serious disease is seen more commonly in males and may result from inflammation of the hepatobiliary system. Biliary atresia may affect the intrahepatic or extrahepatic ducts and may or may not involve the gallbladder, although the latter is the most common form with absence of the gallbladder.

The clinical features of biliary atresia in the neonate include persistent jaundice, **acholic** stools, dark urine, and distended abdomen from hepatomegaly. Early surgical intervention may lead to the prevention of serious complications, which include cirrhosis, liver failure, and subsequent death.

Sonographic findings in a neonate with biliary atresia may vary depending on the type and the severity of the disease (Figure 22-7). The liver size may be normal or enlarged. The echogenicity of the liver parenchyma may be normal or increased with slight decrease in visualization of the peripheral portal venous vasculature (indicative of fibrosis). The intrahepatic ducts are not dilated, although a remnant duct may be identified with some types of atresia. A small triangular structure may be seen superior to the porta hepatis, which is a hypoplastic remnant of the biliary structure.

A normal sized gallbladder may be seen when the **atretic** common bile duct is distal to the insertion of the cystic duct. The finding of a small (less than 1.5 cm) gallbladder is nonspecific and may be seen with either hepatitis or biliary atresia. A change in the gallbladder size after a milk feeding suggests patency of the common hepatic and common bile ducts and is seen only with neonatal hepatitis.

The presence of polysplenia should also be made if the suspicion is biliary atresia because there is a high association of this abnormality. The abdomen should be examined for end-stage liver disease (i.e., ascites, hepatofugal flow, and collateral venous channels).

Choledochal cyst.   A choledochal cyst is an abnormal cystic dilation of the biliary tree, which most frequently affects the common bile duct. There are five types of choledochal cysts, fusiform dilation of the common bile duct (CBD) being the most common:

1. Fusiform dilation of the CBD
2. One or more diverticula of the CBD
3. Dilation of the intraduodenal portion of the CBD (choledochocele)
4. Dilation of the intrahepatic and extrahepatic ducts
5. Caroli's disease with dilation of intrahepatic ducts

The patient clinically presents with jaundice and pain. A palpable mass may be felt in the right upper quadrant. Sonog-

TABLE 22-2 PEDIATRIC ABDOMINAL FINDINGS

Clinical Findings	Sonographic Findings	Differential Considerations
Neonatal Hepatitis		
Hepatomegaly Jaundice when obstruction is present	Liver normal or enlarged Liver parenchyma echogenic with decreased vascularization of peripheral portal venous structures When severe, gallbladder may be small in size	
Biliary Atresia		
Persistent jaundice Acholic stools Dark urine Distended abdomen	Liver may be enlarged Echogenicity of liver parenchyma may be normal or increased with slight decrease in visualization of portal structures Intrahepatic ducts not dilated Polysplenia may be present	
Choledochal Cyst		
Jaundice Pain Palpable mass may be present Hemangioendothelioma First six months of life Rapid growing benign tumor Hepatomegaly Congestive heart failure Cutaneous hemangioma Serum alpha-fetoprotein level may be elevated	Fusiform dilatation of the common bile duct with associated intrahepatic ductal dilatation Multiple hypoechoic lesions in liver Hepatomegaly Tumor is heterogeneous or isoechoic with cystic components Calcification may be present Well circumscribed to poorly marginated Doppler may show AV shunt	Duplicated gallbladder Liver cyst Fluid in duodenum Adenoma Focal nodular hyperplasia Cirrhosis—regenerating nodules Hepatoblastoma Biliary rhabdoma/sarcoma Lymphoma Metastasis
Hepatoblastoma		
Most common malignant tumor <5 years of age Palpable abdominal mass Elevated serum alpha-fetoprotein levels Fever Pain	Hepatomegaly Calcification may occur Solitary heterogeneous mass Area around mass is hyperechoic R/P portal vein thrombosis Doppler shows high-velocity, low-resistance flow	Adenoma Focal nodular hyperplasia Cirrhosis—regenerating nodules Hemangioendothelioma Biliary rhabdoma/sarcoma Lymphoma Metastasis
Hypertrophic Pyloric Stenosis		
Male infants Projectile vomiting Dehydration and weight loss	Distended stomach Hypertrophied pyloric muscle with a canal >16 mm Pyloric wall muscle >3.5 mm	Pseudoechogenic muscle secondary to beam angulation Antropyloric canal posteriorly oriented Pylorospasm with minimal muscular hypertrophy Prostaglandin-induced HPS
Appendicitis		
RLQ pain Nausea, vomiting Increased WBC Fever	Noncompressible appendix Diameter >6 mm Rebound pain	Meckel's diverticulum Pelvic mass Mesenteric adenitis
Intussusception		
Colicky abdominal pain Vomiting Bloody stools Abdominal mass	Alternating hypoechoic and hyperechoic rings surrounding an echogenic center ("target sign") Free peritoneal fluid	Intestinal wall thickening Inflammatory bowel Colitis Perforated appendicitis Viral disease Lymphoma Benign tumors

Figure 22-6   Liver size and texture should be evaluated in a patient with hepatitis. The liver may appear normal or enlarged. **A,** Sagittal liver/aorta. **B,** Sagittal liver/inferior vena cava. **C,** Sagittal liver. **D,** Transverse liver/right kidney. **E,** Transverse liver. **F,** Transverse liver.

raphy is used to differentiate the presence or absence of a gallbladder, dilation of the ductal system, and the presence or absence of a mass (Figure 22-8). When a choledochal cyst is present, there is usually fusiform dilation of the common bile duct with associated intrahepatic ductal dilation.

Causes and Diagnosis of Pediatric Jaundice. There are several causes of jaundice in the pediatric patient, including hepatocellular disease, hepatic neoplasms, cholelithiasis and choledocholithiasis, and cirrhosis. Only hepatitic neoplasms will be presented. The reader is referred to the Abdominal Section, as well as Liver and Gallbladder chapters for further discussion of the other abnormalities.

Hepatic neoplasms.   The two most common neoplasms in the pediatric population are the hemangioendothelioma and the hepatoblastoma.

Hemangioendothelioma. Infantile hepatic hemangioendothelioma is the most common benign vascular liver tumor of early childhood, occurring usually within the first six months of life (Figure 22-9). The mass is usually diagnosed in the first months of life as the mass grows rapidly, causing abdominal distention.

The clinical presentation for infants with hemangioendothelioma is hepatomegaly, which may be accompanied by congestive heart failure and cutaneous hemangioma. The serum alpha-fetoprotein level may be elevated. This benign tumor usually spontaneously regresses by 12 to 18 months of age.

The most common sonographic appearance of hemangioendothelioma is that of multiple hypoechoic lesions and hepatomegaly. The tumor is usually heterogeneous or isoechoic and contains cystic components from the vascular-stroma

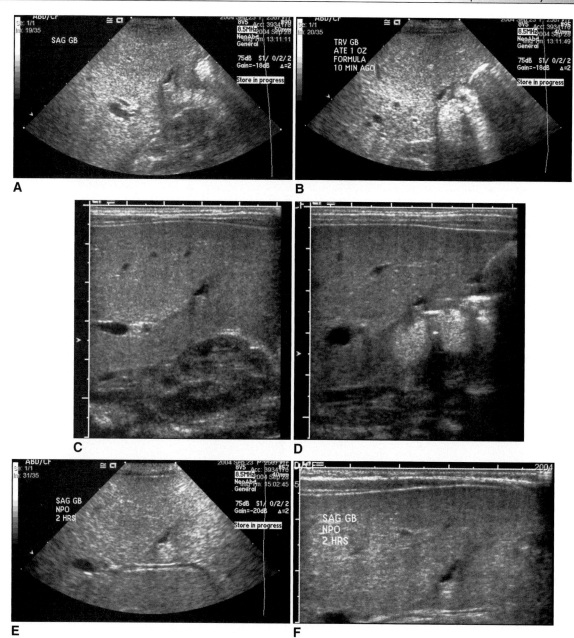

Figure 22-7 Biliary atresia. A 5-day-old infant with direct hyperbilirubinemia of unknown origin with liver congestion, inflammation, and ductal blockage. The liver is enlarged with a fairly homogeneous appearance. The neonate had eaten just before the study and the gallbladder was contracted and measured less than 1 cm. The patient was scanned after 2 hours and the gallbladder did not change in appearance. The common bile duct was not identified. **A,** Sagittal gallbladder. **B,** Transverse gallbladder after 1 oz formula. **C,** Sagittal gallbladder. **D,** Sagittal gallbladder. **E,** Sagittal gallbladder; NPO for 2 hours. **F,** Sagittal gallbladder; NPO for 2 hours.

Figure 22-8   Choledochal cyst. The gallbladder is folded upon itself without evidence of gallstones or wall thickening. Adjacent to the gallbladder, to the right and extending posteriorly, is a thin-walled fluid collection, which measures 2 × 3 cm. The mass is separate from the gallbladder and does not demonstrate flow. It may represent choledochal cyst (Type II) or less likely a duplicated gallbladder. **A,** Transverse liver/hepatic veins. **B,** Transverse liver with two cystic areas. **C,** Transverse liver. **D,** Sagittal gallbladder. **E,** Sagittal gallbladder with fold or separate cystic mass. **F,** Two cystic structures in area of gallbladder. **G,** Transverse gallbladder. **H,** Color shows common bile duct separate from vascular structures.

Figure 22-8, cont'd   I, Right sagittal gallbladder. **J,** Right sagittal gallbladder with fold. **K,** Right sagittal gallbladder. **L,** Right sagittal gallbladder shows two separate cystic structures *(arrows)*.

structure (Figure 22-10). Speckled areas of calcification may be seen within the mass. The tumor may be well circumscribed or poorly marginated. The mass may be solitary or multicentric. Color Doppler shows high flow in the dilated vascular spaces and may be used to show the arteriovenous shunting that accompanies this lesion (Figure 22-11). The aortic caliper decreases in size inferior to the origin of the celiac artery. When arteriovenous shunting is severe, the celiac axis, hepatic artery, and veins are dilated and the infraceliac aorta is small.

Hepatoblastoma. Hepatoblastoma is the most common primary malignant disease of the liver and occurs most frequently in children under 5 years of age, with the majority occurring in children under 2 years of age. The tumor is the third most common abdominal malignancy in children after **nephroblastoma (Wilms' tumor)**. This tumor is sometimes considered the infantile form of hepatocellular carcinoma. The tumor may be familial. Hepatoblastoma has been associated with **Beckwith-Widemann syndrome, hemihypertrophy,** familial adenomatous polyposis, and precocious puberty.

Pathologically the tumor is single, solid, large, or mixed echogenicity, and poorly marginated, with small cysts and rounded or irregularly shaped deposits of calcium. The tumor may show areas of necrosis, hemorrhage, and calcification (Figure 22-12). It usually does not show diffuse infiltration; the remaining liver may be normal. The intrahepatic vessels are displaced and/or amputated by the mass. Color Doppler is useful to detect high velocity flow in the malignant neovasculature.

Clinical findings include a palpable abdominal mass and an elevated serum alpha-fetoprotein level. Patients may be symptomatic with fever, pain, anorexia, and subsequent weight loss. The prognosis of the tumor is dependent on the resectability of the mass.

The sonographic appearance of the hepatoblastoma shows hepatomegaly with a solitary mass that may show some calcification (Figure 22-13). The heterogeneous mass is predominantly solid; however, there may be hypoechoic areas with necrosis and/or hemorrhage. The fleshy areas around the mass are often mildly hyperechoic. It becomes important to identify the hepatic vessels and hepatic veins. Portal vein thrombosis may be present. The Doppler flow pattern in the lesion shows a high-velocity, low-resistant flow pattern.

COMMON SURGICAL CONDITIONS

Hypertrophic Pyloric Stenosis. The **pyloric canal** is located between the stomach and duodenum. In some infants, the pyloric muscle can become hypertrophied, resulting in significantly delayed gastric emptying. Hypertrophy of the circular muscle of the pylorus is an acquired condition that narrows the pyloric canal (Figure 22-14). The pyloric canal itself is not intrinsically stenotic or narrowed, but it functions as if it were as a result of the abnormally thickened surrounding muscle.

Hypertrophic pyloric stenosis (HPS) appears most commonly in male infants between 2 and 6 weeks of age. Rarely, it becomes apparent at birth or as late as 5 months of age. The incidence of HPS is approximately 3 in 1000 neonates. Bile-free vomiting in an otherwise healthy infant is the most

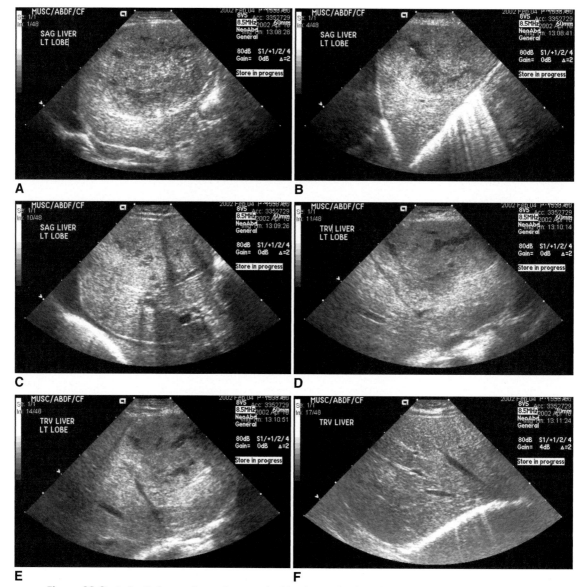

Figure 22-9   Infantile hemangioma. A 2-month-old infant with a liver hemangioma shows a well-circumscribed heterogeneous mass with focal areas of calcium in the left lobe of the liver. There is predominant flow around the mass. There were normal wave forms in both the main portal vein and left hepatic artery. **A,** Sagittal left lobe liver with large heterogeneous mass. **B,** Sagittal left lobe liver with mass. **C,** Sagittal liver with mass; right pleural effusion superior to diaphragm. **D,** Transverse left lobe of liver with large mass. **E,** Transverse left lobe of liver with mass. **F,** Transverse liver inferior to the mass.

A   **B**   **C**

Figure 22-10   Sagittal views of infantile hemangioma. The mass often shows areas of calcification that appear echogenic on sonography. **A-C,** Mass with areas of calcification.

A   **B**

Figure 22-11   Infantile hemangioma. Color Doppler helps to define the vascularity of the mass and the relationship of the portal and hepatic veins to the mass lesion. **A,** Power Doppler shows increased vascularity within the mass. **B,** Power Doppler over the mass.   *Continued*

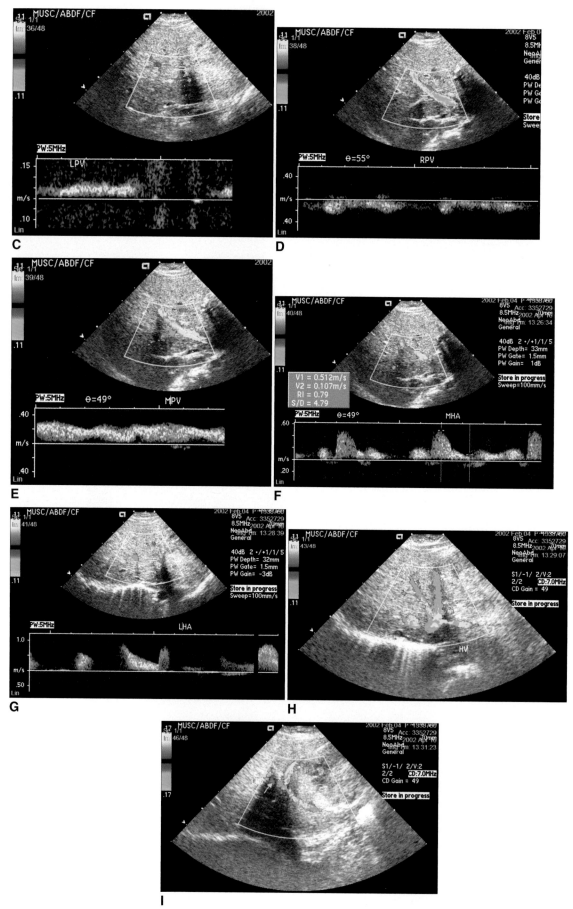

Figure 22-11, cont'd **C,** Left portal vein flow. **D,** Right portal vein flow. **E,** Main portal vein flow. **F,** Right hepatic artery flow. **G,** Left hepatic artery flow. **H,** Hepatic venous flow. **I,** Color flow in portal vein around the mass.

Figure 22-12 Hepatoblastoma. Lobular tumor with areas of necrosis. (From Damjanov I, Linder J: *Pathology: a color atlas,* St Louis, 2000, Mosby.)

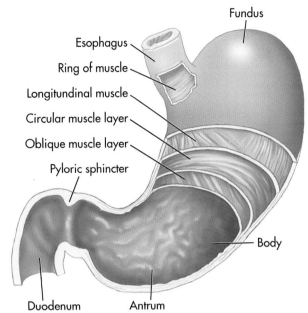

Figure 22-14 Diagram of hypertrophic pyloric stenosis. The pylorus muscle (sphincter) connects the antrum of the stomach with the duodenum of the small intestine.

Figure 22-13 Hepatoblastoma. The portal veins are displaced by the large mass. (From Henningsen C: *Clinical guide to ultrasonography,* St Louis, 2004, Mosby.)

Figure 22-15 Transverse image of the right upper quadrant using the liver as an acoustic window in a 5-week-old boy with hypertrophic pyloric stenosis shows a longitudinal view of an elongated thickened pyloric muscle *(arrows)*. The antrum *(an)* is filled with fluid. The gallbladder *(gb)* is anterior to the pyloric muscle, whereas the right kidney *(k)* is posterior and lateral.

frequent clinical sign. As the pyloric muscle thickens and elongates, the stomach outlet obstruction increases and vomiting is more constant and projectile. Dehydration and weight loss may ensue. Peristaltic waves and reverse peristaltic waves crossing the upper abdomen may be observed during or after feeding as the stomach attempts to force its contents through the abnormal canal (projectile vomiting). In these infants, palpation of an olive-shaped mass in the right upper quadrant is diagnostic and is treated by surgical pyloromyotomy. In infants with a suggestive history or an equivocal physical examination, diagnostic imaging is required to provide direct visualization of the pyloric muscle (Figure 22-15).

In pediatric imaging departments and in other ultrasound departments where there is appropriate expertise, sonography is the imaging method of choice to establish the diagnosis of HPS. If HPS is not a primary diagnostic consideration or if the sonogram is not diagnostic, conventional contrast radiography of the upper gastrointestinal tract is necessary to assess for other potential causes of vomiting (e.g., gastrointestinal

reflux, antral web, pylorospasm, hiatal hernia, and malrotation of the bowel) (Figure 22-16).

The neonate with projectile vomiting frequently is sent directly from the physician's office or the hospital emergency room. If the stomach is empty and HPS is not readily apparent, an oral feeding (i.e., glucose water or Pedialyte) is given to facilitate comprehensive visualization of the pyloric area (Figure 22-17). Conversely an overly distended stomach can displace the pyloric muscle posteriorly, making sonographic

Figure 22-16 **A,** Transverse image of the right upper quadrant using the liver as an acoustic window in a 4-week-old boy with projectile vomiting. There was to-and-fro peristalsis in the fluid-filled duodenal bulb *(db)* and descending duodenum *(dd)*. The descending duodenum tapered abruptly *(arrows)* and could not be traced distally. The right kidney *(k)* is posterior to the descending duodenum. A hypertrophied pyloric muscle was not identified. **B,** Right lateral view from a barium examination in the same patient shows the stomach, antrum *(an)*, duodenal bulb *(db)*, and descending duodenum *(dd)*. The descending duodenum tapers abruptly *(arrows)* and then spirals inferiorly. The barium examination delineates the surgically emergent malrotation, which could not be identified on the sonogram.

Figure 22-17 **A,** Transverse view of the right upper quadrant in a 5-week-old boy. The antrum *(arrows)* is collapsed and contains a linear echogenic centrum representing the interface between the lumen and mucosa. **B,** Transverse view of the right upper quadrant shows the antrum *(arrows)* in the same patient after administration of glucose water by bottle. The antrum *(an)* is now filled with fluid and is easy to differentiate from a hypertrophied pyloric muscle.

delineation virtually impossible (Figure 22-18). In this instance, aspiration of gastric contents via a nasogastric tube may be required.

The infant is usually examined first in the supine and then in the right lateral decubitus position, which aids in the visualization of the pylorus. A preliminary survey of the abdomen is performed to exclude abnormalities such as hydronephrosis or adrenal hemorrhage. Real-time imaging is then performed

using a high-frequency linear array transducer (5 to 12 MHz). Longitudinal images of the pyloric muscle are obtained by placing the transducer transversely across the right upper quadrant, just below the level of the xiphoid process. The transducer is then rotated obliquely until the pyloric muscle is visualized in its long axis (Figure 22-19). The muscle is thickened and elongated and extends into the antrum; this appearance has been called the "cervix" sign. If fluid passes

Figure 22-18   Transverse view of the right upper quadrant in a 5-week-old boy with hypertrophic pyloric stenosis. The fluid-distended antrum *(an)* has pushed the elongated pyloric muscle *(arrows)* posteriorly, precluding accurate measurement of the length of the pyloric canal. The kidney *(k)* is lateral and slightly posterior to the pyloric muscle.

Figure 22-20   Coronal view of the right upper quadrant shows the hypertrophied pyloric muscle in transverse section. The diameter of the muscle *(arrows)* is measured from the outer borders. The muscle thickness *(left arrow to arrowhead)* is measured from the outer border to the mucosal-muscle interface. The portal vein *(pv)* is posterior to the pyloric muscle in this plane.

Figure 22-19   Transverse view of the right upper quadrant shows the longitudinal extent of the hypertrophied pyloric muscle *(arrows)*. The calipers measure the length of the pyloric muscle, which is 20 mm. The kidney *(K)* is posterior and lateral to the pyloric muscle. Gas *(arrowhead)* in the antrum is causing a reverberation artifact.

form echo pattern, with the near and far fields appearing more echogenic.

If the diagnosis has not been established, the patient is then placed in a right lateral decubitus position and the transducer placed transversely in the right upper quadrant. This allows maximum visualization of the stomach and pyloric canal and is most advantageous for documenting the transit of gastric contents into the duodenum. The sonographer should determine the location of the superior mesenteric artery and vein to assess for malrotation, especially in the case of patients with negative findings of HPS.

If there is not enough residual gastric fluid present, 60 to 120 ml of water may be administered either through a bottle or through a nasogastric tube. The stomach should not be overfilled because this displaces the pylorus posteriorly, making visualization more difficult.

Measurements. Sonographic measurement of pyloric muscle thickness enables the diagnosis of HPS. Pyloric muscle measurements can be made in both the short- and the long-axis planes. If the image is oblique, measurements will be overestimated. A muscle thickness of 3.5 mm or greater on the long-axis view, a channel length of 17 mm or greater, and pyloric muscle length of 20 mm or greater is a reliable indicator of HPS.

Individual muscle wall thickness, total diameter, and length of the pyloric canal are measured. The thickness is measured from the periphery of the hypoechoic muscle to its junction with the echogenic central canal. Diameter is measured between the peripheral margins of the hypoechoic muscle layer. Length is measured from the proximal to the distal extremes of the echogenic central canal.

Sonographic Findings. The sonographic diagnosis of HPS depends upon the following findings: (1) visualization of a hypertrophied pyloric muscle with a canal measuring 17 mm or greater, (2) individual pyloric muscle wall thickness of

through the pyloric canal, it is often seen as a "double-track" in the crevices of the compressed mucosa. Other secondary signs include exaggerated gastric peristalsis and delayed gastric emptying.

Transverse short-axis images of the pyloric muscle are obtained from the right coronal plane. The gallbladder is initially identified, after which the transducer is angled medially until the "bull's eye" or "target" appearance of the hypertrophied pyloric muscle and echogenic central canal is noted (Figure 22-20). The pyloric muscle frequently has a nonuni-

3.5 mm or greater, or (3) a pyloric muscle length of 20 mm or greater. An additional significant finding is the presence of active antegrade and reverse gastric peristalsis.

The differential considerations include pylorospasm, gastrointestinal reflux, and duodenal obstruction caused by stenosis or malrotation with bands or volvulus.

Appendicitis. After gastroenteritis, **appendicitis** is the most common acute abdominal inflammatory process in children. Appendicitis occurs when the appendiceal lumen becomes obstructed and subsequently infected. In infants and young children, the progression of acute appendicitis to perforation is more rapid than in older children and adults, sometimes occurring within 6 to 12 hours. Classical physical and laboratory findings may be absent or confusing, making the diagnosis difficult.

Right lower quadrant pain and vomiting are a common clinical presentation. In addition to appendicitis, diagnostic considerations include enteritis, inflammatory bowel disease, and lymphoma. In girls the differential broadens to include gynecologic processes, such as ovarian cysts and neoplasms and ovarian torsion.

Sonography has proven to be very accurate in confirming appendicitis. As in virtually all conditions, a survey examination of the abdomen is first performed to assess the upper abdomen and the kidneys and bladder. In girls the adnexal areas should be examined with the patient having a distended urinary bladder. The bladder should then be emptied to allow gradual graded compression over the area of the appendix with the linear or curved array transducer. The right flank and right lower quadrant are reexamined using a 5 to 12 MHz linear array transducer. The transducer is moved slowly over the abdomen using the graded compression technique. This technique allows the sonographer to carefully apply gentle pressure with the transducer over the region of the appendix. Be sure to explain to the patient what you are going to do before beginning the compression technique. This technique enables the sonographer to visualize the appendix by displacing adjacent bowel loops. The appendix is usually seen anterior and medial to the psoas muscle and lateral to the iliac vessels.

Nonvisualization of the appendix may occur for multiple reasons and is not a definite indication of a normal appendix. Appendiceal nonvisualization may result from any of the following: (1) being obscured by overlying bowel; (2) retrocecal position of the appendix; (3) overdistention or nondistention of the urinary bladder, which alters the position of the appendix and overlying bowel; or (4) lack of sonographer experience. Changing the patient's position and emptying or filling the urinary bladder may facilitate visualization of both the normal and abnormal appendix.

The normal appendix appears as a blind-ending, long, tubular structure in the longitudinal plane and as a bull's-eye in the transverse plane.

Sonographic Findings. Peristalsis is not seen in the appendix, allowing differentiation of normal appendix and small bowel. The appendix may be tortuous and therefore difficult to visualize in its entirety. The walls are not thickened, and the normal appendix compresses easily.

Sonographically the acutely inflamed appendix is noncompressible (Figure 22-21). The appendix is measured in the transverse plane, across the short axis, using the maximum diameter. An outer diameter greater than 6 mm with compression is consistent with appendicitis both in children and adults. An increase in echogenicity has been shown in the surrounding mesentery secondary to the inflammation. Localized pain produced by overlying transducer pressure is an additional finding consistent with appendicitis. Color Doppler is useful to document increased blood flow (hyperemia). Other findings in appendicitis may include free peritoneal fluid or a loculated fluid collection in the lower abdomen. Confirmation of an appendicolith in a symptomatic patient is virtually diagnostic (Figure 22-22). An **appendicolith** is hyperechoic, produces a classic acoustic shadow, may be single or multiple, and may be intraluminal or surrounded by a periappendiceal phlegmon or abscess. The right kidney may at times be hydronephrotic because of ureteral inflammation.

The perforated appendix may or may not be visualized. If decompressed, an abnormally thick bowel wall may be apparent. A localized, well-defined right lower quadrant phlegmon or abscess with or without an appendicolith may be present (Figure 22-23). Free peritoneal fluid may be the lone abnormal sonographic finding. An abscess far removed from the right lower quadrant is another potential intraabdominal complication of an appendiceal perforation.

Enlarged lymph nodes may be a pitfall in diagnosing appendicitis. Patients with mesenteric lymphadenitis may present with prominent lymph nodes and symptoms of appendicitis with flulike symptoms previous to their illness. Color Doppler imaging may help the sonographer to determine the increased flow in the inflamed appendix from the enlarged node.

Intussusception. Intussusception is the most common acute abdominal disorder in early childhood. This condition occurs when the bowel prolapses into a more distal bowel and is propelled in an antegrade fashion. Telescoping of bowel in this manner causes obstruction. The ileum may invaginate into a more distal ileum, causing an ileoileal intussusception. If there is further progression through the ileocecal valve, an ileocecal intussusception results.

Prolapse of the ileum into the cecum or beyond produces an ileocolic intussusception. Intussusception is usually seen in children between the ages of 6 months and 2 years. A higher incidence has been reported in males (2:1), along with a seasonal prevalence. Frequently, there is a history of an antecedent upper respiratory tract infection. Associated inflammation of lymphoid tissue in the ileocolic region may act as a lead point for the telescoping phenomenon.

Children may present with colicky abdominal pain, vomiting, and bloody (currant jelly) stools. Abdominal distention or a mass may also be palpable. In patients with this classic clinical presentation, in whom there are no peritoneal symptoms or fever, preliminary abdominal radiographs followed by a barium or air enema are rapidly undertaken for both diagnos-

Figure 22-21   **A,** Longitudinal view of an inflamed appendix using the graded compression technique. The bulbous tip *(arrowheads)* is clearly defined. **B,** Longitudinal view of a fluid-filled inflamed appendix in a different child. The bulbous tip *(arrows)* is less easily seen. **C,** Longitudinal image of the right lower quadrant in a boy with appendicitis. The rectus abdominis muscle *(ra)* of the anterior abdominal wall is being compressed with the transducer to delineate the longitudinal extent of the appendix to its blind-ending tip *(arrows).* The curved arrows demonstrate the alternating hyperechoic and hypoechoic bowel wall layers. The central echogenic band *(top curved arrow)* represents the interface between the lumen and mucosa. The most peripheral echogenic band *(bottom curved arrow)* represents the interface between the peripheral bowel wall muscle layer and the bowel wall covering. **D,** Transverse image of the right lower quadrant in the same patient demonstrates the inflamed appendix *(arrowheads)* in the transverse plane. The iliac artery *(ia)* and vein course parallel to the appendix. They can be differentiated from the bowel by using Doppler imaging or tracing their course in the longitudinal plane.

Figure 22-22   **A,** Longitudinal image of an inflamed appendix containing multiple echogenic foci *(arrowheads)* consistent with appendicoliths, which cast acoustical shadows. The blind-ending tip *(arrows)* confirms that the echogenic foci are within the appendix and are not gas moving through the small bowel. **B,** Transverse image of an inflamed appendix in a different patient. There is a solitary appendicolith *(white arrows)* located centrally within the lumen. The hypoechoic periphery *(black arrows)* results from edema.

A   **B**

Figure 22-23 **A,** Midline sagittal image in a boy with an appendiceal abscess *(arrows)* posterior to the urinary bladder *(bl).* The appendiceal abscess appears heterogeneous in echogenicity and is well demarcated from the surrounding bowel, which was actively peristaltic on real-time examination. **B,** Coronal image of the right kidney *(arrows)* in the same patient shows moderate hydronephrosis because of distal ureteral inflammation from the abscess. A fluid-filled right renal pelvis *(rp)* may be a secondary sign of a right lower quadrant or pelvic process.

A   **B**

Figure 22-24 **A,** Transverse image of an intussusception *(arrowheads)* showing a target sign. There are several circumferential layers of increased and decreased echogenicity *(arrows)* because of the telescoping bowel. The lumen *(curved arrow)* contains fluid. **B,** In an image at a more superior level in the same patient, intussusception *(arrows)* is identified. The target sign is present, but, instead of being round, it is more C-shaped because the bowel loop is coiled on itself.

tic confirmation and to attempt therapeutic reduction. Failure to reduce an intussusception mandates immediate surgical intervention.

Likewise, surgical intervention is indicated in patients with a classical clinical presentation of intussusception who have developed fever and peritoneal signs. In patients with a vaguer clinical presentation, in whom intussusception remains suspect, an ultrasound examination is a helpful diagnostic undertaking.

Sonographic Findings. The patient is examined in the supine position. A survey of the entire abdomen is performed, followed by an examination focusing on the bowel using a 5 to 12 MHz linear or curved array transducer.

The sonographic appearance of intussusception is of alternating hypoechoic and hyperechoic rings surrounding an echogenic center as seen in a short-axis view of the involved area. This is known as the **target sign** or **donut** (Figure 22-24). In the long axis view, hypoechoic layers on each side of the echogenic center result in a "pseudokidney" or "sandwich" sign appearance (Figure 22-25). The sonolucent ring is believed to represent the edematous infolded loop of the intussusceptum, whereas the echogenic central area represents its compressed mucosa. Other concentric rings are present resulting from visualization of additional bowel wall layers within the intussusception. Free peritoneal fluid is not an uncommon finding with uncomplicated intussusception.

Figure 22-25 **A,** Longitudinal image of the right lower quadrant demonstrates a pseudokidney appearance of an intussusception *(arrows)*. A normal kidney is present in each renal fossa, so this is not a pelvic kidney. **B,** Transverse image of the right lower quadrant in a different patient with intussusception *(arrows)*. The intussusception has a sandwich appearance.

Color Doppler may help to determine the success of an air reduction enema; if there is good color flow to all areas of the telescoping bowel, the chances are better for a reduction. Poor color Doppler may indicate ischemia to the area of affected bowel.

When an intussusception is documented sonographically, an associated cause, though relatively uncommon, should be sought. A double target sign has been reported as being diagnostic of intussuscepted Meckel's diverticulum. Other causes, such as a small bowel tumor or duplication cyst, may likewise be identified. Consideration of barium or air enema versus surgical intervention is as discussed earlier (Figure 22-26). Intussusception may be reduced with hydrostatic pressure or by air reduction. An edematous ileocecal valve may be seen on fluoroscopy that may mimic a residual intussusception. Sonography may be helpful in distinguishing between persistent intussusception and an edematous ileocecal valve. The edematous valve appears as a small sonolucent rim with an echogenic center. It is distinguishable from intussusception in that its cross-sectional diameter is smaller than that of an intussusception, and it lacks the concentric rings frequently seen in intussusception.

In addition to intussusception, conditions that can produce a targetlike sonographic appearance include primary bowel tumors, such as lymphoma, and thickened bowel wall in post-stem cell transplant or bone marrow transplant patients and in patients with inflammatory bowel disease.

Other Surgical Conditions. In addition to hyperpyloric stenosis, appendicitis, and intussusception, other conditions that may lead to surgical correction may be less frequently seen in the neonate. These conditions include mesenteric or omental cysts (often large in size), duplication cysts of the bowel, duodenal atresia, and meconium peritonitis. Older children may also present with duplication cysts of the bowel and hematomas of the bowel resulting from trauma.

Figure 22-26 There are multiple, dilated fluid-filled bowel loops, *(B)* located anterior to the intussusception *(arrowheads)*. The intussusception could not be reduced, a frequent occurrence when an ileocolic intussusception is encountered on contrast enema, mandating surgical intervention.

SELECTED BIBLIOGRAPHY

Bhisitkul DM, Listernick R, Shkolnik A and others: Clinical application of ultrasonography in the diagnosis of intussusception, *J Pediatr* 121:182, 1992.

Bisset GS III, Kirks DR: Intussusception in infants and children: diagnosis and therapy, *Radiology* 168:141, 1988.

Blumhagen JD: The role of ultrasonography in the evaluation of vomiting in infants, *Pediatr Radiol* 16:267, 1986.

Bowen AD: The vomiting infant: recent advances and unsettled issues in imaging, *Radiol Clin North Am* 26:377, 1988.

Breaux CW Jr, Georgeson KE, Royal SA and others: Changing patterns in the diagnosis of hypertrophic pyloric stenosis, *Pediatrics* 81:213, 1988.

Haller JO, Cohen HL: Hypertrophic pyloric stenosis: diagnosis using US, *Radiology* 161:335, 1986.

Herman TE, Siegel MJ: Infantile hepatic hemangioendothelioma, *J Perinatol* 20:447-449, 2000.

Ikeda S and others: Gallbladder contraction in biliary atresia: a pitfall of ultrasound diagnosis, *Pediatr Radiol* 28:451-453, 1998.

Itagaki A, Uchida M, Ueki K and others: Double targets sign in ultrasonic diagnosis of intussuscepted Meckel diverticulum, *Pediatr Radiol* 21:148, 1991.

Jeffrey RB Jr, Laing FC, and Lewis FR: Acute appendicitis: high resolution real-time US findings, *Radiology* 163:11, 1987.

Kendrick A and others: Making the diagnosis of biliary atresia using the triangular cord sign and gallbladder length, *Pediatr Radiol* 30:69-73, 2000.

Lee HC, Yeh HJ, Leu YJ: Intussusception: the sonographic diagnosis and its clinical value, *J Pediatr Gastroenterol Nutr* 8:343, 1989.

Lee HC and others: Dilation of the biliary tree in children: sonographic diagnosis and its clinical significance, *J Ultrasound Med* 19:177-182, 2000.

Mollitt DL, Golladay ES, Williamson S and others: Ultrasonography in the diagnosis of pyloric stenosis, *South Med J* 80:47, 1987.

O'Keeffe FN, Stansberry SD, Swischuk LE and others: Antropyloric muscle thickness at US in infants: what is normal? *Radiology* 178:827, 1991.

Pracros JP, Tran-Minh VA, Morin De Finfe CH and others: Acute intestinal intussusception in children. Contribution of ultrasonography (145 cases), *Ann Radiol* 30:525, 1987.

Puylaert JB: Acute appendicitis: US evaluation using graded compression, *Radiology* 158:355, 1986.

Quillin SP, Siegel MJ, Coffin CM: Acute appendicitis in children: value of sonography in detecting perforation, *Am J Roentgenol* 159:1265, 1992.

Rioux M: Sonographic detection of the normal and abnormal appendix, *Am J Roentgenol* 158:773, 1992.

Sato M and others: Liver tumors in children and young patients: sonographic and color Doppler findings, *Abdom Imaging* 25:596-601, 2000.

Siegel MJ: Acute appendicitis in childhood: the role of US, *Radiology* 185:341, 1992.

Sivit CJ: Diagnosis of acute appendicitis in children: spectrum of sonographic findings, *Am J Roentgenol* 161:147, 1993.

Sivit CJ, Newman KD, Boenning DA and others: Appendicitis: usefulness of US in diagnosis in a pediatric population, *Radiology* 185:549, 1992.

Stringer MD, Capps SNJ, Pablot SM: Sonographic detection of the lead point in intussusception, *Arch Dis Child* 67:529, 1992.

Swischuk LE, Hayden CK, Boulden T: Intussusception: indications for ultrasonography and an explanation of the doughnut and pseudokidney signs, *Pediatr Radiol* 15:388, 1985.

Swischuk LE, Stansberry SD: Ultrasonographic detection of free peritoneal fluid in uncomplicated intussusception, *Pediatr Radiol* 21:350, 1991.

Verschelden P, Filiatrault D, Garel L and others: Intussusception in children: reliability of US in diagnosis\Ma prospective study, *Radiology* 184:741, 1992.

Vignault F, Filiatrault D, Brandt ML and others: Acute appendicitis in children: evaluation with US, *Radiology* 176:501, 1990.

Weinberger E, Winters WD: Intussusception in children: the role of sonography, *Radiology* 184:601, 1992.

CHAPTER 23

The Neonatal and Pediatric Kidneys and Adrenal Glands

Sandra L. Hagen-Ansert

OBJECTIVES

- Understand the sonographic approach to imaging neonatal/pediatric kidneys and adrenal glands
- Describe the causes of hydronephrosis in the neonate/pediatric patient
- Distinguish between multicystic dysplastic kidney and polycystic renal disease
- Discuss the sonographic findings in renal vein thrombosis
- Describe the sonographic findings in renal and adrenal tumors

EXAMINATION PREPARATION

NORMAL ANATOMY AND SONOGRAPHIC FINDINGS
KIDNEYS
ADRENAL GLANDS
BLADDER

PATHOLOGY OF RENAL AND ADRENAL ENLARGEMENT
HYDRONEPHROSIS
PRUNE BELLY SYNDROME
MULTICYSTIC DYSPLASTIC KIDNEY
AUTOSOMAL RECESSIVE POLYCYSTIC KIDNEY DISEASE
AUTOSOMAL DOMINANT POLYCYSTIC KIDNEY DISEASE
RENAL VEIN THROMBOSIS
RENAL/ADRENAL TUMORS
ADRENAL HEMORRHAGE

KEY TERMS

adrenal hemorrhage – occurs when the fetus is stressed during a difficult delivery or a hypoxic insult (lack of oxygen)

arcuate arteries – lie at the base of the medullary pyramids and appear as echogenic structures

autosomal dominant polycystic kidney disease (ADPKD) – congenital polycystic kidney disease that usually presents during middle age. Sometimes asymptomatic, the severity of the disease varies widely. Presents with hypertension, hematuria, and enlarged kidneys. Cysts can also form in the liver, spleen, and pancreas.

autosomal recessive polycystic kidney disease (ARPKD) – rare, congenital polycystic renal disease also known as infantile polycystic disease; typically presents with diffuse enlargement, sacculations, and cystic diverticula of the medullary portions of the kidneys

congenital mesoblastic nephroma – most common benign renal tumor of the neonate and infant

cortex – the outer rim of the kidney; the cortex is thin in the neonate, with an echogenicity similar or slightly greater than that of the normal liver parenchyma

ectasia – dilatation of any tubular vessel

ectopic ureterocele – occurs more commonly in females (on left side); ectopic insertion and cystic dilation of distal ureter of duplicated renal collecting system

hydronephrosis – dilation of the renal collecting system

medullary pyramids – large and hypoechoic in the neonate

multicystic dysplastic kidney (MCDK) – most common cause of renal cystic disease in the neonate; multiple cystic masses within the kidney; may have contralateral ureteral pelvic junction obstruction

nephroblastomatosis – abnormal persistence of fetal renal blastema (potential to develop into Wilms' tumor)

neuroblastoma – malignant tumor usually found in the adrenal glands

polycystic renal disease – poorly functioning enlarged kidneys

posterior urethral valves – most common cause of bladder outlet obstruction in the male neonate

Potter facies – classification of cystic renal disease

prune belly syndrome – triad of hypoplasia or deficiency of the abdominal musculature, cryptorchidism, and urinary tract anomalies

pulmonary hypoplasia – underdevelopment of the lung tissue that occurs in utero (secondary to oligohydramnios)

renal vein thrombosis – kidney becomes enlarged and edematous as a result of obstruction of the renal vein

ureteropelvic junction obstruction – most common neonatal obstruction of the urinary tract; results from intrinsic narrowing or extrinsic vascular compression

VACTERL – adds *c*ardiac and *l*imb anomalies to the VATER syndrome

VATER – *v*ertebral, *a*nal, *t*racheo*e*sophageal fistula and *r*enal anomalies

Wilms' tumor (nephroblastoma) – most frequent malignant tumor in the neonate and infant

------

Sonography is the first diagnostic imaging method of choice when a renal or adrenal abnormality is suspected in the neonate or pediatric patient. There are numerous indications for renal imaging in the newborn period. One major indication is a renal abnormality detected during prenatal sonography. Some of the conditions or findings in the newborn associated with renal abnormalities are flank masses, abdominal distention, anuria, oliguria, hematuria, sepsis or urinary tract infection, meningomyelocele, **VATER** and **VACTERL** anomalies, abnormal external genitalia, and prune belly syndrome. Still other indicators include skin tags (usually near the ear and associated with cardiac anomalies) and a two-vessel umbilical cord. These conditions usually indicate the renal study is for screening the kidneys with no particular renal symptoms present.

EXAMINATION PREPARATION

General aspects of the ultrasound examination of the neonate and pediatric patient are described in Chapter 22. Maintaining body temperature in the neonate is very important because small infants can lose a potentially dangerous amount of body heat quickly. Whenever possible, scanning through the portholes of an Isolette provides an optimal environment for the premature or otherwise fragile neonate. When the examination is performed outside of the Isolette, body heat loss can be minimized by the use of heat lamps and by exposing only the area of the body being interrogated.

Imaging of the urinary bladder, which includes assessment for distal ureteral dilation, is considered an important part of the renal sonographic examination (Figure 23-1). Because of the infant's tendency to urinate spontaneously, scanning is gently initiated over the suprapubic region. If the urinary bladder is not distended at this time, or if voiding occurs before adequate detail can be obtained, this area can be examined after imaging of the kidneys and perirenal areas. Refilling of the urinary bladder is usually relatively rapid if the infant is fed and also when parenteral fluids are being administered.

Long- and short-axis views of the kidneys and of the perirenal areas are initially obtained by scanning via the flanks to obtain coronal and axial images, via the anterior abdomen for longitudinal and transverse images, or both. When necessary, additional transverse and longitudinal views can be obtained with the infant in a prone position. Renal scanning before and after the infant voids may provide useful information. For example, development of, or increase in, **hydronephrosis** after voiding would be very suggestive of high-grade vesicoureteral reflux.

NORMAL ANATOMY AND SONOGRAPHIC FINDINGS

KIDNEYS

In the second trimester, the kidney develops from small renunculi that are composed of a central large pyramid with a thin peripheral rim of cortex. As the renunculi fuse progressively, their adjoining cortices form a column of Bertin. The former renunculi are at that point called "lobes." Remnants of these lobes with somewhat incomplete fusion, often termed "fetal lobulation," should not be confused with renal abnormalities or scars when imaging the kidney. These pyramids remain large even after birth in comparison with the thin rim of cortex that surrounds them. The glomerular filtration rate is low right after term birth, but increases rapidly thereafter. The cortex continues to grow throughout childhood, whereas the pyramids become smaller in size. The larger amount of cortical fat is not present in the neonate and pediatric patient, thus allowing for clear distinction of the cortical-medullary junction.

A   **B**

Figure 23-1   **A,** Transverse image of the pelvis in a 2-day-old infant with bilateral primary megaureter (nonobstructive dilation of the distal ureter). The urinary bladder *(bl)* is well distended. Bilateral dilation of the distal ureter *(ur)* is seen posterior to the bladder. **B,** Longitudinal view of the same patient shows the distal ureter *(ur)* entering the urinary bladder *(bl).*

The normal kidney in the neonate is characterized by a distinct demarcation of the cortex and medullary pyramids. The **medullary pyramids** are large and hypoechoic and should not be mistaken for dilated calyces or cysts. The surrounding **cortex** is quite thin, with echogenicity essentially similar to or slightly greater than that of normal liver parenchyma (Figure 23-2). Renal cortical echogenicity normally decreases to less than that of liver parenchyma usually by 4 to 6 months of age.

The pediatric renal anatomy varies with the pediatric patient, depending on the age of the child. The adolescent and teenager has a sonographic renal anatomy similar to an adult anatomy. The renal parenchyma consists of a peripheral cortex, the glomeruli, and several extensions to the edge of the renal sinus (column of Bertin). The medulla is more central and adjacent to the calices. The normal cortex produces low-level, back-scattered echoes.

The medullary pyramids are relatively hypoechoic and arranged around the central, echo-producing renal sinus. The arcuate vessels are seen as intense specular echoes at the corticomedullary junction. The increased cortical echogenicity may result from glomeruli occupying a larger proportion of cortical volume and the location of 20% of the loops of Henle within the cortex as opposed to the medulla. In neonates and infants the medullary pyramids are prominent and hypoechoic, and corticomedullary definition is accentuated (from a larger medullary volume).

The surrounding cortex is quite echogenic and thick, with the echogenicity essentially similar to or slightly greater than that of normal liver or splenic parenchyma (see Figure 23-2). Because of a paucity of fat in the renal sinus of the neonate, this area is generally hypoechoic and therefore indistinct. The **arcuate arteries,** which lie at the bases of the medullary pyramids, appear as punctate, intensely echogenic structures.

The contour of the neonatal kidney is usually lobulated from residual fetal lobulations. At the site of this fetal lobulation, a parenchymal triangular defect may be identified in the anterosuperior or inferoposterior aspect of the kidney at the junctional parenchymal defect.

Normal renal length varies with the age of the infant (Figure 23-3).

Renal anomalies of number include renal agenesis and supernumerary kidney. Anomalies of position, form, and orientation include pelvic kidney, horseshoe kidney, crossed

Figure 23-2   **A,** Coronal view of a normal right kidney *(arrowheads)* in a 3-day-old male with a left multicystic dysplastic kidney. The medullary pyramids appear as triangular hypoechoic areas. The cortex has the same echogenicity as the liver. **B,** Transverse view of the same kidney *(arrowheads)*. The hypoechoic psoas muscle *(ps)* is located posteromedial to the kidney. The nondilated renal pelvis *(P)* contains anechoic fluid. **C,** Normal kidney *(arrowheads)* in 13-day-old female. The increased echogenicity of the renal cortex compared with the normal liver parenchyma can be normal. The medullary pyramids appear large and hypoechoic *(arrows)*.

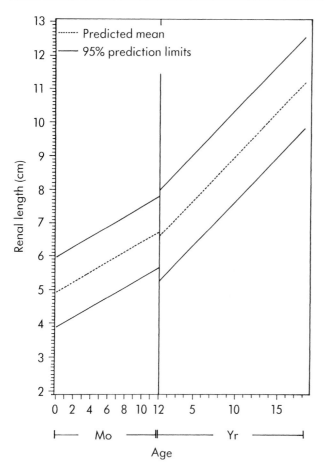

Figure 23-3 Normal renal length versus age. (From Rumack C, Wilson S, Charboneau W: *Diagnostic ultrasound,* ed 3, St Louis, 2005, Mosby.)

ectopy, and renal duplication. The reader is referred to Chapter 10 for further discussion of these anomalies.

ADRENAL GLANDS

The normal adrenal glands are relatively larger and therefore more easily identified in the neonate than in the older infant or young child. Each gland lies immediately superior to the upper pole of the kidney. The left adrenal gland extends slightly medial. Sonographically the gland has an inverted V or Y shape in the longitudinal plane (Figure 23-4, A). In the transverse plane, the portion of the gland delineated has a linear or curvilinear outline (Figure 23-4, B). The adrenal medulla in the neonate is relatively thin, appearing as a distinctly echogenic stripe, surrounded by the more prominent and less echogenic adrenal cortex. When the kidney is absent or ectopic, the ipsilateral adrenal gland remains in the renal fossa, but as a result it may have an altered configuration (Figure 23-5).

BLADDER

The normal urinary bladder is thin-walled in the distended state and should measure less than 3 mm. When empty, the wall thickness increases, but is still less than 5 mm. The distal ureters may be seen at the bladder base if the child is well hydrated. The use of color Doppler may aid in the visualization of the distal ureter as it enters the posterior wall of the bladder.

PATHOLOGY OF RENAL AND ADRENAL ENLARGEMENT

The more common causes of renal and adrenal enlargement that can present as a palpable mass in the neonate are discussed. Table 23-1 lists the clinical and sonographic renal findings and differential considerations for the pathology discussed here.

A   B

Figure 23-4   A, Coronal view of a normal adrenal gland *(arrowheads)* in a 1-day-old infant with ambiguous genitalia. The adrenal medulla *(arrows)* appears as a central echogenic stripe, surrounded by the less echogenic cortex. The adrenal gland has an inverted Y configuration. **B,** Transverse view through a portion of adrenal gland *(arrowheads)* demonstrating the curvilinear shape in this plane.

Figure 23-5 **A,** Crossed-fused renal ectopia *(arrows)* in a 1-day-old male with imperforate anus. Sonogram through the right flank demonstrates the renal pelvis *(rp)* of each kidney. **B,** Coronal image through the right flank demonstrates an elongated adrenal gland *(arrows)* resulting from the absence of a kidney in this renal fossa.

Figure 23-6 **A,** Ureteropelvic junction obstruction in a 2-week-old female infant with an abnormal prenatal ultrasound. Marked dilation of the renal pelvis *(RP)* and calyces *(C)* is present. Parenchymal loss is also noted. The distal ureter was not identified. Radionuclide imaging confirmed the diagnosis. **B,** Uteropelvic junction obstruction in a 1-day-old infant. Coronal image of the kidney *(arrows)* identifies marked dilation of the renal pelvis *(RP)*.

HYDRONEPHROSIS

Hydronephrosis means the dilation of the urinary collecting system. There are many causes of dilation of the collecting system, the most common being obstruction, reflux, or abnormal muscle development. Ultrasound is very sensitive in detecting small amounts of fluid in the renal pelvis. Ultrasound is able to determine the severity of the hydronephrosis, whether the condition is unilateral or bilateral, if the ureters and bladder are dilated, and the status of the renal parenchyma.

Sonographic features found in hydronephrosis include visible renal parenchyma surrounding a central cystic component, small peripheral cysts (dilated calyces) budding off a large central cyst (renal pelvis), and visualization of a dilated ureter. This must be distinguished from the noncommunicating cysts of multicystic dysplastic kidneys.

Ureteropelvic Junction Obstruction. The most common type of obstruction of the upper urinary tract is called **ureteropelvic junction obstruction;** it most often results from intrinsic narrowing or extrinsic vascular compression at the level of the ureteropelvic junction. Bilateral involvement may occur along with a contralateral multicystic dysplastic kidney or vesicoureteral reflux. The obstruction produces proximal dilation of the collecting system; however, the ureter is normal in caliber. There is an increased incidence of abnormalities of the contralateral kidney.

Sonographic Findings. Sonographically, there is pelvocalyceal dilation without ureteral dilation (Figure 23-6, *A*). When the obstruction is pronounced, the dilated renal pelvis extends inferiorly and medially (Figure 23-6, *B*). If vesicoureteral reflux or primary megaureter is present, the ureter

TABLE 23-1 RENAL FINDINGS

Clinical Findings	Sonographic Findings	Differential Considerations
Hydronephrosis		
Flank pain	Pelvocalyceal dilation Ureter is dilated when vesicoureteral reflux or primary megaureter is present	Parapelvic cyst Extrarenal sinus Congenital megacystis Multiple renal cysts Multicystic renal disease Functional dilation Duplicated collecting system
Posterior Urethral Valves		
Decreased urine output	Thickened bladder wall ("keyhole") Hydronephrosis Hydroureter	Megaureter
Multicystic Dysplastic Kidney		
	Unilateral multicystic mass in kidney Contralateral ureteropelvic junction	Hydronephrosis
Polycystic Renal Disease		
Pulmonary hypoplasia Potter's facies	Enlarged kidneys Echogenic kidneys	
Prune Belly Syndrome		
Absence of abdominal muscle Undescended testes Dilated bladder, ureter, prostatic urethra	Kidney is normal, hydronephrotic, or dysplastic Dysplastic enlarged kidneys Dilated ureters Dilated bladder	Posterior urethral valves
Congenital Mesoblastic Nephroma		
Found in children <1 yr	Hyperechoic or hypoechoic or mixed	Adrenal tumor Neuroblastoma Benign renal tumor Abscess
Nephroblastomatosis		
Abnormal persistence of fetal renal blastoma	Bilateral renal enlargement	Adrenal tumor Neuroblastoma
Neuroblastoma		
Nystagmus Unsteady gait	Mass usually in adrenal gland Echogenic Calcification Look for metastasis to liver	Adrenal tumor Benign renal tumor Abscess
Wilms' Tumor		
Hypertension Palpable abdominal or flank mass Weight loss, fever, anemia, pain	Complex mass in kidney Well-circumscribed mass Isoechoic to echogenic May have calcification Look for tumor extension into renal vein or inferior vena cava	Mesoblastic nephroma Renal cell carcinoma Retroperitoneal sarcoma Adrenal cortical carcinoma Multicystic renal hamartoma
Adrenal Hemorrhage		
Abdominal mass Jaundice Anemia	Ovoid enlargement of the gland Anechoic to hyperechoic	Adrenal neuroblastoma Adrenal cyst Adrenal neoplasm

Figure 23-7 **A,** Posterior urethral valves in a male infant. Transverse view of the urinary bladder shows the thickened bladder wall *(arrowheads)*. Dilated distal ureters *(arrows)* are identified posterior to the bladder. **B,** Coronal view of the left kidney shows moderate pelvocalectasis *(rp)*. A urinoma *(arrows)* is seen superior to the kidney.

Figure 23-8 **A,** Sonogram of urinoma *(arrows)* in a 5-week-old with bilateral ureterovesical obstruction. Moderate pelvocalectasis *(rp)* and dilation of the ureter *(ur)* are seen. **B,** Transverse image in the same patient identifies septations within the urinoma *(arrows)*.

may be dilated. The best way to demonstrate the dilated ureters at the ureteropelvic junction is with a coronal scan plane.

Bladder Outlet Obstruction. Bilateral hydronephrosis is frequently caused by obstruction at the level of the bladder or bladder outlet. The bladder may be obstructed by a neurogenic bladder, a pelvic mass, or a congenital anomaly, such as posterior urethral valves. **Posterior urethral valves** are the most common cause of bladder outlet obstruction in the male neonate.

Sonographic Findings. The wall of the urinary bladder appears thickened and trabeculated (Figure 23-7, *A*). Midline sagittal imaging with caudal angulation through the bladder may allow visualization of the distended posterior urethra. Alternatively the posterior urethra can be imaged directly from a perineal approach. The resultant hydronephrosis and hydroureter are usually bilateral. Urinary ascites or a perirenal urinoma can result from high-pressure vesicoureteral reflux, rupturing a calyceal fornix or tearing the renal parenchyma (Figure 23-7, *B*). The perirenal urinoma is usually anechoic; however, septations may be noted. Other potential causes of perirenal urine extravasation include ureteropelvic junction obstruction, ureterovesical junction obstruction, and pelvic masses that obstruct the bladder or ureter (Figure 23-8).

Ectopic Ureterocele. **Ectopic ureterocele** occurs more commonly in females and more often on the left side. It results from an ectopic insertion and cystic dilation of the distal ureter of the upper moiety of a completely duplicated renal collecting system.

Sonographic Findings. The ectopic ureterocele, seen as a fluid mass within the urinary bladder, is located inferomedially to the ureteral insertion of the lower pole ureter (Figure 23-9, *A,B*). Postoperatively, following the incision of the ureterocele, the structure may be seen in a collapsed state. The sonographic delineation of an upper pole fluid mass, in continuity with a dilated ureter and the aforementioned ureterocele, is diagnostic of this entity (Figure 23-9, *C*). Distention and effacement or contraction of the ureterocele may be evident during the real-time study.

PRUNE BELLY SYNDROME

The **prune belly syndrome** (or abdominal muscle deficiency syndrome) is the triad of hypoplasia or deficiency of the abdominal musculature, cryptorchidism, and urinary tract anomalies. This anomaly includes congenital absence or deficiency of the abdominal musculature, large hypotonic dilated tortuous ureters, a large bladder, a patent urachus, bilateral cryptorchidism, and a dilated prostatic urethra. The severely affected patients have urethral atresia and bilateral cystic renal

Figure 23-9   **A,** Transverse image of the urinary bladder *(bl)* in a 2-month-old female with pyelonephritis. A large, thin-walled ureterocele *(arrows)* is seen in the posterior aspect of the bladder. **B,** Longitudinal view of the bladder in the same patient shows the dilated ureter *(ur)* and ureterocele *(arrows)*. Low-level echoes seen in the ureter and ureterocele represent debris. **C,** Coronal view of the kidney in the same patient demonstrates a duplicated kidney with notable pelvocalectasis of the upper pole segment *(urp)* and moderate pelvocalectasis of the lower pole segment *(lrp)*. The ureter from the upper pole segment *(arrows)* is located medial to the lower pole renal pelvis.

dysplasia secondary to obstruction. Resultant pulmonary hypoplasia is fatal. The less severely affected neonates have a bladder with poor contractility without obstruction; however, the ureters may be ectatic and dilated. Reflux is a common problem with the prune belly syndrome.

Sonographic Findings. The sonographic findings vary depending on the severity of the syndrome. The most severely affected neonates show dysplastic echogenic kidneys. In the less severely affected, nonhydronephrotic kidneys with dilated ureters and a huge bladder are seen. This appearance may be similar to that of a neonate with posterior urethral valves. Physically the wrinkled "prunelike" abdomen aids in the clinical diagnosis.

MULTICYSTIC DYSPLASTIC KIDNEY

Multicystic dysplastic kidney (MCDK) is the most common cause of renal cystic disease in the neonate; when hydronephrosis is excluded, it is the most common cause of an abdominal mass in the newborn. The MCDK is a congenital, usually sporadic, renal dysplasia, which is thought to be secondary to severe, generalized interference with ureteral bud function during the first trimester. The malformation results from ureteral obstruction; high ureteral atresia and pyelocalyceal occlusion are almost always present.

In utero the obstruction interferes with ureteral bud division and inhibits the maturation of nephrons in the kidney. Thus the collecting tubules enlarge, becoming cystic and

grossly distorting the shape of the kidney. The remaining renal parenchyma becomes virtually nonfunctioning. Nearly half of the cases have contralateral abnormalities (i.e., ureteropelvic junction obstruction and vesicoureteral reflux).

Sonographic Findings. Sonographically the classic appearance of MCDK is of a unilateral mass resembling a bunch of grapes, which represents a cluster of discrete noncommunicating cysts, the largest of which are peripheral. There is no identifiable renal pelvis (Figure 23-10). A less common hydronephrotic form of MCDK has been described in which a renal pelvis has been identified. The association with contralateral uteropelvic junction obstruction has been noted. Bilateral occurrence of MCDK is fatal.

At times, sonographic differentiation of MCDK from severe uteropelvic junction obstruction may be difficult. In such instances, radionuclide documentation of renal function usually indicates severe hydronephrosis. The use of ultrasound has led to conservative management of MCDK. These abnormal kidneys most often involute and disappear completely or result in a small dysplastic kidney. If there is evidence of growth, resection is usually undertaken.

AUTOSOMAL RECESSIVE POLYCYSTIC KIDNEY DISEASE

Polycystic renal disease identified in the neonatal period is most often **autosomal recessive polycystic kidney disease (ARPKD),** also known as *infantile polycystic disease.* This disease is not very common, occurring in 1 in 6000 to 14,000

Figure 23-10 Multicystic dysplastic kidney *(arrows)* in a 3-week-old male. Axial view of the left flank demonstrates multiple, noncommunicating cysts of varying sizes. There was no apparent renal pelvis. Radionuclide imaging confirmed the diagnosis.

Figure 23-11 Gross pathology of autosomal-recessive polycystic kidney disease demonstrated bilateral renal enlargement with diffuse cyst replacing the tubules and collecting ducts. (From Damjanov I, Linder J: *Pathology: a color atlas,* St. Louis, 2000, Mosby.)

births with a female predominance 2:1. It is transmitted by autosomal recessive inheritance. The typical pathologic presentation is diffuse enlargement, sacculations, and cystic diverticula of the medullary portions of the kidneys (Figure 23-11).

ARPKD is associated with biliary ectasia and hepatic fibrosis (the severity is proportional to the degree of renal involvement). The most severe form is seen in the neonatal stage, whereas the least severe form is seen in the infantile to juvenile stage. In the third trimester of pregnancy, the dilated kidneys occupy nearly the entire abdomen and cause the abdomen to protrude. The perinatal form is the most common and is characterized by varying degrees of renal tubular dilation and hepatic fibrosis. The kidneys are hyperechoic and enlarged with a hypoechogenic outer rim, which represents the cortex compressed by the expanded pyramids. The degree of renal cystic disease determines the severity of renal dysplasia

which can lead to renal failure and eventual liver failure. Pulmonary hypoplasia with respiratory distress and Potter facies may also be associated findings.

In the juvenile form of ARPKD, symptoms can occur later in childhood. The renal tubular ectasia and the resultant renal symptomatology are overshadowed by hepatic fibrosis leading to portal hypertension and gastrointestinal bleeding. In this condition the dilated renal collecting tubules produce an accentuated medullary echogenicity, and the renal cortex has an essentially normal appearance. Increased liver echogenicity reflects hepatic fibrosis.

Sonographic Findings. The most striking feature is bilateral renal enlargement with diffuse increased echogenicity and loss of definition of the renal sinus, medulla, and cortex. The less severe cases may show hepatosplenomegaly and portal hypertension, with the renal parenchyma normal to echogenic. In utero, oligohydramnios and nonvisualization of the bladder will also be apparent. (The lack of amniotic fluid volume in turn leads to the development of pulmonary hypoplasia.) This diagnosis may be made as early as 16 to 18 weeks of gestation in the presence of severe oligohydramnios and nonvisualization of the bladder.

The macroscopic cystlike appearance throughout both kidneys actually reflects dilated renal tubules that are generally less than 2 mm in diameter. The innumerable acoustic interfaces that present because of this morphologic abnormality result in notable echogenicity, obscuring corticomedullary demarcation. A thin, peripheral, hypoechoic renal rim may be demonstrated, representing either a compressed renal cortex or elongated thin-walled cystic spaces (Figure 23-12). Associated mild hepatic fibrosis and ductal hyperplasia can produce a heterogeneous increase in echogenicity of liver parenchyma.

AUTOSOMAL DOMINANT POLYCYSTIC KIDNEY DISEASE

More than 90% of patients with **autosomal dominant polycystic kidney disease (ADPKD)** have a gene locus on the short arm of chromosome 16. There is a wide variation in the severity of the disease. The adult dominant form of polycystic kidney disease usually appears during middle age. On rare occasions, however, it has been reported in a young infant. More typically the disease becomes manifest during the fourth decade of adulthood, with hypertension, hematuria, and enlarged kidneys. Cysts are macroscopic and of varying size and can also form in the liver, spleen, and pancreas. Cerebral berry aneurysms are also known to occur in 10% to 15% of patients with ADPKD. There is an increased incidence of renal cell carcinoma in patients with ADPKD. Sonography of parents and siblings of patients with ADPKD has proven helpful in identifying this abnormality in afflicted persons who are asymptomatic.

Sonographic Findings. On sonography the findings are similar to that of ARPKD. However, a lack of significant renal impairment, normal amniotic fluid volume (in utero), family history, or histological sampling allows differentiation. The well-defined cysts affect both kidneys. The cysts are of varying sizes and can be identified in the kidneys in the adult as the tubular and ductal cells become engorged.

Figure 23-12   **A,** Autosomal-recessive polycystic kidney disease (ARPKD) in a 1-day-old male with abdominal distention. Transverse image of the upper abdomen using the liver as an acoustic window shows that the kidneys are enlarged and echogenic with a hypoechoic peripheral rim *(arrows)*. *sp,* Spine. This appearance is typical for ARPKD. **B,** A 7-MHz linear image of the kidney *(arrowheads)* in the same patient reveals multiple small cysts *(arrows)*. The high frequency allows resolution of the cysts.

Figure 23-13   Renal vein thrombosis in a 5-day-old term newborn with hematuria. Coronal sonogram of the left flank demonstrates an enlarged kidney *(arrows)* with patchy areas of increased echogenicity.

RENAL VEIN THROMBOSIS

Renal vein thrombosis is most likely to occur in the dehydrated or septic infant and is more prevalent in infants of diabetic mothers. One or both kidneys may be involved. There is renal enlargement, hematuria, proteinuria, and a low platelet count.

Sonographic Findings. Thrombosis occurs initially in the small intrarenal venous branches, and at this stage the enlarged kidney has a nonspecific disordered heterogeneous internal echogenicity corresponding to the extent and severity of the process (Figure 23-13). If the thrombus reaches the renal vein or inferior vena cava, it may be directly visualized within these vascular structures. There may be coexistent adrenal hemorrhage, particularly on the left side where the adrenal vein drains directly into the renal vein. Calcification within the involved veins may eventually result. The use of color Doppler helps the

sonographer to identify whether the flow is present, reversed, or obstructed.

Renal/Adrenal Tumors

Congenital Mesoblastic Nephroma. The most common renal tumor of the neonate and young infant is **congenital mesoblastic nephroma** (also known as *fetal renal hamartoma* or *congenital Wilms' tumor*). This tumor is rare, occurring with a prevalence of 8:1,000,000 births. The mesoblastic nephroma consists of connective tissue elements that can completely replace renal tissue. This tumor is benign but is indistinguishable from a Wilms' tumor by any method of imaging. Because the tumor may invade adjacent structures, nephrectomy is indicated.

Sonographic Findings. Sonographically, as with Wilms' tumor, this lesion is solid, but may have a complex texture that includes hyperechoic, hypoechoic, or mixed echogenicity (Figure 23-14). The mass may extend through the renal capsule into the retroperitoneum. It is seen in children less than 1 year of age, whereas Wilms' tumor commonly occurs in children more than 1 year old.

Nephroblastomatosis. Nephroblastomatosis is an abnormal persistence of fetal renal blastema, which has the potential to develop into a Wilms' tumor. A rare cause of bilateral renal enlargement in the neonate is diffuse nephroblastomatosis. It can occur in up to one third of kidneys with a Wilms' tumor. An increased incidence of this abnormality is present in patients with Beckwith-Widemann and hemihypertrophy syndromes, and in patients with some major chromosomal abnormalities.

Sonographic Findings. In addition to renal enlargement, the involved areas may be hypoechoic, hyperechoic, or isoechoic compared with normal renal parenchyma. Although

Figure 23-14 **A,** Mesoblastic nephroma in an 11-week-old infant with a renal mass *(arrows)*. Coronal image of the right flank identifies that the mass is predominantly solid, with some cystic areas, and arises from the right kidney *(k)*. **B,** Transverse view shows the mass *(arrows)* posterior to the liver and anterior and lateral to the spine *(sp)*. Nephrectomy and pathologic evaluation confirmed the diagnosis of mesoblastic nephroma. **C,** Wilms' tumor in a 7-month-old with an abdominal mass. Sonogram reveals a large mass with multiple cystic areas occupying the renal fossa *(arrows)*. This represents an unusual presentation of a Wilms' tumor; more frequently a large solid component is present in these masses.

this abnormality may be evident sonographically, computed tomography or magnetic resonance imaging has been shown to be more accurate.

Nephroblastoma (Wilms' Tumor). Wilms' tumor is the most common intraabdominal malignant renal tumor in young children. The incidence of this tumor peaks between 2 and 5 years of age. This tumor is usually unilateral, although in a small percentage it may occur bilaterally. Wilms' tumor is bulky and expands within the renal parenchyma, resulting in distortion and displacement of the collecting system and capsule. Sonography is used for periodic renal monitoring in those at risk of developing **Wilms' tumor,** including patients with a previous Wilms' tumor or a family history of Wilms' tumor. Periodic sonographic monitoring is also performed in patients with either proven or potential nephroblastomatosis described previously. It is important to note that Wilms' tumor may occur spontaneously, and many pediatric laboratories will monitor both types of patients (those predisposed to the tumor and those with a history of Wilms' tumor) with ultrasound. In addition, ultrasound may be used to monitor the size of the tumor while the patient is treated with chemotherapy drugs to shrink the tumor. Therefore, the size of the tumor is docu-

mented and the appropriate time for surgery is chosen. Early surgical removal and treatment yield a favorable prognosis.

Sonographic Findings. The sonographic appearance of a Wilms' tumor is variable, extending from homogeneous to complex texture (Figure 23-15). The mass usually has areas of echogenicity and may have calcifications within. The liquefaction may represent necrosis and hemorrhage. The borders are sharply marginated and well defined, but bulky, with a hypoechoic to hyperechoic rim surrounding the mass (Figure 23-16). The adjacent renal tissue becomes compressed with the growth of the mass. The large solid mass generally is seen to completely distort the renal sinus, pyramids, cortex, and contour of the kidney. The mass may be so large as to protrude into the hepatic capsule. Resultant hydronephrosis may be present.

Sonography is valuable in detecting Wilms' tumor extension into the renal vein, inferior vena cava, right atrium, and contralateral kidney. The tumor spreads through direct extension into the renal sinus and peripelvic soft tissues, the lymph nodes in the renal hilum, and the paraaortic areas. Careful evaluation of the renal vein, inferior vena cava, and right atrium of the heart are important to document the possible extension of the tumor. Documentation of tumor extension can have a significant bearing on the surgical approach to the patient.

Figure 23-15 Gross pathology of a Wilms' tumor demonstrating the multinodular tumor replacing a large portion of the renal parenchyma. (From Damjanov I, Linder J: *Pathology: a color atlas,* St Louis, 2000, Mosby.)

When the tumor extends into the right atrium, cardiopulmonary bypass may be necessary to resect the tumor completely.

Neuroblastoma. Neuroblastoma, a malignant tumor that arises in the sympathetic chain ganglia and adrenal medulla, may be detected on antenatal sonography or at birth. This is the second most common abdominal tumor of childhood, occurring between the age of 2 months and 2 years. About half of these tumors arise in the medulla of the adrenal gland, although tumors have also been found in the neck, mediastinum, retroperitoneum, and pelvis. Clinical findings depend upon the location of the tumor. Tumors that arise within the adrenal gland show an abdominal mass, hypertension, diarrhea, and bone pain if metastasis is involved.

Sonographic Findings. Neuroblastoma is usually highly echogenic. Intrinsic calcification may be identified (Figure 23-17). The smaller tumors may appear homogeneous and hyperechoic, whereas the large tumors are more complex in

Figure 23-16 **A,** Transverse view of the right upper quadrant demonstrates a large mass in the area of the kidney displacing the liver anteriorly. **B,** The large mass representing a Wilms' tumor is heterogeneous and echogenic. **C,** Evaluation of the inferior vena cava shows extension of the tumor into the IVC.

Figure 23-17   A, Adrenal hemorrhage in a 2-week-old male with a history of neonatal infections, increased bilirubin, and an abdominal mass. Coronal sonogram demonstrates a cystic mass *(arrows)* superior to the kidney. A normal adrenal gland was not identified. The psoas muscle *(ps)* is located posteriorly. **B,** Adrenal hemorrhage in a jaundiced 3-week-old female. Coronal view of the right upper quadrant reveals an echogenic mass *(arrows)* superior to the kidney *(K)* and posterior to the liver *(L).*

appearance. A cystic form of neuroblastoma has also been described. The adjacent kidney is displaced inferiorly and at times laterally. Doppler evaluation may help to differentiate the tumor from an adrenal hemorrhage because there is increased vascularity within the neoplastic growth.

The disease spreads early and widely, so the majority of patients present with metastases. Careful sonographic evaluation of the liver should be made for evidence of metastatic disease. The mass also spreads around the aorta, celiac, and superior mesenteric arteries. This spread of tumor helps to distinguish a neuroblastoma from a Wilms' tumor because this tumor is well encapsulated, although it is somewhat homogeneous and heterogeneous. The neuroblastoma is poorly defined and heterogeneous with irregular hyperechoic areas caused by calcifications. Because intraspinal extension is reported to occur in as many as 15% of patients and because ultrasonography can successfully define the spinal canal in young infants, such examination should be considered in the initial assessment of the infant with suspected neuroblastoma.

ADRENAL HEMORRHAGE

Difficult delivery, large size, infants of diabetic mothers, stress and hypoxia at delivery, septicemia, and shock all predispose the neonate to the development of an adrenal hemorrhage. The newborn with **adrenal hemorrhage,** however, may have none of these associated factors, but still present with abdominal mass, jaundice, and anemia. Usually the hemorrhage is found secondary to other complications, such as uncontrolled bleeding, jaundice, intestinal obstruction, hypertension, adrenal abscess, or impaired renal function.

Sonographic Findings. Sonographically, adrenal hemorrhage results in ovoid enlargement of the gland or a portion of the gland. The appearance of the hemorrhagic gland can range from anechoic to hyperechoic or may be a mixture of

Figure 23-18 Adrenal neuroblastoma in a 1-week-old female with history of a left kidney mass on a fetal sonogram. Coronal image through the left flank reveals a large heterogeneous mass *(arrows)* displacing the left kidney inferiorly.

echogenicities, depending on the extent, age, and severity of the process (Figure 23-18). When enlargement is significant, a characteristic blunting of the superior pole of the underlying kidney is produced, along with inferior displacement of the kidney. The initial appearance of adrenal hemorrhage may render it indistinguishable from an adrenal neuroblastoma. Follow-up sonography can differentiate these two entities. Unlike a neoplasm, a hemorrhagic adrenal gland does not enlarge but rather decreases in size. Generally within 4 to 6 weeks, the lesion becomes appreciably smaller and subsequent calcification may be identified on the sonogram or radiographically.

SELECTED BIBLIOGRAPHY

Avni EF and others: Multicystic dysplastic kidney: natural history from in utero diagnosis and postnatal follow-up, *J Urol* 138:1420, 1987.

Blane CE and others: Single system ectopic ureters and ureteroceles associated with dysplastic kidney, *Pediatr Radiol* 22:217, 1992.

Fang SB and others: Prenatal sonographic detection of adrenal hemorrhage confirmed by postnatal surgery, *J Clin Ultrasound* 27:206-209, 1999.

Feinstein KA, Fernbach SK: Septated urinomas in the neonate, *Am J Roentgenol* 149:997, 1987.

Gordon AC and others: Multicystic dysplastic kidney: is nephrectomy still appropriate? *J Urol* 140:1231, 1988.

Gray DL, Crane JP: Practical pediatric nephrology: prenatal diagnosis of urinary tract malformation, *Pediatr Nephrol* 2:326, 1988.

Hayden CK Jr, Swischuk LE: *Pediatric ultrasonography,* ed 2, Baltimore, 1992, Williams & Wilkins.

Lee W, Comstock CH, Jurcak-Zaleski S: Prenatal diagnosis of adrenal hemorrhage by ultrasonography, *J Ultrasound Med* 11:369, 1992.

Luckens JN: Neuroblastoma in the neonate, *Semin Perinatol* 23:263-273, 1999.

Margraf LR and others: Diagnosis and discussion: autosomal recessive polycystic kidney disease, *Am J Dis Child* 147:77, 1993.

Nadler EP, Barksdale EM Jr: Adrenal masses in the newborn, *Semin Pediatr Surg* 9:156-164, 2000.

Orazi C and others: Renal vein thrombosis and adrenal hemorrhage in the newborn: ultrasound evaluation of 4 cases, *J Clin Ultrasound* 21:163, 1993.

Shkolnik A: Ultrasonography of the urogenital system. In Kelalis PP, King LR, Belman AB, editors: *Clinical pediatric urology,* vol I, ed 3, Philadelphia, 1992, WB Saunders.

Stark JE, Weinberger E: Ultrasonography of the neonatal genitourinary tract, *Appl Radiol* 22:50, 1993.

Strife JL and others: Multicystic dysplastic kidney in children: US follow-up, *Radiology* 186:785, 1993.

Teele RL, Share JC: Evaluating an abdominal mass. In Teele RL, Share JC, editors: *Ultrasonography of infants and children,* Philadelphia, 1991, WB Saunders.

CHAPTER 24

Pediatric Congenital Anomalies of the Female Pelvis

Sandra L. Hagen-Ansert

KEY TERMS

bicornuate uterus – duplication of the uterus and uterine horn or branches

hematometrocolpos – blood-filled vagina and uterus

hydrocolpos – fluid-filled vagina

hydrometrocolpos – fluid-filled vagina and uterus

isosexual – concerning or characteristic of the same sex

oocytes – the early or primitive ovum before it has developed completely

oogonium – a cell produced at an early stage in the formation of an ovum

paramesonephric ducts – (müllerian ducts) either of the paired ducts that form adjacent to the mesonephric ducts in the embryo

unicornuate uterus – anomaly of the uterus in which only one horn develops

uterus didelphys – complete duplication of the uterus, cervix, and vagina

The development of the female genital system and the role embryology plays in congenital abnormalities of the female reproductive tract are presented in this chapter. Sonography has become an important imaging modality for the evaluation of the pelvis in the neonatal, pediatric, and adolescent patient. Frequently, uterine anomalies are associated with abnormalities of the urinary tract. The distended urinary bladder is used as a landmark to image the uterus, ovaries, and adnexal structures in the pelvis.

EMBRYOLOGY OF THE FEMALE GENITAL TRACT

DEVELOPMENT OF THE GONADS

The first parts of the genital system to develop are the gonads. The gonads arise from the parts of the urogenital ridges, called gonadal ridges. This ridge enlarges and frees itself from the mesonephros by developing a mesentery that becomes the mesovarium. At the same time, the coelomic epithelium covering the gonadal ridges grows and forms cords of cells, called primary sex cords, that grow into the mesenchyme of the developing gonads. The primordial germ cells originate in the wall of the yolk sac and migrate into the embryo and enter the primary sex cords to give rise to the ova.

DEVELOPMENT OF THE OVARIES

In embryos with a double "X" chromosome (female), differentiation of the gonads occurs later than in males. The primary sex cords converge to form a network of canals called the *rete ovarii*, which soon disappear with the primary sex cords. At the same time, the surface epithelium of the developing ovary gives rise to secondary sex cords, or cortical cords (Figure 24-1). As these cords grow in the ovary, *primordial germ cells* are incorporated into them. At about 16 weeks of gestation, the cortical cords break up into isolated cell clusters called primordial follicles, each of which contains an **oogonium** derived from the primordial germ cell. Each oogonium is surrounded by a layer of flattened follicular cells derived from the surface epithelial cells in the cortical cord. The oogoniums multiply rapidly by mitosis, producing thousands of these primitive germ cells. Before birth, all oogoniums enlarge to form primary

oocytes and most of them have entered the first meiotic prophase, but this process remains in an arrested state until puberty.

DEVELOPMENT OF THE GENITAL DUCTS

All embryos have identical pairs of genital ducts in the beginning. The female or **paramesonephric ducts** (see Figure 24-1) develop into the female reproductive system. During the indifferent state of sexual development, both pairs of genital ducts are present. Even though the genetic sex of an embryo is determined at fertilization by the kind of sperm that fertilizes the ovum, there are no morphologic indications of maleness or femaleness until the 9th gestational week.

DEVELOPMENT OF THE FEMALE GENITAL DUCTS

The paramesonephric ducts form most of the female genital tract. Their cranial parts form the uterine tubes and their caudal parts fuse to form the *uterovaginal primordium* or canal, which develops into the uterus and part of the vagina. Contact of the uterovaginal primordium with the urogenital sinus induces paired endodermal outgrowths, called *sinovaginal bulbs*, to form. These bulbs fuse to form a solid vaginal plate. The central cells of this plate break down to form the *vagina*; the peripheral cells form the *vaginal epithelium*.

DEVELOPMENT OF THE EXTERNAL GENITALIA

Early in development, both sexes appear similar until the 9th week of gestation. External organs are fully developed by the 12th week. Both the urethra and vagina open into the *urogenital sinus*, which becomes the vestibule of the vagina. The

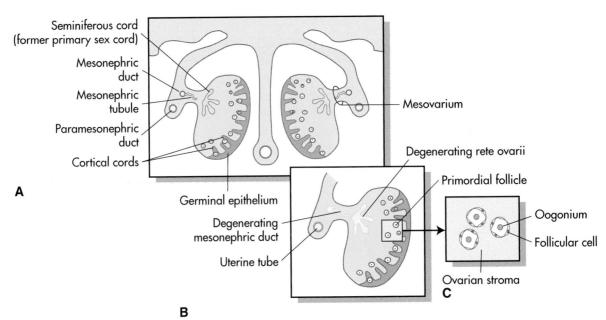

Figure 24-1 **A,** Fetus at 12 weeks of gestation shows the ovary beginning to develop. **B,** Ovary at 20 weeks, showing the primordial follicles formed from the cortical cords. **C,** Section from the ovarian cortex of a 20-week fetus showing three primordial follicles.

urogenital folds become the *labia minora*, the labioscrotal swellings become the *labia majora*, and the *phallus* becomes the *clitoris* (Figure 24-2).

PEDIATRIC GYNECOLOGIC SONOGRAPHY

The sonographic evaluation of the neonatal and pediatric pelvic cavity requires a distended urinary bladder because only the transabdominal ultrasound technique is used. It may be necessary to catheterize and fill the bladder with sterile water if there is difficulty in obtaining a distended urinary bladder. The use of sterile water as a contrast agent may be used to outline the vagina (hydrosonovaginography) in a pediatric patient with a pelvic mass or complex congenital abnormality of the genitourinary tract. The endovaginal approach is reserved for the mature, sexually active, teenage girl when specific definition of the pelvic anatomy is required.

BLADDER

The normal urinary bladder should have a smooth, thin wall. When the bladder is distended (the top of the bladder exceeds the fundus of the uterus), the bladder wall thickness should measure less than 3 mm, with a mean of 1.5 mm. When the bladder is empty or partially full, the wall will appear thicker, but should not measure greater than 5 mm. The distal ureters are not routinely visualized unless they are dilated. Color Doppler allows adequate visualization of the ureters as they empty into the bladder. To image the ureteral jets, angle the probe caudally towards the base of the bladder, turn the color Doppler on with the gain slightly high, but not so high as to see extraneous color "ghost" echoes in the background. Hold the probe still for a several seconds and the jet flow should be noted, first on one side, then on the other.

The bladder neck and urethra may be demonstrated in either sex by angling the transducer inferiorly. The perineum or transrectal approach may also prove useful to image a urethral abnormality. Hydrosonourethrography is used with anterior urethral abnormalities, such as strictures, calculi, urethral valves, diverticula, and trauma.

The postvoid scan may be useful to provide information about the bladder emptying capability; sometimes it is necessary to demonstrate a change in bladder size to separate it from a pelvic cyst.

UTERUS

In the newborn female, the uterus is prominent and thickened with a brightly echogenic endometrial lining caused by the hormonal stimulation received in utero. The uterus is pear-shaped in configuration with the length, approximately 3.5 cm with a fundus-to-cervix ratio of 1:2 (fundus is smaller than the cervix).

The maternal hormones stimulate the initial size of the uterine cavity after birth; as these hormones decrease, so does the uterine size. The uterus assumes a teardrop shape, with the cervix consuming more area than the uterus (Figure 24-3). At 2 to 3 months of age, the uterus regresses to a prepubertal size and tubular configuration with the length measuring 2.5 to 3 cm, the fundus-to-cervix ratio 1:1, and the endometrial stripe echoes not visualized. There may be some endometrial fluid present.

The uterus increases in size after the age of 7 years, with the greatest increase in size occurring after the onset of puberty, when the fundus becomes much larger than the cervix (Table 24-1). It is not until puberty that the uterine shape and size dramatically change. The uterine length increases to 5 to 7 cm, and the fundus-to-cervix ratio becomes 3:1 (fundus is now greater than the cervix). The echogenicity and thickness of the endometrial lining vary according to the phase of the menstrual cycle.

The uterus is supplied by the bilateral uterine arteries, which are branches of the internal iliac arteries. Color flow Doppler may demonstrate flow in the myometrial tissue with little or no flow in the endometrium.

Figure 24-2   Development of the female external genitalia at 11 weeks.

Glans clitoris
Labium minus
Labium majus
Posterior labial commissure

Figure 24-3   Neonatal uterus well seen within the pelvic cavity with ascitic fluid surrounding the teardrop-shaped uterine wall. The cervix consumes the majority of the total uterine length at this stage.

TABLE 24-1	UTERINE MEASUREMENTS	
Age	Uterine Length	Fundus-Cervix Ratio
Newborn	3.5 cm	1:2
Prepubertal (>2 months)	2.5-3 cm	1:1
Postpubertal	5-7 cm	3:1

Data from Comstock CH, Boal DK: Pelvic sonography of the pediatric patient, *Semin Ultrasound* 5:54-67, 1984.

TABLE 24-2	OVARIAN VOLUME MEASUREMENTS	
Premenarchal Age	Mean Ovarian Volume cm³ Menstrual	
0-5 yr	<1 cm³	
6-8 yr	1.2 cm³	
9-10 yr	2.1 cm³	
11 yr	2.5 cm³ (±1.3)	
12 yr	3.8 cm³ (±1.4)	
13 yr	4.2 cm³ (±2.3)	
Menstrual	9.8 cm³ (±5.8)	

Data slightly modified from Cohen HL, Shapiro MA, Mandel FS, and others: Normal ovaries in neonates and infants: a sonographic study of 77 patients 1 day to 24 months old, *AJR* 160:583-586, 1993.

VAGINA

The physical examination of the uterus and vagina is difficult in the young patient and often is only performed under general anesthesia when an anomaly is suspected. The vagina is best imaged on the midline longitudinal image when the bladder is very distended. The vagina appears as a tubular structure posterior to the bladder and is in continuity with the uterine cervix. The mucosal walls cause a bright central echo within the tubular structure.

OVARY

Depending upon the location, size, and age of the patient, evaluation of the ovary in the young patient may be a challenge. In the neonatal patient, the ovary may be found anywhere between the lower pole of the kidneys and the true pelvis. The evaluation of ovarian size is most accurate when the volume is determined by using the prolate-ellipse formula:

$$\text{Volume in cubic centimeters} = \text{Length} \times \text{Height} \times \text{Width} \times 0.523$$

The mean ovarian volume is stable up to 5 years of age and ranges from 0.75 to 0.86 cm³ (Table 24-2). Ovarian volume gradually increases until puberty is reached. Usually the ovarian texture is homogeneous; however, small follicles may be seen with ultrasound.

The appearance of the ovary in the neonatal period is heterogeneous secondary to tiny cysts. The larger cysts in the ovary are more commonly seen in female patients after their

first year of life. The blood supply to the ovary is from the ovarian artery (originates directly from the aorta) and from the uterine artery, which supplies an adnexal branch to each ovary.

PATHOLOGY OF THE PEDIATRIC GENITAL SYSTEM

CONGENITAL ANOMALIES OF THE UTERUS AND VAGINA

The definitive diagnosis and classification of a congenital anomaly of the uterine cavity requires the visualization of the uterine cavity or cavities and the serosal margin(s). Before ultrasound, hysterosalpingography with laparoscopy was used to define the uterine cavity in the teenage and adult patient. With transabdominal and endovaginal ultrasound, the uterine cavities can now be defined. A newer technique in the older patient, sonohysterosalpingography, requires the injection of a small amount of contrast material into the cavity through a catheter threaded into the vagina and cervix to differentiate the uterine cavity and septa.

The uterus provides the endometrial canal for the site of implantation and growth for the intrauterine pregnancy. Developmental problems, interference with blood supply, or distortion of the uterine cavity may result in infertility or spontaneous abortion. Congenital uterine abnormalities occur in approximately 0.5% of females and are associated with an increased incidence of abortion and other obstetric complications later in life.

Congenital anomalies of the uterus and vagina in children are not very common and usually present as an abdominal or pelvic mass secondary to obstruction. There is a very high association of renal anomalies that are found when abnormalities of the uterine cavity are discovered.

The uterus and upper third of the vagina are derived from the embryonic müllerian (paramesonephric) ducts. These ducts must elongate, fuse, and form lumens between the 7th and 12th weeks of embryonic development. When this sequence fails to occur, one of the following three types of müllerian abnormality results: improper fusion, incomplete development of one side, or incomplete vaginal canalization.

Sonographic Findings. If müllerian anomalies are encountered, the kidneys should be examined for ipsilateral renal agenesis or morphologic abnormalities (Figure 24-4) because these conditions are commonly associated with müllerian anomalies. Uterine malformations may be suspected on the basis of abnormal configuration of the uterus on pelvic sonograms.

MÜLLERIAN ANOMALIES

The congenital abnormalities have been classified into six groups based on their prognosis for future fertility and their surgical correction (Figure 24-5).

Class I. Segmental müllerian agenesis or incomplete vaginal canalization is suspected when a young girl reaches puberty without menstruation. This condition produces a transverse vaginal septum or vaginal atresia. **Vaginal atresia** is diagnosed by the development of **hydrocolpos** (fluid-filled vagina), **hydrometrocolpos** (fluid-filled vagina and uterus), or **hematometrocolpos** (blood-filled vagina and uterus) (Figure 24-6). On sonographic examination, the cervix may be absent with or without blood in the uterine and/or cervical cavities. This condition either presents in the neonatal period as a large cystic pelvic-abdominal mass because of stimulation from maternal hormones or is discovered at puberty. These findings also result from an imperforate hymen.

Class II. Unicornuate uterus is related to infertility and pregnancy loss. Sonography demonstrates a uterus that is long and slender (cigar-shaped) and deviated to one side. Usually, renal agenesis is apparent on the contralateral side. This is difficult to differentiate from the normal uterus by sonography,

Figure 24-4 A pelvic kidney is seen adjacent to the bicornuate uterus on this sagittal transabdominal scan.

but is suspected when the uterus appears small and laterally positioned.

Classes III through V. Classes III through V are more difficult to diagnose because they all have two uterine cavities, and their correct classification and treatment depend on the appearance of the external contour of the uterine fundus. In the nonpregnant state, a congenital malformation is often difficult to demonstrate and may mimic a fibroid.

Class III. Uterus didelphys is a complete duplication of the uterus, cervix, and vagina. This condition is not usually associated with fertility problems and does not generally require treatment. Sonography detects two endometrial echo complexes, which are best demonstrated during the secretory phase of the menstrual cycle when the endometrium is most prominent. Then the external contour of the uterus is helpful in distinguishing between the septate and the bicornuate uterus.

Class IV. Bicornuate uterus is a duplication of the uterus with a common cervix (Figure 24-7). This bilobed uterine cavity has wide-spaced cavities and a low incidence of fertility complications and is usually not treated. The exception is when one of the horns is rudimentary and noncommunicating. If an embryo implants in this rudimentary cavity, it may grow until about 12 to 16 weeks, when rupture of the uterine cavity occurs. In many cases the bicornuate uterus is diagnosed incidentally in early pregnancy, when a gestational sac is present in one horn and decidual reaction in the other. The bicornuate uterus is best identified on the transverse sonogram through the superior portion of the two horns of the uterus. The image looks heart-shaped on the transverse plane.

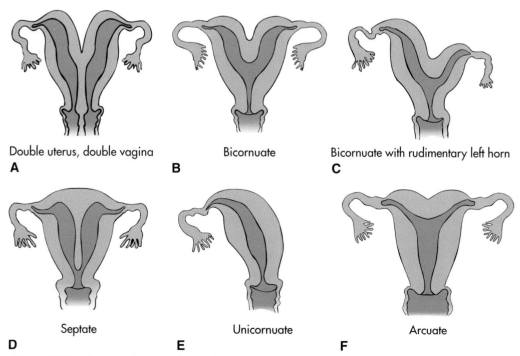

Double uterus, double vagina
A

Bicornuate
B

Bicornuate with rudimentary left horn
C

Septate
D

Unicornuate
E

Arcuate
F

Figure 24-5 Congenital uterine abnormalities. **A,** Uterus didelphys: double uterus and vagina. **B,** Bicornuate uterus. **C,** Bicornuate uterus with a rudimentary left horn. **D,** Septate uterus. **E,** Unicornuate uterus. **F,** Arcuate uterus.

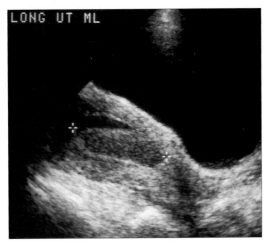

Figure 24-6 Transabdominal image along the midline of the pelvic cavity shows the distended urinary bladder anterior to the uterine cavity. A complex area within the endometrial canal represents both blood and fluid in the uterus and vagina (hematometrocolpos).

Figure 24-7 Transabdominal image of the bicornuate uterus showing two endometrial canals within the bilobed uterine horns.

Class V. Class V involves a septate uterus in which two uterine cavities are seen closely spaced, with one fundus and sometimes two cervical canals or a vaginal septum. This condition has the highest incidence of fertility problems, and the septum may be hysteroscopically removed.

Class VI. Class VI is related to the exposure to the drug diethylstilbestrol (DES) in utero. DES is a synthetic preparation drug that possesses estrogenic properties. The drug is several times more potent than natural estrogens. This drug was once used extensively in the 1970s during pregnancy to treat threatened and habitual abortion. An estimated 5 to 10 million Americans received the drug during pregnancy. The drug was later found to cause vaginal malignancies in the daughters of mothers who were given the drug. The uterus is normal in size and shape externally; however, the cavity is T-shaped with an irregular contour. This condition may be difficult to diagnose with ultrasound.

AMBIGUOUS GENITALIA

The embryo has the potential to develop as a male or female. Errors in sexual development result in ambiguous genitalia or hermaphroditism. True hermaphrodites have both ovarian and testicular tissue. The internal and external genitalia are variable, although most true hermaphrodites have a 46,XX karyotype, but some are mosaics (46,XX/46,XY).

Female pseudohermaphrodites have a 46,XX karyotype. The most common cause is congenital virilizing adrenal hyperplasia. An increased production of androgens leads to masculinization of the external genitalia (enlarged clitoris, abnormalities of the urogenital sinus, and partial fusion of the labia majora).

The external genitalia may also be masculinized by androgenic hormones, which reach it via the placenta from the maternal circulation. These hormones may be present in excessive amounts if the mother's suprarenal cortices are overactive or if she has received hormone therapy involving androgenic substances.

Sonographic Findings. Ultrasonography may be helpful in identifying the presence or absence of the uterus, vagina, and ovaries in utero or in neonates with ambiguous genitalia. However, the in utero cases can be difficult if a clear image cannot be made of the genital area. Sex assignment is based on results of karyotype analysis, gonadal biopsy, and knowledge of genital anatomy.

PRECOCIOUS PUBERTY

Precocious pubertal development may be classified as true precocious puberty or precocious pseudopuberty. True precocious puberty is always **isosexual** (same sex) and involves the development of secondary sexual characteristics and an increase in the size and activity of the gonads. The uterus has an enlarged, postpubertal configuration (fundus to cervix ratio is 2:1 and 3:1), with an echogenic endometrial canal. The ovarian volume is enlarged (greater than 1 cubic cm), and functional cysts are often present.

Precocious pseudopuberty involves the maturation of secondary sexual characteristics, but not the gonad, as there is no activation of the hypothalamic-pituitary-gonadal axis. Excessive exogenous synthesis of gonadal steroids (by the adrenal gland, tumors, or cysts) is the most common cause of precocious pseudopuberty; prolonged exposure to exogenous gonadal hormones may mature the central nervous system and cause true precocious puberty in some children. Sonography is useful to detect the presence of a pelvic mass and a mature uterus.

Sonographic Findings. Ultrasound is used to determine the volume and size of the ovaries, uterus, and cervix, and to exclude an ovarian neoplasm. The liver and the adrenal gland should also be assessed in these patients to rule out the presence of a lesion causing the precocious puberty.

PATHOLOGY OF THE PEDIATRIC OVARY

The development of the ovary begins in the fetal gestational period and continues during childhood. The growth process is dynamic. The neonatal ovaries are similar in function and anatomy to the pubertal and adult ovaries. Only the more common pathologies of the pelvis will be presented, including the ovarian cyst, ovarian torsion, and ovarian teratoma development (Table 24-3).

The typical neonatal and infant ovary is heterogeneous and cystic on ultrasound. Most cysts are less than 9 mm in diameter with the mean diameter of the largest cyst measuring 7.5 mm. Ovarian cysts develop from ovarian follicles. The difference between a pathologic cyst and a physiologic mature follicle is primarily size, with cysts larger than 2 cm considered to be pathologic.

Factors that contribute to the follicular growth in utero include follicle-stimulating hormone (FSH), maternal estrogens, and human chorionic gonadotropin (hCG). The primary stimulus is FSH. This hormone is secreted by the pituitary gland and causes the increase in both the number and size of the small follicles. During the third trimester, the other hormones contribute to further follicular growth. At birth the maternal estrogens and hCG levels fall with the separation of the placenta from the neonate. FSH levels decline secondary to the inhibitory mechanism of the hypothalamus pituitary ovary axis.

Neonatal Ovarian Cysts. The origin of the neonatal cyst may be the result of disordered folliculogenesis occurring in the fetal ovary. Most fetal cysts resolve spontaneously, but they may persist into the neonatal period. Small follicular cysts of 3 to 7 mm are a common and normal finding in neonatal ovaries. Pathologic evaluation of the cysts reveals follicular, corpus luteum, and theca lutein cysts. Their development may be the result of excessive stimulation of the fetal ovary by both placental and maternal hormones. There is a higher incidence of larger ovarian cysts in infants of mothers with toxemia, diabetes, and Rh isoimmunization, all of which are associated with a greater than normal release of placental chorionic gonadotropin.

Follicular cysts have been described in maternal and congenital hypothyroidism. Nonspecific pituitary glycoprotein hormone synthesis has been cited as the explanation for the follicular cysts seen in patients with juvenile hypothyroidism.

Complications. Most ovarian cysts regress spontaneously; however, if they persist complications may arise. The most common primary complications are hemorrhage and salpingotorsion. Torsion is more common in the larger cysts; clinically, patients present with pain, vomiting, fever, abdominal distention, leukocytosis, and peritonitis.

Hemorrhage may result from torsion or may occur spontaneously in a nontwisted cyst. If rupture occurs, hemorrhagic ascites and/or peritonitis may be seen.

If the cyst is large, complications such as bowel obstruction, thorax compression with pulmonary hypoplasia, urinary tract obstruction, or incarceration with an inguinal hernia may occur.

Sonographic Findings. As discussed previously, the size of the ovarian cyst varies greatly with the larger cysts occupying nearly the entire abdomen, thus compressing the normal organs (Figure 24-8). The cyst may appear to be completely anechoic with well-defined borders or may have internal echoes if hemorrhage has occurred. The complicated cyst may contain fluid-debris level, a retracting clot, or septa, or may be completely filled with echoes producing a solid masslike appearance.

Differential Considerations. Ultrasound is able to characterize the mass, but not histologically confirm the diagnosis without a biopsy specimen. It may be difficult to separate an ovarian cyst from a mesenteric or enteric duplication cyst if the cyst is large and the normal ovary becomes displaced or distorted. Other abnormalities that should be considered include hydrometrocolpos, cystic meconium peritonitis, urachal cysts, and anterior meningocele. Neoplastic lesions, such as cystadenoma, cystic teratomas, and granulosa cell tumors, are very rare in the neonate.

OVARIAN TORSION

Torsion of the ovary may occur at any age, from the neonate to the adult; however, most torsion problems occur within the

TABLE 24-3	COMMON NEONATAL PATHOLOGIC CONDITIONS		
	Clinical Findings	Sonographic Findings	Differential Diagnosis
Ovarian cyst	Asymptomatic palpable mass; complications include hemorrhage or torsion	Anechoic well-defined borders Internal echoes with hemorrhage	Mesenteric or duplication cyst Hydrometrocolpos Cystic meconium peritonitis Urachal cysts Anterior meningocele
Ovarian torsion	Severe abdominal pain	Enlarged ovary Fluid in cul-de-sac Fluid/debris secondary to hemorrhage	Appendicitis Gastroenteritis Pyelonephritis Pelvic inflammatory disease
Ovarian teratomas	Asymptomatic; increased size of tumor may cause abdominal pain or distention	Central complex/cystic cavity with debris Dermal plug Fat-fluid levels Calcifications	Appendicitis

Figure 24-8   Sagittal image of the neonatal abdomen shows a large, well-defined anechoic structure anterior to the right kidney and inferior to the liver. This proved to be an ovarian cyst.

Figure 24-9   Sagittal image of an adolescent girl who presented with a severe onset of lower abdominal pain. The enlarged left ovary was shown just posterior to the distended urinary bladder. Color Doppler showed decreased flow around the ovary.

first two decades of life. The normal adnexa in young girls may be very mobile, allowing torsion at the mesosalpinx with changes in intraabdominal pressure or body position. The ovary is extrapelvic in the neonate and infant, whereas in the older child the mass may be in the adnexal area. Torsion occurs more commonly when ovarian cysts or tumors are present. Torsion of the ovary and fallopian tube results from partial or complete rotation of the ovary on its vascular pedicle. This results in compromise of arterial and venous flow, congestion of the ovarian parenchyma, and ultimately, hemorrhagic infarction.

Clinical symptoms include severe onset of abdominal pain. In the infant this symptom may go unrecognized, which in turn may lead to necrosis of the ovary if surgical intervention is not performed quickly. Other causes of lower abdominal pain include appendicitis, gastroenteritis, pyelonephritis, or pelvic inflammatory disease.

Sonographic findings may be nonspecific, but may show enlargement of the affected ovary (Figure 24-9), fluid in the cul-de-sac, and other adnexal pathologic findings, such as cyst or tumor. A predominantly cystic or complex adnexal mass with a fluid-debris level or septa correlates with pathologic evidence of ovarian hemorrhage or infarction. The demonstration of multiple prominent follicles (greater than 8 to 12 mm) in the cortical (peripheral) portion of a unilaterally enlarged ovary has been reported as a specific sonographic sign of torsion. Color Doppler was not specific as the arterial blood flow was variable, depending on the extent of the torsion (complete or incomplete). Fluid in the cul-de-sac was found in the late manifestation of ovarian torsion.

If the ovary shows torsion and subsequent amputation, the ovary is seen to detach from the adnexa and migrate to the other sites in the abdomen. This mass is pedunculated with mesentery and omentum within the pedicle. Eventually these masses calcify and may be seen on a radiograph later in life.

OVARIAN TERATOMAS

Ovarian tumors are uncommon in the neonate and adolescent. When found, germ cell tumors account for 60% of ovarian neoplasms in patients under 20 years of age. The spectrum of

Figure 24-10   Gross pathology of a dermoid tumor filled with sebaceous debris representing teeth and fat.

germ cell tumors range from benign mature teratomas through the malignant varieties, which include the dysgerminomas, embryonal carcinomas, endodermal sinus tumors, immature teratomas, choriocarcinomas, and mixed tumors. The most common pediatric germ cell tumor is the benign mature teratoma or dermoid cyst.

Benign teratomas have a wide spectrum of sonographic characteristics. They can have a central cystic cavity filled with sebaceous debris that is surrounded by a variety of skin appendages, a squamous epithelial layer, and a thick capsule (Figure 24-10). A nubbin of tissue, called the dermal plug or mural nodule, is frequently found in the wall of a teratoma. Other findings may include a solid or complex mass with fat-fluid levels, hair-fluid levels, and calcification. Most dermoid tumors range between 5 and 15 cm in size.

Clinically, most patients with a dermoid tumor are asymptomatic. When the tumor becomes large, abdominal pain or distention may occur. The most frequent complication of a teratoma is torsion, which may occur in 16% to 40% of cases. The pain may mimic appendicitis if located on the right side of the abdomen.

Sonographic Findings. Sonography recognizes the dermoid tumor as a complex mass with a heterogeneous appearance (Figure 24-11). Mural nodules and echogenic foci

Figure 24-11   Endovaginal image of the dermoid tumor seen in a teenage girl. The tumor is filled with bright echogenic material representing the fat, bone, and teeth.

with acoustic shadowing are typical findings on ultrasound. In the neonatal period, there is less shadowing seen in the lesion than in adolescent girls.

SELECTED BIBLIOGRAPHY

Balen A, Dunger D: Pubertal maturation of the internal genitalia, *Ultrasound Obstet Gynecol* 6(3):164-165, 1995.

Blask ARN, Sanders RC, Gearhart JP: Obstructed uterovaginal anomalies: demonstration with sonography, I, Neonates and infants, *Radiology* 179:79, 1991.

Brown RT, Hewitt GD: Chronic pelvic pain and recurrent abdominal pain in female adolescents, *Endocr Dev* 7:213-224, 2004.

Estroff JA: Emergency obstetric and gynecologic ultrasound, *Radiol Clin North Am* 35(4):921-957, 1997.

Gare L, Dubois J, Grignon A and others: US of the pediatric female pelvis: a clinical perspective, *Radiographics* 21(6):1393-1407, 2001.

Hamel-Teillac D: Vulvo-vaginal disorders, *Endocr Dev* 7:39-56, 2004.

Holland-Hall CM, Brown RT: Evaluation of the adolescent with chronic abdominal or pelvic pain, *J Pediatr Adolesc Gynceol* 17(1):23-27, 2004.

Mendelson B and others: Endometrial abnormalities: evaluation with transvaginal sonography, *Am J Roentgenol* 150:139, 1988.

Moore KL: *The developing human,* Philadelphia, 1982, WB Saunders.

Pennes DR, Bowerman RA, Silver TM: Congenital uterine anomalies and associated pregnancies: findings and pitfalls of sonographic diagnosis, *J Ultrasound Med* 4:531, 1985.

Pokorny S: Pediatric & adolescent gynecology, *Compr Ther* 23(5):337-344, 1997.

Porcu E: Imaging in pediatric and adolescent gynecology, *Endocr Dev* 7:9-22, 2004.

Reuter KL, Daly DC, Cohen SM: Septate versus bicornuate uteri: errors in imaging diagnosis, *Radiology* 172:749, 1989.

Schmahmann S and Haller JO: Sonography of the neonatal ovary. In *textbook of neonatal ultrasound,* New York, 1998, Parthenon Publishing Group.

Siegel MJ, Surratt JT: *Obstet Gynecol Clin North Am* 19(1):103-127, 1992.

Sultan C: Pediatric and adolescent gynecology. Evidence-based clinical practice, *Endocr Dev* 7:1:IX-X, 2004.

Thibaud E: Gynecologic clinical examination of the child and adolescent, *Endocr Dev* 7:1-8, 2004.

Thurmond AS: *Imaging of infertility and müllerian abnormalities: women's imaging symposium,* San Diego, 1991, University of California at San Diego.

Weir J, Murray AD: *Mosby's atlas and text of clinical imaging,* St Louis, 1998, Mosby.

CHAPTER 25

The Neonatal Hip

Sandra L. Hagen-Ansert

OBJECTIVES

- List the anatomy of the upper leg
- Describe the three categories of muscle of the upper thigh
- Describe the anatomy of the hip joint
- List the bones of the hip joint
- Compare adduction to abduction of the hip
- Describe the sonographic anatomy of the hip
- Explain the sonographic protocol to image the neonatal hip
- Describe the Barlow maneuver
- Differentiate between subluxation of the hip and dislocation of the hip
- Define Ortolani maneuver

KEY TERMS

abduction – to move away from the body

adduction – to move toward the body

Barlow maneuver – the patient lies in the supine position with the hip flexed 90 degrees and adducted. Downward and outward pressure is applied. If the hip is dislocated, the examiner will feel the femoral head move out of the acetabulum.

developmental displacement of the hip (DDH) – abnormal condition of the hip that results in congenital hip dysplasia; includes dysplastic, subluxated, dislocatable, and dislocated hips

fascia lata – deep fascia of the thigh

femoral triangle – description of a region at the front of the upper thigh, just below the inguinal ligament

frank dislocation – the hip is laterally and posteriorly displaced to the extent that the femoral head has no contact with the acetabulum and the normal "U" configuration cannot be obtained on ultrasound

Galeazzi sign – the knee is lower in position on the affected side when the patient is supine and the knees are flexed. On physical examination, the knee is lower in position on the affected side of the neonate with DDH when the patient is supine and the knees are flexed.

hip joint – formed by the articulation of the head of the femur with the acetabulum of the hip bone

Ortolani maneuver – patient lies in the supine position. The examiner's hand is placed around the hip to be examined with the fingers over the femoral head. The hip is flexed 90 degrees and the thigh is abducted.

pelvic girdle – formation of the hip bones by the ilium, ischium, and pubis

saphenous opening – gap in the fascia lata, which is found 4 cm inferior and lateral to the pubic tubercle

sciatic nerve – largest nerve in the upper thigh

subluxed – occurs when the femoral head moves posteriorly and remains in contact with the posterior aspect of the acetabulum

Ultrasound evaluation of the neonatal hip is continuing to gain clinical acceptance as a diagnostic tool. There are specifically two conditions in which sonography offers advantages over other imaging modalities (i.e., developmental dislocation and/or dysplasia of the hip and hip pain).

Indications for sonography of the neonatal hip:

• Rule out developmental displacement of the hip
• Septic arthritis and/or joint effusion
• Proximal focal femoral deficiency

ANATOMY OF THE HIP

The anatomy of the upper leg consists of many parts, including bones and joints, nerves, arteries, superficial veins, and muscles (Figure 25-1). The thigh is the upper part of the lower extremity. The anterior surface of the thigh is continuous with the inguinal region of the abdomen. The posterior surface of the thigh is inferior to the gluteal region, which is at the back of the pelvis and **hip joint**.

BONES AND JOINTS

The sacroiliac joints unite the two hip bones with the sacral part of the vertebral column. The pubic symphysis is where the two hip bones unite with each other anteriorly.

The hip bones are the fusion of three separate bones: ilium, ischium, and pubis; all together these form the **pelvic girdle**. The bone of the upper thigh is the femur. The femur is surrounded by muscles, ligaments, and tendons. The upper part of the femur, the head, articulates with the hip bone to make the hip joint.

FEMORAL ARTERY

The femoral artery is the principal artery of the upper thigh. This artery is a continuation of the external iliac artery and enters the thigh beneath the inguinal ligament. The femoral artery branches into the profunda femoris artery, which is the main artery supply for the thigh muscles.

SCIATIC NERVE

The sciatic nerve is the largest nerve in the upper thigh. This nerve enters the gluteal region from the pelvis to run caudally down the back of the thigh.

FASCIA LATA

The deep fascia of the thigh, the **fascia lata**, forms a tough connective tissue surrounding the muscles. The part of the fascia on the lateral part of the thigh is the *iliotibial* tract as it extends from the iliac crest to the lateral condyle of the tibia. The **saphenous opening** is a gap in the fascia lata that is found about 4 cm inferior and lateral to the pubic tubercle. The great saphenous vein passes through the saphenous opening to enter the femoral vein.

MUSCLES

The muscles of the thigh fall into three categories: anterior or extensor, medial or adductor, and posterior or hamstring (Table 25-1).

Figure 25-1 Coronal section, looking from the front toward the back. (From McMinn: *Functional and clinical anatomy,* St Louis, 1999, Mosby.)

1. External iliac artery	8. Vastus lateralis
2. Psoas major	9. Shaft of femur
3. Iliacus	10. Vastus medialis
4. Iliac crest	11. Neck of femur
5. Gluteus medius	12. Head of femur
6. Gluteus minimus	13. Acetabular labrum
7. Greater trochanter	14. Rim of acetabulum

FEMORAL TRIANGLE

The **femoral triangle** describes a region at the front of the upper thigh, just below the inguinal ligament. One side of the triangle is formed by the inguinal ligament, whereas the other two sides are formed by adductor longus (medially) and sartorius (laterally) (see Figure 25-1). The contents of the femoral triangle include the *femoral canal, femoral vein* and *artery,* and

TABLE 25-1	MUSCLES	
Muscle Group	Supplied By	Muscles
Anterior compartment/ extensor muscles (front of thigh)	Femoral nerve	**Quadriceps femoris** (rectus femoris plus three vastus muscles)—insert into patella, which is attached to patellar ligament • The vastus muscles arise from the femur • The rectus femoris arises from the hip bone above the acetabulum—acts as a flexor of the hip and extensor of the knee **Sartorius** muscle with longest fibers in the body, crosses the front of the thigh obliquely from the anterior superior iliac spine laterally to the upper medial side of the tibia
Medial compartment/ adductor muscles (inner thigh)	Obturator nerve	**Adductor longus** muscle **Adductor magnus** muscle
Posterior compartment/ hamstring muscles	Sciatic nerve	**Biceps femoris**—outer hamstring **Vastus lateralis**—part of quadriceps

femoral nerve. The femoral vein and artery and the femoral canal are enclosed in a connective tissue sleeve called the femoral sheath.

The contents of the femoral triangle are separated from the more deeply lying hip joint by muscles; the *pectineus* is medial and the *iliacus* is lateral. In the middle is the psoas major muscle (found at the middle of the head of the femur). The *psoas major* becomes tendinous and separates the femoral artery from the capsule of the joint at this point.

GLUTEAL REGION

The gluteal region (buttock) extends from the iliac crest to the gluteal fold and from the midline over the sacrum to the greater trochanter of the femur (Figure 25-2). It includes the area at the back of the hip joint. The large *gluteus maximus* muscle overlies other muscles superior and posterior to the hip joint. The gluteus maximus is a powerful extensor of the hip.

The *gluteus medius* and *gluteus minimus* pass from the outer surface of the hip bone to the greater trochanter. Together they act as abductors of the hip joint. Their most important function is to prevent adduction and keep the pelvis level during walking.

The tensor fasciae latae is a smaller muscle arising from the outer, front part of the iliac crest. The tensor fasciae latae is inserted into the iliotibial tract of the fascia lata. With this attachment, it assists the gluteus maximus in extension of the knee.

Below the lower borders of the gluteus medium and minimus the following muscles are found: piriformis, obturator externus with the gemelli at its upper and lower borders, and quadratus femoris (see Figure 25-2). The **sciatic nerve** and most other structures that leave the pelvis to enter the gluteal region do so by passing under the border of the piriformis. These muscles together act as a lateral rotator of the femur.

HIP JOINT

The articulation of the head of the femur with the acetabulum of the hip bone forms the **hip joint** (Figure 25-3). The joint is not directly palpable because it is surrounded and protected by muscles of the upper thigh. The greater trochanter of the femur forms a palpable knob at the side of the region. The psoas tendon crosses the center of the hip joint just inferior to the inguinal ligament at the top of the femoral triangle. The *pectineus muscle* is medial to the tendon. The femoral vein and canal are anterior to the pectineus muscle. Lateral to the tendon is the *iliacus* muscle, with the femoral nerve anterior. The gluteus minimus muscle is the immediate cover for the upper part of the hip joint, whereas the obturator externus is found winding below it from front to back. The piriformis muscle is immediately posterior to the joint, whereas the obturator internus and the gemelli and quadratus femoris are lower down (see Figure 25-2).

Bones of the Hip Joint. The rounded shape of the femur and the cup shape of the acetabulum form the "ball and socket" hip joint (see Figure 25-3). The acetabulum is made deeper by a rim of fibrocartilage called the **acetabular labrum**. The bony deficiency at the lower part of the acetabulum (*acetabular notch*) is covered by a band of fibrous tissue called the *transverse ligament*. From this point, a rounded ligament (*ligament teres*) passes upwards inside the joint to be attached to the pit or fovea in the head. In the younger child, this ligament contains an artery to supply the femoral head. The artery usually disintegrates by 7 years of age.

Ligaments of the Hip Joint. The hip joint is surrounded by a tough capsule. Anteriorly to the femur, it is attached to the intertrochanteric line (Figure 25-4). Posteriorly, it does extend as far as the intertrochanteric crest but only to halfway along the neck of the femur (Figure 25-5). Therefore, the posterior part of the neck is inside the capsule or *intracapsular* and part of the neck is outside or *extracapsular*.

The outside of the capsule is reinforced by ligaments. The most important is the *iliofemoral ligament*, which blends with the front of the capsule (see Figure 25-1). This ligament is the shape of an inverted "y" or "V" passing from the anterior inferior iliac spine to each end of the intertrochanteric line. It is one of the strongest ligaments in the body and is very important in standing and maintaining correct upright balance.

Figure 25-2 Left gluteal region (after most of the gluteus muscle and all veins have been removed). (From McMinn: *Functional and clinical anatomy,* St Louis, 1999, Mosby.)

1. Gluteus maximus
2. Gluteus medius
3. Superior gluteal artery
4. Superior gluteal nerve
5. Piriformis
6. Inferior gluteal nerve
7. Inferior gluteal artery
8. Sciatic nerve
9. Posterior femoral cutaneous nerve
10. Superior gemellus
11. Obturator internus
12. Inferior gemellus
13. Greater trochanter
14. Obturator externus
15. Quadratus femoris
16. Nerve to obturator internus (11)
17. Internal pudendal artery
18. Pudendal nerve
19. Sacrotuberous ligament
20. Ischial tuberosity

MOVEMENTS OF THE HIP

The movements of the hip are somewhat limited in range because of the tight fit between the femur and acetabulum and because the hip bone is immobile (Figure 25-6). Following are the hip movements and their actions:

1. Flexion—bending forward
2. Extension—bending backwards
3. Abduction—moving sideways outwards
4. Adduction—moving sideways inwards
5. Medial rotation
6. Lateral rotation

The primary flexors of the hip are the psoas major, iliacus, and rectus femoris. Extension is limited to 20 degrees by tension in the iliofemoral ligament and the flexor muscles, and is brought about by the hamstrings and gluteus maximus.

An example of hip adduction is crossing your legs when in a seated position, an action performed by the adductor group of muscles. In abduction the limbs are opened by the gluteus medius and minimus muscles. The more important function of these muscles, however, is to prevent adduction, which is the function they perform during walking.

Recall that the head and shaft of the femur lie at an angle to one another (about 120 degrees), and the axis about which rotation movements take place is not along the line of the shaft of the femur, but along a line drawn from the head of the femur to the lower end of the bone between the condyles. Medial and lateral rotation is related to this principle. When the trochanter moves forward, the femur rotates medially, and when the trochanter moves backwards, the femur rotates laterally. Thus the medial rotators are the anterior fibers of gluteus medius and minimus. The lateral rotators are the small muscles at the back of the joint—piriformis, obturator internus, and quadratus femoris, with assistance of the gluteus maximus.

SONOGRAPHIC EVALUATION OF THE HIP

Sonography has the advantage over conventional radiography in imaging the fine detail of the neonatal hip. The cartilaginous femoral head, the cartilaginous acetabular rim, and labrum are well seen with sonography. The size, shape, and position of the femoral head can be assessed sonographically

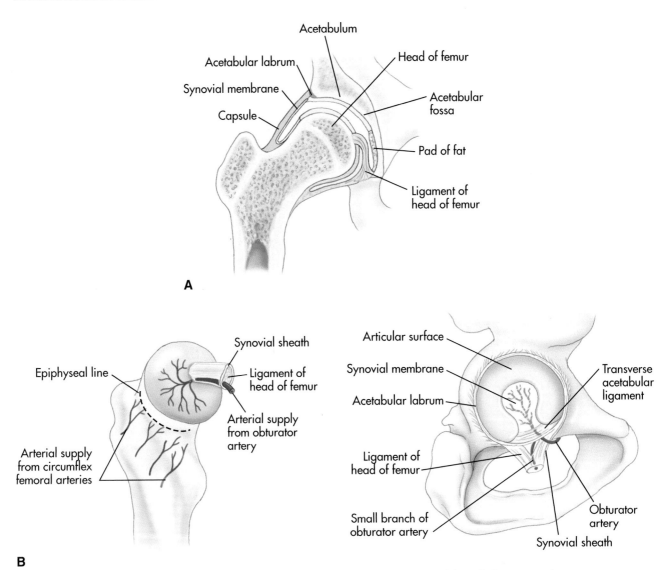

Figure 25-3   Coronal section of the right hip joint (**A**) and articular surfaces of the right hip joint and arterial supply of the head of the femur (**B**).

well before the bones are ossified enough to be seen on radiography. The motion of the femoral head in the acetabulum under stress can also be tested. The shape of the acetabulum can be evaluated. With sonography, the morphologic development of the cartilaginous and bony acetabulum, labrum, and femoral head; the degree to which the femoral head is covered by the labrum; and the position of the femoral head in the acetabulum at rest are assessed during motion and stress.

Indications for neonatal hip sonography include the presence of risk factors for **developmental displacement of the hip**, an abnormal hip examination, and the need to evaluate the response to treatment.

Sonography can be performed until the femoral head ossifies. Ossification of the femoral head begins between 2 and 8 months of age, occurs earlier in girls than boys, and is often complete by 1 year of age. Once the femoral head is completely ossified, it is difficult to obtain adequate sonographic images because of artifact.

SONOGRAPHIC TECHNIQUE

Sonography of the neonatal hip is performed with a linear-array transducer. For average weight neonates up to 3 months of age, a high-frequency transducer of at least 7.5 MHz is used. Infants to age 7 months may be imaged with a 5.0-MHz transducer; and after 7 months, a 3-MHz transducer can be used. The premature infant may be imaged with a 12-MHz transducer.

To achieve a satisfactory examination, the infant should be relaxed and as comfortable as possible. Feeding before or during the examination helps to soothe the infant. Make sure the room is warm and keep blankets close for warmth. Toys and other distractions help to quiet the infant so the examination may be performed. Parental assistance is often helpful, with the mother or father sitting on the bed or next to the infant to help keep the infant calm.

Sonographically the femoral head is hypoechoic because it is cartilaginous and contains a focal echogenic ossification nucleus (Figure 25-7). The femoral head sits within the

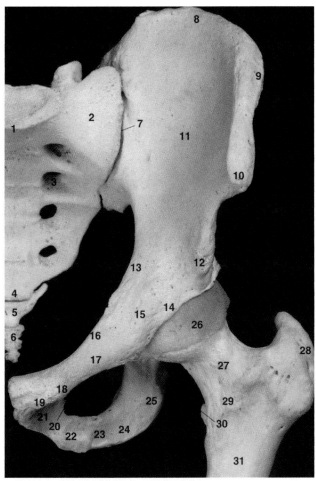

Figure 25-4 Anterior view of left hip bone and femur, with sacrum and coccyx. (From McMinn: *Functional and clinical anatomy,* St Louis, 1999, Mosby.)

Figure 25-5 Posterior view of left hip bone and femur with sacrum and coccyx. (From McMinn: *Functional and clinical anatomy,* St Louis, 1999, Mosby.)

1. Sacral promontory
2. Ala of sacrum
3. Second anterior sacral foramen
4. Apex of sacrum
5. First coccygeal vertebra, with transverse process
6. Fused coccygeal vertebrae
7. Sacroiliac joint
8. Iliac crest
9. Tubercle of iliac crest
10. Anterior superior iliac spine
11. Iliac fossa
12. Anterior inferior iliac spine
13. Arcuate line of ilium
14. Rim of acetabulum
15. Iliopubic eminence
16. Pectineal line (pectin) of pubis
17. Superior ramus of pubis
18. Pubic tubercle
19. Pubic crest
20. Obturator foramen
21. Body of pubis
22. Inferior ramus of pubis
23. Site of union of pubic and ischial rami (22 and 24)
24. Ramus of ischium
25. Ischial tuberosity
26. Head of femur
27. Neck
28. Greater trochanter
29. Intertrochanteric line
30. Tip of lesser trochanter
31. Shaft of femur

acetabulum, which is echogenic and has a deep concave configuration. Two thirds of the head should be covered by the labrum. The labrum is narrow and has a triangular shape. The labrum is composed of hyaline cartilage and is hypoechoic, except at its tip, which is echogenic due to its fibrous content. The femoral head should be stable within the acetabulum with stress after 4 weeks of age. During the neonatal period (i.e., the first 4 weeks of life), there is physiologic laxity of the ligaments about the hip that makes the hip unstable.

Figure 25-6   Anatomic terms used in relation to movement of the hip.

Figure 25-7   Normal ultrasound images of the neonatal hip. **A,** Right hip coronal: flexion/abduction. **B,** Left hip coronal: flexion/abduction. **C,** Right hip transverse: neutral. **D,** Right hip transverse: flexion/adduction/push.

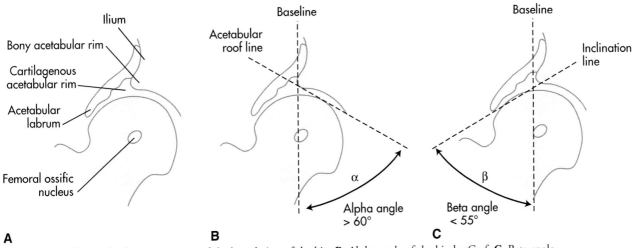

Figure 25-8   **A,** Anatomy of the lateral view of the hip. **B,** Alpha angle of the hip by Graf. **C,** Beta angle of the hip by Graf.

<table>
<tr><td>

BOX 25-1   GRAF'S CLASSIFICATION OF NEONATAL HIPS

- A normal hip has an alpha angle of less than 60 degrees and is classified as a type I hip.
- A type II hip has an alpha angle between 43 and 60 degrees.
- A type III hip has an alpha angle of less than 43 degrees and a beta angle greater than 77 degrees.
- A type IV hip has an alpha angle less than 43 degrees and the beta angle is immeasurable.

</td></tr>
</table>

SONOGRAPHIC PROTOCOL

The basic hip anatomy is imaged in four different views: (1) coronal/neutral, (2) coronal/flexion, (3) transverse/flexion, and (4) transverse/neutral. A two-word combination is used to label the views according to the plane of the body (coronal or transverse) and the position of the hips (neutral or flexed). The primary objective of the dynamic hip assessment is to determine the position and stability of the femoral head and the development of the acetabulum.

Graf's Alpha and Beta Angles. Graf used a series of lines and angle measurements to evaluate the morphology of the acetabulum (Box 25-1).

1. The baseline connects the osseous acetabular convexity to the point where the joint capsule and perichondrium unite.
2. The inclination line connects the osseous acetabular convexity to the labrum.
3. The acetabular roof line connects the lower edge of the medially acetabular roof to the osseous acetabular convexity.

Based on the above lines, the alpha and beta angles are measured. The alpha angle is the angle between the baseline and the acetabular roof line and represents the osseous acetabulum (Figure 25-8). The alpha angle is normally greater than 60 degrees. The beta angle is the angle between the baseline and the

inclination line. This angle evaluates the formation and size of the cartilaginous acetabulum and is normally less than 55 degrees. The alpha angle reflects changes in the osseous portion of the acetabulum, which occur gradually. The beta angle reflects changes in the cartilaginous acetabulum, which occur more quickly than do changes in the osseous acetabulum and may therefore be more sensitive than the alpha angle (Figure 25-9).

Coronal/Neutral View. This view is performed with the infant in the supine position from the lateral aspect of the hip joint, with the plane of the transducer oriented coronally with respect to the hip joint (Figure 25-10). The femur is stabilized with a physiologic amount of flexion. The plane must demonstrate the midportion of the acetabulum with the straight iliac line superiorly and the inferior tip of the os ilium medially within the acetabulum (Figure 25-11). The echogenic tip of the labrum should also be visualized. The alpha and beta angles may be measured from this view. A stability test can be performed in this view by gently pushing and pulling the infant's leg. This helps to verify deformity of the acetabulum and to identify craniodorsal movement of the femoral head under pressure (Table 25-2).

In the normal coronal/neutral view, the femoral head is resting against the bony acetabulum. The acetabular roof should have a concave configuration and cover at least half of the femoral head. The hypoechoic cartilage of the acetabular roof extends lateral to the acetabular lip, terminating in the echogenic labrum. When a hip becomes **subluxed** or dislocated, the femoral head gradually migrates laterally and superiorly with progressively decreased coverage of the femoral head (Figure 25-12).

In hip dysplasia, the acetabular roof is irregular and angled, and the labrum is defected superiorly and becomes echogenic and thickened. When the hip is frankly dislocated, the labrum may be deformed. Echogenic soft tissue is interposed between the femoral head and the bony acetabulum. A combination of deformed labrum and fibrofatty tissue prevents the hip from being reduced.

Coronal/Flexion View. The transducer is maintained in the lateral position while the hip is moved into a 90-degree

Figure 25-9   **A,** Normal hip in the coronal/neutral view. The femoral head sits deep within the bony acetabulum. **B,** In comparison, an abnormal hip shows the femoral head *(H)* positioned laterally and superiorly. **C,** Beta angle of the hip by Graf. (From Henningsen C: *Clinical guide to ultrasonography,* St Louis, 2004, Mosby.)

angle of flexion. During this assessment, the transducer is moved in an anteroposterior direction with respect to the body to visualize the entire hip (Figure 25-13). The curvilinear margin of the body femoral shaft is identified anterior to the femoral head. In the midportion of the acetabulum, the femoral head is surrounded by echoes from the bony acetabular components (Figure 25-14). Superiorly the lateral margin of the iliac bone is seen, and the transducer position should be adjusted so that it becomes a straight horizontal line on the monitor. A normal hip gives the appearance of a "ball on a spoon" in the midacetabulum. The femoral head is the ball, the acetabulum forms the spoon, and the iliac line is the handle (Table 25-3).

In subluxation, the femoral head is displaced laterally, posteriorly, or both, with respect to the acetabulum. Soft tissue echoes are seen between the femoral head and the bony reflections from the medial acetabulum. In dislocation, the femoral head is completely out of the acetabulum. With superior dislocations, the femoral head may rest against the iliac bone. In posterior dislocations, the femoral head is seen lateral to the posterior lip of the triradiate cartilage. The acetabulum is usually not visualized in a dislocation because the bony shaft of the femur blocks the view.

There are two components to this view. The first involves a "push and pull" maneuver. In many clinical sites, this examination is performed by the pediatric orthopedist, the radiolo-

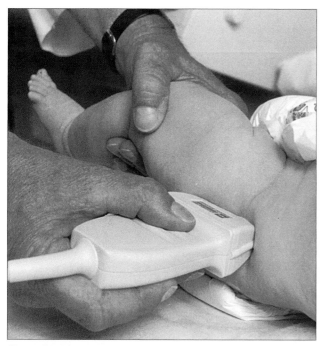

Figure 25-10   Coronal/neutral view. The transducer is coronal with respect to the hip. The femur is in physiologic neutral for the infant (slight hip flexion). (From Rumack CM: *Diagnostic ultrasound,* ed 2, St Louis, 1998, Mosby.)

TABLE 25-2	NEONATAL HIP TECHNIQUE: CORONAL/NEUTRAL VIEW
View: Coronal/ Neutral	Sonographic Findings
Normal	• Femoral head rests against the bony acetabulum • Acetabular roof has concave configuration, covers half of femoral head • Hypoechoic cartilage acetabular roof extends lateral to the acetabular lip, terminates in echogenic labrum
Subluxed/dislocated	• Femoral head gradually migrates laterally and superiorly with decreased coverage of femoral head
Hip dysplasia	• Acetabular roof is irregular and angled • Labrum is defected superiorly; becomes echogenic and thickened
Frankly dislocated	• Labrum may be deformed

A   **B**

Figure 25-11   A, Normal hip sonogram shows sonolucent femoral head resting against the bony acetabulum. Note: fibrocartilaginous tip of labrum *(solid arrow)* and junction of bony ilium and triradiate cartilage *(open arrow).* **B,** Normal hip sonograph with alpha, *a,* and beta, *b,* angles used in measurement. (From Rumack CM: *Diagnostic ultrasound,* ed 2, St Louis, 1998, Mosby.)

Figure 25-12 **A,** Disolocated hip sonogram shows displacement of femoral head laterally with deformity of labrum *(curved arrow).* **B,** Dislocated hip sonogram with abnormal alpha and beta angles. *H,* Femoral head; *L,* lateral; *S,* superior, *I,* iliac line; *m,* femoral metaphysis. (From Rumack CM: *Diagnostic ultrasound,* ed 2, St Louis, 1998, Mosby.)

Figure 25-13 Coronal/flexion view. Transducer is coronal to flexed femur (A). (From Rumack CM: *Diagnostic ultrasound,* ed 2, St Louis, 1998, Mosby.)

Figure 25-14 **A,** Normal coronal/flexion view is identified with femoral head resting against acetabulum. **B,** Disolocated hip shows soft tissue echoes in acetabulum that may prevent hip from being reduced without surgical intervention. *A,* Acetabulum; *H,* femoral head; *I,* iliac line; *L,* lateral; *S,* superior; *arrows,* labrum. (From Henningsen: *Clinical guide to ultrasonography,* St Louis, 2004, Mosby.)

gist, or the experienced pediatric sonographer. In the normal hip, the femoral head is never seen over the posterior lip of the acetabulum (Figure 25-15). When instability is present, a portion of the femoral head appears over the posterior lip of the triradiate cartilage as the femur is pushed. With a pull, the head disappears from the plane. In a dislocated hip, the femoral head may be located over the posterior lip and may or may not move out of the plane with traction.

The second component of the dynamic examination is performed over the midacetabulum. **Barlow maneuver** is performed with adduction and gentle pushing against the knee (Figure 25-16). In the normal hip, the femoral head will remain in place against the acetabulum. With subluxation or

dislocation, the head will migrate laterally and posteriorly, and there will be echogenic soft tissue between the femoral head and the acetabulum.

Transverse/Flexion View. The transverse transducer is rotated 90 degrees and moved posteriorly into a posterolateral position over the hip joint (Figure 25-17). The bony shaft of the femur gives off bright reflected echoes anteriorly, adjacent to the femoral head. The echoes from the bony acetabulum appear posteriorly to the femoral head, and in the normal hip, a U configuration is produced (Figure 25-18). The relationship of the femoral head to the acetabulum is observed during flexion of the hip from adduction to abduction. The deep U configuration is produced with maximum abduction; in adduction the V appearance is seen. Be careful that the transducer is posterior enough to image the medial acetabulum or the hip may appear falsely displaced (Table 25-4).

The hip is then stressed with a gentle posterior push (Barlow maneuver). In the normal hip, the femoral head will remain deeply in the acetabulum in contact with the ischium with stress. In subluxation, the hip will be normally positioned or mildly displaced at rest and there will be further lateral displacement from the medial acetabulum with stress, but the femoral head will remain in contact with a portion of the ischium.

With **frank dislocation**, the hip will be laterally and posteriorly displaced to the extent that the femoral head has no contact with the acetabulum, and the normal U configuration cannot be obtained (Figure 25-19). The process of dislocation and reduction is able to be visualized in unstable hips in the transverse/flexion view. With abduction, the dislocated hip may be reduced, and this represents the sonographic counterpart of the **Ortolani maneuver**.

Transverse/Neutral View. From the transverse/flexion view the leg is brought down into a neutral position. The transducer is now horizontal to the acetabulum from the lateral aspect of the hip (Figure 25-20). The plane passes through the femoral head into the acetabulum at the center of the triradiate cartilage. The exam is begun caudally over the bony shaft of the femur. Moving cephalad, the transition from bone to cartilage in the proximal femur becomes apparent, and the circular cross section of the spherical femoral head is identified (Table 25-5).

In the normal hip, the sonolucent femoral head is positioned against the bony acetabulum over the triradiate cartilage (see Figure 25-20, *B*). The images of the sonogram represent the parts of a flower. The femoral head is the flower; the echoes from the ischium posteriorly and pubis anteriorly represent the leaves at its base. The stem is formed by echoes that pass through the triradiate cartilage into the area of acoustic shadowing created by the osseous structures.

In this view malpositioned hips show soft tissue echoes between the femoral head and acetabulum (see Figure 25-20, *C*). The width and configuration of the gap depend on the nature of the displacement. With subluxation, the femoral head usually moves posteriorly, and remains in contact with the posterior aspect of the acetabulum. With more severe cases, the lateral displacement accompanies posterior migration. Most dislocations are lateral, posterior, and superior.

TABLE 25-3   NEONATAL HIP TECHNIQUE: CORONAL/FLEXION VIEW

View: Coronal/Flexion	Sonographic Findings	Maneuver Changes
Normal	• Curvilinear margin of the body femoral shaft anterior to the femoral head • In midacetabulum, the femoral head is surrounded by echoes from the bony acetabular components • Superiorly seen is lateral margin of the iliac bone; transducer position adjusted to become straight horizontal line • A normal hip gives the appearance of a "ball on a spoon" in the midacetabulum	**"Push and pull":** the femoral head is never seen over the posterior lip of the acetabulum **Barlow:** • Femoral head remains in place in acetabulum
Subluxed/dislocated	Subluxation: • Femoral head displaced laterally, posteriorly, or both, with respect to acetabulum • Soft-tissue echoes seen between femoral head and bony reflections from medial acetabulum Dislocation: • Femoral head completely out of acetabulum • With superior dislocations, femoral head may rest against iliac bone • In posterior dislocations, femoral head seen lateral to posterior lip of triradiate cartilage • Acetabulum not visualized in a dislocation	**"Push and pull":** portion of femoral head appears over the posterior lip of the triradiate cartilage as femur is pushed; with pull, femur may or may not disappear from the plane **Barlow:** • Head migrates laterally and posteriorly; echogenic soft tissue between femoral head and acetabulum

A   B

Figure 25-15   **A,** Push maneuver shows displacement of femoral head over posterior acetabular lip. **B,** Pull maneuver reveals head no longer positioned over triradiate cartilage *(arrowhead)* of posterior lip of acetabulum. *H,* Femoral head; *L,* lateral, *S,* superior line; *a,* acetabulum, *I,* iliac line. (From Rumack CM: *Diagnostic ultrasound,* ed 2, St Louis, 1998, Mosby.)

PATHOLOGY OF THE NEONATAL HIP

DISLOCATION OF THE HIP

Neonatal hip dislocation can be acquired, teratogenic, or developmental. Acquired causes of hip dislocation can be traumatic or nontraumatic (i.e., neuromuscular diseases). Teratogenic dislocations occur in utero and are associated with neuromuscular disorders. Developmental dislocation of the hip was formerly known as *congenital hip dysplasia*. The term *congenital hip dysplasia* covered a very wide spectrum of pathology that usually occurs after birth. Therefore the term has been replaced by *developmental displacement of the hip (DDH)*. This new term includes dysplastic, subluxated, dislocatable, and dislocated hips.

A

Figure 25-16   Barlow maneuver.

Figure 25-17   Transverse/flexion view. The transducer is in the axial plane posterolaterally over the hip joint with the hip flexed. (From Rumack CM: *Diagnostic ultrasound*, ed 2, St Louis, 1998, Mosby.)

B

Figure 25-18   **A,** Normal transverse/flexion view shows U-shaped configuration that is not present in (**B**) dislocated hip. *H,* Femoral head; *I,* ischium; *m,* femoral metaphysic; *L,* lateral; *P,* posterior. (From Henningsen: *Clinical guide to ultrasonography,* St Louis, 2004, Mosby.)

The sonographic appearance of the femoral head is described as normal, subluxed, or dislocated. Stability testing is reported as normal, lax, subluxable, dislocatable, and reducible or irreducible. Sonographic description of the acetabulum is assessed visually and is described as normal, immature, or dysplastic.

DEVELOPMENTAL DISPLACEMENT OF THE HIP

A displacement of the hip is a relatively common congenital abnormality, which can be diagnosed in the early neonatal period. Before sonography, plain film radiographs were used to confirm the diagnosis of a dysplastic hip. Today sonography has replaced radiography because it does not require the neonate to be sedated, no ionizing radiation is used, and the soft tissues are well defined with high-frequency ultrasound. Moreover, the ultrasound examination may be repeated as often as necessary to follow the progression of treatment.

TABLE 25-4   NEONATAL HIP TECHNIQUE: TRANSVERSE/FLEXION VIEW

View: Transverse/Flexion	Sonographic Findings	Maneuver Changes
Normal	• Bony shaft of femur gives bright reflected echoes anteriorly, adjacent to the femoral head • Echoes from the bony acetabulum appear posteriorly to the femoral head, and in the normal hip, a U configuration is produced • Relationship of the femoral head to the acetabulum observed during flexion of hip from adduction to abduction • Deep U configuration produced with maximum abduction; in adduction the V appearance is seen	Barlow: Femoral head will remain deeply in the acetabulum in contact with the ischium with stress
Subluxed/dislocated		Subluxation: Hip normally positioned or mildly displaced at rest; further lateral displacement from medial acetabulum with stress, but femoral head will remain in contact with portion of ischium
Frankly dislocated	Hip will be laterally and posteriorly displaced to the extent that the femoral head has no contact with the acetabulum, and the normal U configuration cannot be obtained	

A   **B**

Figure 25-19   **A,** Normal hip sonogram shows echolucent femoral head surrounded by metaphysis (anterior) and ischium (posterior), forming a U around femoral head. **B,** Dislocated hip sonogram shows sonolucent femoral head displaced posterolaterally. The U configuration of normal metaphysis and ischium is not seen. *H,* Femoral head; *L,* lateral; *P,* posterior; *I,* ischium; *m,* metaphysis. (From Rumack CM: *Diagnostic ultrasound,* ed 2, St Louis, 1998, Mosby.)

Figure 25-20   Transverse/neutral view. **A,** Transducer is perpendicular to neutral femoral head in the plane of acetabulum. **B,** Normal hip sonogram shows sonolucent femoral head centered over triradiate cartilage with pubis (anterior) and ischium (posterior). **C,** Subluxed hip sonogram shows sonolucent femoral head displaced posterolaterally with gap between pubis and femoral head *(arrow). H,* Femoral head; *L,* lateral; *P,* posterior; *I,* ischium; *arrowhead,* triradiate cartilage; *p,* pubis. (From Rumack CM: *Diagnostic ultrasound,* ed 3, St Louis, 2003, Mosby.)

TABLE 25-5	NEONATAL HIP TECHNIQUE: TRANSVERSE/NEUTRAL VIEW	
View: Transverse/Neutral	Sonographic Findings	
Normal	• Sonolucent femoral head is positioned against the bony acetabulum over the triradiate cartilage	
Subluxed/dislocated	• Femoral head usually moves posteriorly, and remains in contact with the posterior aspect of the acetabulum	

Incidence of Developmental Displacement of the Hip. The incidence of DDH is small, ranging between 1.5 and 1.7 per 1000 live births. When lesser degrees of abnormality such as subluxation are included, as many as 10 infants per 1000 live births may show some features of the disorder.

Multiple risk factors may contribute to the condition. It usually affects the firstborn child, with females affected more frequently than males. The left hip is most commonly affected with only a small number of cases affecting both hips. The condition affects Caucasians more than the black population. A breech birth is also a risk factor in DDH, as is low birth

Dislocation of the hip

Normal   Subluxed   Dislocated

Figure 25-21   Dislocation of the hip.

Early signs (dislocation of right hip)

Limitation of abduction   Asymmetry of skin folds   Shortening of femur
                              Prominence of trochanter

Figure 25-22   Physical signs of developmental displacement of the hip.

weight. Other risk factors include maternal hypertension, fetal growth restriction, oligohydramnios, premature rupture of membranes, prolonged gestation, increased birth weight, Potter's syndrome, and neonatal intensive care.

Causes of Developmental Displacement of the Hip. The primary cause of DDH is thought to be a gradual migration of the femoral head from the acetabulum because of the loose, elastic joint capsule. In addition, other factors—such as genetic, mechanical, and physiologic—are thought to play a role.

In the newborn period, the femoral head may dislocate in a lateral and posterosuperior position relative to the acetabulum (Figure 25-21). When this occurs, the femoral head can usually be reduced without deformity to the joint. However, when the dislocation is not recognized early, the muscles tighten and limit movement. This causes the acetabulum to become dysplastic because it lacks the stimulus of the femoral head. In turn, the ligamentous structures stretch and fibrofatty tissue occupies the acetabulum, making it impossible to return the femoral head into the acetabulum.

Genetic factors show that there is a 6% chance that a child will be affected if a sibling has DDH and a 36% chance if one sibling and one parent are affected. There is a 12% chance that an affected individual will have a child with DDH.

As for the mechanical causes of DDH, oligohydramnios, breech presentation, and the primigravid uterus are considered risk factors because each limits the mobility of the hip in its own way. Oligohydramnios limits mobility because there is less than a normal amount of amniotic fluid present for the fetus to move freely within the amniotic sac. In breech presentation, the fetus's hip rests against the maternal sacrum and is usually flexed, which limits movement. This usually affects the left hip. The frank breech presentation of the fetus is the highest risk because the hips are maximally flexed and the knees are extended. The primigravid uterus is smaller than the multigravida uterus and is therefore more confining and thus limits mobility.

PHYSICAL EXAMINATION FOR DEVELOPMENTAL DISPLACEMENT OF THE HIP

A careful physical examination is critical for the diagnosis of developmental displacement of the hip (Figure 25-22). By visual inspection, the dislocated hip shows asymmetric skin folds and shortening of the affected thigh. The knee is lower in position on the affected side when the patient is supine and the knees are flexed (**Galeazzi sign**).

If the physical examination is abnormal at birth, sonography of the hip should be done within 1 to 2 weeks of age. Hip instability may resolve on its own. Newborns with a risk factor for DDH can be examined at 4 to 6 weeks.

There are two basic maneuvers that are helpful in the diagnosis of DDH. The Barlow maneuver determines if the hip can

Figure 25-23   Ortolani maneuver.

be dislocated. The Ortolani maneuver determines if the dislocated femoral head can be reduced back into the acetabulum.

The Barlow Maneuver. This maneuver is performed by having the patient lie in the supine position with the hip flexed 90 degrees and adducted (see Figure 25-16). Downward and outward pressure is then applied. If the hip can be dislocated, the examiner will feel the femoral head move out of the acetabulum with his fingers.

The Ortolani Maneuver (Figure 25-23). The patient lies in the supine position. The examiner's hand is placed around the hip to be examined, with the fingers over the femoral head. The examiner's middle finger lies over the greater trochanter and the thumb is over the lesser trochanter. The hip is flexed 90 degrees and the thigh is abducted. Movement in the normal hip should feel smooth. In cases of DDH, a "clunk" is appreciated as the femoral head returns into the acetabulum. A "click" does not imply DDH. Each hip should be examined individually.

SONOGRAPHIC TECHNIQUE FOR DEVELOPMENTAL DISPLACEMENT OF THE HIP

There are two sonographic techniques used in the diagnosis of DDH: static (morphologic) and dynamic. Although the dynamic approach is more commonly used and preferred, the techniques are not mutually exclusive. Results from these procedures will be presented below.

Static Technique. This technique was introduced by Graf, an Austrian orthopedic surgeon, in 1980. The standard sonographic image is acquired in the coronal plane at the midacetabular level. This image includes the femoral head,

acetabulum, labrum, and the iliac bone as it meets the triradiate cartilage. This produces a coronal image of the hip, which has a configuration of a lazy "Y."

Graf's classification of neonatal hips. According to Graf, there are four types of neonatal hip displacements (Box 25-1). The neonatal hip is classified according to its alpha and beta angles.

Type I hips are normal and require no further evaluation. Type II hips must be monitored and follow-up studies are required. Type III and IV hips must be treated.

Sonographic signs of developmental displacement of the hip include a shallow dysplastic acetabulum, delayed ossification of the femoral head (in either a lateral or posterior direction), increased thickness of the acetabular cartilage, an alpha angle greater than 60 degrees, and a beta angle of less than 55 degrees. A "normal" sonogram does not absolutely exclude DDH, although the sensitivity and specificity of sonography approach 100%.

Dynamic Technique. Harcke and Graf formulated basic standards for dynamic hip sonography, which is currently used in most clinical situations today. All scanning is performed from the lateral or posterolateral aspect of the hip. The hip is imaged in orthogonal planes: coronal (longitudinal) and transverse (axial). Images of the hip are obtained in the coronal-extension/flexion and transverse-extension/flexion positions.

With the hip flexed, the femur is moved through a range of abduction and adduction, with stress views performed in the flexed position.

The infant is lying in a supine position with the feet toward the sonographer. It is wise to leave the diaper on through the examination and expose only the side of the hip being examined. The sonographer should hold the left leg with the left hand and hold the transducer in the right hand. When the right hip is examined, the sonographer should hold the transducer in the left hand and use the right hand to manipulate the leg.

The examination begins with a coronal-neutral or coronal-flexion image. For the coronal-neutral image, the hip is held in 15 to 20 degrees of flexion. This is considered physiological. For the coronal-flexion image, the hip is held in 90 degrees of flexion. The images in the standard or midacetabular plane include the iliac bone as it meets the triradiate cartilage, which should be in the middle of the field. The tip of the labrum must be included in this image.

The sonographic images differ in that the echogenic femoral metaphysis is seen in the coronal-neutral position, but not in the coronal-flexion position. Both images are obtained with the transducer held in the coronal axis of the hip. In both cases, the femoral head should rest against the osseous acetabulum. Approximately two thirds of the femoral head should be covered by the labrum. Stress can be applied in the coronal-flexion position through piston action of the hip. This is accomplished by pushing and pulling the hip in an anterior and posterior direction. If the hip is unstable, the femoral head will be identified posterior to the acetabulum. A coronal-extension image may also be obtained.

The transverse-flexion position is made with the transducer held in the axial plane while the hip is held in 90 degrees of

Figure 25-24   Sonographic images of hip dysplasia.

flexion. The hip is pushed posteriorly and adducted in an attempt to dislocate the hip. This is analogous to the Barlow maneuver. If the hip dislocates, the examiner should be able to feel the femoral head dislocate. The hip is then pulled and abducted to attempt to reduce a dislocatable hip. This is analogous to the Ortolani maneuver. The transverse-extension can also be obtained (Figure 25-24).

If the femoral head dislocates laterally, the center of the femoral head does not line up with the iliac wing. A line drawn through the iliac wing will pass through the medial aspect of the femoral head. If the femoral head dislocates posteriorly, only an echogenic arc (which represents one side of the head) is seen.

A stress view can be obtained with a "piston maneuver." The hip is placed in 90 degrees of flexion and pressure is applied in the anterior and posterior direction. The transducer is held in the axial plane along the posterior and lateral aspect of the hip.

Hips are classified according to their behavior under stress as normal, unstable, or dislocated. The normal neonatal femoral head cannot be displaced out of the acetabulum, but can have up to 6 mm of motion on the left and 4 mm of motion on the right during abduction and adduction due to physiologic laxity.

Unstable hips are further divided into subluxable and dislocatable. A subluxable hip is one in which the proximal femur moves (more than 6 mm on the left and 4 mm on the right) within the acetabulum, but cannot be displaced out of it. A dislocatable hip is one in which the proximal femur can be displaced out of the acetabulum, but can be reduced. A dislocated hip is one in which the femoral head is displaced out of the acetabulum and cannot be reduced.

TREATMENT OF DEVELOPMENTAL DISPLACEMENT OF THE HIP

The initial treatment of uncomplicated DDH is closed reduction. This may be accomplished either by placing two diapers on the neonate or by using a spica cast, Pavlik harness (Figure 25-25), or brace. The hip should be positioned in flexion, with abduction and external rotation.

The position of the femoral head relative to the acetabulum can be determined with sonography. If the patient has a cast, a "window" must be cut into the cast so that the transducer can be placed directly on the skin.

Causes of failure of closed reduction include inversion of the labrum or capsule and invagination of the iliopsoas muscle, which can be imaged most efficiently by sonography and MRI. If closed reduction fails or if the dislocation is teratogenic, the patient usually requires open reduction.

SCREENING

Development of both sides of the neonatal hip (the acetabulum and femoral head) requires the femoral head to be seated normally within the acetabulum. If the femoral head and acetabulum are not in their normal position, both sides of the hip will develop abnormally. This will cause abnormal morphology and function. If the diagnosis is made early and treatment is instituted promptly, a potentially abnormal hip may develop normally.

Figure 25-25   Pavlik harness may be used in the treatment of hip dysplasia.

The most important factor influencing outcome is the age at which the diagnosis is made and treatment initiated. Treatment should begin before the patient walks. Sonography has been found to be more sensitive than physical examination in the detection of DDH. The goal of screening sonography of the neonatal hip is to establish an early diagnosis so that treatment can be instituted as early as possible. Currently sonography is used in the neonatal period if the physical examination is abnormal, or if risk factors or associated congenital anomalies are present.

SELECTED BIBLIOGRAPHY

Cook MA: Developmental displacement of the neonatal hip. In Haller JO, editor: *Textbook of neonatal ultrasound,* New York, 1998, The Parthenon Publishing Group.

Gerscovich EO: Infant hip in developmental dysplasia: facts to consider for a successful diagnostic ultrasound examination, *Appl Radiol* March:18-25,1999.

Graf R: The diagnosis of congenital hip joint dislocation by the ultrasonic compound treatment, *Archiv Orthop Traumat Surg* 97:117-133, 1980.

Graf R: Fundamentals of sonographic diagnosis of infant hip dysplasia, *J Pediatr Orthop* 4:735-740, 1984.

Grissom LE and Harcke HT: The pediatric hip. In Rumack C, Wilson S, Charboneau JW: *Diagnostic ultrasound,* ed 2, St Louis, 1998, Mosby.

Harcke HT, Grissom LE: Performing dynamic sonography of the infant hip, *Am J Roentgenol* 155:837-844, 1990.

Harcke HT: Screening newborns for developmental displacement of the hip: the role of sonography, *Am J Roentgenol* 152:395-397, 1994.

Harcke HT, Grissom LE: Infant hip sonography: current concepts, *Semin Ultrasound CT MRI* 15:256-263, 1994.

Henningsen C: *Clinical guide to ultrasonography,* St Louis, 2004, Mosby.

McMinn RMH, Gaddum-Rosse P, Hutchings RT and others: *McMinn's functional & clinical anatomy,* St Louis, 1995, Mosby.

Weintroub S, Grill F: Ultrasonography in developmental dysplasia of the hip, *J Bone Joint Surg* 82A:1004-1018, 2000.

The Neonatal Spine

Sandra L. Hagen-Ansert

KEY TERMS

cauda equina – bundle of nerve roots from the lumbar, sacral, and coccygeal spinal nerves that descend nearly vertically from the spinal cord until they reach their respective openings in the vertebral column

conus medullaris – the caudal end of the spinal cord

diastematomyelia – a congenital fissure of the spinal cord, frequently associated with spina bifida cystica

dysraphic – refers to the anomalies associated by incomplete embryologic development

filum terminale – slender tapering terminal section of the spinal cord

hydromyelia – dilation of the central canal of the spinal cord

lipoma – common benign tumor composed of fat cells

meningocele – protrusion of the meninges through the gap in the spine, the skin covering being vestigial

myelomeningocele – the spinal cord and nerve roots are exposed, often adhering to the fine membrane that overlies them

myeloschisis – cleft spinal cord resulting from failure of the neural tube to close

spina bifida aperta – open (non–skin-covered lesions) neural tube defects, such as myelomeningocele and meningocele

spina bifida occulta – closed (skin-covered lesions) neural tube defects, such as spinal lipoma and tethered cord

tethered spinal cord – fixed spinal cord that is positioned in an abnormal position

The spinal canal and its contents can be demonstrated sonographically with great clarity in the neonatal period. Conditions such as an occult **tethered spinal cord,** various **dysraphic** conditions, and the relationship of back masses and midline cutaneous deformities to the spinal canal are among the indications for spine sonography. High-resolution ultrasound imaging of the spinal canal has been a clinically acceptable tool for examining the neonate. Clinically the infant may present with a dimple on the posterior surface of the body along the spinal canal. Although it is not uncommon for the buttocks to contain a shallow dimple near the anus, at times the dimple appears unusually deep or asymmetric. Other indications that an abnormality may be present include a hemangioma or a raised midline area, a hairy patch, or even a tail-like projection from the lower spine. The dimple may also be suspicious if it is more than 1 inch from the anus. These findings may suggest the possibility of an underlying maldevelopment of the spinal cord or the adjacent elements, known as *occult dysraphic lesions.* Spinal dysraphism includes disorders of the spine involving absent or incomplete closure of the neural tube. The severity of the defect ranges from mild **spina bifida occulta** to severe **spina bifida aperta.** Failure to recognize these abnormalities early may lead to difficulty in walking or other neurological problems in infancy or childhood.

Advantages of sonography include the ability to perform the procedure easily and at the bedside without ionizing radiation. The availability of high-frequency transducers now leaves operator inexperience as the main reason for unsuccessful neonatal spinal sonography. The sonographer may observe the spinal cord as it pulsates normally within the spinal canal. The vascular supply to the spinal canal may be evaluated with color Doppler ultrasound. The development of fluid collections, cysts, or fatty tumors (lipomas) is easily seen. Malformations of the spinal cord may be imaged and will be presented in this chapter.

EMBRYOGENESIS

The defects of the spinal canal occur in the first 8.5 weeks of life as the fetal nervous system develops. The neural tube and the subsequent spinal cord arise from ectodermal cells. The surface ectoderm separates from the neural tube, with the mesoderm coming to lie between the neural tube and the ectoderm. The mesoderm forms the bony spine, meninges, and muscle. Incomplete separation of the neural tube from the ectoderm may result in cord tethering, **diastematomyelia,** or a dermal sinus. Premature separation of the cutaneous ectoderm from the neural tube can result in abnormal mesenchymal elements, such as lipomas forming between the neural tube and skin. If the neural tube fails to fold and fuse in the midline, defects such as **myelomeningocele** occur. Disorders of the distal cord may lead to fibrolipomas of the **filum terminale.**

ANATOMY OF THE VERTEBRAL COLUMN AND SPINAL CORD

The vertebral column extends from the base of the skull to the tip of the coccyx along the posterior surface of the body. The vertebral column is the central bony stabilizer of the body. Within the vertebral cavity lie the spinal cord, the roots of the spinal nerves, and the covering meninges, which provide protection for the vertebral column.

The vertebral column consists of 33 vertebrae: 7 cervical, 12 thoracic, 5 lumbar, 5 sacral (fused to form the sacrum), and 4 coccygeal fused bones (Figure 26-1). The pads of fibrocartilage, called intervertebral disks, are found between each vertebra and allow flexibility in the spine.

VERTEBRAE

Each vertebra consists of a rounded body anteriorly and a vertebral arch posteriorly (Figure 26-2). These enclose a space called the vertebral foramen, through which run the spinal cord and its coverings. The vertebral arch consists of a pair of cylindrical pedicles, which form the sides of the arch, and a pair of flattened laminae, which complete the arch posteriorly.

The vertebral arch gives rise to seven processes: one spinous, two transverse, and four articular. The two superior articular processes of one vertebral arch articulate with the two inferior articular processes of the arch above, forming two synovial joints.

The pedicles are notched on their upper and lower borders, forming the superior and inferior vertebral notches. On each side, the superior notch of one vertebra and the inferior notch of an adjacent vertebra together form the intervertebral foramen. These foramina serve to transmit the spinal nerves and blood vessels.

In the neonate, problems typically occur in the lower back near the area of the lumbar vertebrae and the sacrum. Characteristics of the lumbar vertebrae may be described as follows:

- The body is large and oval.
- The pedicles are strong and directed posterior.
- The laminae are thick.
- The vertebral foramina are triangular.
- The transverse processes are short, flat, and quadrangular and project backward.
- The articular surfaces of the superior articular processes face medially, and those of the inferior articular processes face laterally.

SACRUM

The sacrum consists of five bones fused together. The upper border articulates with the fifth lumbar vertebra. The narrow inferior border articulates with the coccyx. Laterally the sacrum articulates with the two iliac bones to form the sacroiliac joints. The anterior and upper margin of the first sacral vertebra bulges forward as the posterior margin of the pelvic inlet and is known as the sacral promontory.

The vertebral foramina are present and form the sacral canal. The laminae of the fifth sacral vertebra, and sometimes those of the fourth also, fail to meet in the midline and form the sacral hiatus (Figure 26-3). The sacral canal contains the anterior and posterior roots of the sacral and coccygeal spinal nerves, the filum terminale, and fibrofatty material. It also contains the lower part of the subarachnoid space down as far as the lower border of the second sacral vertebra.

The anterior and posterior surfaces of the sacrum each have four foramina on each side for the passage of the anterior and posterior rami of the upper four sacral nerves.

INTERVERTEBRAL DISKS

The intervertebral disks are responsible for one fourth of the length of the vertebral column. They are thickest in the cervical and lumbar regions where the movements of the vertebral column are greatest. Each disk consists of a peripheral part, the *annulus fibrosus,* and a central part, the *nucleus pulposus* (Figure 26-4). The annulus fibrosus consists of fibrocartilage. The

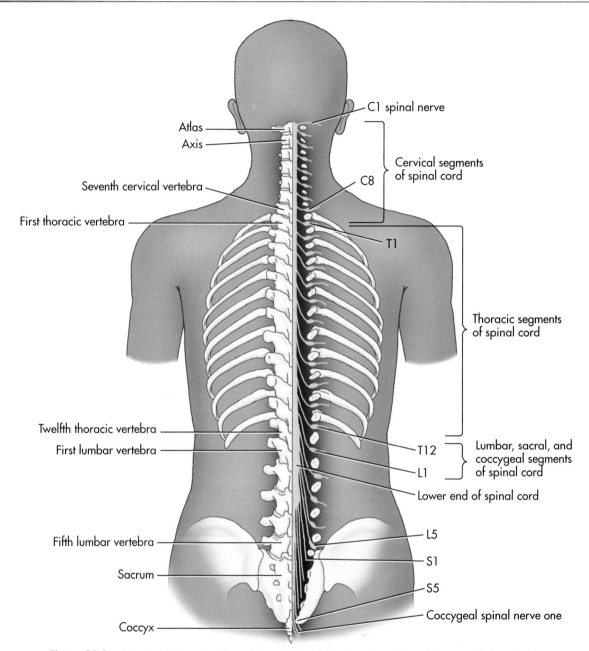

Figure 26-1   Spinal cord. Posterior view of the spinal cord showing the origins of the roots of the spinal nerves. On the right, the laminae have been removed to expose the right half of the spinal cord and the nerve roots.

nucleus pulposus is an ovoid mass of gelatinous material containing a large amount of water, a small number of collagen fibers, and a few cartilage cells. It is normally under pressure and situated slightly nearer to the posterior than to the anterior margin of the disk.

LIGAMENTS AND NERVES
The anterior and posterior longitudinal ligaments run as continuous bands down the anterior and posterior surfaces of the vertebral column from the skull to the sacrum. The joints between the vertebral bodies are innervated by the small meningeal branches of each spinal nerve.

SPINAL CORD
The spinal cord is a cylindrical, grayish white structure that begins above at the foramen magnum, where it is continuous with the medulla oblongata of the brain. It terminates below in the adult at the level of the lower border of the first lumbar vertebra. In the younger child, it is relatively longer and ends at the upper border of the third lumbar vertebra (Figure 26-5).

Inferiorly the cord tapers off into the conus medullaris, from the apex of which a prolongation of the pia mater, the filum terminale, descends to be attached to the back of the coccyx. The cord has a deep longitudinal fissure in the midline

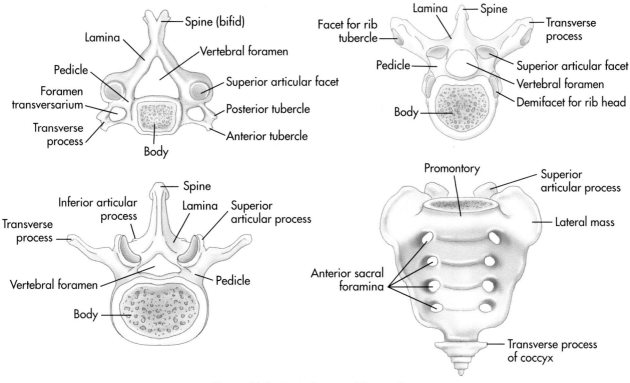

Figure 26-2   Basic features of the vertebrae.

anteriorly, the anterior median fissure, and on the posterior surface a shallow furrow, the posterior median sulcus.

ROOTS OF THE SPINAL NERVES

Along the length of the spinal cord are attached 31 pairs of spinal nerves. The spinal nerve roots unite to form a spinal nerve. The lower nerve roots together are called the cauda equina.

MENINGES OF THE SPINAL CORD

The spinal cord is surrounded by three meninges: the dura mater, the arachnoid mater, and the pia mater (see Figure 26-5).

The dura mater is the most external membrane and is a dense strong, fibrous sheet that encloses the spinal cord and cauda equina. It is continuous through the foramen magnum with the meningeal layer of dura covering the brain. Inferiorly, it ends on the filum terminale at the level of the lower border of the second sacral vertebra.

The arachnoid mater is a delicate impermeable membrane covering the spinal cord and lying between the pia mater internally and the dura mater externally. It is separated from the dura by the subdural space, which contains a thin film of tissue fluid. The arachnoid is separated from the pia mater by a wide space, the subarachnoid space, which is filled with cerebrospinal fluid.

The pia mater is a vascular membrane that closely covers the spinal cord. It is continuous above the neck through the foramen magnum with the pia covering the brain; below it fuses with the filum terminale.

SONOGRAPHIC EVALUATION OF THE NEONATAL SPINAL COLUMN

The incomplete ossification of the posterior spinal elements allows sonography to provide a broad panoramic view of the neonatal spinal canal and its contents. A posterior approach is used with the patient prone or lateral decubitus, but the examination could be performed with the baby in an upright (against the mother's abdomen) or sitting position. It is crucial that the spine be flexed enough to separate the posterior spinal elements. When prone, this is accomplished by having the baby lie over a small pillow or a rolled towel. Slight elevation of the upper part of the body will better distend the caudal aspect of the thecal sac. Care must be taken that flexion is not so extreme as to compromise the infant's breathing. This consideration is amplified if the baby has been sedated. The infant usually falls asleep during the procedure once the warm coupling gel is applied and the transducer is gently rubbed along the spine canal.

The sonographer should use the highest frequency transducer available to obtain the greatest soft tissue detail. Small neonates will require a higher frequency (7 to 10 MHz) than a chunky baby, who would require perhaps a 5- to 7-MHz transducer. The linear array transducer works the best to completely scan along the spinal canal. The curved array or sector transducers are best used in special situations where the body surface is curved, such as the craniocervical junction or at the margin of a **meningocele.**

Scanning is performed in the midline sagittal (longitudinal) and axial (transverse) planes, the latter mainly between the

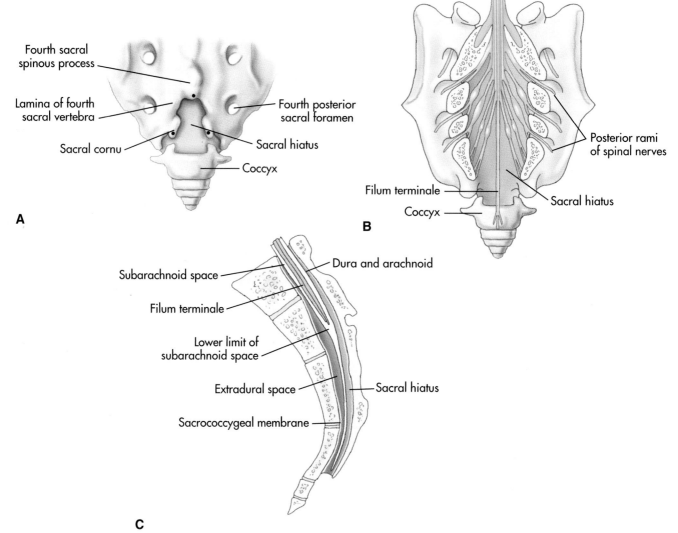

Figure 26-3 **A,** The sacral hiatus. The black dots indicate the position of the important bony landmarks. **B,** The dural sheath (thecal sac) around the lower end of the spinal cord and spinal nerves in the sacral canal; the laminae have been removed. **C,** Longitudinal section through the sacrum.

spinous processes. Sagittal images are oriented with the baby's head toward the left on the viewing screen, similar to conventional abdominal images. On transverse scans, the patient's right side is to the left of the monitor.

Since most examinations are performed to exclude an occult tethered spinal cord, determining the vertebral level of the tip of the *conus medullaris* is most important, and accordingly the lumbar spinal canal receives the most attention. The entire spinal canal is examined, however, at multiple levels.

The depth of field is adjusted so the vertebral bodies are at the bottom of the image. The spinal canal is usually easily identified, and the depth of the image is adjusted accordingly. It is helpful to scan the sacral region first, where the canal is easily identified by the stepwise ascent of the sacral vertebral elements, and then follow the spinal canal craniad. A stand-off pad may be used between the transducer and the skin surface to examine the soft tissue dorsal to the spine, such as looking

for a sinus tract. Oscillations of the spinal cord and roots of the *cauda equina* are observed best when the image persistence or frame averaging is minimized.

SONOGRAPHIC ANATOMY OF THE SPINAL CANAL

With sonography, the spinal canal is defined anteriorly by the echogenic posterior vertebral body surfaces and posteriorly by the posterior dorsal spinal elements, some of which might be incompletely ossified (Figure 26-6). The dura is visible as an echogenic line just internal to these osseous borders. The spinous processes appear as inverted "Us." Laminae are seen when scanning slightly off midline and appear similar to overlapping roof tiles. The coccyx is mostly or completely unossified and therefore hypoechoic.

The spinal cord is hypoechoic with slightly echogenic borders and an echogenic line extending longitudinally along its midline. This central echo complex represents or is close to the cord's central canal (Figure 26-7).

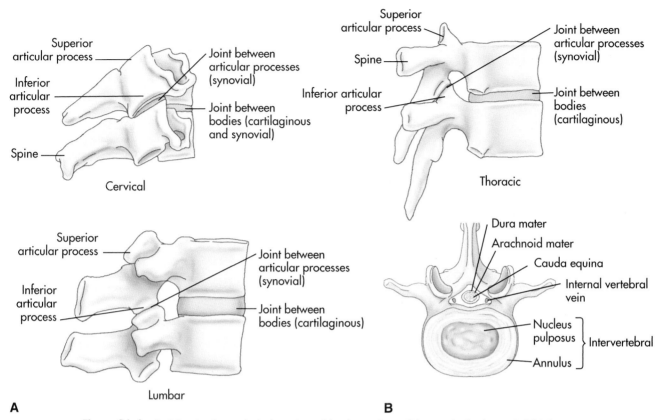

Figure 26-4   **A,** Joints in the cervical, thoracic, and lumbar regions of the vertebral column. **B,** Third lumbar vertebra seen from above, showing the relationship between intervertebral disk and cauda equina.

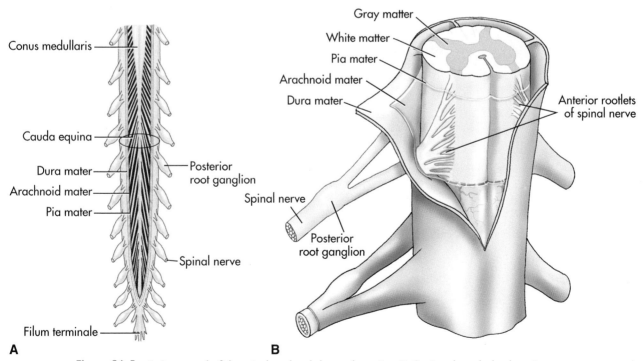

Figure 26-5   **A,** Lower end of the spinal cord and the cauda equina. **B,** Section through the thoracic part of the spinal cord showing the anterior and posterior roots of the spinal nerves and meninges.

The size and shape of the spinal cord vary along its length. Its diameter is narrowest in the midthoracic and thoracolumbar junctions. Transverse dentate ligaments of the cord are sometimes visible. The cord tapers caudally at the conus medullaris.

The nerve roots that surround the spinal cord are echogenic (Figure 26-8). They are especially noticeable at and below the conus forming the cauda equina. Dorsal and ventral nerve roots can have a spiderlike configuration at the tip of the conus in the transverse view. Clusters of normal nerve roots might be mistaken for an echogenic *intracanalicular* mass. Nerves, however, will be observed to move and change configuration as one scans

Figure 26-6 Normal spinal canal—sagittal view. Normal ultrasound of the neonatal spinal canal defined anteriorly by the echogenic posterior body surfaces and posteriorly by the posterior dorsal spinal elements. *1,* Posterior elements or spinous processes; *2,* posterior arachnoid-dural layer bordering spinal canal; *3,* subarachnoid space filled with cerebrospinal fluid; *4,* posterior margin of the spinal cord; *5,* spinal cord with central echo complex; *6,* anterior margin of the spinal cord.

along the canal in real time. In transverse views, nerve roots might appear as an echogenic clump in the middle of the spinal canal or as bilateral clusters, sometimes in an upside down "V" configuration. Another potential false-positive finding is the bilateral dorsal and ventral roots at the very tip of the conus that can superficially mimic a split cord, *diastematomyelia.* Although they appear similar on the sonographic image, they are readily distinguished during real-time scanning in both projections, above and below the area of concern.

The spinal cord and roots of the cauda equina are normally observed to move. This is best seen with minimal frame persistence. Dorso-ventral oscillations occur at the frequency of the heartbeat, and there is also a superimposed motion, which occurs with respirations. These movements are variably present in neonates, but are almost always seen after 1 or 2 months of age.

Level of the Conus Medullaris. The single most important determination is usually the level of the tip of the tapered conus medullaris (Figure 26-9). The normal level is in the upper lumbar canal, above the superior endplate of L3, with most cords ending above L2.

The level of the lumbar vertebral level may be determined by looking at the baby's back during the scanning examination. A transverse projection across the midline from the lowest palpable rib end is often L2. A similar projection from the palpated apex of the iliac crest is often L5. One can count vertebral levels on ultrasound by counting caudad from the lowest rib-bearing vertebra or by counting cranial from the caudal end of the thecal sac (usually S2), from the coccyx, or from the lumbosacral junction.

One can also sonographically identify the lowest rib over each kidney and follow it medially to its vertebral body. That

A   **B**

Figure 26-7   Thoracic **(A)** and lumbar **(B)** spine of normal 5-day-old cord. The spinal cord is hypoechoic with slightly echogenic borders and an echogenic line extending longitudinally along its midline *(central echo complex).* (From Rumack CM: *Diagnostic ultrasound,* ed 2, St Louis, 1998, Mosby.)

Figure 26-8 Level of conus—transverse view. The nerve roots are echogenic as they surround the spinal cord. *1,* Paravertebral muscles; *2,* laminae of vertebral arches; *3,* subarachnoid space filled with cerebrospinal fluid; *4,* spinal cord with central echo complex; *5,* paired dorsal and ventral nerve roots; *6,* vertebral body.

Figure 26-9 Normal conus medullaris—sagittal view. The tapered conus medullaris shows the end of the spinal cord. 1, Posterior elements or spinous processes; 2, cauda medullaris, 3, filum terminale; 4, cauda equina and nerve roots.

level can be assigned as T12, although it could be off by a level if the patient has 11 or 13 pairs of ribs. If the conus tip is mid-lumbar, its exact level might therefore need to be determined by a correlative radiograph. The conus tip is carefully noted in both longitudinal and transverse sonographic projections and this position is marked on the skin by a radiopaque marker, such as a nipple "B-B" marker.

Most tethered cords are unquestionably low and correlative radiographs are not usually necessary. Sometimes the conus tip is obscured by an overlying posterior spinal element, but this is more often a problem in older infants and children. In those cases the conus level is inferred to be lying between the lowest level showing cord and the adjacent caudal level, which contains only the cauda equina.

PATHOLOGY OF THE NEONATAL SPINAL COLUMN

Spinal sonography is performed primarily to study the contents of the spinal canal. The most common request is to search for the occult tethered cord. Other problems, such as

lipoma, hydromyelia and diastematomyelia, cysts of the spinal cord, and myelomeningocele, are presented. For more extensive discussion of spinal anomalies, the reader is referred to Chapter 55. See Table 26-1 for clinical findings, sonographic findings, and differential considerations for spinal anomalies.

TETHERED SPINAL CORD

The tethered spinal cord is a pathologic fixation of the spinal cord in an abnormal caudal location, so that the cord suffers mechanical stretching, distortion, and ischemia with daily activities, growth, and development. The tethered spinal cord, in addition to being in a more caudal location, is often fixed eccentrically within the canal (Figure 26-10). Spinal cord oscillations might be diminished in the tethered cord. If cord oscillations are present distant from the site of tethering, they are often dampened or absent closer to the point of fixation. This normal brisk oscillation of the cord is not as apparent in normal neonates as it is in older infants; therefore, looking for dampened or absent oscillations in neonates with tethered cords has limited usefulness (false positives). Most nonoscillating cords in neonates are normal and are not due to tethering. These oscillations usually diminish as the child grows, presumably because the cord is anchored and is being stretched.

LIPOMA

The tethered cord is usually associated with a mass of the lower cord or *filum terminale.* This anomaly comprises 20% to 50% of the spinal dysplasias. This mass often has lipomatous elements and can be continuous with the subcutaneous tissues and present as a fatty lump on the lower back. Lipomas can be isolated to the filum terminale or extend to and infiltrate the spinal cord and conus medullaris to varying degrees. Lipomas are usually echogenic and may present as a small or large mass (Figure 26-11).

HYDROMYELIA AND DIASTEMATOMYELIA

Hydromyelia is another sonographically observable abnormality of the spinal cord that can be seen in variable degrees. One should be aware that slight prominence of the central canal at the caudal end of the cord is a common finding in neonates. Focal hydromyelia is often present just cephalad to the site of tethering in dysraphic conditions such as myelomeningocele or lipomyelomeningocele. Hydromyelia might also accompany diastematomyelia (Figure 26-12), a condition in which the cord is split at one or more sites by an osseous, cartilaginous, or fibrous septum. The two segments of the cord can be seen most clearly on transverse views. They might rejoin caudal to the cleft. The vertebral column is virtually always abnormal on plain radiography in patients with diastematomyelia.

CYSTS OF THE SPINAL CORD

Small cysts in the filum terminale might be remnants of a terminal ventricle or an arachnoid pseudocyst and have no significance. A cyst in the cauda equina region may be seen with a thick filum terminale.

TABLE 26-1	SPINAL ANOMALIES	
Abnormality	Definition/Clinical Findings	Sonographic Findings
Tethered spinal cord	Tethered cord is a group of complicated developmental malformations of the spinal cord Benign; terrible consequences if not treated As children grow, the spinal cord is not able to grow because of the abnormal structures holding onto the cord Children may have pain or lose function of legs, bowel, or bladder Fatty mass may be present on mid to lower back Increased areas of pigmentation Dimples on back Large collections of hair on back	Cord fixed centrally within spinal canal Decreased cord oscillations
Lipoma	Fatty lump on lower back	Echogenic small to large mass
Hydromyelia	Increased fluid in the central canal of the spinal cord	Prominence of central canal at caudal end of cord Focal hydromyelia present cephalad to site of tethered cord
Diastematomyelia	A congenital fissure of the spinal cord, frequently associated with spina bifida cystica	Cord split at one or more sites by osseous cartilaginous or fibrous septum Vertebral column is always abnormal
Cysts of spinal cord	Well-marginated mass	Anechoic mass in cauda equina region
Myelomeningocele	Spina bifida with a portion of the spinal cord and membranes protruding	Flat nontubulated cord with nerve roots extending into the defect
Meningocele	Congenital hernia in which the meninges protrude through a defect in the skull or spinal column	Shows only fluid within the sac May have fine lacelike strands into the sac Cord may be eccentric or tethered

Figure 26-10 Tethered spinal cord. **A** and **B,** Longitudinal scans of the lumbosacral spine show how the spinal cord extends below the L3 vertebra before tapering into a conus. **C,** Transverse lumbar spine. The tethered spinal cord shows the cord is fixed eccentrically within the canal.

Figure 26-11 **A,** Longitudinal images of the echogenic leptomyelolipoma. **B,** MRI. The cord (*arrows* in A, *c* in B) extends to the lumbosacral *(LS)* junction, where it is tethered by the mass, *m.* (From Rumack CM: *Diagnostic ultrasound,* ed 2, St Louis, 1998, Mosby.)

Figure 26-12 Diastematomyelia. Transverse scan of the lumbar spinal canal shows left and right hemicords. Each hemicord has an eccentric central canal.

MYELOMENINGOCELE OR MYELOSCHISIS

The primary reason for studying the cord in cases of clinically obvious myelomeningocele or **myeloschisis** is to exclude additional cord pathology, such as diastematomyelia.

Intraoperative sonography has been successfully used to detect the margin of the skin defect. The anatomy of the cord, adhesion of the cord to the dorsal aspect of the spinal canal cephalad to the defect, and the appearance of the neural placode and nerve roots in the defect can all be seen on a sonogram.

Sonography is used to distinguish a meningocele from a myelomeningocele or if the dysraphic defect is skin-covered (Figure 26-13). Myelomeningocele shows a flat nontubulated cord (neural placode) with nerve roots extending into the defect. The nerve roots rise from the neural placode with dorsal roots lateral and ventral roots medial. In contrast, a meningocele shows nothing but fluid within the sac. However, a meningocele can also contain fine lacelike strands extending into the sac. These fibers are finer than nerve roots and are strands of lining tissue, such as arachnoid. Although the spinal cord is tabulated and does not enter the sac in a meningocele, the cord might be focally eccentric in the canal and even be tethered by a focal adhesion.

OTHER INDICATIONS AND ASSOCIATIONS

Midline cutaneous abnormalities over the lower back have been the most common reason for requesting neonatal spinal sonography. Midline dimples over the lower back occur in approximately 2% to 4.3% of newborns. Most are low sacral or coccygeal pits without an associated tethered cord. A tract can sometimes be seen and followed, especially if it is fluid filled or if it disrupts normal soft tissue planes. The soft tissue interfaces are continuous echogenic lines between skin, subcutaneous fat, muscle, and fascia. A sinus tract will disrupt the echogenic line with possible extension to the dura. However, dural penetration is difficult to ascertain or exclude on sonography. The neonatal coccyx is usually of very low echogenicity and should not be mistaken for a cyst or fluid collection.

During the first month of gestation, the neural tube is closing, whereas neural and epithelial tissues are differentiating from the overlying ectoderm. The concurrence of these events might explain the coincidence of midline cutaneous and spinal defects. Midline hair patches, fatty lumps, skin tags, pigmented nevi, lumbar dimples, aplasia cutis, and hemangiomas over the back should prompt a search for an occult tethered spinal cord. Hemangiomas seem to have a high association with tethered spinal cord. Tethered cord has an association with neonates with imperforate anus.

Meningomyelocele   Myelomeningocele

A   **B**

Figure 26-13 **A,** Meningomyelocele is a hernia of the spinal cord and membranes through a defect in the vertebral column. **B,** Myelomeningocele is seen in patients with spina bifida with a portion of the spinal cord and membranes protruding through the defect.

SELECTED BIBLIOGRAPHY

Beek FJA, Bax KMA, Mali WFTM: Sonography of the coccyx in newborns and infants, *J Ultrasound Med* 13:629-634, 1994.

Dick EA, Patel K, Owens CM: Spinal ultrasound in infants, *British Journal of Rad* 75:384-392, 2002.

DiPiertro MA: The conus medullaris: normal US findings throughout childhood, *Radiology* 188:149-153, 1993.

DiPiertro MA, Garver KA: Sonography of the neonatal spinal canal. In Haller JO, editor: *Textbook of neonatal ultrasound,* New York, 1998, Parthenon Publishing Group.

Glasier CM, Chadduck WM, Leithiser RE Jr and others: Screening spinal ultrasound in newborns with neural tube defects, *J Ultrasound Med* 9:339-343, 1990.

Kriss VM, Desai NS: Occult spinal dysraphism in neonates: assessment of high-risk cutaneous stigmata on sonography, *AJR* 171;4:1687-1692, 1998.

Kriss VM, Kriss TC, Babcock DS: The ventriculus terminalis of the spinal cord in the neonate: a normal variant on sonography, *Am J Radiol* 165:1491-1493, 1995.

Rypens F, Avni EF, Matos C and others: Atypical and equivocal sonographic features of the spinal cord in neonates, *Pediatr Radiol* 25:429-432, 1995.

Unsinn KM, Geley T, Freund MC and others: US of the spinal cord in newborns: spectrum of normal findings, variants, congenital abnormalities, and acquired diseases, *Radiographics* 20;4:923-938, 2000.

Ziegler M, Dorr U: Pediatric spinal sonography. Part I: anatomy and examination technique, *Pediatri Radiol* 18:9-13, 1988.

Glossary

abdominal aortic aneurysm – permanent localized dilation of an artery, with an increase in diameter of 1.5 times its normal diameter.

abdominal circumference (AC) – measurement at the level of the stomach, left portal vein, and left umbilical vein.

abduction – to move away from the body.

abruptio placenta – premature detachment of the placenta from the maternal wall.

abscess – localized collection of pus.

absorption – process of nutrient molecules passing through wall of intestine into blood or lymph system.

acardiac anomaly – a rare anomaly in monochorionic twins in which one twin develops without a heart and often without an upper half of the body.

accessory spleen – results from the failure of fusion of separate splenic masses forming on the dorsal mesogastrium; most commonly found in the splenic hilum or along the splenic vessels or associated ligaments.

achondrogenesis – lethal autosomal-recessive short-limb dwarfism marked by long bone and trunk shortening, decreased echogenicity of the bones and spine, and "flipperlike" appendages.

achondroplasia – a defect in the development of cartilage at the epiphyseal centers of the long bones producing short, square bones.

acidic – a type of solution that contains more hydrogen ions than hydroxyl ions.

acini cells – cells that perform exocrine function.

acinus (acini) – glandular (milk producing) component of the breast lobule (see terminal ductal-lobular unit, or TDLU). Each breast contains hundreds of lobules that each contain one or a few small glands (acini) along with the surrounding stromal connective tissue elements, the small ducts, a variable amount of fat, and Cooper's ligaments. The TDLU (a terminal duct and its corresponding acinus) is the site of origin of nearly all pathologic processes of the breast.

acoustic emission – occurs when an appropriate level of acoustic energy is applied to the tissue, the microbubbles first oscillate and then rupture; the rupture of the microbubbles results in random Doppler shifts appearing as a transient mosaic of colors on a color Doppler display.

acoustic impedance – measure of a material's resistance to the propagation of sound; expressed as the product of acoustic velocity of the medium and the density of the medium ($Z = pc$).

acrania – condition associated with anencephaly in which there is complete or partial absence of the cranial bones.

acrocephalopolysyndactyly – congenital anomaly characterized by a peaked head and webbed fingers and toes.

acromioclavicular joint (AC) – the joint found in the shoulder that connects the clavicle to the acromion process of the scapula.

acute tubular necrosis – acute damage to the renal tubules; usually due to ischemia associated with shock.

Addison's disease – condition caused by hyposecretion of hormones from the adrenal cortex.

adduction – to move toward the body.

adenoma – tumor of the glandular tissue.

adenomyomatosis – small polypoid projections.

adenomyosis – benign invasive growth of the endometrium that may cause heavy, painful menstrual bleeding.

adenopathy – enlargement of the lymph nodes.

adenosis – disease of the glands. In the breast, overgrowth of the stromal and epithelial elements of the small glands (acini) within the breast lobule. Adenosis is one component of fibrocystic condition, recognized by characteristic histopathologic changes in a breast biopsy specimen. Adenosis can exist by itself or in conjunction with other manifestations of fibrocystic conditions, such as fibrosis (e.g., sclerosing adenosis combines adenosis with surrounding fibrosis), and is often mistaken for possible breast cancer.

adrenal hemorrhage – hemorrhage that occurs when the fetus is stressed during a difficult delivery or a hypoxic insult.

afferent arteriole – arteriole that carries blood into the glomerulus of the nephron.

alimentary canal – also known as the gastrointestinal tract; includes the mouth, pharynx, esophagus, stomach, duodenum, and small and large intestines.

alkaline – a type of solution that contains more hydroxyl ions than hydrogen ions.

allantoic duct – elongated duct that contributes to the development of the umbilical cord and placenta during the first trimester.

alobar holoprosencephaly – most severe form of holoprosencephaly, characterized by a single common ventricle and malformed brain; orbital anomalies range from fused orbits to hypotelorism, with frequent nasal anomalies and clefting of the lip and palate.

alpha-fetoprotein (AFP) – protein manufactured by the fetus, which can be studied in amniotic fluid and maternal serum. Elevations of alpha-fetoprotein may indicate fetal anomalies (neural tube, abdominal wall, gastrointestinal), multiple gestations, or incorrect patient dates. Decreased levels may be associated with chromosomal abnormalities.

amaurosis fugax – transient partial or complete loss of vision in one eye.

American College of Radiology (ACR) – a national professional organization of physicians who specialize in radiology. Agency that first began voluntary accreditation of facilities performing screening mammography and that created the BI-RADS system of reporting and classifying mammograms that was later made mandatory by federal legislation (Mammography Quality Standards Act of 1994).

amniocentesis – aspiration of a sample of amniotic fluid through the mother's abdomen for diagnosis of fetal maturity and/or disease by assay of the constituents of the fluid.

amnion – smooth membrane enclosing the fetus and amniotic fluid; it is loosely fused with the outer chorionic membrane.

amniotic band syndrome – rupture of the amnion that leads to entrapment or entanglement of the fetal parts by the "sticky" chorion.

amniotic bands – multiple fibrous strands of amnion that develop in utero that may entangle fetal parts to cause amputations or malformations of the fetus.

amniotic cavity – cavity in which the fetus exists that forms early in gestation and surrounds the embryo; amniotic fluid fills the cavity to protect the embryo and fetus.

amniotic fluid – produced by the umbilical cord and membranes, and by the fetal lung, skin, and kidneys.

amniotic fluid index (AFI) – sum of the four quadrants of amniotic fluid. The uterus is divided into four quadrants; each "quadrant" is evaluated with the transducer perpendicular to the table in the deepest vertical pocket without fetal parts; the four quadrants are added together to determine the amniotic fluid index.

amplitude – strength of the ultrasound wave measured in decibels.

ampulla of Vater – small opening in the duodenum in which the pancreatic and common bile duct enter to release secretions.

amylase – enzyme secreted by the pancreas to aid in the digestion of carbohydrates.

amyloidosis – metabolic disorder marked by amyloid deposits in organs and tissue.

anaplastic carcinoma – rare, undifferentiated carcinoma occurring in middle age.

androgen – substance that stimulates the development of male characteristics, such as the hormones testosterone and androsterone.

anechoic – without echoes; simple cyst on ultrasound should be anechoic.

anembryonic pregnancy (blighted ovum) – ovum without an embryo.

anemia – abnormal condition in which blood lacks either a normal number of red blood cells or normal concentration of hemoglobin.

anencephaly – neural tube defect characterized by the lack of development of the cerebral and cerebellar hemispheres and cranial vault; this abnormality is incompatible with life.

angle of incidence – angle at which the ultrasound beams strike the interface between two types of tissue.

angle of reflection – the amplitude of the reflected wave depends on the difference between the acoustic impedances of the two materials forming the interface.

anisotropy – the quality of comprising varying values of a given property when measured in different directions.

anomaly – an abnormality or congenital malformation.

anophthalmia – absent eyes.

anophthalmos – absence of one (cyclops) or both eyes.

anorectal atresia – complex disorder of the bowel and genitourinary tract.

anterior cerebral artery (ACA) – smaller of the two terminal branches of the internal carotid artery.

anterior communicating artery (AcoA) – a short vessel that connects the anterior cerebral arteries at the interhemispheric fissure.

anterior pararenal space – space located between the anterior surface of the renal fascia and the posterior area of the peritoneum.

anterior tibial artery – artery that begins at the popliteal artery and travels down the lateral calf in the anterior compartment to the level of the ankle.

anterior tibial veins – veins that drain blood from the dorsum of the foot and anterior compartment of the calf.

anteverted – position of the uterus when the fundus is tipped slightly forward.

antiradial – plane of imaging on ultrasound of the breast that is perpendicular to the radial plane of imaging. The radial plane of imaging uses the nipple as the center point of an imaginary clock face imposed on the breast, such that the radial 12 o'clock plane is a line extending upward toward the top of the breast. Similarly, the radial 9 o'clock plane extends straight out to the right aspect of the breast, and so on. Three-dimensional measurements of a breast mass can be recorded using sagittal transverse or radial/antiradial planes.

aorta – largest arterial structure in the body; arises from the left ventricle of the heart to supply blood to the head, upper and lower extremities, and abdominopelvic cavity by descending into the abdominal cavity to branch into iliac vessels at the level of the umbilicus.

apex of prostate – inferior region of the prostate.

apex of ventricle – the ventricles of the heart come to a point called the *apex*; normally the apex is directed toward the left hip.

aphasia – inability to communicate by speech or writing.

apical – position of the transducer located over cardiac apex (at the point of maximal impulse).

apocrine metaplasia – in the breast, an increase in the number and activity of the lining cells of the breast acini (glands). These lining cells normally secrete only a small amount of fluid in the nonlactating breast. Fluid production can often increase with apocrine metaplasia, which is one of the conditions thought to be responsible for the formation of benign fluid-filled breast cysts.

aponeurosis – band-like flat tendons connecting muscle to the bone.

appendicitis – inflammation of the appendix.

appendicolith – echogenic structure within the appendix.

aqueductal stenosis – blockage of the duct connecting the third and fourth ventricles.

arcuate arteries – arteries that lie at the bases of the medullary pyramids and appear as echogenic structures.

arcuate vessels – small vessels found along the periphery of the uterus.

arcuate arteries – small vessels found at the bases of the renal pyramids.

areola – the pigmented skin surrounding the breast nipple.

arhinia – absence of the nose.

Arnold-Chiari malformation – defect in which the cerebellum and brainstem are pulled toward the spinal cord (banana sign); frontal bossing, or "lemon head," is also evident on ultrasound.

arteries – vascular structures that carry blood away from the heart.

arteriosclerosis – thickening and hardening of arterial walls.

arteriovenous fistula – communication between an artery and vein.

ascites – accumulation of serous fluid in the peritoneal cavity.

asphyxiating thoracic dystrophy – significantly narrow diameter of the chest in a fetus.

asplenia – no development of splenic tissue.

assisted reproductive technology (ART) – technologies employed to assist the infertility patient to become pregnant. These methods include in vitro fertilization, gamete intrafallopian transfer, zygote intrafallopian transfer, and artificial insemination.

asymptomatic – without symptoms.

ataxia – impaired ability to coordinate movement, especially disturbances of gait.

atrial fibrillation – condition in which the atria beat more than 400 beats per minute and the ventricular rate is 120 to 200 beats per minute.

atrial septal defect – communication between the right and left atrium that persists after birth.

atrioventricular block – block of transmission of the electrical impulse from the atria to the ventricles (may be 2:1 or 3:1 block).

atrioventricular node – area of specialized cardiac muscle that receives the cardiac impulse from the sinoatrial node and conducts it to the atrioventricular bundles.

atrioventricular septal defect – defect that occurs when the endocardial cushion fails to fuse in the center of the heart.

atrioventricular valve – valve located between the atria and ventricle.

atrium (trigone) of the lateral ventricles – the ventricle is measured at this site (junction of the anterior, occipital, and temporal horn) on the axial view.

attenuation – reduction in the amplitude and intensity of a sound wave as it propagates through a medium; attenuation of ultrasound waves in tissue is caused by absorption and by scattering and reflection.

atypical ductal hyperplasia (ADH) – see atypical hyperplasia.

atypical hyperplasia – abnormal proliferation of cells with atypical features involving the TDLU, with an increased likelihood of evolving into breast cancer; in atypical ductal hyperplasia (ADH), the pathologist recognizes some, but not all, of the features of ductal carcinoma in situ (DCIS); atypical lobular hyperplasia (ALH) shows some, but not all, of the features of lobular carcinoma in situ (LCIS); ALH and LCIS are now grouped by some authors under the term lobular neoplasia.

atypical lobular hyperplasia (ALH) – see atypical hyperplasia; lobular neoplasia.

augmentation – increase in blood flow velocity with distal limb compression or with the release of proximal limb compression.

auscultation – procedure of listening to the heart sounds with a stethoscope.

autoimmune hemolytic anemia – anemia caused by antibodies produced by the patient's own immune system.

autonomy – self-governing or self-directing freedom and especially moral independence; the right of persons to choose and to have their choices respected.

axial plane – placement of the transducer above the ear (above the canthomeatal line).

axilla – armpit.

axillary artery – continuation of the subclavian artery.

axillary vein – vein that begins where the basilic vein joins the brachial vein in the upper arm and terminates beneath the clavicle at the outer border of the first rib.

banana sign – the shape of the cerebellum when a spinal defect is present (cerebellum is pulled downward into the foramen magnum).

bare area – area superior to the liver that is not covered by peritoneum so that the inferior vena cava may enter the chest.

Barlow maneuver – the patient lies in the supine position with the hip flexed 90 degrees and adducted. Downward and outward pressure is applied. If the hip is dislocated, the examiner will feel the femoral head move out of the acetabulum.

basal body temperature – the morning body temperature taken orally before the patient does any activity.

base – superior region of the prostate.

basilar artery – artery formed by the union of the two vertebral arteries.

basilic vein – vein that originates on the small finger side of the dorsum of the hand.

battledore placenta – marginal or eccentric insertion of the umbilical cord into the placenta.

Beckwith-Wiedemann syndrome – group of disorders having in common the coexistence of an omphalocele, macroglossia, and visceromegaly.

beneficence – quality or state of being beneficent (doing good, such as performing acts of kindness).

benign prostatic hypertrophy – enlargement of the glandular component of the prostate.

bicornuate uterus – duplication of the uterus (two horns and one vagina).

bicuspid aortic valve – two leaflets instead of the normal three leaflets with asymmetric cusps.

bile – bile pigment, old blood cells, and the by-products of phagocytosis are known together as *bile*.

bilirubin – yellow pigment in bile formed by the breakdown of red blood cells.

biophysical profile (BPP) – assessment of fetus to determine fetal well-being; includes evaluation of cardiac non-stress test, fetal breathing movement, gross fetal body movements, fetal tone, and amniotic fluid volume.

biparietal diameter (BPD) – measurement of the fetal head at the level of the thalamus and cavum septum pellucidum.

blood urea nitrogen (BUN) – laboratory measurement of the amount of nitrogenous waste, along with creatinine; waste products accumulate in the blood when kidneys malfunction.

body of the pancreas – located in the midepigastrium anterior to the superior mesenteric artery and vein, aorta, and inferior vena cava.

bowel herniation – extrusion of the bowel outside the abdominal cavity; during the first trimester normally occurs between 8 and 12 weeks.

Bowman's capsule – the cup-shaped end of a renal tubule enclosing a glomerulus; site of filtration of the kidney; contains water, salts, glucose, urea, and amino acids.

brachial artery – continuation of the axillary artery.

brachycephaly – fetal head is elongated in the transverse diameter and shortened in the anteroposterior diameter.

brainstem – comprises the midbrain, pons, and medulla oblongata.

branchial cleft cyst – remnant of embryonic development that appears as a cyst in the neck.

Braxton-Hicks contractions – spontaneous painless uterine contractions described originally as a sign of pregnancy; they occur from the first trimester to the end of pregnancy.

breast – differentiated apocrine sweat gland with a functional purpose of secreting milk during lactation.

breast cancer (breast carcinoma) – breast cancer involves two main types of cells: ductal and lobular. Ductal cancer, accounting for approximately 85% of the breast cancer cases, also includes many subtypes, such as medullary, mucinous, tubular, apocrine, or papillary types. In addition, very early or preinvasive breast cancer is generally ductal in type. This preinvasive breast cancer is also called *in situ*, *noninvasive*, or *intraductal* breast cancer. Another commonly used term for this early type of cancer is *ductal carcinoma in situ*, or *DCIS*.

breast cancer screening – screening for breast cancer involves annual screening mammography (starting at age 40), monthly breast self-examination (BSE), and self-breast examination (SBE).

Breast Imaging Reporting and Data System (BI-RADS) – trademark system created by the American College of Radiology (ACR) to standardize mammographic reporting terminology, categorize breast abnormalities according to the level of suspicion for malignancy, and facilitate outcome monitoring. This system of classification of breast imaging results has now been made a mandatory part of mammogram reports by federal legislation (Mammography Quality Standards Act of 1994).

breast self-examination (BSE) – part of breast cancer screening; every woman is encouraged to perform breast self-examination monthly starting at age 20; BSE is usually best performed at the end of menses.

breech – indicates the fetal head is toward the fundus of the uterus.

bronchogenic cyst – most common lung cyst detected prenatally.

bronchopulmonary sequestration – extrapulmonary tissue is present within the pleural lung sac (intralobar) or connected to the inferior border of the lung within its own pleural sac (extralobar).

bruit – noise caused by tissue vibration produced by turbulence.

Budd-Chiari syndrome – thrombosis of the hepatic veins.

buffer – chemical compound that can act as a weak acid or a base to combine with excess hydrogen or hydroxyl ions to neutralize the pH in blood.

bulbus cordis – primitive chamber that forms the right ventricle.

bulk modulus – amount of pressure required to compress a small volume of material a small amount.

bull's eye (target) lesion – hypoechoic mass with echogenic central core (abscess, metastasis).

bursa – a saclike structure containing thick fluid that surrounds areas subject to friction, such as the interface between bone and tendon.

calcitonin – a thyroid hormone that is important for maintaining a dense, strong bone matrix and regulating the blood calcium level.

caliectasis – rounded calyces with renal pelvis dilation measuring greater than 10 mm in the anteroposterior direction.

calyx – part of the collecting system adjacent to the pyramid that collects urine and is connected to the major calyx.

capillaries – minute vessels that connect the arterial and venous systems.

cardiac orifice – entrance of the esophagus into the stomach occurs at the cardiac orifice.

cardiomyopathy – disease of the myocardial muscle layer of the heart that causes the heart to dilate secondary to regurgitation and also affects cardiac function.

cardiosplenic syndromes – sporadic disorders characterized by symmetric development of normally asymmetric organs or organ systems.

cartilage interface sign – echogenic line on the anterior surface of the cartilage surrounding the humeral head.

cauda equina – bundle of nerve roots from the lumbar, sacral, and coccygeal spinal nerves that descend nearly vertically from the spinal cord until they reach their respective openings in the vertebral column.

caudal pancreatic artery – branch of the splenic artery that supplies the tail of the pancreas.

caudal regression syndrome – lack of development of the lower limbs (may occur in the fetus of a diabetic mother).

caudate lobe – small lobe of the liver situated on the posterosuperior surface of the left lobe; the ligamentum venosum is the anterior border.

caudate nucleus – area of the brain that forms the lateral borders of the anterior horns, anterior to the thalamus.

cavernous transformation of the portal vein – periportal collateral channels in patients with chronic portal vein obstruction.

cavum septum pellucidum – prominent structure best seen in the midline filled with cerebrospinal fluid in the premature infant.

cebocephaly – form of holoprosencephaly characterized by a common ventricle, hypotelorism, and a nose with a single nostril.

celiac axis – first major anterior artery to arise from the abdominal aorta inferior to the diaphragm; it branches into the hepatic, splenic, and left gastric arteries.

central zone – portion of the prostate that surrounds the urethra; site of benign prostatic hypertrophy.

centripetal artery – terminal intratesticular arteries arising from the capsular arteries.

cephalic vein – vein that begins on the thumb side of the dorsum of the hand.

cephalocele – protrusion of the brain from the cranial cavity.

cerebellum – area of the brain that lies posterior to the brainstem below the tentorium.

cerebral vasospasm – vasoconstriction of the arteries.

cerebrum – two equal hemispheres; largest part of the brain.

cervical polyp – hyperplastic protrusion of the epithelium of the cervix; may be broad based or pedunculated.

cervical stenosis – acquired condition with obstruction of the cervical canal.

cervix – inferior segment of the uterus; more than 3.5 cm long during normal pregnancy, decreases in length during labor.

cholangitis – inflammation of the bile duct.

cholecystectomy – removal of the gallbladder.

cholecystitis – acute or chronic inflammation of the gallbladder.

cholecystokinin – hormone secreted into the blood by the mucosa of the upper small intestine; stimulates contraction of the gallbladder and pancreatic secretion of enzymes.

choledochal cyst – cystic growth of the common bile duct that may cause obstruction.

choledocholithiasis – stones in the bile duct.

cholelithiasis – gallstones.

cholesterosis – variant of adenomyomatosis; cholesterol polyps.

choriocarcinoma – malignant invasive form of gestational trophoblastic disease.

chorion – cellular, outermost extraembryonic membrane, composed of trophoblast lined with mesoderm; it develops villi about 2 weeks after fertilization, is vascularized by allantoic vessels a week later, gives rise to the placenta, and persists until birth.

chorion frondosum – the portion of the chorion that develops into the fetal portion of the placenta.

chorionic cavity – surrounds the amniotic cavity; the yolk sac is between the chorion and amnion.

chorionic plate – that part of the chorionic membrane that covers the placenta.

chorionic villi – vascular projections from the chorion.

choroid plexus – echogenic cluster of cells important in the production of cerebrospinal fluid that lie along the atrium of the lateral ventricles.

circle of Willis – vascular network at the base of the brain.

circummarginate placenta – condition in which the chorionic plate of the placenta is smaller than the basal plate, with a flat interface between the fetal membranes and the placenta.

circumvallate placenta – condition in which the chorionic plate of the placenta is smaller than the basal plate; the margin is raised with a rolled edge.

cistern – reservoir for cerebrospinal fluid.

clapper-in-the-bell sign – hypoechoic hematoma found at the end of a completely retracted muscle fragment.

claudication – walking-induced muscular discomfort of the calf, thigh, hip, or buttock.

clinical breast examination (CBE) – examination of the breast by a health care provider; part of breast cancer screening. Every woman is encouraged to have a thorough CBE in conjunction with her routine health care assessment. Between ages 20 and 40, CBE is advised every 3 years. From age 40 on, CBE should be performed by the woman's regular health care provider annually.

cloacal exstrophy – defect in the lower abdominal wall and anterior wall of the urinary bladder.

C-loop of the duodenum – forms the lateral border of the head of the pancreas.

coagulopathy – a defect in blood-clotting mechanisms.

coarctation of the aorta – discrete or long segment narrowing in the aortic arch, usually at the level of the left subclavian artery near the insertion of the ductus arteriosus.

coccygeus muscles – muscles that form the floor of the pelvis.

collateral circulation – circulation that develops when normal venous channels become obstructed.

collateral vessels – ancillary vessels that develop when portal hypertension occurs.

color flow mapping (CFM) – ability to display blood flow in multiple colors depending on the velocity, direction of flow, and extent of turbulence.

column of Bertin – bands of cortical tissue that separate the renal pyramids; a prominent column of Bertin may mimic a renal mass on sonography.

comet tail artifact (ring-down) – posterior linear equidistant artifact created when sound reverberates between two strong reflectors, such as air bubbles, metal, and glass.

common bile duct – duct that extends from the point where the common hepatic duct meets the cystic duct; drains into the duodenum after it joins with the main pancreatic duct.

common carotid artery (CCA) – artery that rises from the aortic arch to supply blood to the head and neck.

common duct – refers to common bile or hepatic ducts when cystic duct is not seen.

common femoral arteries – arteries originating from the iliac arteries and seen in the inguinal region into the upper thigh.

common femoral vein – vein formed by the confluence of the profunda femoris and the superficial femoral vein; also receives the greater saphenous vein.

common hepatic artery – artery arising from the celiac trunk to supply the liver.

common hepatic duct – bile duct system that drains the liver into the common bile duct.

common iliac arteries – a division of the abdominal aorta at the level of the umbilicus to supply blood to the lower extremities.

common iliac vein – vein formed by the confluence of the internal and external iliac veins.

complete abortion – complete removal of all products of conception, including the placenta.

complete atrioventricular septal defect – large ventricular and atrial septal defect with a single, undivided, free-floating leaflet that stretches between both ventricles.

complete mole – trophoblastic parts without a fetus; forms when the sperm fertilizes an empty egg.

confidentiality – the nondisclosure of certain information except to another authorized person.

confluence of the splenic and portal veins – junction of the splenic and portal veins that occurs in the midabdomen and serves as the posterior border of the pancreas.

congenital bronchial atresia – pulmonary anomaly that results from the focal obliteration of a segment of the bronchial lumen.

congenital mesoblastic nephroma – most common benign renal tumor of the neonate and infant.

conjoined twins – monozygotic twins physically joined by varying degrees; condition that occurs when the division of the egg occurs after 13 days.

continuous wave probe – probe with which sound is continuously emitted from one transducer and continuously received by a second transducer.

contrast-enhanced sonography – sonography in which an agent is used to reduce or eliminate some of the current limitations of ultrasound imaging and Doppler blood flow detection.

conus medullaris – the caudal end of the spinal cord.

Cooper's ligaments – connective tissue septae that connect perpendicularly to the breast lobules and extend out to the skin; are considered to be the fibrous "skeleton" supporting the breast glandular tissue.

coronal – horizontal plane through the longitudinal axis of the body to image structures from anterior to posterior.

coronal plane – transducer is perpendicular to the anterior fontanelle in the coronal axis of the head.

corpus callosum – prominent group of nerve fibers that connect the right and left sides of the brain; found superior to the third ventricle.

corpus luteum – yellow body formed from the Graafian follicle after ovulation that produces estrogen and progesterone.

corpus luteum cyst – small endocrine structure that develops within a ruptured ovarian follicle and secretes progesterone and estrogen. It may persist until the 20th to 24th week of pregnancy.

cortex – outer parenchyma of an organ. Liver cortex is thin in the neonate, with echogenicity similar to or slightly greater than that of the normal liver parenchyma.

cran- – helmet; *cranial*: pertaining to the portion of the skull that surrounds the brain.

craniosynostoses – premature closure of the cranial sutures.

creatinine (Cr) – a product of metabolism; laboratory test measures the ability of the kidney to get rid of waste; waste products accumulate in the blood when the kidneys are malfunctioning.

cremasteric artery – small artery arising from the inferior epigastric artery (a branch of the external iliac artery), which supplies the peritesticular tissue, including the cremasteric muscle.

cremasteric muscle – an extension of the internal oblique muscle that descends to the testis with the spermatic cord; contraction of the cremasteric muscle shortens the spermatic cord and elevates the testis.

critical aortic stenosis – abnormal thickening and closure of the aortic leaflets in the second or third trimester causes the left ventricle to "balloon" from increased pressure.

Crohn's disease – inflammation of the bowel, accompanied by abscess and bowel wall thickening.

crossed renal ectopia – condition that occurs when the kidney is located on the opposite side of its ureteral orifice.

crown-rump length (CRL) – most accurate measurement for determining gestational age in the first trimester.

crus of the diaphragm – muscular structure in the upper abdomen at the level of the celiac axis.

cryptorchidism – failure of the testes to descend into the scrotum; testicles remain within the abdomen or groin and fail to descend into the scrotal sac.

crystal – special material in the ultrasound transducer that has the ability to convert electrical impulses into sound waves.

culling – process by which the spleen removes nuclei from the red blood cells as they pass through.

Cushing's syndrome – condition caused by hypersecretion of hormones from the adrenal cortex.

cycle – measurement of the vibration of the crystal in frequency per second.

cyclopia – severe form of holoprosencephaly characterized by a common ventricle, fusion of the orbits with one or two eyes present, and a proboscis (maldeveloped cylindrical nose).

cyst – fluid-filled sac of variable size.

cyst aspiration – common breast procedure (both diagnostic and interventional) that involves placing a needle through the skin of the breast into a cystic mass and pulling fluid out of the cystic mass through the needle. In the case of a palpable cyst, this procedure can be performed in a physician's office. In the case of a small, complex, or nonpalpable cyst, image guidance (usually with ultrasound) can be used to facilitate the aspiration.

cystadenocarcinoma – a malignant tumor that forms cysts.

cystadenoma – benign adenoma containing cysts.

cystic adenomatoid malformation – abnormality in the formation of the bronchial tree with secondary overgrowth of mesenchymal tissue from arrested bronchial development.

cystic duct – duct that connects the gallbladder to the common hepatic duct.

cystic fibrosis – inherited disorder of the exocrine glands; symptoms include mucus build-up within the lungs and other areas of the body.

cystic hygroma – dilation of jugular lymph sacs (may occur in axilla or groin) because of improper drainage of the lymphatic system into the venous system. Large, septated hygromas are frequently associated with Turner's syndrome, congestive heart failure, and death of the fetus in utero; isolated hygromas may occur as solitary lesions at birth.

cystic medial necrosis – weakening of the arterial wall.

dacryocystocele – cystic dilation of the lacrimal sac at the nasocanthal angle.

Dandy-Walker syndrome – displacement of the fourth ventricle, often accompanied by hydrocephalus.

dartos – layer of muscle underneath the scrotal skin.

decibel (dB) – unit used to quantitatively express the ratio of two amplitudes or intensities; decibels are not absolute units, but express one sound level or intensity in terms of another or in terms of a reference (e.g., the amplitude 10 cm from the transducer is 10 dB lower than the amplitude 5 cm from the transducer).

decidua basalis – the part of the decidua that unites with the chorion to form the placenta.

decidua capsularis – the part of the decidua that surrounds the chorionic sac.

deep femoral vein – vein that travels with the profunda femoris artery to unite with the superficial femoral vein to form the common femoral vein.

deep venous thrombosis (DVT) – blockage of the venous circulation (upper or lower) by a blood clot.

deferential artery – arises from the vesicle artery (a branch of the internal iliac artery) and supplies the vas deferens and epididymis.

DeQuervain's thyroiditis – inflammatory condition of the thyroid, sometimes occurring after a viral respiratory infection.

dermoid – benign tumor comprised of hair, muscle, teeth, and fat.

developmental displacement of the hip – abnormal condition of the hip that results in congenital hip dysplasia; includes dysplastic, subluxated, dislocatable, and dislocated hips.

diagnostic breast imaging – also called "consultative," "workup," or "problem-solving" mammography or breast imaging. This type of breast imaging examination is more intensive than routine screening mammography. Diagnostic breast imaging is usually directed toward a specific clinical symptom of possible breast cancer, or an abnormal finding on a screening mammogram. The goal of diagnostic breast imaging is to categorize the abnormality according to the level of suspicion for cancer (see Breast Imaging and Reporting System [BI-RADS]).

diamniotic – multiple pregnancy with two amniotic sacs.

diaphragmatic hernia – opening in the pleuroperitoneal membrane that develops in the first trimester.

diastematomyelia – a congenital fissure of the spinal cord, frequently associated with spina bifida cystica.

diastole – part of the cardiac cycle in which the ventricles are filling with blood; the tricuspid and mitral valves are open during this time.

dichorionic – multiple pregnancy with two chorionic sacs.

diffuse hepatocellular disease – disease that affects hepatocytes and interferes with liver function.

diffuse nontoxic goiter – condition that occurs as a compensatory enlargement of the thyroid gland resulting from thyroid hormone deficiency; also known as colloid goiter.

diplopia – double vision.

dissecting aneurysm – tear in the intima and/or media of the abdominal aorta.

dizygotic – twins that arise from two separately fertilized ova.

dolichocephaly – fetal head is shortened in the transverse plane and elongated in the anteroposterior plane.

Doppler effect – change in the frequency of a sound wave when either the source or the listener is moving relative to one another; the difference between the received echo frequency and the frequency of the transmitted beam is the Doppler shift; pulsed wave Doppler is used in most fetal examinations; this means that the transducer has the ability to send and receive Doppler signals.

Doppler sample volume – the sonographer selects the exact site to record Doppler signals and sets the sample volume (gate) at this site.

Doppler shift in frequency – change in frequency as red blood cells move from a lower-frequency sound source at rest toward a higher-frequency sound source; change in frequency.

dors- – back; *dorsal*: position toward the back of the body.

dorsal pancreatic artery – branch of the splenic artery that supplies the body of the pancreas.

dorsalis pedis artery – continuation of the anterior tibial artery on the top of the foot.

dorsiflexion – upward movement of the hand or foot.

double decidual sac sign – interface between the decidua capsularis and the echogenic, highly vascular endometrium.

double outlet right ventricle – ventricular septal defect with the overriding aorta directed more to the right ventricular outflow tract than the left (more than 50% override toward the right).

dromedary hump – normal variant that occurs on the left kidney as a bulge of the lateral border.

duct of Santorini – small accessory duct of the pancreas found in the head of the gland.

duct of Wirsung – largest duct of the pancreas that drains the tail, body, and head of the gland; it joins the common bile duct to enter the duodenum through the ampulla of Vater.

ductus arteriosus – communication between the pulmonary artery and descending aorta that closes after birth.

ductus venosus – fetal vein that connects the umbilical vein to the inferior vena cava and runs at an oblique axis through the liver.

duodenal atresia – complete blockage at the pyloric sphincter.

duodenal bulb – first part of the duodenum.

duodenal stenosis – narrowing of the pyloric sphincter.

dynamic range – ratio of the largest to smallest signals that an instrument or component of an instrument can respond to without distortion.

dysarthria – difficulty with speech because of impairment of the tongue or muscles essential to speech.

dysphagia – inability or difficulty in swallowing.

dysraphic – refers to the anomalies associated by incomplete embryologic development.

dysuria – painful or difficult urination.

Ebstein's anomaly – abnormal apical displacement of the septal leaflet of the tricuspid valve.

eclampsia – coma and seizures in the second- and third-trimester patient secondary to pregnancy-induced hypertension.

ectopia cordis – condition in which the ventral wall fails to close and the heart develops outside the thoracic cavity.

ectopic kidney – kidney located outside of the normal position, most often in the pelvic cavity.

ectopic pregnancy – pregnancy occurring outside the uterine cavity.

ectopic ureterocele – ectopic insertion and cystic dilation of distal ureter of duplicated renal collecting system; occurs more commonly in females (on left side).

efferent arteriole – arteriole that supplies the peritubular capillaries of the kidneys, which also supply the convoluted tubules.

ejaculatory ducts – ducts that connect the seminal vesicle and the vas deferens to the urethra at the verumontanum.

electrocardiography – study of the heart's electrical activity.

embryo – conceptus to the end of the ninth week of gestation.

embryo transfer – a technique that follows IVF in which the fertilized ova are injected into the uterus through the cervix.

embryologic age (conceptual age) – age since the date of conception.

embryonic period – time between 6 and 12 weeks.

encephalocele – protrusion of the brain through a cranial fissure.

endocardium – inner layer of the heart wall.

endocrine – process of cells that secrete into the blood or lymph circulation that has a specific effect on tissues in another part of the body.

endometrial carcinoma – condition that presents with abnormal thickening of the endometrial cavity; usually presents with irregular bleeding in perimenopausal and postmenopausal women.

endometrial hyperplasia – condition that results from estrogen stimulation to the endometrium without the influence of progestin; frequent cause of bleeding (especially in postmenopausal women).

endometrial polyp – pedunculated or sessile well-defined mass attached to the endometrial cavity.

endometrioma – localized tumor of endometriosis most frequently found in the ovary, cul-de-sac, rectovaginal septum, and peritoneal surface of the posterior wall of the uterus.

endometriosis – condition that occurs when functioning endometrial tissue invades sites outside the uterus.

endometritis – infection within the endometrium of the uterus.

endometrium – inner lining of the uterine cavity that appears echogenic to hypoechoic on ultrasound, depending on the menstrual cycle.

epicardium – outer layer of the heart wall.

epididymal cyst – cyst filled with clear, serous fluid located in the epididymis.

epididymis – anatomic structure that lies posterior and lateral to the testes in which the spermatozoa accumulate.

epididymitis – infection and inflammation of the epididymis.

epigastric – above the umbilicus and between the costal margins.

epigastrium – area between the right and left hypochondrium that contains part of the liver, duodenum, and pancreas.

epignathus – teratoma located in the oropharynx.

epineurium – the covering of a nerve that consists of connective tissue.

epiploic foramen – opening to the lesser sac.

epitheliosis – overgrowth of cells lining the small ducts of the terminal ductal-lobular unit; one of the common components of most varieties of fibrocystic condition.

erythroblastosis fetalis – hemolytic disease marked by anemia, enlargement of liver and spleen, and hydrops fetalis.

erythrocyte – red blood cell.

erythropoiesis – production of red blood cells.

esophageal atresia – congenital hypoplasia of the esophagus; usually associated with a tracheoesophageal fistula.

esophageal stenosis – narrowing of the esophagus, usually in the distal third segment.

estimated fetal weight (EFW) – estimation based on incorporation of all fetal growth parameters (biparietal diameter, head circumference, abdominal circumference, femur and humeral length).

estrogen – the female hormone produced by the ovary.

ethics – discipline dealing with what is good and bad and with moral duty and obligation.

euthyroid – refers to a normal functioning thyroid gland.

exencephaly – abnormal condition in which the brain is located outside the cranium.

exocrine – process of secreting outwardly through a duct to the surface of an organ or tissue or into a vessel.

exophthalmia – abnormal protrusion of the eyeball.

exstrophy of the bladder – protrusion of the posterior wall of the urinary bladder, which contains the trigone of the bladder and the ureteric orifices.

external carotid artery (ECA) – smaller of the two terminal branches of the common carotid artery.

external iliac vein – vein that drains the pelvis along with the internal iliac vein.

extracorporeal shock-wave lithotripsy – a device that breaks up kidney stones; the shock waves are focused on the stones, disintegrating them and permitting their passage in the urine.

extrahepatic – outside the liver.

falciform ligament – ligament that attaches the liver to the anterior abdominal wall and undersurface of the diaphragm.

false knots of the umbilical cord – condition that occurs when blood vessels are longer than the cord; they fold on themselves and produce nodulations on the surface of the cord.

false pelvis – portion of the pelvic cavity that is above the pelvic brim, bounded posteriorly by the lumbar vertebrae, laterally by the iliac fossae and iliacus muscles, and anteriorly by the lower anterior abdominal wall.

falx cerebri (interhemispheric fissure) – echogenic fibrous structure separating the cerebral hemispheres.

fascia lata – deep fascia of the thigh.

fasciculi – term describing a small bundle of muscles, nerves, and tendons.

febrile – has a fever.

fecalith – calculus that may form around fecal material associated with appendicitis.

femoral triangle – description of a region at the front of the upper thigh, just below the inguinal ligament.

femoral veins – upper part of the venous drainage system of the lower extremity that empties into the inferior vena cava at the level of the diaphragm.

femur length (FL) – measurement from the femoral head to the distal end of the femur.

fetal cystic hygroma – malformation of the lymphatic system that leads to single or multiloculated lymph-filled cavities around the neck.

fetal goiter (thyromegaly) – enlargement of the thyroid gland.

fetal hydronephrosis – dilated renal pelvis.

fetus papyraceous – fetal death that occurs after the fetus has reached a certain growth that is too large to resorb into the uterus.

fever – elevation of normal body temperature (above 98.6° F).

fibroadenoma – most common benign solid tumor of the breast, consisting predominantly of fibrous and epithelial (adenomatous) tissue elements. These masses tend to develop in young women (even teenagers), tend to run in families, and can be multiple. The usual appearance of a fibroadenoma is a benign-appearing mammographic mass (round, oval, or gently lobular and well circumscribed) with a correlating sonographic mass that is well defined and demonstrates homogeneous echogenicity.

fibrocystic condition (FCC) – also called *fibrocystic change* or *fibrocystic breast*, this condition represents many different tissue processes within the breast that are all basically normal processes that over time can get exaggerated to the point of causing symptoms or mammographic changes that raise concern for breast cancer. The main fibrocystic tissue processes are adenosis, epitheliosis, and fibrosis. These processes can cause symptoms such as breast lumps and pain. These processes can cause mammographic changes such as cysts, microcalcifications, distortion, and mass-like densities. Pathologic changes of fibrocystic condition include apocrine metaplasia, microcystic adenosis, blunt ductal adenosis, epithelial ductal hyperplasia, lobular hyperplasia, and sclerosing adenosis. Only a few fibrocystic tissue processes are associated with an increased risk of subsequent development of breast cancer. These include atypical ductal hyperplasia and lobular neoplasia (formerly called lobular carcinoma in situ).

filum terminale – slender tapering terminal section of the spinal cord.

fine needle aspiration – the use of a fine-gauge needle to obtain cells from a mass.

first generation agents – agents containing room air (i.e., Albunex).

focal nodular hyperplasia – liver tumors with an abundance of Kupffer cells; sonographically, they are isoechoic to the surrounding normal liver tissue.

focal zone – the region over which the effective width of the sound beam is within some measure of its width at the focal distance.

focused assessment with sonography for trauma – limited examination of the abdomen or pelvis to evaluate free fluid or pericardial fluid.

follicle-stimulating hormone (FSH) – hormone produced in the pituitary that influences the ovaries.

follicular carcinoma – occurs as a solitary mass within the thyroid gland.

follicular cyst – benign cyst within the ovary that may occur and disappear on a cyclic basis.

fontanelle – soft space between the bones; the space is usually large enough to accommodate the ultrasound transducer until the age of 12 months.

foramen of Bochdalek – type of diaphragmatic defect that occurs posterior and lateral in the diaphragm; usually found in the left side.

foramen of Morgagni – diaphragmatic hernia that occurs anterior and medial in the diaphragm and may communicate with the pericardial sac.

foramen ovale – opening between the free edge of the septum secundum and the dorsal wall of the atrium; also termed *fossae ovale*.

four chamber – view that transects the heart approximately parallel with dorsal and ventral surfaces of body.

four-dimensional (4-D) ultrasound – ability to reconstruct the 3-D image and see it in real time.

frame rate – rate at which images are updated on the display; dependent on frequency of the transducer and depth selection.

frank dislocation – the hip is laterally and posteriorly displaced to the extent that the femoral head has no contact with the acetabulum and the normal "U" configuration cannot be obtained on ultrasound.

free hand – system that uses a smooth sweeping motion in a single plane of acquisition.

fremitus – refers to vibrations produced by phonation and felt through the chest wall during palpation; a technique used in conjunction with power Doppler to identify the margins of a lesion.

frequency – number of cycles per second that a periodic event or function undergoes; number of cycles completed per unit of time; the frequency of a sound wave is determined by the number of oscillations per second of the vibrating source.

frontal bossing – slight indentation of the frontal bones of the skull; also known as "lemon head."

functional cyst – cyst resulting from the normal function of the ovary.

fusiform dilation – enlargement with tapering at both ends.

gain – measure of the strength of the ultrasound signal; can be expressed as a simple ratio or in decibels; overall gain amplifies all signals by a constant factor regardless of the depth.

Galeazzi sign – the knee is lower in position on the affected side when the patient is supine and the knees are flexed. On physical examination, the knee is lower in position on the affected side of the neonate with DDH when the patient is supine and the knees are flexed.

gallbladder – storage pouch for bile.

gamete intrafallopian transfer (GIFT) – a human fertilization technique in which male and female gametes are injected through a laparoscope into the fimbriated ends of the fallopian tubes. Recently, this has been performed under ultrasound guidance.

Gartner's duct cyst – small cyst within the vagina.

gastrin – endocrine hormone released from the stomach (stimulates secretion of gastric acid).

gastrocnemius veins – paired veins that lie in the medial and lateral gastrocnemius muscles and terminate into the popliteal vein.

gastroduodenal artery – branch of the common hepatic artery that supplies the stomach and duodenum.

gastrophrenic ligament – ligament that helps support the greater curvature of the stomach.

gastroschisis – congenital fissure that remains open in the wall of the abdomen just to the right of the umbilical cord; bowel and other organs may protrude outside the abdomen from this opening.

gastrosplenic ligament – one of the ligaments between the stomach and spleen that helps hold the spleen in place.

Gaucher's disease – one of the storage diseases in which fat and proteins are deposited abnormally in the body.

germinal matrix – fragile periventricular tissue (includes the caudate nucleus) that easily bleeds in the premature infant.

Gerota's fascia – another term for the renal fascia; the kidney is covered by the renal capsule, perirenal fat, Gerota's fascia, and pararenal fat.

gestational age – age of embryo since the date of conception.

gestational sac – structure that is normally within the uterus that contains the developing embryo.

gestational sac diameter – measurement used in the first trimester to estimate appropriate gestational age with menstrual dates.

gestational trophoblastic disease – trophoblastic tissue that has overtaken the pregnancy and has propagated throughout the uterine cavity; these tumors arise from the placental chorionic villi.

glomerulus – part of the filtration process in the kidney.

glucagon – hormone that stimulates the liver to convert glycogen to glucose; produced by alpha cells.

goiter – any enlargement of the thyroid, focal or diffuse, regardless of cause.

gonadotropin – a hormonal substance that stimulates the function of the testes and ovaries.

Graves' disease – syndrome characterized by a diffuse toxic goiter, ophthalmopathy, and cutaneous manifestations.

gravidity – total number of pregnancies.

gray scale – B-mode scanning technique that permits the brightness of the B-mode dots to be displayed in various shades of gray to represent different echo amplitudes.

grayscale harmonic imaging – allows detection of contrast-enhanced blood flow and organs with grayscale ultrasound; in the harmonic-imaging mode, the echoes from the oscillating microbubbles have a higher signal-to-noise ratio than found in conventional ultrasound; regions with microbubbles (e.g., blood vessels and organ parenchyma) are better visualized.

greater omentum – double fold of the peritoneum attached to the duodenum, stomach, and large intestine; helps support the greater curve of the stomach; known as the "fatty apron."

greater sac – primary compartment of the peritoneal cavity; extends across the anterior abdomen from the diaphragm to the pelvis.

greater saphenous vein – originates on the dorsum of the foot and ascends anterior to the medial malleolus and along the anteromedial side of the calf and thigh; joins the common femoral vein in the proximal thigh.

growth-adjusted sonar age (GASA) – method whereby the fetus is categorized into small, average, or large growth percentile.

gutters – most dependent areas in the flanks of the abdomen and pelvis where fluid collections may accumulate.

Guyon's canal or tunnel – a fibrous tunnel that contains the ulnar artery and vein, ulnar nerve, and some fatty tissue.

gynecomastia – hypertrophy of residual ductal elements that persist behind the nipple in the male, causing a palpable, tender lump. There is generally no lobular (glandular) tissue in the male. A breast mass resulting from gynecomastia must be distinguished from male breast cancer.

harmonic imaging – in the HI mode, the ultrasound system is configured to receive only echoes at the second harmonic frequency, which is twice the transmit frequency.

Hartmann's pouch – small part of the gallbladder that lies near the cystic duct where stones may collect.

Hashimoto's thyroiditis – chronic inflammation of the thyroid (goiter).

haustra – normal segmentation of the wall of the colon.

head of the pancreas – portion of the pancreas that lies in the C-loop of the duodenum; the gastroduodenal artery is the anterolateral border and the common bile duct is the posterolateral border.

Heister's valves – tiny valves found within the cystic duct.

hemangioma of the cord – vascular tumor within the umbilical cord.

hematocele – blood within the sac surrounding the testes.

hematochezia – passage of bloody stools.

hematocrit – the percent of the total blood volume containing the red blood cells, white blood cells, and the platelets.

hematometrocolpos – blood-filled vagina and uterus.

hematopoiesis – blood-cell production.

hemifacial microsomia – abnormal smallness of one side of the face.

hemiparesis – unilateral partial or complete paralysis.

hemoglobin – oxygen-binding protein found in red blood cells.

hemolytic anemia – anemia resulting from hemolysis of red blood cells.

hemoperitoneum – collection of bloody fluid in the abdomen or pelvis secondary to trauma or surgical procedure.

hemopoiesis – formation of blood.

hemorrhage – collection of blood.

hemosiderin – pigment released from hemoglobin process.

hepatic artery (HA) – common hepatic artery arises from the celiac trunk and courses to the right of the abdomen and branches into the gastroduodenal artery and proper HA.

hepatic flexure – point at which the ascending colon arises from the right lower quadrant to bend at this point to form the transverse colon.

hepatic veins – largest tributaries that drain the liver and empty into the inferior vena cava at the level of the diaphragm.

hepatocellular carcinoma – a common liver malignancy related to cirrhosis; the carcinoma may present as a solitary massive tumor, multiple nodules throughout the liver, or diffuse infiltrative masses in the liver; HCC can be very invasive.

hepatofugal – flow away from the liver.

hepatopetal – flow toward the liver.

hermaphroditism – condition in which both ovarian and testicular tissues are present.

hertz (Hz) – unit for frequency, equal to 1 cycle per second.

heterotopic pregnancy – simultaneous intrauterine and extrauterine pregnancy.

heterozygous achondroplasia – short-limb dysplasia that manifests in the second trimester of pregnancy; conversion abnormality of cartilage to bone affecting the epiphyseal growth centers; extremities are markedly shortened at birth with a normal trunk and frequent enlargement of the head.

hilus – area of kidney where vessels, ureter, and lymphatics enter and exit.

hip joint – formed by the articulation of the head of the femur with the acetabulum of the hip bone.

Hirschsprung's disease – congenital megacolon.

holoprosencephaly – congenital defect caused by an extra chromosome which causes a deficiency in the forebrain.

homeo- – same.

homeostasis – maintenance of a stable internal environment.

homozygous achondroplasia – short-limb dwarfism affecting fetuses of achondroplastic parents.

horseshoe kidney – congenital malformation in which both kidneys are joined together, most commonly at the lower poles.

human chorionic gonadotropin (hCG) – hormone within the maternal urine and serum; hCG is elevated during pregnancy; laboratory test that indicates pregnancy when values are elevated.

humeral length – measurement from the humeral head to the distal end of the humerus.

hydatidiform mole – benign form of gestational trophoblastic disease in which there is partial or complete conversion of the chorionic villi into grapelike vesicles; villia are avascular and there is trophoblastic proliferation; condition may result in malignant trophoblastic disease.

hydranencephaly – congenital absence of the cerebral hemispheres because of an occlusion of the carotid arteries; midbrain structures are present, and fluid replaces cerebral tissue.

hydrocele – fluid within the sac surrounding the testes.

hydrocephalus – ventriculomegaly in the neonate; abnormal accumulation of cerebrospinal fluid within the cerebral ventricles, resulting in compression and frequently destruction of brain tissue.

hydrocolpos – fluid-filled vagina.

hydrometrocolpos – collection of fluid in the vagina and uterus.

hydromyelia – dilation of the central canal of the spinal cord.

hydronephrosis – dilation of the renal collecting system.

hydrops – massive enlargement of the gallbladder.

hydrops fetalis – fluid occurring in at least two areas in the fetus: pleural effusion, pericardial effusion, ascites, or skin edema.

hydrosalpinx – fluid within the fallopian tube.

hydroureters – dilated ureters.

hyperechoic – echo texture that is more echogenic than the surrounding tissue. Hyperechoic masses in the breast are nearly always benign.

hyperemesis gravidarum – excessive vomiting that leads to dehydration and electrolyte imbalance.

hyperglycemia – uncontrolled increase in glucose levels in the blood.

hyperlipidemia – congenital condition in which there are elevated fat levels that may cause pancreatitis.

hyperplasia – enlargement of the adrenal glands.

hypertelorism – abnormally wide-spaced orbits usually found in conjunction with congenital anomalies and mental retardation.

hypertension – elevation of maternal blood pressure that may put fetus at risk.

hyperthyroidism – overactive thyroid gland.

hypertrophic pyloric stenosis (HPS) – thickened muscle in the pylorus that prevents food from entering the duodenum; occurs more frequently in males.

hyperventilation – deficiency of carbon dioxide.

hypochondrium – area of the duodenum in the upper zone on both sides of the epigastric region beneath the cartilages of the lower ribs.

hypoechoic – echo texture that is less echogenic than the surrounding tissue. Most solid breast masses (including cancer) are hypoechoic.

hypoglycemia – deficiency of glucose in the blood.

hypophosphatasia – congenital condition characterized by decreased mineralization of the bones resulting in "ribbonlike" and bowed limbs, underossified cranium, and compression of the chest; early death often occurs.

hypoplastic left heart – underdevelopment of the mitral valve, left ventricle, and aorta.

hypoplastic right heart – underdevelopment of the tricuspid valve, right ventricle, and pulmonary artery.

hypospadias – abnormal congenital opening of the male urethra on the undersurface of the penis.

hypotelorism – abnormally closely spaced orbits; association with holoprosencephaly, chromosomal and central nervous system disorders, and cleft palate.

hypotension – low blood pressure.

hypothyroidism – underactive thyroid gland.

hypoventilation – abnormal condition of the respiratory system of insufficient ventilation resulting in an excess of carbon dioxide.

iliac arteries – arteries that originate from the bifurcation of the aorta at the level of the umbilicus.

iliacus muscles – paired muscles that form the lateral wall of the pelvis.

ileus – dilated loops of bowel without peristalsis; associated with various abdominal problems, including pancreatitis, sickle cell crisis, and bowel obstruction.

incarcerated hernia – confinement of a part of the bowel; the visceral contents cannot be reduced.

incompetent cervix – cervix dilation that can result in the membranes bulging and rupturing so that fetus drops out; occurs silently in the second trimester.

incomplete abortion – retained products of conception.

incomplete atrioventricular septal defect – membranous septal defect, abnormal tricuspid valve, primum atrial septal defect, and cleft mitral valve.

induced acoustic emission – After the injection of the tissue-specific UCA Sonazoid, the reflectivity of the contrast-containing tissue increases; when the right level of acoustic energy is applied to tissue, the contrast microbubbles eventually rupture, resulting in random Doppler shifts; these shifts appear as a transient mosaic of colors on the color Doppler display; masses that have destroyed or replaced normal Kupffer cells will be displayed as color-free areas.

infantile polycystic kidney disease – autosomal recessive disease that affects the fetal kidneys and liver; the kidneys are enlarged and echogenic on ultrasound.

inferior mesenteric artery (IMA) – artery that arises from the anterior aortic wall at the level of the third or fourth lumbar vertebra to supply the left transverse colon, descending colon, sigmoid colon, and part of the rectum.

inferior mesenteric vein – vein that drains the left third of the colon and upper colon and joins the splenic vein.

inferior vena cava – largest venous abdominal vessel, formed by the union of the common iliac veins; supplies the right atrium of the heart along the posterior lateral wall.

infiltrating (invasive) ductal carcinoma – cancer of the ductal epithelium; most common general category of breast cancer, accounting for around approximately 85% of all breast cancers. This cancer usually arises in the terminal duct in the TDLU. If the cancerous cells remain within the duct without invading the breast tissue beyond the duct wall, this is ductal carcinoma in situ (DCIS). If the cancerous cells invade breast tissue (i.e., invasive ductal carcinoma or IDC), the cancer may spread into the regional lymph nodes and beyond. Of the many subtypes of IDC, the most common is infiltrating ductal carcinoma, not otherwise specified (IDC-NOS).

infiltrating (invasive) lobular carcinoma (ILC) – cancer of the lobular epithelium of the breast, arises at the level of the TDLU; accounts for 12% to 15% of all breast cancers.

informed consent – consent to surgery by a patient or to participation in a medical procedure or experiment by a subject after achieving an understanding of what is involved.

infracristal septal defect – defects found below the crista supraventricularis ridge in the membranous or muscular area.

inguinal ligament – ligament between the anterior superior iliac spine and the pubic tubercle.

innominate artery – first branch artery from the aortic arch.

innominate veins – veins that follow these courses: on the right, courses vertically downwards to join the left innominate vein below the first rib to form the superior vena cava; on the left, courses from left chest beneath the sternum to join the right innominate vein; the left innominate vein is longer than the right.

insulin – hormone that allows circulating glucose to enter tissue cells; failure to produce insulin results in diabetes mellitus.

interface – surface forming the boundary between media having different properties.

internal carotid artery – larger of the two terminal branches of the common carotid artery that arises from the common carotid artery to supply the anterior brain and meninges.

internal os – inner surface of the cervical os.

international normalized ratio – a method developed to standardize prothrombin time (PT) results among laboratories by accounting for the different thromboplastin reagents used to determine PT.

interstitial pregnancy – pregnancy occurring in the cornu of the uterus.

intertubercular plane – lowest horizontal line joins the tubercles on the iliac crests.

intrahepatic – within the liver.

intramural leiomyoma – most common type of leiomyoma; deforms the myometrium.

intraperitoneal – within the peritoneal cavity.

intrauterine contraceptive device (IUD, IUCD) – device inserted into the endometrial cavity to prevent pregnancy.

intrauterine growth restriction (IUGR) – decreased rate of fetal growth, usually a fetal weight below the tenth percentile for a given gestational age; may be symmetric (all growth parameters are small) or asymmetric (maybe caused by placental problem; head measurements correlate with dates; body disproportionately smaller); formerly referred to as intrauterine growth retardation.

intrauterine insemination – the introduction of semen into the vagina or uterus by mechanical or instrumental means rather than by sexual intercourse.

intravenous injection – a hypodermic injection into a vein for the purpose of injecting a contrast medium.

intravenous urography – procedure used in radiography wherein contrast is administered intravenously to help visualize the urinary system.

intussusception – bowel prolapses into distal bowel (telescoping) and is then propelled in an antegrade fashion.

invasive mole – tumor that penetrates into and through the uterine wall.

in vitro fertilization (IVF) – a method of fertilizing the human ova outside the body by collecting the mature ova and placing them in a dish with a sample of spermatozoa.

ischemic rest pain – critical ischemia (lack of blood) of the distal limb when the patient is at rest.

islets of Langerhans – portion of the pancreas that has an endocrine function and produces insulin, glucagon, and somatostatin.

isoechoic – echo texture that resembles the surrounding tissue. Isoechoic masses can be difficult to identify.

isthmus – small piece of thyroid tissue that connects the lower lobes of the gland.

IUP – intrauterine pregnancy.

jaundice – excessive bilirubin accumulation causes yellow pigmentation of the skin; first seen in the whites of the eyes.

jejunoileal atresia – blockage of the jejunum and ileal bowel segments that appears as multiple cystic structures within the fetal abdomen.

junctional fold – small septum within the gallbladder, usually arising from the posterior wall.

juxtathoracic – near the chest wall (thorax).

kilohertz (kHz) – 1000 Hz.

Klatskin's tumor – cancer at the bifurcation of the hepatic ducts; may cause asymmetric obstruction of the biliary tree.

Kupffer cells – special hepatic cells that remove bile pigment, old blood cells, and the by-products of phagocytosis from the blood and deposit them into the bile ducts.

large for gestational age (LGA) – fetus measures larger than would be expected for dates (diabetic fetus).

lateral arcuate ligament – thickened upper margin of the fascia covering the anterior surface of the quadratus lumborum muscle.

left atrium – filling chamber of the heart.

left crus of the diaphragm – tendinous connection of the diaphragm that arises from the sides of the bodies of the first two lumbar vertebrae.

left gastric artery – artery that arises from the celiac axis to supply the stomach and lower third of the esophagus.

left hypochondrium – left upper quadrant of the abdomen that contains the left lobe of the liver, spleen, and stomach.

left lobe of the liver – lobe that lies in the epigastrium and left hypochondrium.

left portal vein – the main portal vein branches into the left and right portal veins to supply the liver.

left renal artery – artery that arises from the posterolateral wall of the aorta directly into the hilus of the kidney.

left renal vein – leaves the renal hilum, travels anterior to the aorta and posterior to the superior mesenteric artery to enter the lateral wall of the inferior vena cava.

left ventricle – pumping chamber of the heart.

leiomyoma – most common benign gynecologic tumor in women during their reproductive years.

lemon sign – seen on sonography, sign of frontal bones collapsing inward; occurs with spina bifida.

lesser omentum – membranous extension of the peritoneum that suspends the stomach and duodenum from the liver; helps to support the lesser curvature of the stomach.

lesser sac – peritoneal pouch located behind the lesser omentum and stomach.

lesser saphenous vein – vein that originates on the dorsum of the foot and ascends posterior to the lateral malleolus and runs along the midline of the posterior calf; vein terminates as it joins the popliteal vein.

leucopoiesis – white blood cell formation stimulated by presence of bacteria.

leukocyte – white blood cell; primary function is to defend the body against infection.

leukocytosis – increase in the number of leukocytes.

leukopenia – abnormal decrease of white blood corpuscles; may be drug induced.

levator ani muscles – a pair of muscles that form the floor of the pelvis.

lienorenal ligament – ligament between the spleen and kidney that helps hold the spleen in place and supports the greater curvature of the stomach.

ligament – fibrous band of tissue connecting bone or cartilage to bone that aids in stabilizing a joint.

ligamentum teres – termination of the falciform ligament; seen in the left lobe of the liver.

ligamentum venosum – transformation of the ductus venosus in fetal life to closure in neonatal life. It separates left lobe from caudate lobe; shown as echogenic line on the transverse and sagittal images.

limb–body wall complex – anomaly with large cranial defects, facial cleft, large body wall defects, and limb abnormalities.

linea alba – fibrous band of tissue that stretches from the xiphoid to the symphysis pubis.

linea semilunaris – line that extends from the ninth costal cartilage to the pubic tubercle.

lipase – pancreatic enzyme that acts on fats; enzyme is elevated in pancreatitis and remains increased longer than amylase.

lipoma – common benign tumor composed of fat cells.

liver function tests – specific laboratory tests that look at liver function (aspartate or alanine aminotransferase, lactic acid dehydrogenase, alkaline phosphatase, and bilirubin).

lobular carcinoma in situ (LCIS) – see lobular neoplasia.

lobular neoplasia – term preferred by many authors to replace LCIS (not considered a true cancer nor treated as such) and atypical hyperplasia.

long axis – plane that transects heart perpendicular to dorsal and ventral surfaces of body and parallel with long axis of heart.

loop of Henle – portion of a renal tubule lying between the proximal and distal convoluted portions; reabsorption of fluid, sodium, and chloride occurs in the proximal convoluted tubule and the loop of Henle.

lower uterine segment – thin expanded lower portion of the uterus at the junction of the internal os and sacrum that forms in the last trimester of pregnancy.

lymph – alkaline fluid found in the lymphatic vessels.

lymphangiectasia – dilation of a lymph node.

lymphoma – malignancy that primarily affects the lymph nodes, spleen, or liver.

macrocephaly – enlargement of the fetal cranium as a result of ventriculomegaly.

macroglossia – hypertrophied tongue.

macrosomia – birth weight greater than 4000 g or above the 90th percentile for the estimated gestational age; these infants have fat deposition in the subcutaneous tissues.

main lobar fissure – boundary between the right and left lobes of the liver; seen as hyperechoic line on the sagittal image extending from the portal vein to the neck of the gallbladder.

main portal vein – vein formed by union of the splenic vein and superior mesenteric vein; enters the liver at the porta hepatis.

main pulmonary artery – main artery that carries blood from the right ventricle to the lungs.

major calyces (also known as the **infundibulum**) – area of the kidneys that receives urine from the minor calyces to convey to the renal pelvis.

malpighian corpuscles – small, round, deep red bodies in the cortex of the kidney, each communicating with a renal tubule.

mammary layer – middle layer of the breast tissue (one of three layers recognized on breast ultrasound between the skin and the chest wall) that contains the ductal, glandular, and stromal portions of the breast.

Marfan's syndrome – hereditary disorder of connective tissue, bones, muscles, ligaments, and skeletal structures.

maternal serum alpha-fetoprotein (MSAFP) – antigen present in the fetus; the maternal serum is tested between 16 and 18 weeks of gestation to detect abnormal levels; can also be tested directly from the amniotic fluid from amniocentesis.

maternal serum quad screen – a blood test conducted during the second trimester (15 to 22 weeks) to identify pregnancies at a higher risk for chromosomal anomalies (trisomy 21 and trisomy 18) and neural tube defects.

maximum or **deep vertical pocket** – method to determine the amount of amniotic fluid; pocket less than 2 cm may indicate oligohydramnios; greater than 8 cm indicates polyhydramnios. This method is used more often in multiple gestation pregnancy.

McBurney's point – site of maximum tenderness in the right lower quadrant; usually with appendicitis.

mean velocity – velocity based on the time average of the outline velocity (maximum velocity envelope).

mechanical index – an index that defines the low acoustic output power that can be used to minimize the destruction of microbubbles by energy in the acoustic field; when the microbubbles in microbubble-based ultrasound contrast agents are destroyed, contrast enhancement is lost.

Meckel's diverticulum – congenital sac or blind pouch found in the lower portion of the ileum; a remnant of the proximal part of the yolk stalk.

meconium ileus – small-bowel disorder marked by the presence of thick echogenic meconium in the distal ileum.

medial arcuate ligament – thickened upper margin of the fascia covering the anterior surface of the psoas muscle. It connects the medial borders of the two diaphragmatic crura as they cross anterior to the aorta.

mediastinum testis – linear structure within the midline of the testes.

medulla of the adrenal – central tissue of the adrenal gland that secrets epinephrine and norepinephrine.

medulla of the kidney (also known as the **pyramid**) – inner portion of the renal parenchyma that contains the loop of Henle.

medullary carcinoma – neoplastic growth that accounts for 10% of thyroid malignancies.

medullary pyramids – large and hypoechoic in the neonate.

megahertz (MHz) – 1,000,000 Hz.

Meigs' syndrome – benign tumor of the ovary associated with ascites and pleural effusion.

membranous or velamentous insertion of the cord – insertion of the cord into the membranes before it enters the placenta.

menarche – onset of menstruation; state after reaching puberty in which menses occur normally every 27 to 28 days.

meninges – linings of the brain.

meningocele – open spinal defect characterized by protrusion of the spinal meninges.

meningomyelocele – open spinal defect characterized by protrusion of meninges and spinal cord through the defect, usually within a meningeal sac.

menopause – cessation of menstruation.

menses – monthly flow of blood from the endometrium.

menstrual age – gestational age of the fetus determined from the first day of the last normal menstrual period (LMP) to the point at which the pregnancy is being assessed.

mesentery – a fold from the parietal peritoneum that attaches to the small intestine anchoring it to the posterior abdominal wall.

mesosalpinx – free margin of the upper portion of the broad ligament where the oviduct is found.

mesothelium – tissue that lines the body cavities of the embryo, part of which develops into the peritoneum.

meta- – change.

metabolism – physical and chemical changes that occur within the body.

metastatic disease – tumor that develops away from the site of the organ; most common form of neoplasm of the liver; most common primary sites are colon, breast, and lung.

microcephaly – head smaller than the body.

micrognathia – abnormally small chin; commonly associated with other fetal anomalies.

microphthalmos – small eyes.

middle cerebral artery (MCA) – large terminal branch of the internal carotid artery.

midline echo complex (the falx) – widest transverse diameter of the skull; proper level to measure the biparietal diameter.

minor calyces – area of the kidneys that receives urine from the renal pyramids; form the border of the renal sinus.

mitral atresia – thickened, underdeveloped mitral apparatus.

mitral regurgitation – failure of the leaflets to close completely, allowing blood to leak backward into the left atrium.

mitral valve – atrioventricular valve between the left atrium and left ventricle.

molar pregnancy – also known as gestational trophoblastic disease; abnormal proliferation of trophoblastic cells in the first trimester.

molecular imaging agents – agents include Optison, Definity, Imagent, Levbovist, and Sono Vue.

monoamniotic – multiple pregnancy with one amniotic sac.

monochorionic – multiple pregnancy with one chorionic sac.

monozygotic – twins that arise from a single fertilized egg that divides to produce two identical fetuses.

Morison's pouch – right posterior subphrenic space that lies between the right lobe of the liver, anterior to the kidney and right colic flexure, where fluid may lie or an abscess may develop.

MSD – mean sac diameter.

mucinous cystadenocarcinoma – malignant tumor of the ovary with multilocular cysts.

mucinous cystadenoma – benign tumor of the ovary that contains thin-walled, multilocular cysts.

mucosa – mucous membrane; thin sheet of tissue that lines cavities of the body that open to the outside; it is the first layer of bowel.

multicentric breast cancer – breast cancers occurring in different quadrants of the breast that are at least 5 cm or more apart; multicentric cancers are more likely to be of different histologic types than is a multifocal cancer.

multicystic dysplastic kidney disease (MCDK) – multiple cysts replace normal renal tissue throughout the kidney; usually causes renal obstruction; most common cause of renal cystic disease in the neonate; may have contralateral ureteral pelvic junction obstruction.

multifocal breast cancer – breast cancer occurring in more than one site within the same quadrant or the same ductal system of the breast.

multinodular goiter – nodular enlargement of the thyroid associated with hyperthyroidism.

multiplanar imaging – ability to collect data from axial, coronal, and sagittal planes for reconstruction into 3-D format.

Murphy's sign – positive sign implies exquisite tenderness over the area of the gallbladder upon palpation.

muscle – a type of tissue consisting of contractile cells or fibers that affects movement of an organ or part of the body.

muscularis – third layer of bowel.

myelin – substance forming the sheath of Schwann cells.

myeloschisis – cleft spinal cord resulting from failure of the neural tube to close.

myocardium – thickest muscle in the heart wall.

myometritis – infection within the myometrium of the uterus.

myometrium – middle layer of the uterine cavity that appears very homogeneous with sonography.

nabothian cyst – benign tiny cyst within the cervix.

naked tuberosity sign – the deltoid muscle is on the humeral head; seen with a full-thickness tear of the rotator cuff.

neck of the pancreas – small area of the pancreas between the head and the body; anterior to the superior mesenteric vein.

neonate – infant during the early newborn period.

neoplasm – refers to any new growth (benign or malignant).

nephroblastomatosis – abnormal persistence of fetal renal blastema (potential to develop into Wilms' tumor).

nephron – functional unit of the kidney; includes a renal corpuscle and a renal tubule.

neuroblastoma – malignant adrenal mass that is seen in pediatric patients.

nonimmune hydrops (NIH) – group of conditions in which hydrops is present in the fetus but not a result of fetomaternal blood group incompatibility.

nonmaleficence – refrain from harming oneself or others.

nonpalpable – cannot be felt on clinical examination; nonpalpable breast mass is one that is usually identified on screening mammogram and is too small to be felt as a breast lump on BSE or CBE.

nonresistive – vessels that have high diastolic component and supply organs that need constant perfusion (internal carotid artery, hepatic artery, and renal artery).

Non-Stress Test (NST) – test that utilizes Doptone (a brand of Doppler instrumentation used in obstetric examinations) to record the fetal heart rate and its reactivity to the stress of uterine contraction.

normal situs – indicates normal position of the abdominal organs (liver on right, stomach on left, heart apex to the left).

nuchal cord – condition that occurs when the cord is wrapped around the fetal neck.

nuchal lucency – increased thickness in the nuchal fold area in the back of the neck associated with trisomy 21.

obstructive disease – blockage of bile excretion within the liver or biliary system.

obturator internus muscle – arises from the anterolateral pelvic wall surrounding the obturator foramen to insert on the greater trochanter of the femur.

oculodentodigital dysplasia – underdevelopment of the eyes, fingers, and mouth.

oligohydramnios – insufficient amount of amniotic fluid.

-ology – study of; *physiology*: study of body functions.

omphalocele – anterior abdominal wall defect in which abdominal organs (liver, bowel, stomach) are atypically located within the umbilical cord and protrude outside the wall; highly associated with cardiac, central nervous system, renal, and chromosomal anomalies. It develops when there is a midline defect of the abdominal muscles, fascia, and skin.

omphalomesenteric cyst – cystic lesion of the umbilical cord.

oophoritis – infection within the ovary.

ophthalmic artery – first branch of the internal carotid artery.

Ortolani maneuver – patient lies in the supine position. The examiner's hand is placed around the hip to be examined with the fingers over the femoral head. The hip is flexed 90 degrees and the thigh is abducted.

osteogenesis imperfecta – metabolic disorder affecting the fetal collagen system that leads to varying forms of bone disease; intrauterine bone fractures, shortened long bones, poorly mineralized calvaria, and compression of the chest found in type II forms.

otocephaly – underdevelopment of the jaw that causes the ears to be located close together toward the front of the neck.

ovarian carcinoma – malignant tumor of the ovary that may spread beyond the ovary and metastasize to other organs via the peritoneal channels.

ovarian cyst – cyst of the ovary that may be found in the fetus; results from maternal hormone stimulation and is usually benign.

ovarian hyperstimulation syndrome (OHS) – a syndrome that presents sonographically as enlarged ovaries with multiple cysts, abdominal ascites, and pleural effusions. Often seen in patients who have undergone ovulation induction post administration of follicle-stimulating hormone or a GnRH analogue followed by hCG.

ovulation induction therapy – controlled ovarian stimulation with clomiphene citrate or parenterally administered gonadotropins.

ovarian torsion – partial or complete rotation of the ovarian pedicle on its axis.

Paget's disease of the breast – surface erosion of the nipple that results from direct invasion of the skin of the nipple from underlying breast cancer.

palpable – can be felt on clinical examination; palpable breast lump is one that is identified on CBE or BSE.

pampiniform plexus – multiple veins that drain the testicles; when a varicocele is present, dilation and tortuosity may develop.

pancreatic ascites – fluid accumulation caused by a rupture of a pancreatic pseudocyst into the abdomen; free-floating pancreatic enzymes are very dangerous to surrounding structures.

pancreatic duct – duct that travels horizontally through the pancreas to join the common bile duct at the ampulla of Vater.

pancreatic pseudocyst – "sterile abscess" collection of pancreatitis enzymes that accumulate in the available space in the abdomen (usually in or near the pancreas).

pancreaticoduodenal arteries – arteries that help supply blood to the pancreas along with the splenic artery.

pancreatitis – inflammation of the pancreas; may be acute or chronic.

papillary carcinoma – most common form of thyroid malignancy.

paralytic ileus – dilated, fluid-filled loops of bowel without peristalsis secondary to obstruction, decreased vascularity, or abnormal metabolic state.

parametritis – infection within the uterine serosa and broad ligaments.

paraovarian cyst – cystic structure that lies adjacent to the ovary.

parasternal – transducer placement over the area bounded superiorly by left clavicle, medially by sternum, and inferiorly by apical region.

pariet- – wall; *parietal membrane*: membrane that lines the wall of a cavity.

parietal peritoneum – layer of the peritoneum that lines the abdominal wall.

parity – number of live births.

partial mole – condition that develops when two sperm fertilize an egg.

partial situs inversus – reversal of the heart or the abdominal organs (dextrocardia or liver on the left, stomach on the right).

partial thromboplastin time – laboratory test that can be used to evaluate the effects of heparin, aspirin, and antihistamines on the blood clotting process; PTT detects clotting abnormalities of the intrinsic and common pathways.

patent ductus arteriosus – open communication between the pulmonary artery and descending aorta that does not constrict after birth.

peau d'orange – French term that means "skin of the orange"; descriptive term for skin thickening of one breast that, on clinical breast examination, resembles the skin of an orange. Such an appearance can result from an inflammatory breast condition (mastitis), simple edema, or skin involvement from underlying breast cancer.

pelv- – basin; *pelvic cavity*: basin-shaped cavity enclosed by the pelvic bones.

pelvic girdle – formation of the hip bones by the ilium, ischium, and pubis.

pelvic inflammatory disease (PID) – all-inclusive term that refers to all pelvic infections (endometritis, salpingitis, hydrosalpinx, pyosalpinx, and tuboovarian abscess).

pelvic kidney – location of the kidney when the kidney does not migrate upward into the retroperitoneal space.

pelviectasis – dilated renal pelvis measuring 5 to 9 mm in the anteroposterior direction.

pennate – featherlike pattern of muscle growth.

pentalogy of Cantrell – rare anomaly with five defects: omphalocele, ectopic heart, lower sternum, anterior diaphragm, and diaphragmatic pericardium.

perforating veins – veins that connect the superficial and deep venous systems.

pericardium – sac surrounding the heart, reflecting off the great arteries.

perineurium – the surrounding connective tissue of muscle.

period – duration of a single cycle of a periodic wave or event.

peripheral occlusive arterial disease – narrowing or stenosis of the peripheral arteries.

peripheral zone – posterior and lateral aspect of the prostate.

perirenal space – located directly around the kidney; completely enclosed by renal fascia.

peristalsis – rhythmic dilatation and contraction of the gastrointestinal tract as food is propelled through it.

peritoneal cavity – potential space between the parietal and visceral peritoneal layers.

peritoneal lavage – invasive procedure that is used to sample the intraperitoneal space for evidence of damage to viscera and blood vessels.

peritoneal recess – slitlike spaces near the liver; potential space for fluid to accumulate.

peritonitis – inflammation of the peritoneum.

periventricular leukomalacia – echogenic white matter necrosis best seen in the posterior aspect of the brain or adjacent to the ventricular structures.

peroneal veins – veins that drain blood from the lateral lower leg.

phagocytosis – process by which cells engulf and destroy microorganisms and cellular debris; "cell-eating"; for example, the red pulp destroys the degenerating red blood cells.

Phalen's sign (Phalen's test, Phalen's maneuver, or Phalen's position) – an increase in wrist compression due to hyperflexion of the wrist for 60 seconds; this test is done with the patient holding the forearms upright and pressing the ventral side of the hands together.

phenylketonuria (PKU) – hereditary disease caused by failure to oxidize an amino acid (phenylalanine) to tyrosine, because of a defective enzyme; if PKU is not treated early, mental retardation can develop.

pheochromocytoma – benign adrenal tumor that secretes hormones that produce hypertension.

phlegmasia alba dolens – swollen, painful white leg.

phlegmasia cerulea dolens – swollen, painful cyanotic leg.

phrenocolic ligament – one of the ligaments between the spleen and splenic flexure of the colon.

phrygian cap – gallbladder variant in which part of the fundus is bent back on itself.

Pierre Robin syndrome – micrognathia and abnormal smallness of the tongue usually with a cleft palate.

piezoelectric effect – generation of electric signals as a result of an incident sound beam on a material that has piezoelectric properties; in the converse (or reverse) piezoelectric effect, the material expands or contracts when an electric signal is applied.

piriformis muscle – muscle that arises from the sacrum between the pelvic sacral foramina and the gluteal surface of the ilium.

pitting – process by which the spleen removes abnormal red blood cells.

placenta – organ of communication (nutrition and products of metabolism) between the fetus and the mother; forms from the chorion frondosum with a maternal decidual contribution.

placenta accreta – growth of the chorionic villi superficially into the myometrium.

placenta increta – growth of the chorionic villi deep into the myometrium.

placenta percreta – growth of the chorionic villi through the myometrium.

placenta previa – placental implantation that encroaches upon the lower uterine segment; the placenta comes first and bleeding is inevitable.

placental grade – technique of grading the placenta for maturity.

placental grading – arbitrary method of classifying the maturity of the placenta with a grading scale of 0 to 3.

placental insufficiency – abnormal condition of pregnancy manifested by a restricted rate of fetal and uterine growth. One or more placental abnormalities cause dysfunction of maternal-placental or fetal-placental circulation.

placental migration – movement of the placenta as the uterus enlarges the placenta; a low-lying placenta may move out of the uterine segment in the second trimester.

planar reconstruction – movement of the intersection point (point of rotation) of the three orthogonal image planes throughout the 3-D volume and rotating the image planes; the sonographer or physician has the liberty to generate anatomic views from an infinite number of perspectives.

plantar flexion – pointing of the toes toward the plantar surface of the foot.

pleur – rib; *pleural membrane*: membrane that encloses the lungs within the rib cage.

pleural effusion (hydrothorax) – accumulation of fluid within the thoracic cavity.

pneumothorax – a collection of air or gas in the pleural cavity.

polycystic kidney disease – poorly functioning enlarged kidneys.

polycystic ovarian disease – endocrine disorder associated with chronic anovulation.

polycythemia – excess of red blood cells.

polycythemia vera – chronic, life-shortening condition of unknown etiology involving bone marrow elements; characterized by an increase in red blood cell mass and hemoglobin concentration.

polydactyly – anomalies of the hands or feet in which there is an addition of a digit; may be found in association with certain skeletal dysplasias.

polyhydramnios – excessive amount of amniotic fluid.

polyp of gallbladder – small, well-defined soft tissue projection from the gallbladder wall.

polysplenia – condition where there is more than one spleen; associated with cardiac malformations.

popliteal artery – artery that begins at the opening of the adductor magnus muscle and travels behind the knee in the popliteal fossa.

popliteal vein – vein that originates from the confluence of the anterior tibial veins and posterior and peroneal veins.

porta hepatis – central area of the liver where the portal vein, common duct, and hepatic artery enter.

portal confluence – see confluence of the splenic and portal veins.

portal vein – vein formed by the union of the superior mesenteric vein and splenic vein near the porta hepatis of the liver.

portal venous hypertension – results from intrinsic liver disease; may cause flow reversal to the liver, thrombosis of the portal system, or cavernous transformation of the portal vein.

portal-splenic confluence – junction of the splenic and main portal vein; posterior border of the body of the pancreas.

postcoital test (PCT) – a clinical test done within 24 hours after intercourse to assess sperm motility in cervical mucus.

posterior arch vein – main tributary of the greater saphenous vein.

posterior cerebral artery (PCA) – artery that originates from the terminal basilar artery and courses anteriorly and laterally.

posterior communicating artery (PCoA) – courses posteriorly and medially from the internal carotid artery to join the posterior cerebral artery.

posterior pararenal space – space found between the posterior renal fascia and the muscles of the posterior abdominal wall.

posterior tibial veins – veins that originate from the plantar veins of the foot and drain blood from the posterior lower leg.

posterior urethral valve – the presence of a valve in the posterior urethra; occurs only in male fetuses; most common cause of bladder outlet obstruction in the male neonate.

postterm – fetus born later than the 42-week gestational period.

Potter's syndrome – condition characterized by renal agenesis, oligohydramnios, pulmonary hypoplasia, abnormal facies, and malformed hands and feet.

Pourcelot resistive index – Doppler measurement that takes the highest systolic peak minus the highest diastolic peak divided by the highest systolic peak.

preeclampsia – also known as *pregnancy-induced hypertension (PIH)*. A complication of pregnancy characterized by increasing hypertension, proteinuria, and edema.

premature atrial and ventricular contractions – fetal cardiac arrhythmia resulting from extra systoles and ectopic beats.

premature rupture of the membranes (PROM) – leaking or breaking of the amniotic membranes causing the loss of amniotic fluid, which may lead to premature delivery or infection.

premenarche – time period in young girls before the onset of menstruation.

preterm – fetus born earlier than the normal 38- to 42-week gestational period.

primary yolk sac – first site of formation of red blood cells that will nourish the embryo.

proboscis – a cylindrical protuberance of the face that in cyclopia or ethmocephaly represents the nose.

profunda femoris artery – artery posterior and lateral to the superficial femoral artery.

projectile vomiting – condition found in pyloric stenosis in the neonatal period; after drinking, the infant experiences projectile vomiting secondary to the obstruction.

proliferative phase – days 5 to 9 of the menstrual cycle; endometrium appears as a single thin stripe with a hypoechoic halo encompassing it; creates the "three-line sign."

prostate specific antigen – laboratory test that measures levels of the protein prostate specific antigen in the body; elevated levels could indicate prostate cancer.

prothrombin time – laboratory test used to detect clotting abnormalities of the extrinsic pathway; measured against a control sample, PT tests the time it takes for a blood sample to coagulate after thromboplastin and calcium are added to it.

prune-belly syndrome – dilation of the fetal abdomen secondary to severe bilateral hydronephrosis and fetal ascites; fetus also has oligohydramnios and pulmonary hypoplasia.

pseudoaneurysm – perivascular collection (hematoma) that communicates with an artery or a graft and has the presence of pulsating blood entering the collection.

pseudoascites – sonolucent band near the fetal anterior abdominal wall seen in the fetus over 18 weeks (does not outline the falciform ligament or bowel as ascites will).

pseudo-dissection – condition seen in a patient with aortic dissection; there is no intimal flap seen, only hypoechoic thrombus near the outer margin of the aorta with echogenic laminated clot.

pseudogestational sac – decidual reaction that occurs within the uterus in a patient with an ectopic pregnancy.

psoas major muscle – begins at the level of hilum of the kidneys and extends inferiorly along both sides of the spine into the pelvis.

pudendal artery – the internal and external pudendal arteries partially supply the scrotal wall and epididymis and occasionally the lower pole of the testis.

pulmonary embolism – blockage of the pulmonary circulation by a thrombus or other matter; may lead to death if blockage of pulmonary blood flow is significant.

pulmonary hypoplasia – small, underdeveloped lungs with resultant reduction in lung volume; secondary to prolonged oligohydramnios or as a consequence of a small thoracic cavity.

pulmonary stenosis – thickening and narrowing of the pulmonic cusps; causes blood to back up into the right ventricle and atrium.

pulmonary veins – four pulmonary veins bring blood from the lungs back into the posterior wall of the left atrium; there are two upper (right and left) and two lower (right and left) pulmonary veins.

pulsatility index (PI) – Doppler measurement that uses peak systole minus peak diastole divided by the mean.

pulse duration – measure of the ring-down (an artifact that occurs when the ultrasound transducer strikes the ribs) time of a transducer after excitation.

pulsed wave transducer – single crystal that sends and receives sound intermittently; a pulse of sound is emitted from the transducer, which also receives the returning signal.

pyloric canal – canal located between the stomach and duodenum.

pyocele – pus located between the visceral and parietal layers of the tunica vaginalis.

pyogenic – pus producing.

pyogenic abscess – pus-forming collection of fluid.

pyosalpinx – retained pus within the inflamed fallopian tube.

pyramidal lobe – lobe of the thyroid gland that is present in small percentage of patients; extends superiorly from the isthmus.

pyramids – area of the kidneys that convey urine to the minor calyces.

radial – descriptive term used to denote area of the breast relative to a clock.

radial artery – artery that begins at the brachial artery bifurcation.

reactive hyperemia – alternative method to stress the peripheral arterial circulation.

real-time – ultrasound instrumentation that allows the image to be displayed many times per second to achieve a "real-time" image of anatomic structures and their motion patterns.

rectouterine pouch (pouch of Douglas) – area in the pelvic cavity between the rectum and the uterus that is likely to accumulate free fluid.

rectus abdominis muscle – muscle of the anterior abdominal wall.

rectus sheath hematoma – hemorrhage within the anterior rectus sheath muscle usually secondary to trauma.

recurrent rami – terminal ends of the centripetal (intratesticular) arteries that curve backward toward the capsule.

red pulp – tissue composed of reticular cells and fibers (cords of Billroth); surrounds the splenic sinuses.

reducible hernia – capable of being replaced in a normal position; the visceral contents can be returned to normal intraabdominal location.

refractile shadowing (edge artifact) – the bending of the sound beam at the edge of a circular structure, resulting in the absence of posterior echoes.

refraction – change in the direction of propagation of a sound wave transmitted across an interface where the speed of sound varies.

renal agenesis – interruption in the normal development of the kidney resulting in absence of the kidney; may be unilateral or bilateral.

renal artery – artery that arises from the posterolateral wall of the aorta, travels posterior to the inferior vena cava to supply the kidney.

renal artery stenosis – narrowing of the renal artery; historically, this has been very difficult to evaluate sonographically.

renal capsule – first layer adjacent to the kidney that forms a tough, fibrous covering.

renal corpuscle – part of the nephron that consists of Bowman's capsule and the glomerulus.

renal hilum – area in the midportion of the kidney where the renal vessels and ureter enter and exit.

renal pelvis – area in the midportion of the kidney that collects urine before entering the ureter.

renal sinus – central area of the kidney that includes the calyces, renal pelvis, renal vessels, fat, nerves, and lymphatics.

renal vein thrombosis – obstruction of the renal vein resulting in kidney becoming enlarged and edematous.

resistive index – peak systole minus peak diastole divided by peak systole (S-D/S 5 RI); an RI of 0.7 or less indicates good perfusion; an RI of 0.7 or higher indicates decreased perfusion.

resolution – ability of the transducer to distinguish between two structures adjacent to one another.

respect for persons – incorporates both respect for the autonomy of individuals and the requirement to protect those with diminished autonomy.

respiratory phasicity – change in blood flow velocity with respiration.

rete testis – network of the channels formed by the convergence of the straight seminiferous tubules in the mediastinum testis; these channels drain into the head of the epididymis.

reticuloendothelial cells – certain phagocytic cells (found mainly in the liver and spleen) make up the reticuloendothelial system (RES), which plays a role in the defense against infection and synthesis of blood proteins and hematopoiesis.

retromammary layer – deepest of the three layers of the breast noted on breast ultrasound. The retromammary layer is predominantly fatty and can be thin. The retromammary layer separates the active breast glandular tissue from the pectoralis fascia overlying the chest wall muscles.

retroperitoneum – space behind the peritoneal lining of the abdominal cavity.

retroverted – refers to the position of the uterus when the fundus is tipped posteriorly.

Rh blood group – system of antigens that may be found on the surface of red blood cells. When the Rh factor is present, the blood type is Rh positive; when the Rh antigen is absent, the blood type is Rh negative. A pregnant woman who is Rh negative may become sensitized by the blood of an Rh positive fetus. In subsequent pregnancies, if the fetus is Rh positive, the Rh antibodies produced in maternal blood may cross over the placenta and destroy fetal cells, causing erythroblastosis fetalis.

rhabdomyoma – benign cardiac tumor of the heart that is associated with tuberous sclerosis.

right atrium – filling chamber of the heart.

right crus of the diaphragm – arises from the sides of the bodies of the first three lumbar vertebrae.

right gastric artery – artery that supplies the stomach.

right hepatic artery – artery that supplies the gallbladder via the cystic artery.

right hypochondrium – right upper quadrant of the abdomen that contains the liver and gallbladder.

right lobe of the liver – largest of the lobes of the liver.

right portal vein – the main portal vein branches into the right and left portal veins to supply the lobes of the liver.

right renal artery – artery that arises from the posterolateral wall of the aorta and travels posterior to the inferior vena cava to enter the hilum of the kidney.

right renal vein – vein that leaves the renal hilum to enter the lateral wall of the inferior vena cava.

right ventricle – pumping chamber of the heart that sends blood into the pulmonary artery.

ROI – region of interest.

rugae – inner folds of the stomach wall.

saccular aneurysm – localized dilatation of the vessel.

sagittal plane – vertical plane through the longitudinal axis of the body that divides it into two portions.

salpingitis – infection within the fallopian tubes.

saphenous opening – gap in the fascia lata, which is found 4 cm inferior and lateral to the pubic tubercle.

sciatic nerve – largest nerve in the upper thigh.

scoliosis – abnormal curvature of the spine.

scrotum – dependent sac containing the testes and epididymis.

S/D ratio – difference between peak systole and peak diastole.

secondary yolk sac – sac formed at 23 days when the primary yolk sac is pinched off by the extra embryonic coelom.

second generation agents – agents containing heavy gasses (i.e., Optison).

secretin – hormone released from small bowel as antacid; stimulates secretion of bicarbonate.

secretory (early) phase – days 10 to 14 of the menstrual cycle; ovulation occurs; the endometrium increases in thickness and echogenicity.

secretory (luteal) phase – days 14 to 28 of the menstrual cycle; the endometrium is at its greatest thickness and echogenicity with posterior enhancement.

semilunar valve – valve located in the aortic or pulmonic artery.

seminal vesicles – reservoirs for sperm located posterior to the bladder.

sentinel node – represents the first lymph node along the axillary node chain. This is the node chain the surgeon identifies for evidence of metastasis.

sepsis – spread of an infection from its initial site to the bloodstream.

septa testis – multiple septa formed from the tunica albuginea that course toward the mediastinum testis and separate the testicle into lobules.

septicemia – infection in the blood.

septum primum – first part of the atrial septum to grow from the dorsal wall of the primitive atrium; fuses with the endocardial cushions.

septum secundum – part of the atrial septum that grows into the atrium to the right of the septum primum.

seroma – accumulation of serous fluid within tissue.

serosa – fourth layer of bowel; thin, loose layer of connective tissue, surrounded by mesothelium covering the intraperitoneal bowel loops.

serous cystadenocarcinoma – most common type of ovarian carcinoma; may be bilateral with multilocular cysts.

serous cystadenoma – second most common benign tumor of the ovary; unilocular or multilocular.

serum amylase – pancreatic enzyme that is elevated during pancreatitis.

short axis – plane that transects heart perpendicular to dorsal and ventral surfaces of body and perpendicular to long axis of heart.

sickle cell anemia – inherited disorder transmitted as an autosomal recessive trait that causes an abnormality of the globin genes in hemoglobin.

sickle cell crisis – condition in sickle cell anemia in which the malformed red cells interfere with oxygen transport, obstruct capillary blood flow, and cause fever and severe pain in the joints and abdomen.

simple ovarian cyst – smooth, well-defined cystic structure that is filled completely with fluid.

single umbilical artery – condition of one umbilical cord instead of two; it has a high association with congenital anomalies.

single ventricle – condition in which there are two atria with one ventricle.

sinoatrial node – forms in the wall of the sinus venosus near its opening into the right atrium.

situs inversus – heart and abdominal organs are completely reversed.

sludge – low-level echoes found along the posterior margin of the gallbladder; move with change in position.

small for gestational age (SGA) – fetus measures smaller than would be expected for dates.

soleal sinuses – large venous reservoirs that lie in the soleus muscle and empty into the posterior tibial or peroneal veins.

sonohysterography – technique that uses a catheter inserted into the endometrial cavity with the insertion of saline solution or contrast medium to fill the endometrial cavity for the purpose of demonstrating abnormalities within the cavity or uterine tubes.

spatial pulse length – spatial extent of an ultrasound pulse burst.

Spaulding's sign – overlapping of the skull bones; occurs in fetal death.

specific gravity – laboratory tests that measure how much dissolved material is present in the urine.

spectral analysis waveform – graphic display of the flow velocity over period of time.

spectral broadening – change in the spectral width that increases with flow disturbance.

spermatic cord – structure made up of vas deferens, testicular artery, cremasteric artery, and pampiniform plexus that suspends the testis in the scrotum.

spermatocele – cyst within the vas deferens containing sperm.

spherocytosis – condition in which erythrocytes assume a spheroid shape; hereditary.

sphincter of Oddi – small muscle that guards the ampulla of Vater.

sphygmomanometer – device used to measure blood pressure.

spiculation – fingerlike extension of a malignant tumor; usually appears as a small line that radiates outward from the margin of a mass.

spina bifida – neural tube defect of the spine in which the dorsal vertebrae (vertebral arches) fail to fuse together, allowing the protrusion of meninges and/or spinal cord through the defect; two types exist: spina bifida occulta (skin-covered defect of the spine without protrusion of meninges or cord) and spina bifida cystica (open spinal defect marked by sac containing protruding meninges and/or cord).

spina bifida aperta – open (non–skin-covered lesions) neural tube defects, such as myelomeningocele and meningocele.

spina bifida occulta – closed defect of the spine without protrusion of meninges or spinal cord; alpha-fetoprotein analysis will not detect these lesions.

splaying – widening.

splenic agenesis – complete absence of the spleen.

splenic artery – one of the three vessels that arise from the celiac axis to supply the spleen, pancreas, stomach, and greater omentum; forms the superior border of the pancreas.

splenic flexure – the transverse colon travels horizontally across the abdomen and bends at this point to form the descending colon.

splenic hilum – site where vessels and lymph nodes enter and exit the spleen; located in the middle of the spleen.

splenic sinuses – long, irregular channels lined by endothelial cells or flattened reticular cells.

splenic vein – vein that drains the spleen; travels horizontally across the abdomen (posterior to the pancreas) to join the superior mesenteric vein to form the portal vein; serves as the posterior medial border of the pancreas.

splenomegaly – enlargement of the spleen.

spontaneous – flow is present without augmentation.

-stasis – standing still; *homeostasis*: maintenance of a relatively stable internal environment.

strabismus – eye disorder in which optic axes cannot be directed to the same object.

strangulated hernia – an incarcerated hernia with vascular compromise.

subclavian artery – artery that originates at the inner border of the scalenus anterior and travels beneath the clavicle to the outer border of the first rib to become the axillary artery.

subclavian steal syndrome – symptoms of brain stem ischemia associated with a stenosis or occlusion of the left subclavian, innominate, or right subclavian artery proximal to the origin of the vertebral artery.

subclavian vein – continuation of the axillary vein.

subcostal – placement of the transducer located near body midline and beneath costal margin.

subcutaneous layer – most superficial of the three layers of the breast identified on breast ultrasound, the subcutaneous layer is mainly fatty; it is located immediately beneath the skin and superficial to the mammary layer. The subcutaneous layer can be very thin and difficult to recognize.

subependyma – fragile area beneath the ependyma that is subject to bleed in the premature infant.

subhepatic – inferior to the liver.

subjective assessment of fluid – sonographer surveys uterine cavity to determine visual assessment of amniotic fluid present.

subluxed – occurs when the femoral head moves posteriorly and remains in contact with the posterior aspect of the acetabulum.

submandibular window – window formed when transducer is placed at the angle of the mandible and angled slightly medially and cephalad toward the carotid canal.

submucosa – one of the layers of the bowel, under the mucosal layer; contains blood vessels and lymph channels.

submucosal leiomyoma – type of leiomyoma found to deform the endometrial cavity and cause heavy or irregular menses.

suboccipital window – window formed when the transducer is placed on the posterior aspect of the neck inferior to the nuchal crest.

subphrenic – below the diaphragm.

subserosal – type of leiomyoma that may become pedunculated and appear as an extrauterine mass.

subvalvular aortic stenosis – formation of a membrane beneath the aortic leaflets causes left ventricular outflow obstruction.

succenturiate placenta – one or more accessory lobes connected to the body of the placenta by blood vessels.

sulcus – groove on the surface of the brain that separates the gyri.

superficial femoral artery – artery that courses the length of the thigh through Hunter's canal and terminates at the opening of the adductor magnus muscle.

superficial femoral vein – vein that originates at the hiatus of the adductor magnus muscle in the distal thigh and ascends through the adductor (Hunter's) canal.

superficial inguinal ring – triangular opening in the external oblique aponeurosis.

superior mesenteric artery – artery that arises inferior to the celiac axis to supply the proximal half of the colon and the small intestine.

superior mesenteric vein – vein that drains the proximal half of the colon and small intestine, travels vertically (anterior to the inferior vena cava) to join the splenic vein to form the portal veins.

superior vena cava – vessel receiving venous return from the head and upper extremities into the upper posterior medial wall of the right atrium.

superior vesical arteries – after birth the umbilical arteries become the superior vesical arteries.

supracristal septal defect – high membranous septal defect just beneath the pulmonary orifice.

suprapubic – above the symphysis pubis.

suprasternal – transducer placement in the suprasternal notch.

supraventricular tachyarrhythmias – abnormal rhythms above 200 beats per minute with a normal sinus conduction rate of 1:1.

surface mode – in the surface-light mode there are brighter image intensity values to structures that are closer to the viewer and darker image intensity values to structures that are further from the viewer.

synovial sheath – membrane surrounding a joint, tendon, or bursa that secretes a viscous fluid called synovia.

systemic lupus erythematosus (SLE) – inflammatory disease involving multiple organ systems; fetus of a mother with SLE may develop heart block and pericardial effusion.

systole – part of the cardiac cycle in which the ventricles are pumping blood through the outflow tract into the pulmonary artery or the aorta.

systolic to diastolic (S/D) ratio – Doppler determination of the peak systolic velocity divided by the peak diastolic velocity.

tachycardia – heart rate more than 100 beats per minute.

tail of Spence – a normal extension of breast tissue into the axillary or arm pit region.

tail of the pancreas – tapered end of the pancreas that lies in the left hypochondrium near the hilus of the spleen and upper pole of the left kidney.

target (donut) sign – characteristic of gastrointestinal wall thickening consisting of an echogenic center and a hypoechoic rim; frequently associated with sectional areas of the gastrointestinal tract; the muscle is hyperechoic, and the inner core is hypoechoic.

tendinitis (tendinopathy, tendinosis, or tenosynovitis) – inflammation of a tendon.

tendon – fibrous tissue connecting muscle to bone.

tentorium – "tent" structure in the posterior fossa that separates the cerebellum from the cerebrum.

teratoma – solid tumor.

terminal ductal-lobular unit (TDLU) – smallest functional portion of the breast involving the terminal duct and its associated lobule containing at least one acinus (tiny milk-producing gland). The TDLU undergoes significant monthly hormone-induced changes and radical changes during pregnancy and lactation. The TDLU is the site of origin of nearly all significant pathological processes involving the breast, including all elements of fibrocystic condition, fibroadenomas, and in situ and invasive breast cancer (both lobular and ductal).

testicle – male gonad that produces hormones that induce masculine features and production of spermatozoa.

testicular artery – artery arising from the aorta just distal to each renal artery; it divides into two major branches supplying the testis medially and laterally.

testicular vein – the pampiniform plexus forms each testicular vein; the right testicular vein drains directly into the inferior vena cava, whereas the left testicular vein drains into the left renal vein.

tethered spinal cord – fixed spinal cord that is positioned in an abnormal position.

tetralogy of Fallot – a congenital anomaly consisting of four defects: membranous ventricular septal defect, overriding of the aorta, right ventricular hypertrophy, and pulmonary stenosis.

thalamus – portion of the midbrain that serves as two landmarks for the sonographer that abut both sides of the third ventricle.

thalassemia – group of hereditary anemias occurring in Asian and Mediterranean populations.

thanatophoric dysplasia – lethal short-limb dwarfism characterized by a marked reduction in the length of the long bones, pear-shaped chest, soft-tissue redundancy, and frequently clover-leaf skull deformity and ventriculomegaly.

theca-lutein cysts – multilocular cysts that occur in patients with hyperstimulation (hydatidiform mole and infertility patients); appear as multiple cysts within each ovary; complication of hyperstimulation.

Thompson's test – a test used to evaluate the integrity of the Achilles' tendon that involves plantar flexion with squeezing of the calf.

thoracentesis – surgical puncture of the chest wall for removal of fluids; usually done by using a large-bore needle.

thoracic outlet syndrome – changes in arterial blood flow to the arms related to intermittent compression of the proximal arteries.

three-dimensional (3-D) ultrasound – permits collection and review of data obtained from a volume of tissue in multiple imaging planes and rendering of surface features.

thrombocytes – platelets in blood.

thyroglossal duct cyst – congenital anomaly that presents in the midline of the neck anterior to the trachea.

thyroiditis – inflammation of the thyroid.

thyroid-stimulating hormone (TSH) – hormone secreted by the pituitary gland that stimulates the thyroid gland to secrete thyroxine and triiodothyronine.

tibial-peroneal trunk – arterial branch that exits after the anterior tibial artery and bifurcates into the posterior tibial artery and the peroneal artery.

time gain compensation (TGC) – also referred to as *depth gain compensation*; ability to compensate for attenuation of the transmitted beam as the sound wave travels through tissues in the body; usually, individual pod controls allow the operator to manually change the amount of compensation necessary for each patient to produce a quality image.

Tinel's sign (Hoffmann-Tinel sign, Tinel's symptom, or Tinel-Hoffmann sign) – pins-and-needles type tingling felt distally to a percussion site. Sensation can be either an abnormal or a normal occurrence (i.e., hitting the elbow creates a tingling in the distal arm).

TIPS – transjugular intrahepatic portosystemic shunt.

tissue specific ultrasound contrast agent – a type of contrast agent whose microbubbles are removed from the blood and are taken up by specific tissues in the body; one example is the agent Sonozoid

-tomy – cutting; *anatomy*: study of structure, which often involves cutting or removing body parts.

transducer – any device that converts signals from one form to another.

transitional zone – prostate area that is located on both sides of the proximal urethra and ends at the level of the verumontanum.

transorbital window – transducer placement on the closed eyelid.

transparent mode – sometimes called x-ray mode, is best for viewing a relatively low-contrast block of soft tissue.

transposition of the great arteries – failure of the truncus arteriosus to complete its rotation during the first trimester; causes the pulmonary artery to arise from the left ventricle and the aorta to arise from the pulmonary artery (blue baby at birth).

transpyloric plane – horizontal plane that passes through the pylorus, the duodenal junction, the neck of the pancreas, and the hilum of the kidneys.

transtemporal window – transducer placement on the temporal bone cephalad to the zygomatic arch anterior to the ear.

transvaginal transducer – high-frequency transducer that is inserted into the vaginal canal to obtain better definition of first-trimester pregnancy.

transverse lie – description of the fetus lying transversely (horizontally) across the abdomen.

Treacher Collins syndrome – underdevelopment of the jaw and cheek bone and abnormal ears.

tricuspid atresia – underdevelopment of the tricuspid valve (usually associated with hypoplasia of the right ventricle and pulmonary stenosis).

tricuspid valve – atrioventricular valve found between the right atrium and right ventricle.

trigonocephaly – premature closure of the metopic suture.

trimester – pregnancy is divided into three 13-week segments called trimesters.

true knots of the umbilical cord – knots formed when a loop of cord is slipped over the fetal head or shoulders during delivery.

true (minor) pelvis – found below the brim of the pelvis; the cavity of the minor pelvis is continuous at the pelvic brim with the cavity of the major pelvis.

truncus arteriosus – common arterial trunk that divides into the aorta and pulmonary artery.

tuboovarian abscess (TOA) – infection that involves the fallopian tube and the ovary.

tunica adventitia – outer layer of the vascular system.

tunica albuginea – inner fibrous membrane surrounding the testicle.

tunica intima – inner layer of the vascular system.

tunica media – middle layer of the vascular system; veins have thinner tunica media than arteries.

tunica vaginalis – membrane consisting of a visceral layer (adherent to the testis) and a parietal layer (adherent to the scrotum) lining the inner wall of the scrotum; a potential space between these layers is where hydroceles may develop.

Turner's syndrome – congenital endocrine disorder caused by failure of the ovaries to respond to pituitary hormone stimulation; cystic hygroma often seen.

twin-to-twin transfusion – monozygotic twin pregnancy with single placenta and arteriovenous shunt within the placenta; the donor twin becomes anemic and growth restricted with oligohydramnios; the recipient twin may develop hydrops and polyhydramnios.

tympany – predominant sound heard over hollow organs (stomach, intestines, bladder, aorta, gallbladder).

ultrasound contrast agents – agents that can be administered intravenously to evaluate blood vessels, blood flow, and solid organs.

umbilical – around the navel.

umbilical cord – connecting lifeline between the fetus and placenta; it contains two umbilical arteries and one umbilical vein encased in Wharton's jelly.

umbilical herniation – failure of the anterior abdominal wall to close completely at the level of the umbilicus.

uncinate process – small, curved tip of the pancreatic head that lies posterior to the superior mesenteric vein.

unicornuate uterus – anomaly of the uterus in which only one horn and tube develop.

ureteropelvic junction – junction of the ureter entering the renal pelvis; most common site of obstruction.

ureteropelvic junction obstruction – most common neonatal obstruction of the urinary tract; results from intrinsic narrowing or extrinsic vascular compression.

ureterovesical junction – junction where the ureter enters the bladder.

ureters – retroperitoneal structures that exit the kidney to carry urine to the urinary bladder.

urethra – small, membranous canal that excretes urine from the urinary bladder.

urethral atresia – lack of development of the urethra; condition causing a massively distended bladder (prune belly).

urinary amylase – pancreatic enzyme that remains elevated longer than serum amylase in patients with acute pancreatitis.

urinary bladder – muscular retroperitoneal organ that serves as a reservoir for urine.

urinary incontinence – the uncontrollable passage of urine.

urinoma – cyst containing urine.

uterine synechiae – scars within the uterus secondary to previous gynecological surgery.

uterovesical space – anterior pouch between the uterus and bladder.

uterus didelphys – complete duplication of the uterus, cervix, and vagina.

VACTERL – **v**ertebral abnormalities, **a**nal atresia, **c**ardiac abnormalities, **t**racheo**e**sophageal fistula, and **r**enal and **l**imb abnormalities.

vagina atresia – failure of the vagina to develop.

valvulae conniventes – normal segmentation of the small bowel.

varicocele – dilated veins caused by obstruction of the venous return from the testicle.

varicose veins – dilated, elongated, tortuous superficial veins.

vas deferens – tube that connects the epididymis to the seminal vesicle.

vasa previa – condition that occurs when the umbilical cord vessels cross the internal os of the cervix.

vascular ultrasound contrast agents – a type of ultrasound contrast agent whose microbubbles are contained in the body's vascular spaces; examples of this type of agent include Optison, Definity, Imagent, Levovist, SonoVue.

vasovagal – concerning the action of stimuli from the vagus nerve on blood vessels.

veins – collapsible vascular structures that carry blood back to the heart.

velocity – speed of the ultrasound wave; determined by tissue density.

velocity envelope – trace of the peak velocities as a function of time.

ventricular septal defect – communication between the right and left ventricles.

ventriculitis – inflammation or infection of the ventricles that appears as echogenic linear structures along the gyri; may also appear as focal echogenic structures within the white matter.

ventriculomegaly – abnormal accumulation of cerebrospinal fluid within the cerebral ventricles resulting in dilation of the ventricles; compression of developing brain tissue and brain damage may result; commonly associated with additional fetal anomalies.

veracity – truthfulness, honesty.

vertebral artery – branches of the subclavian artery that merge to form the basilar artery.

vertex – position of fetus with head down in the uterus.

vertigo – sensation of having objects move about the person or sensation of moving around in space.

verumontanum – junction of the ejaculatory ducts with the urethra.

villi – inner folds of the small intestine.

visceral peritoneum – layer of peritoneum that covers the abdominal organs.

vital signs – medical measurements used to ascertain how the body is functioning.

volar – the anterior portion of the body when in the anatomical position.

volume rendering – the volume is evaluated by rotating the volume data to a standard orientation and then scrolling through parallel planes. The data may be rotated to assess oblique planes.

wall echo shadow (WES) sign – sonographic pattern found when the gallbladder is packed with stones.

wandering spleen – spleen that has migrated from its normal location in the left upper quadrant.

wave – propagation of energy that moves back and forth or vibrates at a steady rate.

wavelength – distance over which a wave repeats itself during one period of oscillation.

Wharton's jelly – myxomatous connective tissue that surrounds the umbilical vessels and varies in size.

white blood cells – cells that defend the body by destroying invading microorganisms and their toxins.

white pulp – tissue composed of lymphatic tissue and lymphatic follicles.

Wilms' tumor – most frequent malignant tumor in the neonate and infant.

yolk sac – circular structure seen between 4 and 10 weeks that supplies nutrition to the fetal pole (the developing embryo); it lies within the chorion outside the amnion.

yolk stalk – the umbilical duct connecting the yolk sac with the embryo.

zygote – fertilized ovum resulting from union of male and female gametes.

zygote intrafallopian transfer (ZIFT) – a human fertilization technique in which the zygotes are injected through a laparoscope into the fimbriated ends of the fallopian tubes. Recently, this has been performed under ultrasound guidance.

Index

Page numbers followed by *f, t,* or *b* indicate figures, tables, or boxes, respectively. Numbers in **boldface** type are in Volume Two.

Selected Medical and Ultrasound Abbreviations

AAA	abdominal aortic aneurysm	**AVM**	arteriovenous malformation	**DFV**	deep femoral vein
AB	abortion	**AVSD**	artrioventricular septal defect	**DM**	diabetes mellitus
ABI	ankle-brachial index	**BA**	basilar artery	**DOB**	date of birth
AC	abdominal circumference; acromioclavicular (joint)	**BD**	biocular distance	**DVT**	deep vein thrombosis
		Bi-RADS	Breast Imaging and Reporting Data Systems	**DWM**	Dandy-Walker malformation
ACA	anterior cerebral artery			**dx**	diagnosis
AcoA	anterior communicating artery	**BPD**	biparietal diameter	**ECA**	external carotid artery
ACOG	American College of Obstetrics and Gynecology	**BPP**	biophysical profile	**ECG**	electrocardiogram
		BSE	breast self-examination	**EDC**	expected date of confinement
ACR	American College of Radiology	**BUN**	blood urea nitrogen	**EDD**	expected date of delivery
		bx	biopsy	**EFW**	estimated fetal weight
ACTH	andrenocorticotropic hormone	**CA**	calcium; cancer; celiac axis	**ERCP**	endoscopic retrograde cholan-giopancreatography
AD	autosomal dominant	**CABG**	coronary artery bypass graft		
ADPKD	autosomal-dominant poly-cystic kidney disease	**CAD**	coronary artery disease	**ESP**	early systolic peak
		CBD	common bile duct	**ETOH**	alcohol
AE	acoustic emission	**CBE**	clinical breast examination	**FAST**	focused assessment with sonography for trauma
AFAFP	amniotic fluid alpha-fetoprotein	**CBF**	cerebral blood flow		
		CCA	common carotid artery	**FBM**	fetal breathing movements
AFI	amniotic fluid index	**CD**	common duct	**FCC**	fibrocystic condition
AFP	alpha-fetoprotein	**CES**	contrast-enhanced sonography	**FL**	fetal length; falciform ligament
AFV	amniotic fluid volume	**CFA**	common femoral artery	**FM**	fetal movement
AI	aortic insufficiency	**CFI**	color flow imaging	**FMD**	fibromuscular dysplasia
AIDS	acquired immunodeficiency syndrome	**CFM**	color flow mapping	**FNA**	fine needle aspiration
		CHD	congestive heart disease; con-genital heart disease	**FNH**	focal nodular hyperplasia
AIUM	American Institute of Ultrasound in Medicine			**FSH**	follicle-stimulating hormone
		CHF	congestive heart failure	**FT**	fetal tone
ALH	atypical lobular hyperplasia	**CI**	cardiac index; cephalic index	**FUO**	fever of unknown origin
ALK PHOS	alkaline phosphatase	**CK**	creatine kinase	**GASA**	growth-adjusted sonar age
ALT	alanine aminotransferase	**CL**	caudate lobe	**GB**	gallbladder
AMA	American Medical Association; against medical advice	**CNS**	central nervous system	**GDA**	gastroduodenal artery
		CO_2	carbon dioxide	**GI**	gastrointestinal
Amb	ambulatory	**COPD**	chronic obstructive pulmonary disease	**GIFT**	gamete intrafallopian transfer
AP	anteroposterior			**GSHI**	gray scale harmonic imaging
Appy	appendectomy	**Cr**	creatinine	**GSV**	greater saphenous vein
AR	autosomal recessive	**CRL**	crown-rump length	**GSW**	gunshot wound
ARDS	adult respiratory distress syn-drome; acute respiratory dis-tress syndrome	**CSF**	cerebrospinal fluid	**GU**	genitourinary
		CSP	cavum septum pellucidum	**GYN**	gynecology
		CT	computed tomography	**HC**	head circumference
ARPKD	autosomal-recessive polycystic kidney disease	**CVA**	cerebrovascular accident	**HCC**	hepatocellular carcinoma
		CVS	chorionic villus sampling	**hCG**	human chorionic gonadotropin
ART	assisted reproductive technology	**CW**	continuous wave		
AS	aortic stenosis	**Cx**	cervix	**Hgb**	hemoglobin
ASAP	as soon as possible	**D&C**	dilation and curettage	**HI**	harmonic imaging
ASD	atrial septal defect	**dB**	decibel	**HIV**	human immunodeficiency virus
AST	aspartate aminotransferase	**DCIS**	ductal carcinoma in situ		
AT	acceleration time	**DDH**	developmental displacement of hip	**HLHS**	hypoplastic left heart syndrome
ATN	acute tubular necrosis				
AV	atrioventricular	**DFE**	distal femoral epiphyseal (ossification)	**hPL**	human placental lactogen
AVF	arterio-venous fistula			**HPS**	hypertrophic pyloric stenosis